THE FOUNTAIN OF HEALTH

THE FOUNTAIN OF HEALTH

An A-Z of Traditional Chinese Medicine

Dr Charles Windridge
Consultant Editor
Dr Wu Xiaochun

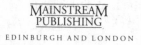

MAINSTREAM
PUBLISHING

EDINBURGH AND LONDON

First published in Great Britain in 1994 by
MAINSTREAM PUBLISHING COMPANY (EDINBURGH) LTD
7 Albany Street
Edinburgh EH1 3UG

ISBN 1 85158 687 3 (cloth)
ISBN 1 85158 635 0 (paper)

A catalogue record for this book is available from the British Library

Typeset in Janson by Litho Link Ltd, Welshpool, Powys, Wales
Printed in Finland by WSOY

Contents

Introduction

This book can be briefly described as a reliable outline guide to the principles, practices and benefits of traditional Chinese medicine, together with the more general aspects of the Chinese approach to health, presented in a simple-to-use, easy-reference dictionary form. But one should note that, here and there, a few of the entries have a characteristically encyclopaedic quality, which is unavoidable because some of the explanations cannot be reduced to terse statements of the kind so beloved of lexicographers, nor is it essential that they should be, for it is desirable that a dictionary should be readable as well as useful, which cannot be realized where elegance of style is completely sacrificed in the cause of brevity. Some of the entries are supplemented with explanatory illustrations.

The prime purpose of this book is to provide for the current interest, and also stimulate further interest, in TCM, or traditional Chinese medicine, which the medical authorities of the West have relegated, in their wisdom – or lack of it – and somewhat disdainfully, to the category of alternative medicine, but which has been clearly shown to be very superior medicine in many respects. It will fully cater for the needs of those who wish to make a sound and rewarding study of TCM, which is by far the finest system of preventive medicine in the world, and one of the major components among the various techniques evolved by the Chinese to accomplish a total mastery of the art of living, which is surely the most important of all the arts, and which they measure in terms of health, longevity and peace of mind. In this connection, it is interesting to note that, nowadays, there is a tendency for Chinese physicians to be trained in both TCM and Western-style medicine, and so they are aware of the advantages – and disadvantages – of both systems, which must be of benefit to their patients in giving them the best – and withholding the worst! – of both worlds.

The information in this book is not confined to herbal remedies and manipulative and surgical techniques – the bare bones of the healing arts, so to speak. This cannot be, for the Chinese set much store by harmonious relationships, and there is almost a complet integration of all their activities in health, medicine, diet, th martial arts, philosophy, law, social conduct, and so forth, and fev are studied or pursued in absolute isolation; and, therefore, to full and properly understand Chinese medicine, one must have som knowledge of the Chinese way of life in general, particularly as i affects their system of medicine. Accordingly, there are reference to the Chinese diet and cuisine, of which herbal medicines are ar offshoot, the martial arts, which have meditative overtones tha promote mental health, and Chinese philosophy, including Taoisn and Confucianism, which provides the key to a clear understanding of the purposes, theories and mysteries of TCM. There are also some historical references, especially in regard to the eminen physicians and the development of medical techniques in botl ancient China and more recent times. Furthermore, definition have been provided for some of those items of medical terminology such as *analgesic*, *melancholia* and *rheumatism*, which are not peculiar to Chinese medicine, but are common to all cultures where the practice of medicine is at an advanced level, though it should be understood that some of the terms used by Chinese physicians have no general currency outside traditional Chinese medical practice.

Any person who wishes to achieve a long and healthy life of vigorous youthfulness would do well to follow the Chinese example in matters of sound diet, adequate exercise, moderate habits. preventive medicine and a wise philosophy of living. This must be good advice, for China has the oldest civilization in the world, its practices have withstood the test of time, and its citizens are remarkably healthy and do live to a very great age.

The Chinese physician has at his disposal a vast repertoire of herbal remedies and manipulative techniques – alleviative, curative and preventive – with all the emphasis being on the preventive. This makes good sense, for many of the ailments which are virtually incurable can be prevented by the application of some forethought. It is certainly no accident that in China there is a low incidence of cancer, diabetes, diseases and defects of the heart and circulation, and many of the other illnesses which commonly afflict the people of the West. But what is particularly noteworthy is that, among these Chinese herbal medicines, there are those which will inhibit or retard the ageing process. In China, it is not uncommon for a woman in her fifties to have all the youthful bloom of a girl of teenage years.

Sensible people hardly need to be persuaded of the importance of health, and so, quite understandably, many readers will want to pply the remedies and other useful directions contained in this book. But they should bear in mind that it is meant to be a work of general and popular interest, and although the information contained herein is accurate, it does not constitute a complete study of materia medica, Chinese or otherwise, nor is it a comprehensive manual of instruction or pharmacopoeia of the kind intended for the use of physicians and pharmacists. Such manuals can be unsafe instruments in the hands of the unskilled. In general, do-it-yourself medicine has severe limitations, and it is not a practice to be greatly encouraged. Before embarking upon a course of self-treatment, one should be fully aware of the attendant risks, which include inaccurate diagnoses and wrong dosages. For this reason, dosages are stated with the remedies in this book only in those instances where it is expressly safe to do so.

Of course, it is not unreasonable that the skilled amateur in the field of the healing arts should consider himself to be adequately qualified to apply simple remedies for minor and run-of-the-mill ailments. In fact, it is sometimes desirable that he should do so, for it frees the qualified physician so that he may attend to more urgent matters. And it could be the case with medical treatments, as it certainly is with many other skills, that the dedicated and enthusiastic amateur will often achieve better results than the uncaring and cynical professional. Nevertheless, self-diagnosis can be very misleading. For example, a headache is generally regarded as a commonplace ailment, but it may be symptomatic of a much more serious condition which only a professional physician can accurately diagnose. Furthermore, there is often a tendency to treat the symptoms rather that the cause of an illness, which is just about as sensible as trying to extinguish a fire by switching off the fire-alarm. It could be argued that no one could know a person's body better than he knows it himself; but it is doubtful if this could really always be the case, for it must sometimes be difficult for a person to make an objective judgement in an essentially subjective situation. The self-diagnosis made by a hypochondriac, who will imagine that every little ache or pain heralds the onset of a terminal illness, is likely to be very different from that of the super-optimist taking the nonchalant view that 'whatever it is, it will soon wear off'.

The best advice that could be given here is to say that the person who has the slightest doubt about his state of health, or the cause, nature or treatment of an illness, especially if it is serious or complicated, should seek professional medical counsel.

Warning

Much of the information in this book has been culled from traditional-type Chinese herbals and similar works, and as these authorities are unquestionably reliable, the suggested remedies should normally be safe to use and without any adverse side-effects. Nevertheless, though mistakes are very unlikely, they are certainly possible, for even the best-regulated systems have their imperfections, and there are always exceptions to a general rule. Furthermore, language is sometimes misleading, and allergic reactions are occasionally produced by seemingly harmless medicines. Therefore, the application of these remedies is a matter for the sole discretion of the reader, and neither the author nor the publisher of this book can accept legal responsibility for any errors which may have inadvertently entered into the text, or those made by the reader himself.

Fortunately, herbal medicines can generally be used with complete safety, and so, unless one happens to be particularly reckless, one is not likely to come to grief in using the remedies in this book.

Herbal medicines are natural, generally non-addictive and have no unpleasant side-effects. Dosages are non-critical more often than not. Many medicines have the same or similar properties, and so, if a patient develops an allergy to a particular medicine, his physician can usually prescribe a more suitable alternative. However, herbal medicines are slow in action, and they must be taken over a long period if they are to be truly effective. On the other hand, cures brought about by herbal medicines tend to be permanent.

A few of the medical scientists of the West have made the criticism that Chinese herbal medicines are unreliable because they have not been laboratory-tested. But this is hardly a valid criticism, for the efficacy and safety of Chinese herbal medicines have been clearly demonstrated by many centuries of valuable experience, whereas some of the laboratory-tested Western-style synthetic medicines have proved to be unreliable, addictive or dangerous, which fact would be readily acknowledged by the victims of thalidomide. One hardly dares to think about the damage done by some of the addictive tranquillizing and soporific drugs which have appeared on the market during recent years. But, in fairness, it must be said that some manufactured medicines contain natural ingredients. For example, digitalis, which is used as a heart stimulant, is extracted from the foxglove. And biochemists assure us that the aspirin (acetylsalicylic acid) derived from coal tar is no different in its medicinal properties from that extracted from the bark of the willow tree.

One should note that many of the proprietary brands of medicine which may be purchased 'off-prescription', and are obtainable at grocery stores and other retail outlets, are dangerous if taken as an overdose, and they certainly are commonly taken in excess, especially by those people who subscribe to the mistaken belief that one cannot have too much of a good thing. But, here, the fault lies more with the user of the medicine than with the medicine itself.

Those persons who intend to collect herbs in order to make their own medicines should remember that some poisonous plants, such as the foxglove and woody nightshade, have very attractive fruits or flowers – they look good enough to eat! – and that some totally different species are of a similar appearance. Therefore, to avoid mishaps, one must identify plants correctly. A good flora guide, such as *The Concise British Flora in Colour*, by W. Keble Martin, would be helpful in this respect. Do NOT eat any part of a plant unless you are quite sure it is safe to do so.

One should also remember that endangered species of plants, which are the ones threatened by extinction, are protected by law. It is an offence to pick them.

Facts and Figures

The following facts and figures will be of assistance in understanding many of the entries in this dictionary.

CHINESE WORDS AND NAMES

There are over a hundred different languages and dialects in China, the main language being Mandarin, which is spoken more in the north than in the south. Cantonese is the main language of the south. But, although people from different parts of China may not be able to understand each other when speaking, they can always understand each other when expressing themselves in writing, for the same written characteristics are used for all the Chinese languages; and, in a slightly modified form, they are also used in Japan.

The written language of China is essentially visual, and in its early stages of development, its characters were pictures of real things – people, animals, plants, objects, etc. At later stages, these pictures were streamlined for ease in writing them, and so they became more symbolic than pictorial. They were also adopted to

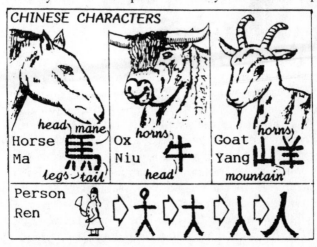

CHINESE CHARACTERS

Horse Ma — head, mane, legs, tail
Ox Niu — horns, head
Goat Yang — horns, mountain
Person Ren

represent abstractions, just as we, in the West, might use a pictur of a ship to represent travel or good fortune, or a fire to represen passion or danger.

Chinese words and names can be written in an Anglicized form but some Chinese word-sounds cannot be precisely expressed with the letters of the English alphabet, which has given rise to severa systems of transcription, together with some apparent inconsisten cies and not a little confusion. Thus, the name of the founder o Taoism may be written as *Lao-Tse*, *Lao-Tze*, *Lao-Tzu* or *Lao Zi*, and *Peking* may also be written as *Beijing*, *Chou dynasty* as *Zhou dynasty* and *Mao Tse-tung* as *Mao Zedong*.

Of course, some of these inconsistencies are due to the Anglicized forms being transcriptions from languages other thar Mandarin. It is interesting to note that the English word *tea* derives from the Fujianese (Fukienese) word *t'e* (pronounced as 'tay'), and the English slang word *char* derives from the Mandarin word *ch'a*.

The policy with this dictionary is to use transcriptions in the most recently developed system, called Hanyu pinyin, which was introduced by the Chinese government in 1979, and which is now the official system of China. Exceptionally, transcriptions are given in the Wade system, which is much older, where they have become firmly established in the English vocabulary, for these will be more familiar to readers. Thus, 'The Book of Changes', which is one of the Confucian classics, is written as *Yijing* in the Hanyu-pinyin system, but it is better known to the people of the West as *I Ching*, which is in the Wade system. Similarly, the largest port in the south of China is well known to us as *Canton*, but its name would be written as *Guangzhou* in Hanyu pinyin.

THE NAMES OF HERBS

All the plants known to man have been given Latinized botanical names, which are precise, and so serve to prevent confusion. They are the names by which they are known to botanists and other scientists throughout the world. Latin – and its latter-day versions – is the lingua franca of the scientific world. These botanical names are also called Linaean names because the Swedish naturalist Carl von Linné (1707–78) devised this binomial nomenclature, in which the first word, spelt with an initial capital letter, is the name of the genus, or family, and the second word is the name of the individual species. Thus, one could say: 'The common oak, *Quercus robur*, and the holm oak, *Quercus ilex*, belong to the genus *Quercus*.'

But, in addition to these botanical names, plants have common names. In fact, some have more than one. The cuckoo-pint, *Arum maculatum*, has over 50 common names, which include wild arum lily, wake-robin, lords-and-ladies, red-hot poker, jack-in-the-pulpit, soldiers-and-sailors, parson-in-his-smock, friar's cowl, jack-by-the-hedgerow and bishop's throne. These common names vary from region to region. What is called heather, *Calluna vulgaris*, in one part of Britain, is called ling in another. Also, the same name is sometimes shared by plants of entirely different species. The corn camomile, ox-eye daisy, feverfew and sneezewort are all loosely described as daisies. This is confusing, and can lead to plants being wrongly identified; and so the person who uses herbs for medicinal purposes should not disregard their botanical names.

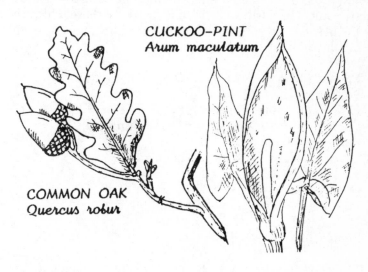

CUCKOO-PINT
Arum maculatum

COMMON OAK
Quercus robur

However, it is the common names with which readers are likely to be more familiar, and so, where a herb constitutes an entry in this dictionary, its common name is given. This, together with its botanical name, is followed by other data – uses, dosage, etc. For example:

marigold *Calendula officinalis* * * *

Many of the herbs indigenous to China will not be known to the people of the West, and some do not have Chinese names which can be satisfactorily translated into English. In these cases, an Anglicized rendering of the Chinese name is given thus:

tienchi *Radix pseudo-ginseng* * * *

UNITS OF MEASUREMENT

In common with the other nations, China has adopted metric units as its official system of measurement, though in China, as in the West, traditional units are still being used for non-scientific or unofficial purposes. In medical work, the usual metric units of measurement are grams (g) and milligrams (mg) for weight, and litres (l) and millilitres (ml) for capacity and volume. Solids, including powders, are measured by weight, and liquids by both weight and volume.

Measurements in herbal medicine are generally not critical, and so there is no reason why simple homely units, such as cups and tablespoons, and imperial units should not be used together with metric units. In this book, the units used are those which seem to be the best for the purpose in hand. The following equivalents will be helpful in this respect.

1 pound (lb) = 0.454 kilograms (kg) = 454 grams
1 ounce (oz) = 28.35 grams (g)
1 kilogram = 1000 grams = 2.2 pounds
1 pint (pt) = 0.568 litres (l) = 568 millilitres (ml)
1 litre = 1000 millilitres = 1.76 pints
1 imperial teaspoon = 1 5-ml spoon
1 imperial dessertspoon = 1 10-ml spoon
1 imperial tablespoon = 1 20-ml spoon
1 breakfast cup = ½ pint = 284 millilitres
1 teacup = ⅓ pint = 227 millilitres
1 millilitre water weighs 1 gram.

Rounded-off values may be used where the amounts are not critical.
Examples: 1 oz = 30 g; 1 kg = 2 lb.
The solidus is used to indicate alternatives. Example: 1 pint/575 ml.

USING HERBAL MEDICINES

Instructions for using herbal medicines are to be found among the entries, but the following general points should be noted.

1. Dosages are always stated as the weight of the dried herb. For most infusions and decoctions, 15 g dried herb per 1 pint/575 ml water is the accepted value. Double the quantity if the fresh herb is used.

2. Fresh herbs may be added to soups, stews and salads, or consumed without any kind of preparation, as with vegetables and fruit, but Chinese physicians would recommend that they be infused, for aqueous solutions are assimilated much more readily than solids.

3. Generally, herbal medicines must not be consumed with alcohol, for it negates their therapeutic effects and is sometimes dangerous.

4. Exercise self-restraint when taking addictive medicines.

5. Most infusions and decoctions may be sweetened with sugar or honey.

Chinese Medicine

Honour a physician with the honour due to him.

Ecclesiasticus 38. 1

The Chinese value health above all else. They recognize that one's own body is one's most precious possession – and perhaps it is the only thing which one truly possesses, and that for only a limited period of time – and that its sound state of health, and not money, property or power, is the real wealth. They regard material wealth as a means to an end, not an end in itself.

The strongly held views of the Chinese in this regard have led to the evolvement of a system of preventive medicine which is not only the oldest in the world but also the finest. It would certainly be a foolish bit of self-deception to assume that the physicians of the West have a monopoly in medical knowledge and skills. Chinese physicians were practising with remarkable success thousands of years ago, long before Hippocrates devised his celebrated oath.

In this connection, one should note that some of the medicines recently 'discovered' by the medical scientists of the West were known to, and were being administered by, Chinese physicians many centuries ago. For example, the alkaloid ephedrine, used in the treatment of asthma, and derived from the Chinese herb *ma huang* (*Ephedra sinica*), was listed in *Huang Di Nei Jing*, or 'The Internal Book of Huang Di' which is a product of the scholar–emperors and physicians of ancient China, but it is a newcomer to the *British Pharmacopoeia*. Another example of this kind is the iodine-rich black ash from burnt seaweed that is used in the treatment of goitre, a morbid enlargement of the thyroid gland due to iodine deficiency, and which often occurs as a pendulous swelling of the neck. By the end of the Han dynasty (206 BC–AD 220), anaesthetics were being used in the excision of tumours, and the circulation of the blood had been discovered.

The Chinese also greatly value wisdom. For them, the virtues of health and wisdom go hand in hand. The former gives them a long life of youthful vigour, and the latter gives them a life which is meaningful, purposeful and serene. Therefore, it is hardly surprising that physicians and teachers are among the most highly respected persons in Chinese society. But, really, this is to be expected in a land where aggressiveness and acquisitiveness are not regarded as cardinal virtues. Elderly persons are also highly esteemed, for the Chinese recognize that age often brings wisdom.

According to the tenets of Taoism and Confucianism, which are the two main religions of China (though, strictly speaking, they are ways of life, and not religions in our sense of the term), a sound state of health, both physical and mental, is the outcome of maintaining harmony with nature, within the body and throughout society. Taoism, which was founded by Lao Zi, who lived during the sixth century BC, lays all the emphasis on harmony with nature, whereas Confucianism, which was founded by Confucius (551–479 BC) lays all the emphasis on harmony in society, which explains why the social life of the Chinese centres around the family, which is close-knit and held together by strong ties of affection and loyalty. Filial duty and family unity are two of the cornerstones of Confucianism. This concept of harmonious relationships enters into and completely permeates not only the Chinese approach to health, which includes their system of medicine, but also all Chinese institutions, and each and every aspect of their thinking and conduct. It is their notion of spirituality and civilized behaviour. It is their *raison d'être*.

Some of the principles of Taoism preceded its founder by hundreds of years, and their origins are shrouded in mystery. This has produced an enigma, for people are enjoined to seek Tao, or 'the Way'; but there is no clear indication of how this might be achieved. Lao Zi himself said: 'Those who say they can explain Tao do not understand it; and those who understand it do not say'. But it is clear that the Tao encourages gentleness, mercy, humility and acceptance of the inexorable laws of nature.

The teachings of Confucius, which stress the virtues of wisdom, justice, sincerity, charity and propriety, are intended to produce the *zhunzi* (*chun-tzu*), or 'true gentleman', who will behave correctly in all situations. His name, as we know it, is a Latinized version of *Kung Fuzi*, his Chinese name, which was contrived for him by the Jesuit missionaries who came to China many centuries after his death. He was a person of profound wisdom, immense benevolence and incisive logic, and there is no doubt that his teachings, in so far as they are rational, free of superstition and inspire self-confidence, and are not enforced by oppressive laws and motivated by unenlightened self-interest, have given the Chinese a sound set of unassailable moral values, and thereby a strong lead, health-wise as well as socio-politically, over the rest of the world.

The gold in one's heart is far more precious than the gold in one's purse.

Analects, Confucius

One could easily believe that life would be far less difficult for many people if they were to practise the Confucian virtues, and there would certainly be a lower incidence of mental and nervous disorders. Many forms of ill health are due to the unregulated way in which we live. Without a doubt, many of the ills of society are due to the twin evils of greed and dishonesty, which are destructive in the extreme.

O what a tangled web we weave,
When first we practise to deceive.

Marmion, Sir Walter Scott

Buddhism, which was founded by Siddhartha Gautama (*c*. 563 – *c*. 483 BC) is the third largest religion of China, but many Chinese view it with suspicion, partly because it has a celibate priesthood, which they consider to be unnatural, and partly because of the belief that the human soul passes from one animal to another in a series of reincarnations, which they consider to be nonsensical. On the other hand, Buddhists are peace-loving people, which makes them a good influence; and since they are opposed to the slaughter of animals they have developed a wide range of delectable and health-giving vegetarian dishes, some of which have medicinal properties, and which have been a great boon to the Chinese, and done much to improve their health. It was the Buddhist monks who popularized the tea-drinking habit; and tea, in Chinese opinion, is beneficial to the health in a variety of ways. They have also devised some forms of kungfu, or martial arts, as a means of self-defence, but which now provide opportunities for keep-fit exercises. These have meditative overtones which are conducive to a sound state of mental health.

The foregoing comments can be summarized quite briefly by saying that the Chinese have thoroughly mastered the art of living, whereas we, in the West, have only mastered the arts of technology, which are much less important by comparison. To the Chinese mind, survival is of paramount importance, and they regard success in the art of living as largely a matter of being as healthy as one can, for as long as one can, and as contentedly as one can – health, a long life and peace of mind. They have a fourth concern, which is respect for their ancestors. Without health, they would fail either to survive or live contentedly. A long life enables them to make more of a life which is already too brief, and they recognize that their ancestors have given them the gift of life, which is the most precious of all gifts, together with many centuries of accumulated wisdom, which has enriched their lives. They are fully aware of the simple genetic principle that like tends to breed like, and that if they are healthy and worthy people it is because their ancestors were healthy and worthy people. They know that their own behaviour will play a major part in determining the destiny of their descendants as yet unborn.

To achieve contentment, the Chinese follow a piece of good advice, often attributed to Confucius and contained in the *I Ching*, a classical work of great antiquity: 'Our main purpose in life should not be to hanker after a heaven in the sky, which probably does not exist, but to create a heaven on earth for each other by effecting complete harmony between the yin and yang forces within us and around us.'

It is sometimes difficult to undo the damage done to the health, whether it is caused by illness or injury; and, in such cases, it often happens that the body will never be quite the same again. With the human body, as with a machine, regular maintenance may prevent a disaster. No doubt it was this realization which prompted the physicians and sages of ancient China to build and perfect a system of prophylactic medicine on the sound principle that damage which cannot be remedied may often be prevented.

> To administer medicines for illnesses which have already developed is akin to the conduct of a man who begins to dig a well after he has become thirsty.
>
> *The Internal Book of Huang Di*

However, TCM is not a single system but a number of different systems, some with several branches, conducted by a variety of practitioners, such as physicians, herbalists, accoucheurs, masseurs and acupuncturists, with training, experience, expertise and specialities at all levels in all fields. To the Western observer, this may seem to be a bit of a hotchpotch; but, in fact, it is a superbly integrated body of knowledge, skills and wisdom which, in one way or another, provides a preventive or curative treatment or some kind of alleviation for each and every one of all the ills to which the human flesh is heir.

When medicine was first practised in China, over 5000 years ago, little was known about the exact functioning of most of the organs of the body. But the Chinese physicians of those far-off times persevered and learned by experience and, over the centuries, they evolved a sound code of practice even though they were often working in the dark. Quite frequently, they were treating illnesses whose exact causes were unknown with medicines whose exact effects were unknown. But they did achieve some good results. To the Western mind, this approach would seem to be most unscientific, but Chinese physicians would argue that experience is a good teacher. As the poet Lord Byron said, 'The Tree of Knowledge is not that of Life.'

TCM differs from Western medicine in a number of respects, its most salient features being emphasis more on the preventive than the curative and the alleviative, the employment of herbal remedies, which are natural and generally without any unpleasant side-effects, a wide variety of manipulative techniques, emphasis on sound diet, adequate exercise and moderate habits, and the deep conviction that health in both body and mind is largely a matter of establishing harmonious relationships on the all-pervading yin-yang principle. To these, one might add the skill, dedication and perseverance of the Chinese physician.

Whatever the nature of an illness, whether serious or a trifling malady, chronic or otherwise, the Chinese physician will treat it with great patience and equanimity, and the occasional touch of genius, and rarely does he fail to succeed in some measure. He also gives advice and institutes treatments that will prolong the lives of his patients and maintain them in a state of youthful vigour.

However, the Chinese physician does have one advantage which is not always readily available to his counterpart in the West. He receives the full co-operation of his patients. As they value their health, so they value the physician, and they are fully supportive of his efforts. Throughout their lives, almost from the day they are born, the Chinese systematically arrange their diet, medicines, physical exercise, and so forth, and regularly consult their medical advisers so that they may prevent or delay the onset of many illnesses, especially those associated with age, such as poor circulation, blood pressure, rheumatism and cataracts.

The Chinese physician's ethical code, imbued with great wisdom, ensures a standard of Chinese medical practice which the whole world could envy. It is largely due to the thorough training of Chinese physicians, which is a paramount aspect of Chinese medicine. Many are trained in the medical schools attached to the universities, where they study medicine in both the Western style and the traditional style of China. But, in the rural areas, many are trained in only the traditional way, which is by serving as assistants or apprentices to an established practitioner, as apothecaries were once trained in Britain, and still are so trained in Spain.

The apprenticeship system is one which has much to commend it, for it involves on-the-job training which is practical and lengthy, unsuitable would-be entrants to the profession are weeded out, there is a close relationship between the teacher and the taught, often with a 1:1 teacher-pupil ratio, and the teacher is a highly skilled practitioner of long and wide experience. Anyone who has been on holiday in Spain and required medical attention will know that apothecaries trained in this way are competent and versatile, giving advice, dispensing medicines, extracting teeth, performing minor operations, and so on.

Chinese medicine is essentially allopathic, as it is in the West. It is a system of medicine by which a treatment is applied to induce a condition that is opposite in nature to that caused by the illness. Do not we, in the West, apply the same principle when we 'starve a fever and feed a cold'?

> Treat hot illnesses with cooling medicines, and treat cold illnesses with warming medicines.
>
> *The Pharmacopoeia of Shen Nong*

Scholars of the period of the Han dynasty attributed the discovery of many medicinal herbs to Shen Nong (*c.* 3500 BC) one of the legendary emperors. It is possible that he suggested that the yin-yang principle of complementary opposites be applied in medical treatments, and that any bodily imbalance due to illness, injury or some other cause could be corrected by a medicine, food or manipulative technique of an opposite character.

All illnesses and medicines, together with foods that have medicinal properties, are broadly classified as yin or yang. As one might expect, yin medicines are used to treat yang illnesses, and vice versa, so maintaining the bodily balance, or harmony. Yang illnesses tend to be positive, manifesting themselves with vigour and hotness, whereas yin illnesses tend to be negative, manifesting themselves less clearly with weakness and coldness.

The procedure in allopathic medicine is quite the reverse of that in homoeopathic medicine, the latter being a system by which minute doses of drugs are administered in order to induce symptoms that are similar to those caused by disease. Its purpose is to activate the immunity system of the body, so making it more resistant to disease. Homoeopathy has no great place in traditional Chinese medicine, but it is used on a small scale and with some degree of success in Western medicine.

Chinese philosophy, and Taoism in particular, in which herbal medicine is an inextricable component, has its roots in the researches made by Shen Nong and the Han physicians, who taught that health may be gained, and even the meaning of life understood, by working with nature.

After many centuries of experience, Chinese physicians came to the conclusion that the human body as a whole is self-regulating and self-healing, and because of the presence of chemical substances, which they call vital essences and humours, it develops immunity to infectious diseases. But nature sometimes needs assistance, and the Chinese physician provides this by administering those herbal medicines which he assumes to contain the same protective substances that are produced naturally within the human body. That this practice is generally sound is confirmed by modern Western science with its researches into vitamins, hormones and the functionings of the endocrine glands.

The Greek physician Hippocrates (c. 460–370 BC), sometimes called the Father of Western Medicine, came to the same conclusion, for he pointed out that it is nature, not the physician, that heals, though the physician may render nature some assistance. But one may wonder just how reliable is the assistance rendered to nature by those addictive and synthetic drugs prescribed so lavishly by some of the physicians of the West.

With their preference for prophylaxis, Chinese physicians would argue that the observance of a few elementary rules of hygiene would prevent the spread of infection, and then there would be less need of curative and alleviative treatments. But they would also argue that this should not become a fetish, as it often is in the West, for too much cleanliness could destroy the effectiveness of the immune system of the body and the natural oil secreted by the skin, which serves as a barrier against infection; and overuse of chemical detergents probably does more damage than the micro-organisms they are intended to eliminate. Certainly, the benefits of hygiene are sometimes more aesthetic than clinical. To the Western mind, white is symbolic of purity; but, although white garments show up dirt better than those which are black or coloured, there is little evidence to indicate that the white coat worn by a pharmacist is basically any cleaner than the black suit worn by a funeral director. And the use of perfumes and other cosmetic preparations is sometimes a case of employing one smell to cover up another. It could well be that many people would think twice about using certain cosmetics if they knew more about the sources and quality of the ingredients.

On the subject of infections and asepsis, it is interesting to note that, for many centuries, the Chinese have used garlic, *Allium sativum*, as an internal antiseptic, which is mild and selective in that it destroys only those minute intestinal flora which are harmful. During the civil war in China, which ended with the establishment of the People's Republic of China in 1949, there was a general shortage of medical supplies, and garlic was used quite effectively as an external antiseptic. In the period of the Song dynasty (960–1279), Chinese physicians were beginning to use the fermented brine of salted vegetables as a penicillin-type antibiotic in the treatment of diseases caused by bacteria of the genus *Streptococcus*. Moreover, Chinese physicians have long been aware that the species of *Penicillium* mould from which the antibiotic penicillin is derived grows naturally on sheep dung and other organic materials, and so the discovery of penicillin by Sir Alexander Fleming (1881–1955) and later developed by Howard Chain and Ernst Florey, was not so new and as novel as people might have thought at the time, for Chinese physicians, many centuries earlier, had conceived of antibiosis being a distinct possibility.

The Chinese have always taken good care of the environment. It is one aspect of the Taoist principle of working with nature. A healthy environment yields clean air, pure water and an abundance of fresh food, without which a lifestyle of quality would not be possible. Nature must not be abused, and so it is important to return to nature a little of what nature has given. A good example of this attitude is to be found in the paddy fields, which are a prominent feature of agriculture in the south of China. When the rice is harvested, the grains, or seeds, are stored until they are required for use as food, the stems are dried to make a straw which is fashioned into mats, hats, shoes, bags and other useful items, and the roots are left in the ground, where they rot to form a compost, or are burnt to make a fertilizer, thereby ensuring a supply of nutrients for the rice plants of the next season.

A further, and most significant, example of this attitude is to be found in the behaviour of Qin Shi Huang Di (259–210 BC), the first emperor of China. He feared that freedom of thought and speech might lead to opposition to his rule, and so he ordered the burning of all books. But he exempted books about agriculture, medicine and divination. Clearly, he had perceived that success in survival and the art of living is largely determined by the food products yielded by sound agricultural policies, an effective system of medicine, and some knowledge of future events as far as that is possible, for to be forewarned is to be forearmed.

Huang Di, or 'the Yellow Emperor', a legendary figure who should not be confused with Qin Shu Huang Di, the first emperor, took a personal interest in diet, medicine and divination, which is not surprising since he wished to achieve immortality. His discoveries are recorded in *Huang Ni Dei Jing*, or 'The Internal Book of Huang Di', which was compiled by a group of scholars during the time of the Han dynasty.

The Chinese diet is related to health and medicine, and it is varied, balanced and mainly vegetarian. It contains an abundance of foods which have health-giving or medicinal properties. They are what we might call health foods, though the term health food as it is used in the West is something of a misnomer, for some of the so-called health foods are, in fact, vitamin supplements, food concentrates and the like, and, in the quantities consumed, they are sometimes unhealthy. Vitamins are essential to the health, but only in small amounts, and, in themselves, they have little or no nutritional value.

One of the important principles of TCM is the belief that a person's health and well-being is largely determined by *qi*, or 'essential life-force', which is energy provided by nature, and which can exist both within and without the body, indicating that there is a relationship between health and the environment. Perhaps *élan vital*, or 'life-force', a concept postulated by the French philosopher Henri Bergson (1859–1941), is a fair definition of *qi*. This notion seems to be far-fetched until we begin to think in terms of enzymes, vitamins, minerals and trace elements, which are vital to the health, and which are contained in foodstuffs, and so are products of the environment. It says much for the perspicacity of the physicians of ancient China that they had discovered by observation and inspired guesswork what modern science has only recently discovered and confirmed by laboratory experiments. Chinese physicians should be forgiven for likening *qi* to a fluid, for chemical substances are digested and assimilated in a liquid form. However, most of the medical scientists of the West adamantly maintain that *qi* does not exist, but they could be wrong.

There are more things in heaven and earth, Horatio,
Than are dreamt of in your philosophy.

Hamlet, William Shakespeare

This difference of opinion could be explained by saying that the thought processes and customs of the people of the East have always been totally different from those of the people of the West. But this is now changing, for improvements in communications are creating a smaller world, which is leading to a sharing of knowledge which, eventually, will be for the greater good of every member of the world community. This is as true of medicine as it is of any other branch of study. It is significant that a few medical scientists in the West are now tending to follow the Chinese example, and are investigating more fully the curative properties of the chemical substances which occur in plants and animals.

An adequate amount of exercise is vital to health. Most Chinese take exercise by practising kungfu, or the martial arts, which, despite the blood-curdling yells and the rapidity of the movements involved, are essentially gentle sports in which all the movements are governed and patterned by certain rules and laid-down procedures, though they were originally developed for self-defence, when it was the exponent's purpose to put his assailant out of action without too much effort on his own part, and with no injury to himself, and even with little or no injury to his assailant.

There is certainly nothing gentle about rugby football, baseball, hockey and some of the other games played in the West. The large numbers of internal injuries, such as contusions, green-stick fractures and pulled muscles and ligaments, which are sustained by the participants, may not be apparent at the time but show up in later life as growths and other deformities, together with cardiac malfunctions. Over-exertion, as in weight-lifting and similar activities, is best avoided.

There are hundreds of different systems of classical kungfu, each with its own style and traditions, but all have certain features in common. *Kungfu* is a Chinese term which means 'skill produced by training', and it could be applied to painting, needlework or any other skilled activity. But, more specifically, it is used to denote the skills of the martial arts, though *wushu* is the proper term.

A system of kungfu which is very gentle, and so suitable for children and elderly people, is the Tai Chi, which has meditative and philosophical aspects. Its slow and graceful movements are an attempt to physically copy the harmonious relationships which emanate from the yin and yang principle. Generally, elderly people do not engage in combat, but are content to practise the movements as a kind of shadow-boxing.

Regular exercise helps to ensure that muscles do not become soft and flabby, that joints do not become stiff, and that the most benefit is derived from the intake of food. Oxygen enters the body via the lungs, but the actual process of respiration occurs in the tissues, and a good circulation of the blood, which is promoted by regular exercise, conveys oxygen and nutrients to the tissues where they are required. It also conveys the waste products of respiration to the kidneys and lungs, where they are excreted.

Exercise is also an aid to the digestion, for the bodily movements assist peristalsis, which is the involuntary contractions and relaxations of the muscular wall of the alimentary canal, so the chyme, which is the food that has undergone gastric digestion, is kept in motion, thereby aiding assimilation and preventing constipation. A little exercise often relieves flatulence, or 'shifts the wind', as this process is described in colloquial terms. However, it is inadvisable to take strenuous exercise immediately after a meal, for it would put too much of a strain on the heart.

Chinese diet is closely related to TCM. Apart from the fact that a sound diet is conducive to health, many of the culinary herbs and spices have medicinal properties, and it is the traditional practice for some medicines to be administered as items of diet – in soups, stews and salads.

Li Shizhen (1517–93), a most dedicated physician of the period of the Ming dynasty (1368–1644), compiled an encyclopaedia of herbs, *Ben Cao Gang Mu*, or 'Outlines and Divisions of Herbal Medicines', a work which occupied him for nearly 30 years. It lists about 2000 remedies. Of these, only 300 are in common use today. Li Shizhen's work was widely distributed throughout China and other countries in the Far East, and was translated into many European languages, which says much for his knowledge and skill as a physician. It is still regarded as an authoritative work.

At an earlier period, Han scholars had listed many herbs in *Shen Nong Ben Cao Jing*, or 'The Pharmacopoeia of Shen Nong'. Shen Nong put all medicines into three main classes: those which support life, those which fortify vitality, and those which are poisons and which are used to treat the most virulent diseases. One should note that some of the medicines listed in a Chinese pharmacopoeia are of animal or mineral origin.

The Chinese do not make a sharp distinction between what is a health food and what is a medicine, for many Chinese foods have medicinal properties, and so they are as much medicines as they are sources of nutrition and pleasure. Chinese physicians take the view that, if one's diet is sound, one should generally have no great need of formal medicines.

Delicious dishes banish potions and pills;
Nourishing food is the cure for most ills.

Chinese Traditional

Chinese herbal medicine began over 5000 years ago, as an offshoot of the culinary arts, when it was first noticed that some plants were not only safe to eat but also had beneficial effects in other directions. Those found to be poisonous, causing nausea, diarrhoea, drowsiness or even death, were avoided. At a later stage, it was noticed that many plants had specifically beneficial effects: some relieved sickness, some eased pain, some had a stimulating effect, and so on. And some of the poisonous plants, which had initially been ignored, were applied externally to destroy skin infections or soothe aching limbs, or were taken internally in small amounts or mild forms as cathartics (to relieve constipation) or emetics (to induce vomiting). There were apparent contradictions, as with those species of nettles whose stinging hairs, which contain formic acid, irritate the skin, sometimes painfully, but which may be infused to make a medicine that can be applied externally to treat rashes or taken internally as an iron tonic to improve the blood.

Chinese herbal medicine is also an offshoot of the quest for immortality which was instituted by some of the emperors of ancient China, who regarded themselves as demigods, and were wont to set their physicians and other learned men the task of searching for herbs and other devices which they might use to achieve immortality. This quest was abandoned when it became evident that its objective could never be realized. But it had not been an entirely unfruitful exercise, for its researches had yielded a wide range of health foods and herbal medicines which improve the general health, increase virility and inhibit the ageing process, so extending the life span, and thereby producing more than a little peace of mind.

And so, although the physicians of ancient China did not find the means of attaining immortality, nor was that likely, they did contrive the means to attain the next best thing, which is a long and healthy life of vigorous youthfulness. They had discovered the secret of Peter Pan, and they began to translate it into action more than 3000 years ago; and youth, like health, is a very precious commodity.

The Chinese are calm by temperament, and of moderate habits, and they try to establish harmony in all their endeavours, which are a few of the reasons why they are healthy and have great peace of mind. It follows that the person who is not reckless in his habits will be less prone to illness and accidents; and, if he has peace of mind, he will surely sleep better, eat better and generally feel better.

In this respect, the Chinese are strongly influenced by the teachings of Lao Zi and Confucius, both of whom advocated a strict adherence to the 'golden mean', which is the principle that one should always take the middle way, and so avoid violent extremes of conduct. Confucius, in his well-known 'golden rule', also indicated the correct form of human relationships.

> What you do not want done to yourself, do not do to others.
>
> *Analects*, Confucius

In the West, excess consumption of tobacco, alcohol and drugs, and gambling and casual sex are recognized as being the cardinal vices, if not the cardinal sins. Perhaps gourmandizing should be added to these vices, for it is certainly the case that more people die from overeating than under-eating. Unfortunately, the people of the West tend to adopt an 'all-or-nothing' approach, so immoderation abounds. With many, it is either total self-indulgence or total abstinence. The Chinese see no virtue in greed; on the other hand, they see no virtue in complete self-denial. Li Shizhen said of wine: 'A beautiful gift from heaven if taken in moderation.'

As one would expect, the Chinese are moderate in their sexual habits, and their attitude towards sex is matter-of-fact and without any sanctimonious humbug. Their principle here is that what is healthy must be moral. But they would certainly not subscribe to the converse view that what is moral must be healthy, for definitions of morality vary from culture to culture. In Western society, there is often a moral justification for conduct which is patently immoral, and it often has a basis in commercial greed. It could seem that some of the laws in Western society have more to do with expediency than with morality, on the principle of 'if you can't beat 'em, join 'em'. Perhaps we, in the West, have developed intelligence at the expense of integrity.

Whatever philosophers may decide about man's destiny, nature has already decreed that his main purpose is to ensure the continuance of the human race, and to that end has provided him with an instinct for self-preservation and a capacity for procreation. It seems that, though there is no immortality for the individual, there is an attempt at immortality for the race, which could offer a little consolation to those who are reluctant – and perhaps afraid –

to accept the harsh finality of death. 'Hope springs eternal in the human breast . . .'

That men and women are intended to love and complement each other is plainly obvious to the Chinese, but it is less obvious to those people of the West who regard unnatural practices as being acceptable.

As far as the Chinese are concerned, it is an inescapable fact that sex is as natural as eating or drinking or any other bodily function. But they also recognize that, with sex, as with food, there is a need for moderation and precautions, for one can have too much – or too little – of a good thing. The consequences of unbridled lust or total celibacy can be just as damaging as those of gluttony or fasting. What is more, a pleasure taken too often ceases to be a pleasure.

The Chinese have an abhorrence of certain sexual practices, such as prostitution and homosexuality, and other sexual deviations which they regard as being unnatural, unhealthy and destructive of stability within the family and society. Contraceptive devices are unnatural, but they accept these as a matter of compromise, for China already has far too many mouths to feed.

The Chinese advocate marriage, not as a sacred institution, nor to earn themselves a place in some kind of paradise, but on a secular basis, and as a practical way of preventing the spread of disease and of providing the security of good parenthood for their offspring. The emphasis is more on planned procreation than reckless recreation.

It cannot be gainsaid that moderate habits are conducive to a sound state of mental health. It must be the case that the person who has a regulated and uncomplicated way of life, in both work and play, will be less prone to stress, and so less likely to succumb to those mental and nervous disorders that are called neuroses, anxiety states, nervous breakdowns, nervous debility, and so forth, which are manifested by irrational anger or acute fear, and which evoke the desire to fight or take flight. These conditions are more likely to be due to malfunctions of the body – tiredness, glandular disturbances, inadequate diet, etc. – than any serious malfunction of the brain or nervous system.

In this respect, some people seem to create difficulties for themselves by overtaxing themselves, both bodily and mentally, as the consequence of cheating, over-ambition, self-deception or becoming involved in perverse pleasures. One is tempted to think that the nervous disorders which arise in this way are really moral disorders. Chinese physicians advise that, with these conditions, laughter and sleep are good medicines.

Chinese physicians would certainly go along with the following quotation from the Roman poet Juvenal (*c.* AD 60–130), for they are of the opinion that mental health and physical health are interdependent, and that the mind, or personality, or soul, or psyche, as it was called by the ancient Greeks, though we may call it what we will, manifests some of the functions of the body, and it can have no separate existence from the body, though the religions of the West have systematically encouraged an erroneous belief which is entirely to the contrary. Obviously, the wise physician, be he Chinese or Western, will understand that, to take care of the mind, one must also take care of the body.

> *Orandum est ut sic mens sans in corpore sano.*
> (Your prayer must be for a healthy mind in a healthy body.)
> *Satires*, Juvenal

The brain may be the organ of reasoning and stored thoughts, but it requires a nervous system if it is to be supplied with data, and a blood supply, provided by the heart, if it is to function at all. It is also influenced by those chemical substances, called hormones, which are secreted by the endocrine glands. Strong feelings of joy, sadness and anger are registered by the brain, but are prompted by the chemistry of the body. It is often the case that what is regarded as an illness of the mind is, in fact, an unfavourable reaction of the mind to an illness of the body. These revealing facts are a product of modern medical research, but they confirm the validity of what Chinese physicians have long suspected.

Chinese physicians have a wide range of sedative and soporific medicines which, in emergencies, may be used to still the aggressions and fears of those persons who have fallen victim to a nervous disorder, but who might have been spared this sorry fate if they had lived more moderately in matters of diet, exercise, rest, sleep, sex, work and play.

In the West, not a few people become nervously ill and mentally disturbed as a consequence of participation in pleasures which are both exotic and erotic. But it is those people who live quietly and stably in a dull routine, or what the Chinese call 'uninteresting times', who are the more likely to be free of illness and accidents.

Those Chinese who feel they have need of a 'salve for sickness of the soul' consult the *I Ching*, which is briefly, but accurately, described in the following quotation:

Semi-sacred, a legacy from ancient China, a classical work of great antiquity, fount of profound wisdom, the most reliable of all divinatory oracles, supportive of the all-important art of living, founded by the Taoists, studied by Confucius and improved by his followers, and, in its inspiration, the oldest and one of the most valuable books in the world, the *I Ching* is amazingly GOOD NEWS!

The *I Ching* is a source of wisdom for the talented and ambitious, consolation for the afflicted and desperate, and encouragement for all who value health, longevity and peace of mind.

The *I Ching* consists essentially of 64 six-line figures, or hexagrams, which have been made by pairing the eight trigrams of the Pa Kua, a mystic symbol, of which a copy is shown below. A complete line is positive (yang) and represents one in the binary system of numbers; and a broken line is negative (yin) and represents zero. Sixty-four is a multiple of two, which is the base number in the binary system. This, of course, is the principle of the electronic computer, and it is one of the many instances where, by over 5000 years, the sages of ancient China anticipated some of the recent scientific and technological developments in the West; from which it may be gathered that those people of the West who consider themselves to be intellectually superior to the Chinese certainly have much to learn.

In this connection, one should note that the nervous system functions in much the same way as an electronic computer, the brain being its memory bank, and the 'messages' it carries are in the

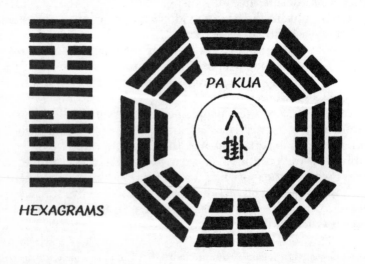

HEXAGRAMS

PA KUA

八
卦

form of electrochemical impulses, or waves of excitation, which transfer energy from a nerve cell to its adjacent nerve cells. Every thought can be expressed as a question requiring an answer which is either 'yes' (positive) or 'no' (negative), though there are degrees of positivity and negativity.

Occasionally, as with a computer, the brain fails to operate correctly. 'The lines get crossed', as we might say in popular parlance. This kind of knowledge should dispel some of the stigma which, in the West, is sometimes ascribed to mental and nervous disorders. There is nothing immoral about having a sprained ankle, and so why should it be thought to be immoral to have a 'sprained brain'? But it must be admitted that a mental illness may stem from immoral behaviour. There is the classic example of the man who revels in deception, but who eventually becomes the victim of self-deception – he has come to believe in his own lies. Cast in this mould are the people who develop fixations as the consequences of romantic attachment, religious belief, political ideology and suchlike. But faith has always been the enemy of reason.

One of the features of the *I Ching* is that, in many of its hexagrams, one of the trigrams in a pair is an exact mirror image of the other. Could this mean that the philosophers of ancient China were aware of the physicist's principle of the lateral inversion and understood the laws of optics? This is an interesting speculation.

Carl Gustav Jung (1875–1961), the eminent Swiss psychiatrist and psychologist, consulted the *I Ching* when applying treatments to his patients, and Baron von Leibnitz (1646–1716), the German mathematician and philosopher, was inspired by the *I Ching* when he invented a mechanical calculator and a form of the calculus, which is a branch of mathematics that is essential to the needs of modern engineering. This is surely a sound testimony to the validity of the *I Ching* as a source of wisdom.

Chinese physicians are very much aware of the perils of suppressing symptoms and treating symptoms rather than the actual illness. The nervous system is, among its many functions, the alarm system of the body, and the various aches and pains which it manifests are nature's way of proclaiming that something is amiss, and they often enable the physician to locate and treat the cause of an illness. It certainly is not enough to merely deaden the pain, which can usually be done with analgesics.

The Chinese physician uses massage in a gentle form, which involves light stroking, as a diagnostic technique to locate growths and other abnormalities, and to examine the nature of those ailments which may be indicated by the temperature of the skin.

Other diagnostic techniques are hearing, smell, sight and knowledge of the patient's habits. The physician uses a stethoscope to listen to the sound made by the patient's heart, lungs and other viscera. By tradition, his stethoscope is a bamboo tube. He observes and examines the eyes, tongue, skin, toe-nails, finger-nails and excretions, and also notices the patient's behaviour and habits in speech, coughing, breathing, perspiration, urination, defaecation, eating, drinking and menstruation. These methods are basically the same as those employed in Western medicine, the essential difference being that they are used more extensively, and probably more skilfully, by the Chinese physician, for he generally has no X-rays, cardiograms and the like to aid him if he is practising in the traditional way.

It takes a Chinese physician many years to learn all the skills of pulse-taking and the other diagnostic techniques. With so much care and complication in diagnosis, it follows that a medical examination in China is always thorough, never cursory.

Chinese physicians employ a wide range of manipulative techniques, which include massage in its many different forms, acupuncture, acupressure, moxibustion, poulticing and blood-letting.

Massage is used in the treatment of sciatica, rheumatism, stiff joints, sprains, pulled muscles and tendons, paralysis, prolapse of internal organs and similar conditions. It stimulates the circulation of the blood, clears the pores of waste and blockages, and increases vitality and resistance to disease. It is thought to tone *qi*, or 'vital energy'.

Massage could be regarded as 'exercise in reverse' because, in so far as it improves the circulation of the blood and tones the muscles and other organs, it provides some of the same benefits as exercise. It has the additional advantage that the work is done by the masseur, not by the subject. It is the lazy person's approach to taking exercise. It is of particular benefit to martial artists, whose muscles and tendons are sometimes severely strained, and also to elderly people who, for one reason or another, cannot indulge in vigorous exercise.

Acupuncture is a system of therapy whereby the brain, nervous system and vital organs are stimulated by the insertion of thin steel needles into vital-energy points, or nerve endings, on the body. The stimulation, which is achieved by rotating the needles, has specific remedial effects on the various organs to which the points are related, and also has a more generalized effect in improving *qi* within the body. It is a painless procedure.

Although many of the medical scientists of the West are sceptical about the efficacy of acupuncture, it has been shown to be effective in the treatment of many ailments, both internal and external, and it is of immense value in the treatment of depression and other nervous disorders. Those who have taken a course of acupuncture claim that the outcome has pleasantly surprised them.

Acupressure is very similar to acupuncture except that the fingertips are used instead of needles, and it is less effective. It is often combined with massage to relieve headaches and painful joints.

Moxibustion is another system of treatment which is similar to acupuncture, but a glowing wick, instead of needles, is the source of stimulation. It is used as a treatment for a wide variety of ailments – including mumps and nosebleeds!

Bian Que (407–310 BC), whom the Chinese regard as being the first professional physician in China, is thought to have been the first person to practice acupuncture.

Blood-letting is employed as a treatment for abscesses, swellings, fever, heat stroke, diarrhoea and apoplexy. Until fairly recent times in the West, leeches (blood-sucking worms) were used for this purpose, but the practice was abandoned when it was realized that leeches can be a source of infection, and that the loss of a large quantity of blood is very weakening. But Chinese physicians have no such problems. A sharp needle, sterilized by being held in a flame, is used to prick a small hole where the treatment is required, and only a little blood is released.

There is certainly no lack of surgical expertise among the medical men of China. During the time of the Song dynasty, anaesthetics were being used in minor surgery. However, the Chinese surgeon is not 'quick on the draw' with his knife, for he would argue that, as far as is possible, patients should be spared the misery of post-operative shock and pain, and that, in any case, crudely performed surgery may do damage to the tissues and organs which is worse than that caused by the illness which it is intended to cure or alleviate.

Chinese physicians use herbal medicines in many situations where Western doctors would use surgery. Fractured bones are mended by applying herbs, and the bones knit and the adjacent tissues heal very quickly without infection or other complications. Boils and tumours, cysts, warts and other growths are not excised, but are painlessly reduced or detached by means of herbal applications.

The Chinese physician will, as a matter of necessity, hospitalize his patients for surgery which requires expensive equipment or special techniques. Otherwise, he prefers that they be treated in their own homes, and on the sound principle that a person who is already in a weakened state should be kept well away from a source of infection; and a hospital is certainly that. The absence of professional nursing skill in a patient's home will be largely offset by the devotion of his family, together with the overall supervision of his physician.

China has the oldest civilization in the world, and so it is hardly surprising that the Chinese always give first priority to the promotion of health and the cultivation of medical knowledge, and they have been enormously successful in that direction. Certainly, we would be most unwise if we were to underestimate their capabilities in other directions.

The information in this section provides the foreknowledge of the Chinese approach to health and medicine without which the newcomer to TCM cannot hope to use this dictionary with complete ease. But only the more salient features have been touched upon, the more in-depth information being contained in the main body.

Eternal Harmony

Earth and sky meet, four seasons merge, wind and rain are gathered in, and Yin and Yang are in harmony.

Chinese Traditional

Fundamental to the proper understanding of all Chinese philosophy and institutions, including TCM, is the yin-yang principle of complementary opposites.

The symbol shown alongside represents the Tai Chi, or Supreme Ultimate. It is the Chinese concept of a deity – and an inanimate one! – and the First Cause of the universe and the origin of life. It embodies the *yin*, which are negative (−) poles, or forces, and the *yang* which are positive (+) poles, or forces. According to Chinese philosophy, order and harmony throughout the universe and within the human body are maintained by keeping these opposing forces in a constant state of delicate balance. Without this balance, there would be chaos. Yin signifies passivity, fragility, night, death and femininity, whereas yang signifies movement, strength, day, birth and masculinity. A yin force and a yang force attract each other, but two yin forces or two yang forces repel each other. 'Like poles repel: unlike poles attract.'

On the Tai Chi symbol, the black yin segment contains a small white yang circle, and the white yang segment contains a small black yin circle. This is a symbolic way of saying that yin contains a little yang, and yang contains a little yin, so that neither yin nor yang can ever be entirely predominant. It also indicates the Chinese notion that the universe is a finely balanced and integrated whole – exemplified by the orderly motion of the planets and the succession of the seasons – as also is the human body when in a sound state of health. The Chinese have so arranged their society that it is a finely balanced and integrated whole, and they perceive the function of the physician as being mainly that of maintaining a harmonious balance within the human body.

The yin-yang principle of complementary opposites and har- monious relationships derives from the Taoist philosophy, which was founded by Lao Zi, who lived during the time of the Zhou dynasty (1100–221 BC), which was the Golden Age of Chinese philosophy, when Chinese society took on the form that it still retains today. The yin-yang principle accounts for all the causes and effects in nature, and explains all the motivations of mankind. In being supportive of the modern scientific theory of cause and effect, the yin-yang principle validates the doctrine of predestination, which is the belief that all events are pre-ordained. It opposes the doctrine of self-determination, or free will, which, until recent times, had long been held as tenable by the philosophers and religionists of the Western world. But free will is an illusion created by our inability to foresee the events which have been preordained for us.

The Chinese belief in the yin-yang principle of universal and eternal harmony is consistent with modern scientific ideas about the structure of matter and the nature of energy. An atomic explosion is a spectacular example of what happens if there is a shift in the fine balance between yin and yang.

The yin-yang principle certainly should not be dismissed as superstition, for modern science has provided us with many examples of complementary opposites in nature: light and shadow, acceleration and deceleration, force and inertia, the north and south poles of magnets, positive and negative charges of electricity, evaporation and condensation, etc. – and the atom itself is a collection of positive and negative charges (protons and electrons). It is awesome to realize that the sages of ancient China anticipated Newton's Third Law of Motion – 'action and reaction are equal and opposite' – by over 3000 years.

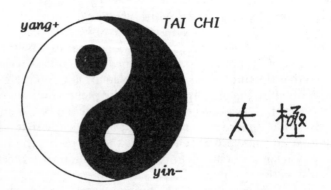

The Chinese Diet

When going to an eating-house, make sure it is one that is full of people.

Chinese Proverb

The Chinese diet is closely health related, and so it follows that, if one wishes to make a study of Chinese medicine, one must have some knowledge of the Chinese diet.

The Chinese cook has two main concerns: health and appetite. He considers that it is not enough that meals should be highly nutritious and possessed of health-giving properties. They should also arouse the appetite or people will not be persuaded to partake of them. What is the good of a nutritious meal which no one particularly wants to eat?

The main features of the Chinese diet are as follows.

1. Meals are made appetizing by harmonious blending, on the yin-yang principle, of complementary opposites in colour, texture, flavour and fragrance – dark with bright, smooth with lumpy, sour with sweet, and so on.
2. The Chinese diet is mainly vegetarian. Red meat is rarely consumed, the main sources of protein being eggs, fish, poultry, beans and cereals. This makes sense, for our nearest relatives, the apes and monkeys, are not meat-eating animals, and so perhaps we should be vegetarians, too.
3. The courses and the contents of the individual dishes are balanced on the yin-yang principle – acid with alkaline or neutral, irritating with smooth, cooked with uncooked, fish with cereal, and so on. The two main categories of food are the *fan* and the *cai*. The former consists of cereals and vegetables, of which rice is the usual mainstay, and the latter consists of meat and fish. *Fan*, which literally means 'cooked grain', provides bulk, and is filling and satisfying. It is easily digested, protective, smooth and not irritating to the alimentary canal, and it absorbs the excess grease and acids in the richly spiced

sauces of the *cai*, whose main function is to provide a savoury send-off for the *fan*, which might otherwise be somewhat insipid.

4. There is great variety, and so one cannot consume too much of what is harmful, nor too little of what is beneficial. Thus, no dietary planning is required, nor are diet sheets, vitamin supplements and similar paraphernalia.

5. There is a distinct preference for fresh ingredients, that is fruits and vegetables in season, freshly slaughtered pigs and poultry, and freshly caught fish.

6. Those food items which are known to he harmful, such as animal fats and synthetic additives, are kept at a minimum or avoided altogether.

7. The ingredients are usually diced, shredded or thinly sliced to create a greater surface area so that they are much more easily blended, cooked and digested.

8. Stir-frying is the main method of cooking. This ensures that the ingredients are cooked quickly so that the nutrients are sealed in and not destroyed.

9. Steaming is another popular method of cooking. It has two advantages. The food never reaches a temperature which is higher than that of boiling water, so it will not burn or be over-cooked. Also, most of the soluble substances it contains are not lost by becoming dissolved in the water, as would occur if it were boiled. We, in the West, have a saying: 'The best part of a cabbage is thrown away with the water.'

10. Porcelain spoons, wooden ladles and chopsticks are preferred to metal cutlery, for food becomes tainted by contact with metals. Also, metals are good conductors of heat, and so one's fingertips are more likely to be burnt by a metal spoon than one made of porcelain or wood.

11. Many of the Chinese foodstuffs and culinary herbs have medicinal properties, and many Chinese medicines are admin-istered as items of diet.

A cursory study of the diet of the Chinese might suggest that some of their culinary techniques are rather pointless. But a deeper study reveals that there is indeed sound purpose in their methods. A good example of this is the inclusion of at least one sweet-and-sour dish in a large meal.

The explanation is that a sweet-and-sour dish contains vinegar, which is ethanoic acid (or acetic acid in the older system of chemical nomenclature), and which augments the hydrochloric acid that occurs naturally in the stomach. This acid has three main purposes. It provides an acid medium without which the gastric enzymes will not function, it destroys some of the micro-organisms which cause stomach upsets, and it dissolves small bones, so rendering them non-injurious and as a soluble source of calcium.

The Chinese practice of cutting or shredding food ingredients into small pieces has much to commend it, for it ensures that a very large surface area is exposed to the action of digestive juices. The Chinese diner busily engaged with his chopsticks is less likely to suffer from indigestion than his European or American counterpart who is hastily swallowing large gobbets of meat.

The wok is another instance of the ingenuity and deep thinking of the Chinese. Of all the tools which are available to the culinary artist, the wok must surely be the most useful and the most versatile. Its nearly hemispherical shape ensures a rapid and even distribution of heat. It is easy to use and keep clean because it has no awkward angles and joints, as is the case with saucepans and frying-pans, features which make for economy in money, time and patience. One can only wonder why this amazingly easy-to-use cooking aid, which was evolved many centuries ago, did not enter the kitchens of the Western world until recent times.

The wok is ideal for stir-frying, for which purpose it is mainly used, because its deep, smooth, sloping sides ensure that the ingredients and the oil remain in its bottom, where the heat is at a maximum, which makes for economy in the use of oil, and prevent the ingredients from spilling over the rim when they are being stirred, as sometimes occurs when a frying-pan is used for this purpose.

The wok is also used for deep-frying, shallow-frying, sautéing, boiling, simmering, steaming, braising and poaching. Only a small quantity of oil is required for deep-frying; and two different items may be fried at the same time, one deep and one shallow.

The Chinese do not make a sharp distinction between medicines and health foods, but if a Chinese physician were asked for definitions, he would probably say that the former are non-nutritious substances with specific or general remedial properties, whereas the latter are foods which, in addition to being nutritious, have health-giving or medicinal properties.

The people of the West would be inclined to define a health food as one which improves the health or does no harm to the health, on the principle that so many of the foodstuffs available in the West are of a deleterious character that those which at least do no harm to the health are considered to be of special merit. For example, both beef and fish are rich in protein, but the latter is to be preferred as an item of diet, and could be regarded as a health food, because its oils are polyunsaturated and do not lead to the formation of cholesterol with all its attendant risks, which include thrombosis and arteriosclerosis (hardening of the arteries).

Chinese physicians and cooks classify foodstuffs according to their medicinal properties – heating, cooling, irritating, nourishing, etc. This is only a rough-and-ready technique, but it works quite well in practice. Here are some examples:

VERY HEATING: mutton, smoked fish, peanut butter.
HEATING: eggs, pig's liver, walnuts, leeks.
NEUTRAL: chicken, pigeon, carrots, rice.
COOLING: fish, duck, mushrooms, cabbage.
VERY COOLING: shellfish, bananas, cucumber, tea.
MILDLY IRRITATING: beef, onions, garlic, wine.
VERY IRRITATING: shellfish, vinegar, aubergines.
NOURISHING: chicken, eels, honey, garlic.
VERY NOURISHING: pigeon, pig's liver, ginseng tea.

The Chinese cook will employ this technique, often with the recommendations of a physician, when preparing dishes for invalids. A person with a fever will be given cooling foods, a person with an upset stomach will not be given irritating foods, and so on.

Of the wide range of health foods that are available to the Chinese, the following are available at high-class provisions dealers and Chinese grocery stores in the West: green tea, honey, royal jelly, gingseng, garlic, Chinese wolfberries, long-grain rice, taro starch, scallions, ginger, soyabean products, abalone, tienchi, sweet potatoes, pig's trotters, winter mushrooms, king prawns, figs, cassia, ginseng tea.

But, in thinking in terms of a healthy diet, knowing what NOT to eat must be as important as knowing what to eat. This list, which is far from being exhaustive, shows some of the dietary items which the Chinese keep at a bare minimum or avoid altogether.

1. Unboiled water.
2. Synthetic additives: acidity regulators, sweeteners, flavourings, colourings, preservatives, emulsifiers, flavour enhancers, etc.
3. Adulterants.
4. Refined sugar.
5. Butter, dripping, lard, cream, suet and other animal fats.
6. Red meat and fatty meat of any kind.

7. Eggs that are not well cooked.
8. Alcohol.
9. Taro root if uncooked or insufficiently cooked.
10. Salt.
11. Cotton-seed oil (which is believed to cause male infertility).
12. Bitter almonds, for they contain prussic acid (hydrogen cyanide), which is a poison.
13. Gingko nuts.
14. Chocolate and other confectionery.
15. Unwashed fruit and vegetables.
16. The 'dead man's fingers' (apron and gills) in crabs.
17. Stock cubes.
18. Stale and tainted food.
19. Preserved foods.
20. Junk food.

In particular, one should avoid using monosodium glutamate (MSG), a substance first isolated from seaweed by a Japanese scientist in 1908. It enhances the flavour of food, and for that purpose it is often added to the food served in Chinese restaurants in the West; but it sometimes produces an allergic reaction, accompanied by a headache, palpitations and severe thirst, which is called 'Chinese restaurant syndrome', and if it is added to food before it is cooked, it is liable to be rendered toxic by the high temperature of cooking – and it is very potent!

The Tang period (618–907) physician Sun Simiao pointed out the health benefits of a sound diet and regular exercise. Since he lived to be 101, he obviously practised what he so ardently preached.

A man may have a long and healthy life if he regularly takes wholesome food and proper exercise and effects an emission twice monthly or twenty-four times annually.

Precious Prescriptions, Sun Simiao

Another Chinese physician, but of more recent times, has made a pertinent observation: 'The roast beef of old England has claimed many victims!' It is certainly true that the diet of the West is such that one could easily believe that its people are intent on committing felo de se.

Water is not a food, for it contains no nutrients, but it is certainly vital to our existence. Whatever its source, all water intended for drinking, even spa water, should be boiled. The water that is available to us on tap is not always as potable as the authorities would have us believe, and though the sparkling spring water coming to us in attractively labelled bottles may contain mineral salts which are beneficial to the health, it may also contain pathogenic micro-organisms which are anything but beneficial to the health, and, in fact, it may be less safe to drink than tap water.

Hot water is a good start for the day if it is drunk immediately before breakfast. It offsets the dehydration caused by perspiration during the night, it has a cleansing effect on the bowel, it provides a solvent for the food which is to follow and, being water in a fairly pure form, it is easily assimilated by the alimentary canal.

Water may be taken medicinally to promote frequent urination, which eliminates waste from the blood.

Rules for Health

There are some unfortunate persons who, as a consequence of an inherited or congenital defect or an injury sustained in an accident, can never hope to attain to a long and healthy life. But, for most people, it is possible to live to a great age, and be healthy and youthful in the process, by adhering to these simple rules:

1. Remember that prevention is better than cure. Consult a physician if you have doubts about your health.
2. Adopt the Chinese diet. Failing that, ensure that your meals are balanced, and consume more cereals, vegetables, fruit and fish, and less red meat, sugar and products containing artificial additives.
3. Think young in all that you say and do.
4. Consume one garlic clove each day – preferably fresh, crushed and chopped.
5. Take a large drink of boiled water before breakfast every day.
6. Take up a gentle form of the martial arts, such as Tai Chi. Failing that, take a long and gentle walk twice daily.
7. Be moderate and regular in all you do – diet, tobacco, alcohol, exercise, rest, sleep, sex, work and play – to prevent illness, injury and social friction.
8. Avoid the vices of casual sex, drug-taking and gambling.
9. Work with, not against, nature. Avoid all unnatural acts.
10. Be clean personally and in handling food, but do not allow it to become a fetish or you are likely to become a hygiene crank, which will not help your body, though it could upset your mind.
11. Worry less, laugh more, and do not miss out on sleep.
12. Abide by Confucius's golden rule: 'What you do not want done to yourself, do not do to others.' And always keep in mind his five cardinal virtues: wisdom, justice, charity, honesty and propriety.

THE FOUNTAIN OF HEALTH

Of course, most people do not wish to be merely healthy. They also want to be youthful.

> Age, I do abhor thee; youth, I do adore thee.
> *Venus and Adonis*, William Shakespeare

The Chinese secret of youth is the realization that, though one cannot arrest the passage of time, one can do much to reduce the speed at which the bodily organs deteriorate. The Chinese do this in a variety of ways, the main ones being those summarized below:

Moderate exercise to ensure that the muscles and other organs do not deteriorate from disuse or become damaged by over-use.

Balanced and varied diet so that the organs do not deteriorate as a consequence of starvation, malfunction or infection.

Preventive medicine to preclude or delay the onset of illness. All illnesses and injuries, even those said to be cured, have physical or psychological after-effects which assist the ageing process, if only to a small degree.

Personal hygiene for a healthy skin and to prevent the spread of infection.

Health foods and herbal medicines to delay or inhibit the ageing process, usually by controlling the hormone levels.

Moderate habits to prevent the misuse or abuse of the bodily organs.

Social harmony to prevent unhappiness, tensions and nervous breakdowns, which assist the ageing process.

The Dictionary

abalone *Haliotis gigantea* Medicine. Distribution: global. Parts: shell (finely ground). Character: cool, salty. Affinity: liver. Effects: sedative to liver, antipyretic. Symptoms: giddiness, headaches, swollen eyes. Treatments: insomnia, cataracts, conjunctivitis. Dosage: 15–25 g. Abalone is a gastropod, and its shell is lined with nacre, or mother-of-pearl. It is particularly abundant in the warm coastal waters of South China and California. It is also called a sea-ear because of its ear-shaped shell. In the Channel Islands, it is known as an ormer. As an item of diet, it is easily cooked and digested, and it is rich in protein, retinol, cobalamine, biotin, iron, copper, sodium, zinc and iodine. It is considered to be a good blood tonic. Boiled with lean pork to make a soup, it is a treatment for liver conditions, giddiness, headaches, insomnia, fevers and tuberculosis. Cooked with a pig's bladder, it is a treatment for women's ailments.

ABALONE

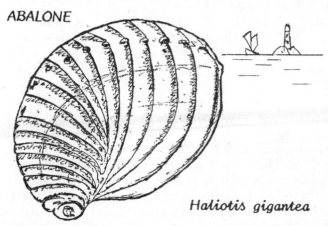

Haliotis gigantea

abdomen Region above the pelvis and below the ribs and diaphragm containing the liver, stomach, pancreas, spleen, kidneys, intestines and bladder. In women, it also contains the uterus and ovaries.

abdominal pain The fresh peel of the mandarin orange, *Citrus reticulata*, eaten in a non-critical dosage of 3–8 g, is considered to be an effective treatment. Massage is also an effective treatment.

abortifacient A drug or instrument used to induce an abortion. Barley, *Hordeum vulgare*, has abortifacient properties, and its dried sprouts may be taken orally to make muscular contractions easier during childbirth.

abortion The termination of pregnancy and the expulsion of the foetus before the time when it is likely to survive birth, which is accepted as being 28 days after the last menstruation. Continual bleeding during early pregnancy generally indicates that an abortion will be inevitable. See **miscarriage**.

abrasion A superficial injury to the skin caused by rubbing or scraping. See **cuts**.

abscess Localized accumulation of pus formed in any part of the body as a consequence of the decay of tissues. TCM internal treatments: infusions of 10–30 g leaves and flowers of dandelion, *Taraxacum officinale*, and 3–9 g flowers of chrysanthemum, *Chrysanthemum morifolium*. TCM external treatments include: a dry compress of gypsum (calcium sulphate) crystals; a wet compress of cloves of garlic, *Allium sativum*; a wet compress of a decoction of flowers of chrysanthemum, *Chrysanthemum morifolium*. Some abscesses can be punctured with a sterilized needle to release the pus. This should be done by a physician. See **cupping** and **cuttlefish**.

absolute values The Chinese are realists, not idealists, and they do not believe in absolute values either in medicine or in social affairs. They are fond of compromise, and they regard all things as being relative and flexible, and nothing is ever completely this or completely that. A balance between what is good and what is bad, what is hot and what is cold, what is strengthening and what is weakening, and so on, is their mode of treatment of illness. Thus, a yang illness is treated with a yin medicine, and vice versa. See **golden mean**.

abstinence The Chinese see no virtue in greed; on the other hand, they see no virtue in complete self-denial. They consider moderation to be one of the ways to maintain a sound state of health, and they regard fasting, celibacy and teetotalism to be just as damaging to the health as gluttony, lust and alcoholism. One can have too little as well as too much of a good thing. See **moderation**.

abulia Lack or absence of will-power. A term used in Western psychiatry. See **will-power**.

a.c. An abbreviation for the Latin words *ante cibum*, meaning 'before food', and used in prescriptions.

accident An accident may be defined as an event which is unexpected or has no apparent cause, though it *will* have a cause, for all events are pre-ordained, and modern scientific opinion is that there can be no effect without a cause. In a narrower sense, it may be defined as an unforeseen occurrence causing injury or damage. The person who values his health, be he European or Chinese, will take care, as far as he is able, to avoid accidents, which have a great variety of causes, including overdoses of medicine, poison, broken glass, sharp tools, unattended fires, highly flammable materials, damaged electrical equipment, faulty ladders and irresponsible behaviour.

accident prone A term applied to those people who are more than normally liable to be involved in accidents, either causing them or as victims. People may be accident prone as the result of a peculiarity of temperament (such as recklessness) or a phobia. Some accidents may be regarded as unavoidable, in so far as they arise from conditions in the natural, industrial, commercial or social environment. Accident-prone individuals would be well advised to follow the Chinese example by adopting moderate habits, avoiding violent extremes of conduct, thinking before acting and accepting the Confucian teaching that patience is a virtue. See **first aid** and **golden mean**.

accommodation The extent to which the eye can adjust its lens to focus on objects at various distances.

acetabulum The cup-shaped socket in the pelvis which holds the ball-shaped head of the thigh-bone, or femur, to form the hip-joint. See **arthritis**.

HIP-JOINT — pelvis — acetabulum — femur. This is a ball-and-socket joint

acetic acid See **ethanoic acid**.

acetone A flammable colourless liquid (CH_3COCH_3) with the characteristic smell of nail varnish, and which is used as a solvent for fats and resins. It is produced by the body in severe diabetes and a few other severely abnormal conditions.

acetonuria The presence of acetone in the urine.

acetylsalicylic acid See **aspirin**.

ache A prolonged and dull pain which is often symptomatic of chronic illness. It is also one of the symptoms of ageing, when joints and muscles become stiff. In the West, it is usually treated with an analgesic, such as aspirin, but the Chinese have shown that massage is sometimes effective as a treatment. Aches are less excruciating than pains, and so they tend to be disregarded, but medical advice should be sought when an ache persists, for it may be an indication of a condition which is more serious than is realized. See **pain**.

achievement See **success**.

Achilles tendon The large tendon which attaches the calf muscles to the heel bone. It is named after Achilles, a hero in Greek legend, whose only vulnerable spot on his body was his heel.

acid Chemists define an acid, in a most complicated way which is not readily understood by the layman, as a solid, liquid or gaseous substance that produces hydrogen ions (H^+), has a sour taste, turns neutral litmus red, has a pH value of less than 7, reacts with certain metals to liberate hydrogen, and reacts with bases, which are oxides and hydroxides of metals, to produce a salt and water. Examples: sulphuric acid + copper oxide → copper sulphate + water; hydrochloric acid + caustic soda → sodium chloride (table salt) + water; citric acid + baking soda → sodium citrate + water. Acids only behave as such when they are dissolved in water. Those which contain little water are said to be concentrated, and those which contain much water are said to be dilute. They are classified as mineral acids when they are of mineral origin, as with hydrochloric, sulphuric and nitric acids, and as organic acids when they are of plant or animal origin, as with citric, oxalic and ethanoic acids. This is a somewhat arbitrary classification, for hydrochloric acid, which is produced by the stomach, could be regarded as being both mineral and organic in origin. Many acids are poisonous or corrosive, and so they must NOT be tasted – to find out if they really do have a sour taste, perhaps – unless you are quite sure that it is safe to do so.

acidity Excessively acid condition of the stomach, which may be manifested by flatulence, heartburn and other discomforts, and may be caused by gastritis, stomach ulcers or a surfeit of spicy foods. Treatment: white rice porridge with the addition of 5 slices ginger or the peel of half an orange, fresh or dried. See **white rice porridge**. Avoid hot, spicy, acid and deep-fried foods, tea, coffee, cocoa and alcohol. Acupressure treatment requires massage of the acupoints in the furrow between the second and third toes, at the middle of the ankle joint on the front of the leg, and at 4 finger-widths below the kneecap on the outside of the shinbone. See **acupressure**. If this condition persists, obtain medical advice.

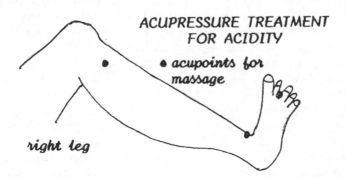

ACUPRESSURE TREATMENT FOR ACIDITY

● acupoints for massage

right leg

acidosis A decrease in the normally alkaline state of the blood and body fluids. This shift in the acid-alkaline balance of the body may arise from diabetes, kidney failure, respiratory problems, severe diarrhoea, starvation and some types of poisons. The Chinese would regard this as an undesirable change in the yin-yang balance, yin being alkaline and associated with cold, internal, descending ailments, and yang being acidic and associated with hot, external, ascending ailments. The appropriate treatment will be decided according to the organs affected, and the nature of the affects.

acid stomach See **acidity**.

acne Blackheads. It is most distressing for adolescents to have to endure the embarrassment of the facial disfigurement due to acne, which is manifested as blackheads, pustules and the like. They are so sensitive about this condition that they are not likely to be consoled by being told that beauty is only skin deep. As John Ruskin said: 'The saying that beauty is but skin deep is but a skin-deep saying.' Generally, it should give no real cause for alarm, for it is, to a large extent, no more than a manifestation of the hormonal changes which are normal to adolescent development. But it should be properly treated; otherwise any scars formed may persist into middle age. Acne is sometimes confused with eczema, but they are different ailments. Acne is essentially a facial condition, though it may affect the shoulders, chest and back, which first appears at puberty. The sebaceous glands produce an excess of sebum, which is an oily substance that is protective to the skin, and become blocked and chronically inflamed, and may even become infected. Pus and sebum build up to form pimples, comedones, or blackheads, and whiteheads, which often result in pitting, scars and patches of dead skin. There are many possible causes: hormonal imbalances, premenstrual tension, impure blood, faulty elimination from the bowel, stress, inadequate diet and lack of personal hygiene. During puberty, the hormone androgen is produced in very large quantities, and this encourages the release of sebum. Fortunately, acne generally clears up in the early twenties. In treating acne, the Chinese physician will give attention to the patient's general health, diet, skin, blood and bowel. He will prescribe eliminatives and alternatives, and ointments and lotions to relieve pruritis, or itchiness. Since the exact causes of acne are sometimes difficult to identify, he will try out a wide range of remedies in the hope of finding one that is completely effective. The acne-sufferer should take care of his general health, drink copious quantities of water as an eliminative, consume one clove of garlic per day and modify his diet, supplementing it with royal jelly, ginseng and wolfberries. Dietary items to be avoided or kept at a minimum: meat, poultry, shellfish, eggs, oily and fatty foods, refined sugar, chocolate, cocoa, tea, coffee, dairy products, bread and cereal foods made from refined flour, nuts, spices, tomatoes and avocadoes. Dietary items to be included: raw vegetables, fresh fruits, unsweetened fruit juices, molasses, honey, fish, wholemeal bread and cereals, brown rice, sunflower seeds and soyabean products. The skin must be kept scrupulously clean, but not with ordinary soap, for it blocks up the skin pores and may contain irritants. But a non-irritant soap can be made by mixing water with oatmeal to make a smooth paste. After the face is washed in hot water, it should be washed in cold water to close up the pores. Blackheads and pimples should not be squeezed, but it is sometimes helpful to paint the affected parts with lemon juice. In China, a popular treatment is an infusion of the flowers of the peach, *Prunus persica*, in cold water taken internally in a daily dosage of 3 g. But peach flowers are not readily obtainable in the United Kingdom. Internal treatments by infusions: stinging nettle, *Urtica dioica*, all parts, 5 g; garden nettle, *Urtica urens*, all parts, 5 g; sage, *Salvia officinalis*, leaves, 6 g; burdock,

Arctium lappa, root, 6 g; dandelion, *Taraxacum officinale*, all parts, 15 g; camomile, *Matricaria chamomilla*, flowers, 6 g; onion, *Allium sepa*, all parts, 50 g. External treatments by lotions: any of the infusions previously listed, together with the following: comfrey, *Symphitum officinale*, leaves or roots, 15 g; thyme, *Thymus vulgare*, leaves, 6 g; marigold, *Calendula officinalis*, petals, 5 g; lady's bedstraw, *Gallium verum*, leaves, 6 g; angelica, *Angelica archangelica*, leaves, 6 g. Note that the sage used by Chinese physicians is not *Salvia officinalis* but *dan shen*, *Salvia miltiorrhiza*, a species indigenous to China, Manchuria and Japan. See **complexion**.

aconite *Aconitum carmichaeli* Herbal medicine. Distribution: China (Sichuan and Shanxi provinces). Parts: roots. Character: very hot, very pungent. Affinity: heart, kidneys, spleen. Effects: cardiotonic, analgesic, stimulates yang energy and warms kidneys and spleen. Symptoms: cold hands and feet, weak pulse, diarrhoea, abdominal pain, bodily aches and pains. Treatments: all yang injuries, yang deficiency in kidneys, wind-cold-damp ailments, dysfunction of spleen. Aconite, which is also the name of the drug derived from this plant, is highly toxic, and so it must be used only under proper medical supervision. Sources of aconite in the West are the two species of monkshood, or wolfsbane, *Aconitum anglicum* and *Aconitum napellus*.

aconitine A poisonous alkaloid derived from aconite.

acoustic Relating to sound or the sense of hearing.

acquired An adjective which describes a permanently poor state of health which is neither hereditary nor congenital.

acquired immune deficiency syndrome See **AIDS**.

acrid See **odour**.

acromegaly A condition, slow to develop, in which the pituitary gland produces an excessive secretion of the growth hormone, which causes enlargement and thickening of the feet, hands and head.

acrophobia Morbid fear of heights.

actinomycosis A fungal infection of the mouth, lungs and intestines. It may cause abscesses.

active exercise See **active movements**.

active ingredient The medicinally active substance in a herb. In the West, drugs manufacturers refine and concentrate active ingredients so that they will act more quickly and the dosage can be accurately regulated. But this is not always a sound practice, for pure and concentrated ingredients sometimes produce unwanted side-effects. A good example of this is ephedrine, which is extracted from the Chinese herb *Ephedra sinica* and used as a treatment for asthma. It over-stimulates the heart muscle, so causing palpitations, hypertension and nervous exhaustion. Chinese physicians, however, use the herb in its natural and untreated form, and so, though it is slower to act, there are no unpleasant side-effects. The other, non-active, substances, in the herb act as a buffer, so causing the active ingredient to be absorbed more slowly.

active movements Voluntary movements of the body, that is, physical actions due to exercise of the will. See **passive movements**.

acupoints Vital-energy points, also called pressure points, which are groups of nerve endings on the meridians. They are the points where needles are inserted in acupuncture treatments, or the fingertips are pressed in acupressure treatments. Anyone who has suffered from shingles, which is an illness in which the nerve endings become very painfully inflamed, would readily testify that these nerve endings do exist and are not a figment of the imagination of some physician in ancient China. As to the number of acupoints, various values are given. An ancient text suggests as few as 365, but the accepted value is somewhere between 800 and 2000, though only about 150 are in common use. No doubt, some practitioners make their own modifications. The diagram shows the acupoints along the liver meridian on the back of the right leg. On charts and models, these points are numbered. Of course, there will be other meridians on that part of the leg. See **meridian**.

LIVER ACUPOINTS ON RIGHT LEG

liver meridian

acupoint

acupressure A combination of massage and acupuncture techniques which originated in China and Japan over 3000 years ago, and in which the fingertips are used instead of needles to exert pain-relieving pressure on the acupoints, which are the same as those used in acupuncture. In the massage techniques, other parts of the body, as well as the fingertips are used, namely the thumbs, palms, elbows, knees and feet. Acupressure improves the immune system, increases vitality and regulates and balances *qi*, or 'vital energy', which flows through invisible channels called meridians. There are several forms of acupressure, including *shiatsu*, *shin tao* and *shin do*, which differ only in the acupoints used and the amount of pressure applied. Before a treatment is begun, the practitioner will take the patient's pulse and investigate his diet and personal habits to make sure that acupressure is a suitable treatment for his condition. Acupressure has been shown to be effective as a treatment for a wide variety of ailments and conditions, including allergies, arthritis, asthma, back pains, circulatory problems, colic in babies, constipation, depression, dyspepsia, headaches, insomnia, menstrual cramps, migraine, nervous tension, painful joints and toothache. One can practise acupressure on oneself or the members of one's family – instruction manuals are available – but one should consult a qualified practitioner when there is any doubt about the nature, cause or treatment of a condition. See **shiatsu**.

acupuncture This is a system of therapy by which the brain, nervous system and vital organs are stimulated by fine stainless-steel needles inserted into acupoints, or vital-energy points, on the meridians. This stimulation, which is achieved by rotating the needles to produce a tingling, tightly twisting sensation, has specific remedial effects on the organs to which the acupoints and meridians relate. It also has a more generalized effect in improving vitality by unblocking, increasing or decreasing the flow of *qi*, or 'vital energy', through the meridians, and so correcting any yin-yang imbalances. It is essentially a painless procedure, and is usually followed by a pleasant feeling of heaviness and relaxation. Needless to say, the needles do need to be properly sterilized to prevent the transmission of blood-borne diseases, such as hepatitis and the HIV virus. Acupuncture is often used in conjunction with herbal remedies. It would be difficult to say exactly when acupuncture began, for the Chinese have been practising medicine for thousands of years, but it was mentioned in *Huang Di Nei Jing Su Wen*, or 'The Yellow Emperor's Canon of Internal Medicine'. According to historians of the period of the Han dynasty (206 BC-AD 220), Bian Que was the first person to practise acupuncture. He brought a patient out of a coma by applying needles. The Chinese regard him as the first truly professional physician. Although some of the medical scientists of the Western world are sceptical about the efficacy of acupuncture, it has been shown to be effective in the treatment of many ailments, both internal and external, and is of great value in the treatment of depression and other nervous disorders. Those who think they might benefit from a course of acupuncture should consult a Chinese physician. The outcome could be one of pleasant surprise. See **involuntary movement**.

acupuncture needles The needles used in acupuncture have a long history. Archaeologists have indicated that a form of acupuncture was practised with slivers of stone, called *bian*, during the New Stone Age. They have been described as 'stone borers' or 'stone piercers'. In *Shan Hai Jing*, or 'Book of Mountains and Seas', which was written over 200 years ago, there is a reference to deposits of jade and a stone, probably flint, suitable for making needles. Later on, needles of bone, bamboo and earthenware came into use. In actual fact, these earthenware needles were no more than bits of broken pottery. By 800 BC, metal needles of iron, bronze, silver and gold had arrived on the scene. In modern times, stainless-steel needles came into use. These are sterilized in an autoclave. Boiling water is not sufficient for this purpose, for some micro-organisms are very heat resistant. The really up-to-date acupuncturist uses disposable needles supplied in sealed, sterilized packs.

acupuncture treatments Acupuncture is used to treat more than 300 ailments and conditions, which include allergies, angina, anxiety, arthritis, asthma, bronchitis, bursitis, cataracts, catarrh, colds, colitis, cramps, deafness, depression, digestive problems, disturbed vision, facial paralysis, glaucoma, haemorrhoids, hay fever, headaches, hepatitis, hypertension, hypoglycaemia, impotence, infertility, influenza, insomnia, measles, neuralgia, otitis media, palsy, poliomyelitis, premenstrual tension, sciatica, sinus problems, sprains, stress, stroke, tinnitus, ulcers, vaginitis, vertigo and whooping cough. The World Health Organisation endorses acupuncture for the treatment of many of these conditions. Acupuncture has been shown to be of some assistance to women in labour, and also effective in treating addiction to drugs, tobacco and alcohol. Anaesthesia by acupuncture was prompted by its successful use in relieving post-operative pain. It is now used for anaesthesia in tonsillectomies, tooth extraction, thyroidectomies, herniotomies and even major surgery. Patients are conscious throughout an operation, and there are no unpleasant after-effects as there are with chemical anaesthesia. The acupuncturist will make a complete investigation of a person's state of health and lifestyle in order to decide whether acupuncture is a suitable treatment. This involves taking the pulse, examining the tongue, skin, hair texture and finger-nails, listening to the breathing and voice, observing posture and movements, and enquiring about the patient's diet, sleeping habits and medical history. But why are acupuncture treatments so successful? Sceptics say that acupuncture functions in much the same way as a placebo. But a placebo has its advantages in so far as it gives the patient some confidence. However, Chinese neurologists have produced evidence to show that acupuncture stimulates the brain into releasing neuropeptides called endorphins and enkephalins, which are morphine-like substances that induce anaesthesia. According to an old Chinese legend, soldiers who had survived arrow wounds sometimes also recovered from their chronic ailments. It seems that the arrow wounds had conferred a kind of immunity. Researchers in Europe have demonstrated that it is possible to 'block' a nerve so that 'pain messages' cannot reach the brain, which is a type of anaesthesia. The fluctuations of the hormones in the body seem to correspond with the movements of *qi* and vital essences, and so, thousands of years ago, the Chinese learned by experience what we, in the West, have learned by scientific experiments only in recent years, which was good thinking on their part. Chinese physicians would contend that acupuncture needling on the appropriate meridian stimulates the vital organ to which it is connected, and the vital organ is then better able to cope with the illness which is afflicting it. Thus, to treat hepatitis, one would need to needle the liver meridian. See **vital organs** and **gate control theory**.

acute A term used to describe an illness that is sudden, brief and generally severe, coming quickly to a crisis, and of an opposite nature to a chronic illness.

adaptogen A medicine which seems to encourage the body to adapt to adverse conditions and so be better able to cope with disease. Siberian ginseng is a good example.

addiction A craving for tobacco, alcohol or a harmful drug, with an increased, but dangerously deceptive, bodily tolerance for larger doses. Acupuncture is considered to be an effective treatment for smoking, alcoholism and some forms of drug addiction. See **drug addiction** and **withdrawal**.

Addison's disease Inadequate secretion of hormones by the adrenal glands. Symptoms: tiredness, weakness, nausea, anaemia, hypotension and dark discolourations of the skin.

additives Substances, usually synthetic, which are added to foodstuffs to preserve them, make them more appetizing or 'improve' them in some other way, and which include preservatives, acidity regulators, flavour enhancers, sweeteners, flavourings, colourings, antioxidants, tenderizers, anti-caking agents, emulsifiers, stabilizers, gelling agents, glazing agents, raising agents and thickeners. In excess, some of these additives can cause hay fever, asthma and other allergy conditions, though some are quite harmless. In the West, these additives are allowed, provided they are within the limits prescribed by law, but food manufacturers are legally bound to indicate the additives in a food product on its container. In China, these synthetic additives are rarely used, if at all, for the Chinese prefer to rely on the preserving and appetizing qualities of natural food products. To the Chinese mind, there is something quite unethical about adding to food what could really be no more than a non-food or a low-grade mild poison.

adenoid A mass of lymphatic tissue in the pharynx, and which prevents infection spreading from the nose and mouth into the trachea and lungs.

adipose Fatty, but only in reference to animal tissue.

adipose tissue Fat-containing connective tissue beneath the skin.

adiposis dolorosa Dercum's disease. An illness, peculiar to women, characterized by scattered and painful nodular deposits of fat.

ad. lib. An abbreviation for the Latin words *ad libitum*, meaning 'as one wishes' or 'freely', and used in prescriptions.

administering medicines In China, medicines are administered externally in much the same way as they are in the West – by means of lotions, liniments, ointments, poultices, compresses, bathing, etc. Many internal medicines are also administered in the same way as in the West – as pills and potions. But most are administered as items of diet, and are added to soups, broths, stews, salads and other dishes. This procedure is easy because dosages of Chinese medicines are generally non-critical, and it has one important advantage, which is that medicines in liquid form are assimilated much more readily than those in solid form. The Chinese make effective use of a wide range of medicinal wines, a practice that is uncommon in the West. Chinese physicians are not very enthusiastic about nasal sprays and similar gadgetry, and take the view that the stomach is the best point of entry for most internal medicines. For example, in China, stems of the joint fir, *Ephedra sinica*, which is a treatment for asthma, are combined with other herbs and swallowed. The medicinal constituents enter the bloodstream, via the digestive tract, whence they are carried, and most effectively, to the bronchial tubes. In the West, ephedrine, the active ingredient in the joint fir, is sprayed into the nose or throat in a concentrated form. Chinese physicians prefer to use the whole herbs in their natural form rather than as concentrated extracts. See **active ingredient**.

adrenal glands Suprarenal glands. These two glands, situated at the upper ends of the kidneys, produce some important hormones, such as adrenalin and corticosteroids.

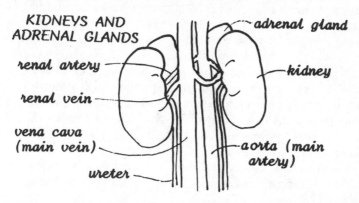

KIDNEYS AND ADRENAL GLANDS

adrenal gland

renal artery

kidney

renal vein

vena cava (main vein)

aorta (main artery)

ureter

adrenalin Epinephrine. A hormone secreted by the adrenal glands. It stimulates the sympathetic nervous system into increasing the action of the heart, blood pressure and the rate of breathing. This hormone is produced at a time of danger or fright, and provides the courage or strength to deal with an emergency.

aerobics This is a vogue word which is used as a collective description of those activities, such as walking, football and swimming, which are involved with the body's need for oxygen. These exercises strengthen the heart and lungs and increase stamina. The Chinese have engaged in breathing and remedial exercises for thousands of years. See **breathing exercises**.

aetiology The study of the causes of diseases.

afebrile Without fever; of normal temperature.

affinity of herbs Herbal medicines have an affinity for certain organs, which may be yin or yang. Thus, the dandelion, *Taraxacum officinale*, which is used to treat abscesses, tumours and blood clots in the lungs, has an affinity for the liver, which is yin, and the stomach, which is yang. See **herbal prescriptions** and **gui jing**.

afterbirth See **placenta**.

afterpains Pain due to the rhythmic contractions of the uterus following childbirth.

agar See **seaweeds**.

age and sex There is a tendency in the West for sexual activity to be associated with youth. People who retain their sexual appetites into old age are considered unusual. The reasons for this may lie in the Western diet and other aspects of life-style. In the West youth generally does not last for long, and the chances are that by the time people have reached late middle-age they will be prone to a range of defects of the circulation and heart and other vital organs. The situation is very different in China, where it is understood that elderly people with a good appetite for both food and sex are also likely to be in a sound state of health and possessed of youthful vigour. But a good appetite in these directions must not be equated with gluttony and promiscuity, practices which are anathema to the Chinese. The Tang period (618–907) physician Sun Simiao, in his 'Precious Prescriptions', points out the benefits of regular and moderate habits in diet, exercise and sex. He lived to be 101! Perhaps one of the lessons to be learned here is that sexual immoderacy in one's youth might lead to sexual impotency in one's old age. See **longevity**.

ageing Ageing is not an illness but a natural process, though it is one from which most of us would want to be spared. Remarkably, and in no small measure, the Chinese are spared from premature ageing and a senile old age – such is their wisdom and mastery of medicine. They realize that, though they cannot arrest the passage of time, they can do much to reduce the speed at which the bodily organs deteriorate. Ageing is caused by a variety of factors, which include each individual's genetic inheritance, a slowing down of the production of hormones, a weakening of the body's immune system so that it becomes less resistant to disease, a lifetime of physical exertion and stress, and exposure to pollution and the sun's ultraviolet rays, together with obesity, unsound diet, lack of exercise and sleep, and over-use of drugs. As consequences, muscles become flabby, limbs and joints become stiff, veins and arteries harden and wrinkles develop, and there is a loss of sexual potency and physical attractiveness and energy. One of the problems of ageing is that organs deteriorate at different speeds. Thus, perfectly healthy kidneys may not function correctly if they are served by a defective heart. Researchers in the West have put forward several theories about the causes of ageing, but the Chinese view that ageing is largely due to a faulty life-style and disharmony within the body must have validity, even though it may seem to be over-simplistic, for the Chinese do have a long and healthy life of youthful vigour. See **cross-linkage**, **cell nutrition**, **free radical** and **longevity**.

ageing-inhibitor One of those many Chinese medicines and health foods which, by toning the vital organs, improving the complexion, cleansing the blood, eliminating waste and reducing stress, inhibit or retard the ageing process. Some common items in this category are Chinese wolfberry, *Lycium chinense*; Asiatic ginseng, *Panax ginseng*; American ginseng, *Panax quinquefolium*; Siberian ginseng, *Eleutherococcus senticosus*; garlic, *Allium sativum*; chrysanthemum, *Chrysanthemum morifolium*, tienchi, *Panax pseudo-gingseng*; burdock, *Arctium lappa*; stinging nettle, *Urtica dioica*; and royal jelly, some of which are used in medicinal wines. There are certain items of diet, including liver, egg yolks, sunflower seeds, molasses, seaweed, wheatgerm, fresh pineapple and certain high-grade proteins, which could also be put into this category. Aerobic exercises and acupuncture may also be applied as ageing-inhibitors.

age spots See **complexion**.

agoraphobia A morbid fear of being alone in open spaces.

agrimony *Agrimonia pilosa* Herbal medicine. Distribution: China, Japan, Europe. Parts: leaves, stems. Character: cool, bitter. Affinity: lungs, liver, spleen. Effects: astringent, haemostatic, cardiotonic, increases thrombocytes and strengthens blood vessels. Symptoms: haemorrhages, skin and membrane inflammations, colic. Treatments: all forms of haemorrhage, ulcers, hyper-acidity, urinary infections, infections of the intestinal tract. Dosage: 4–12 g. *Agrimonia eupatoria*, a European species of agrimony, has somewhat similar medicinal properties.

ah shi Chinese term meaning 'tender points'. Acupoints.

AIDS An abbreviation for 'acquired immune deficiency syndrome'. This condition, which renders the immune system ineffective, is a later development of infection by the HIV, or 'human immunodeficiency virus', which attacks those cells that normally confer immunity to infection. The main sufferers are homosexual and bisexual men who have contracted the virus through homosexual intercourse, haemophiliacs who were infected by contaminated blood prior to 1985 in the United Kingdom, when donated blood began to be subjected to rigid controls, and drug addicts who share needles. HIV is transmitted by sexual contact, including unprotected vaginal and anal intercourse, sharing needles, contact between warm body fluids and open wounds, as could occur, though much less of a probability, with kissing and toilet seats, and, in pregnancy, from mother to child. The symptoms are many, and include fevers, exhaustion, excessive perspiration, a dry cough, diarrhoea, pneumonia, hepatitis, tuberculosis, herpes, thrush, swollen glands, shingles, a dry and itchy skin, and two rare types of cancer. As yet, there is no effective treatment. Recent research in China on the treatment of viral diseases with herbal medicines has been very encouraging, which could offer some hope to AIDS sufferers. AIDS cannot be cured, but its spread can be prevented reasonably easily. It does seem to be the case that the incidence of AIDS in China is low by comparison with other countries.

ailment See **illness**.

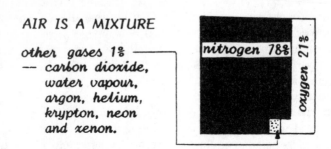

AIR IS A MIXTURE

other gases 1% —
— carbon dioxide,
water vapour,
argon, helium,
krypton, neon
and xenon.

nitrogen 78%

oxygen 21%

air Air is a mixture of gases. About ⅘ of air is nitrogen, and about ⅕ is oxygen. About 1 per cent consists of a mixture of carbon dioxide, water vapour and the inert gases, which are argon, helium, krypton, neon and xenon. There are traces of other gases, such as methane from decaying vegetation, oxides of sulphur, which are industrial waste, and carbon monoxide, an extremely poisonous gas which emanates from the exhausts of motor-cars. Water vapour, which could be described as 'cold steam', is not a true gas, for it liquifies at ordinary temperatures. Oxygen is the most active gas in air, and it supports life and burning, so it is vital to our existence. Until fairly recent times, air was not thought to have any real existence. The ancient Greeks believed that a breeze or a wind is a movement of spiritual forces. One may wonder if the people of ancient China thought in similar terms, and regarded breezes and winds as a transference of *qi*, or 'primordial vital energy'. Certainly, no one could doubt that winds possess energy, and there is something quite primordial about all the forces of nature. See **breathing** and **qi**.

air pollution The atmosphere in some industrial areas of the West is heavily polluted at dangerous levels. The pollutants include soot, smoke, carbon monoxide, motor-car exhaust fumes, asbestos fibres, stone and metal dusts, airborne particles of pesticides and fertilizers, oxides of sulphur and nitrogen, acid rain, gases and vapours from aerosol containers, and radioactive particles; and the destruction of the ozone layer is certainly not helping the environment. This pollution gives great cause for alarm. Pollution is less of a problem in China, where the economy is essentially agricultural, though the situation might change when China becomes more industrialized. It is to be hoped that the Chinese will maintain their traditional attitude towards the environment, for which, as a consequence of the Taoist insistence on harmony with nature, they have always shown tremendous respect. They believe that *qi*, or 'vital energy', is a component of the atmosphere, and they are not likely to be eager to destroy what they regard as being vital to their existence.

air therapy The use of air, as with breathing exercises, to promote health and relaxation and to alter mental states in meditation. Air therapy is one of the components of the *tao* of revitalization, which is one of the Eight Pillars of Taoism. See **breathing exercises** and **revitalization**.

akebia *Akebia quinata* Herbal medicine. Distribution: China, Japan. Parts: stems. Character: cold, bitter. Affinity: lungs, heart, bladder, small intestine. Effects: diuretic, antiphlogistic, galactogogue. Symptoms: murky and scanty urination, swollen feet and legs, reduced lactation, mouth abscesses, sleeplessness, restlessness. Treatments: insomnia, dysmenorrhoea, oedema. Dosage: 4–6 g. See **lactation**.

albinism A hereditary condition in which a person or animal has a congenital absence of the normal body pigment. An albino has a pink skin, white hair and pink eyes. See **hereditary defects**.

albumen The specific name for the albumin contained in the white of an egg.

albumin One of a class of complex, water-soluble proteins contained in egg-white, milk, blood, etc. See **albumen**.

albuminuria A condition in which albumin is present in the urine. It may be indicative of a renal dysfunction.

alchemy In Europe, alchemy was the medieval forerunner of modern chemistry. Its name derives from the Arabic word *alkimia* (*al* meaning 'the'). The alchemists were mainly concerned with trying to find an elixir which would give eternal life, and a philosophers' stone which would transmute base metals into gold. China, also, had its alchemists, who flourished at the time of the Zhou dynasty (*c.* 1100–221 BC), which was a much earlier period in history. It could well be that the alchemical ideas in the West emanated from China, and reached Europe via the Arabs, who had contacts with China. The efforts of the alchemists were not an unfruitful exercise, for they did occasionally make some important discoveries which helped to lay the foundations of modern chemistry. The Chinese alchemists were particularly successful. They produced a wide range of tonic medicines, some of which inhibit or retard the ageing process. A long and healthy life of youthful vigour must surely be the next best thing to eternal life, one would think. And, though they did not succeed in transmuting base metals into gold, they did devise various pills and potions to relieve pain and misery, and so transmute the leaden metal of human existence into the gold of a healthy and serene life.

alcohol Spirit. *Alcohol* is the general name for a series of chemical compounds of similar structure and properties – methanol, ethanol, glycol, etc. It is also commonly used as the everyday name for ethanol, or ethyl alcohol, as it was called in an older system of chemical nomenclature, which is a potable liquid – within certain limits – that is made by fermentation, as in making wine and brewing beer. Yeast, which is a single-celled fungus, feeds on sugar and yields carbon dioxide and alcohol as excretory products. It must NOT be confused with methanol, or methyl alcohol, commonly known as wood spirit, which is made from wood and is poisonous. Methylated spirit, which is used as a fuel and a solvent, contains about 90 per cent ethanol, the remainder being methanol and dye. The methanol renders it unfit for drinking, and so exempts it from excise duty, and the dye, which is mauve or blue, is a warning that it is not potable. The Chinese value alcohol both as a source of pleasure and for its medicinal properties. But, in using it for pleasure, they take the middle way, regarding total abstinence as being almost as great a folly as drunkenness. Li Shizhen (1517–1593), one of the great physicians of the period of the Ming dynasty (1368–1644), said of wine: 'A beautiful gift from heaven which, if not taken immoderately . . . brings great joy and disposes of melancholy. Taken in a large quantity, it injures the nerves . . . and causes catarrh and feverishness.' In its medicinal properties, alcohol could be said to be stimulative, sedative, soporific and antiseptic. And it is good for the health of the mind, as Li Shizhen pointed out. The Chinese use a wide range of medicinal wines, and so, in China, alcohol is bound to be more valued than despised. The medicinal value of alcohol is now beginning to be recognized in the West. In France, where most people are wine drinkers, there is a lower incidence of heart disease than in the United Kingdom, and some British medical experts contend that 4 pints of beer per week considerably reduces the risk of heart disease. See **wine** and **hangover**.

alcoholism Dipsomania. Addiction to and dependence on alcohol, or the diseased condition resulting from the addiction. Acupuncture is often successful as a treatment for alcoholism, with ear acupuncture being the most effective technique. Needles are inserted into special points in the ear, and are allowed to remain there for several weeks at a time, with longer breaks in between, until the addiction is completely broken.

alimentary canal The digestive tract, which extends from the mouth to the anus. The diagram shows the organs and other components which comprise the alimentary canal, together with those which serve it or are served by it. The ingested food is broken down by digestive juices in the mouth, stomach, duodenum and small intestine. Nutrients are assimilated into the bloodstream through the walls of the small intestine. Waste and undigested and unassimilated food are expelled, via the anus, by the rectum.

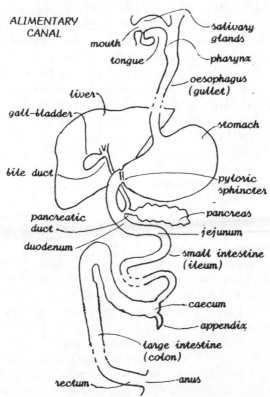

ALIMENTARY CANAL

mouth
tongue
salivary glands
pharynx
oesophagus (gullet)
liver
gall-bladder
stomach
bile duct
pyloric sphincter
pancreatic duct
pancreas
jejunum
duodenum
small intestine (ileum)
caecum
appendix
large intestine (colon)
rectum
anus

alkali A substance that will dissolve in water to form a solution which will turn litmus blue and phenolphthalein pink. An alkali reacts with an acid to form a salt and water. All alkalis are bases. See **acid**.

alkaloid One of a group of nitrogenous-based compounds found in plants. Some examples: caffeine, morphine, codeine, cocaine, ephedrine, quinine, nicotine, mescaline and strychnine. Some are very potent in their pharmacological action.

alkalosis An abnormal increase in the alkaline state of the blood and body fluids, which Chinese physicians would regard as a yin condition. It may cause severe cramps in the muscles. See **acidosis**.

allergen Antigen. One of the substances – for example, dust, pollen, feathers and milk products – which can cause an allergy. See **histamine**.

allergy Hypersensitivity, which is often hereditary, to one or more of certain substances in the environment. Nettle-rash, hay fever and one form of eczema are allergic reactions. Words such as *allergen* and *allergy*, do not exist in TCM; but, quite obviously, Chinese physicians recognize that the body will react unfavourably when it is subjected to certain conditions, which they regard as being either yin or yang. If the symptoms produced by a condition are yin, a yang treatment will be applied and vice versa. Thus, those illnesses which are cold, descending, empty and internal, whether allergies or otherwise, will be treated with yang medicines; and those which are hot, ascending, full and external will be treated with yin medicines. But the Chinese physician will do more than this. He will treat the affected organs so that they are better able to cope with the conditions to which they are being subjected. For example, in cases of asthma, the heart as well as the lungs would be treated. Acupuncture is sometimes effective as a treatment where an allergy is accompanied by stress. Nervous conditions due to allergies will lead to hypertension, for which an infusion or decoction of the seeds of the common plantain. *Plantago asiatica*, in a dosage of 5–8 g, taken internally, is a treatment. In the West, allergy sufferers are enjoined to watch their diet – eliminating those items which are known to be allergens – take regular exercise, try and reduce anxiety and tension, and rest and relax. The Chinese do not need this advice, for their diet is excellent, and they do take regular exercise. Babies should be breast-fed, for the proteins in cow's milk may cause bowel upsets and eczema. The Chinese would contend that nature intended cow's milk for the use of calves, which makes sense. It is sometimes difficult to tell the difference between a true allergy and mere sensitivity or intolerance. One suspects that, in the West, there are occasions when an illness which cannot be accurately diagnosed is regarded as an allergy. See **histamine** and **antihistamine**.

allopathy A system of medicine in which the treatments applied are of an opposite character to the symptoms of illness. TCM is allopathic, yin illnesses being treated with yang medicines and vice versa. See **homoeopathy** and **naturopathy**.

almond oil See **medicinal oils**.

alopecia *Alopecia areata*, to give this condition its full medical name is a patchy baldness occurring mainly in adolescents and young adults. There is uncertainty about its causes, but debility and hormonal changes are the prime suspects. Recovery is generally spontaneous, particularly where there is a change of life-style. The usual treatment is care of the general health, including a sound diet, together with tonic medicines. This is a rare condition among the Chinese, whose diet is sound, and who take tonic medicines regularly.

alpha tocopherol Vitamin E. An antioxidant contained in carrots, sunflower seeds, soya beans and leafy vegetables and is preventive of thrombosis and heart disease. A deficiency of this vitamin may cause anaemia in new-born babies. Carrots and sunflower seeds feature prominently in the tonic soups of the Chinese.

alternative A medicine which alters the metabolic processes so that they are more able to cope with nutritional and eliminative functions. Antioxidants, blood purifiers and laxatives could be regarded as alternatives.

alternative medicine Complementary medicine. A term used to describe those systems of medicine, whatever their source – China, Africa, India, etc. – of which the procedures, in both theory and application, are different from the well-established system in Europe and the United States, and which is known as conventional medicine. Chinese physicians, with the encouragement of the Chinese government, use what they deem to be the best from all systems, an unbigoted approach surely of great benefit to their patients.

aloe *Aloe vera* Herbal medicine. Distribution: India, West Africa, West Indies. Parts: leaves. Character: cold, bitter. Affinity: stomach, liver, large intestine. Effects: antiseptic, sedative, emmenagogue, purgative, laxative. Symptoms: headaches, constipation. Treatments: intestinal parasites, reduced menstrual flow. Dosage: 0.3–0.9 g.

Alzheimer's disease Pre-senile dementia, or premature ageing. The symptoms are the same as those of senile dementia, or senility, but they occur in middle age or even earlier. There is a deterioration of the patient's intellect, personality and physique, and eventually he becomes bedridden and incontinent. There is no cure, but acupuncture and an infusion of rosemary, *Rosmarinus officinalis*, taken internally, may alleviate the symptoms.

amenorrhoea Absence of menstruation. This condition is said to be *primary* when there have never been periods, and *secondary* when they cease after being present initially. TCM treatments include: nut grass, *Cyperus rotundus*; turmeric, *Curcuma longa*; peach, *Prunus persica*.

amentia Mental abnormality, usually congenital.

American ginseng *Panax quinquefolium* Herbal medicine. Distribution: North America. Parts: roots. Character: neutral, sweet. Affinity: spleen, lungs. Effects: sedative, tonic to spleen and lungs, adaptogenic. Symptoms: nervous tension, exhaustion, nausea. Treatments: dyspepsia, anorexia. Dosage: 2–12 g. This herb tones *qi*.

amino acids Organic fatty acids containing the ammonium radical (NH_2), which is a base. They combine together to form proteins, which are more complex. The body can synthesize some amino acids for itself; it derives the others from food. Animals derive nitrogen from amino acids, and green plants synthesize amino acids from nitrates in the soil. See **protein**.

amna An ancient oriental system of massage in which the hands and feet are rubbed and manipulated. See **shiatsu**.

amnesia Loss of memory. TCM treatments include: Chinese wolfberry, *Lycium chinense*; eucommia, *Eucommia ulmoides*; tienchi, *Panax pseudo-gingseng*. But the nature of the treatment will be largely determined by the cause of the amnesia, which is brought on by shock, hysteria, alcoholism or drug addiction or, more rarely, by epilepsy, meningitis, a brain tumour or syphilis. Amnesia must not be confused with mere forgetfulness, which mainly affects elderly people and is not permanent, and which is not an illness but only an indication that the brain has its limitations.

amoeba A single-celled, jelly-like animal which is just visible to the naked eye and lives in the slime at the bottom of ponds and rivers. It is constantly changing its shape, which is its means of locomotion. Its activities are controlled by the nucleus, which is a primitive nervous system. See **amoebic dysentery**.

amoebic dysentery Inflammation of the large intestine due to

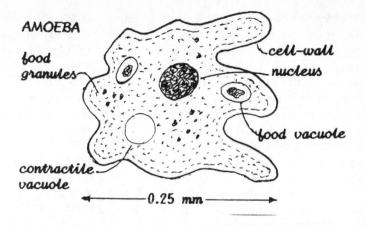

AMOEBA

food granules — cell-wall — nucleus

food vacuole

contractile vacuole

←——— 0.25 mm ———→

infection by parasitic amoebas, and accompanied by pain, severe diarrhoea and evacuation of blood and mucus. See **dysentery**.

amylase See **maltose**.

anaemia A decrease in the number of red blood cells, or erythrocytes, or the haemoglobin they contain, which results in a reduction in the oxygen-carrying ability of the blood. The symptoms are tiredness, giddiness, headaches, paleness, shortness of breath, loss of appetite, palpitations, insomnia and swollen ankles. There are several types of anaemia. The commonest is due to iron deficiency, which results from poor diet, loss of blood, infection or illness. Another common type is due to a deficiency of folic acid, one of the B-complex vitamins, which is abundant in liver and fresh vegetables. Sickle-cell anaemia is an inherited condition found among people of African or Middle Eastern descent. Its symptoms, which first appear in childhood, include weakness, fevers and yellowing of the skin and whites of the eyes. Pernicious anaemia, which mainly affects people in blood group A, can only be treated with regular injections of cobalamin (vitamin B_{12}). See **pernicious anaemia**. As a treatment, both Chinese and Western physicians would recommend a diet containing iron-rich and blood-fortifying foods, such as liver, watercress, eggs, honey, molasses, figs and the raw juices of carrots, spinach, nettles, parsley and horseradish. Chinese physicians would recommend acupuncture and moxibustion as treatments for mild forms of anaemia. Chinese herbal remedies include garlic, *Allium sativum*; ginseng, *Panax ginseng*; stinging nettle, *Urtica dioica*; greater burdock, *Arctium lappa*; dandelion, *Taraxacum officinale*; and tienchi, *Panax pseudoginseng*. Fig wine would be helpful.

anaesthesia The absence of sensation, particularly that which is induced artificially. A general anaesthetic produces a total loss of consciousness, and a local anaesthetic, applied as a liquid, either directly to the skin or injected, produces insensibility in a selected part of the body. In the West, anaesthetics came into use during the nineteenth century. Ether was first used in 1842, and chloroform in 1847. But anaesthesia in China has a longer history than this. Towards the end of the period of the Han dynasty (206 BC-AD 220), anaesthetics were being used in the excision of tumours. This development was mainly due to the pioneering efforts of Hua Tuo (AD 141–208) who used 'narcotic soups' in treating abscesses and skin tumours. The ingredients included, loco weed, *Datura metel*; aconite, *Aconitum carmichaeli*; and rhododendron, *Rhododendron sinense*. By the time of the Song dynasty (960–1279), anaesthetics were well established as a technique in minor surgery. In China, since 1959, acupuncture has been extensively used for anaesthesia in major surgery. See **acupuncture treatments**.

Analects A collection of the sayings of Confucius. See **Lunyu**.

anal fissures A condition often associated with haemorrhoids. Treatment: flowers of the marigold, *Calendula officinalis*, applied in an ointment or wet compress.

analgesic A substance administered to reduce pain, but without any loss of consciousness. Aconite, aspirin and paracetamol are in popular use in the West. The best pain-relievers are extracted from the opium poppy, *Papaver somniferum*. Chinese herbal analgesics include: rhubarb, *Rheum officinale*; liquorice, *Glycyrrhiza glabra*; mugwort, *Artemisia vulgaris*; nut grass, *Cyperus rotundus*; magnolia, *Magnolia liliflora*; chrysanthemum, *Chrysanthemum morifolium*; and mandarin orange, *Citrus reticulata*. Acupuncture is also used to relieve pain. See **aspirin**.

anatomy The Chinese would have no wish to disturb the graves of their ancestors, for whom they have the utmost respect, and so their knowledge of human anatomy has not been obtained by dissection and similar methods. See **zoology** and **physiology**.

ancylostoma See **hookworm**.

ancestor worship The so-called ancestor worship of the Chinese is, in fact, no more than a great respect which borders on reverence. The Chinese are aware that, if they are worthy and healthy people, it is because their progenitors were worthy and healthy people, who have given them the gift of life and many centuries of accumulated wisdom. The application of this simple genetic principle produces many medical and social benefits, and also ensures a continuity of traditional values. Chinese people take good care of their health, and great care when selecting marriage partners so that they will be likely to produce healthy offspring. It was the practice in ancient China for the emperor to choose a bride, who would be the mother of his successor, from among the healthiest and most talented of his concubines. There were occasions when a young and healthy boy from a good family, but totally unrelated to the emperor, would be adopted and trained to be the prince and heir to the imperial throne. Obviously, the Chinese emperors were aware of the genetic damage that could be done by inbreeding. In China, it is the elderly people, and not the children, who have all the privileges and celebrate their birthdays. See **eugenics**.

androgen Testosterone, the male sex hormone, or any other substance capable of developing or maintaining the male characteristics of the body. See **primary sex characteristics**.

aneurin Thiamin. See **vitamin**.

aneurysm The morbid dilation and weakening of an artery.

angelica *Angelica sinensis* Herbal medicine. Distribution: China. Parts: roots. Character: warm, pungent-sweet. Affinity: spleen, liver. Effects: emennagogue, analgesic, sedative, laxative, tonic to blood and circulation. Symptoms: dysmenorrhoea, menorrhagia, amenorrhoea and other menstrual problems, postnatal abdominal and rheumatic pains. Treatments: blood deficiency, rheumatism, scarring. Dosage: 9–14 g. This herb is particularly valuable in the treatment of menstrual disorders. There are several species of angelica used in medicine. Indigenous to China are *Angelica anomala*, used to treat colds, headaches, 'wind-injury' aches and pains, abscesses, swellings, leucorrhoea and snake bites, and *Angelica pubescens*, used as an analgesic to treat rheumatism and arthritis. In the West, there are garden angelica, *Angelica officinalis*, and wild angelica, *Angelica sylvestris*, both of which are used as a carminative and a treatment for debility, impaired digestion, liver conditions, sore throats, coughs, congestion and respiratory ailments generally, including asthma.

anger In TCM, anger is associated with the liver, and it is thought to be due to excessive or heated blood. Fits of anger are damaging to the liver. See **emotion** and **liver**.

angina Angina pectoris, to give this condition its full medical name, which literally means 'breast pang', is characterized by a sharp pain behind the sternum, or breastbone, which may spread to the neck and shoulders. It is caused by an inadequate supply of oxygen to the heart, as occurs when the arteries serving the muscles of the heart are constricted and inelastic. This condition can be prevented in some measure by adopting the Chinese diet and consuming one clove of garlic per day.

angled luffa In China, this gourd is consumed as a vegetable and a health food. Boiled with black soya beans and a fish head, and then consumed as a soup, it is a traditional remedy for poor lactation and aching muscles and joints.

animal-derived medicines Not all Chinese medicines are derived from herbs. A few are animal products, and include organs, tissues and extracts from such animals as the earthworm, cicada, water-buffalo, musk deer, scorpion, centipede, antelope, pangolin, turtle, tortoise and ass. Animal-derived medicines are prominent among the tonics, and they include such exotic items as dried sea-horses, stag horn, rhinoceros horn, ass hide and the dried genitalia of seals. They generally contain male sex hormones. See **plant-derived medicines**.

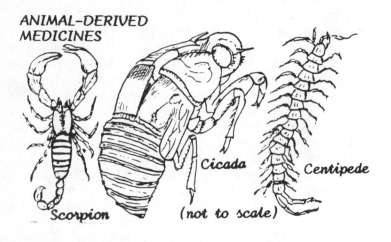

ANIMAL-DERIVED MEDICINES

Scorpion Cicada Centipede (not to scale)

animals and health It is important to remember that some of the diseases of animals, such as anthrax and rabies, can be transmitted to man. See **zoonoses**. Also, some of the micro-organisms which cause diseases in humans are carried by animals. See **vector**. Food intended for human consumption may be contaminated by contact with animals. See **food hygiene**.

animals of the Chinese years See **Chinese years**.

an mu One of the Chinese systems of massage. See **massage**.

anodyne A medicine or other agency which relieves pain or anxiety. Analgesics and sedatives are within this category.

anorexia Loss of appetite.

anorexia nervosa A nervous disorder, mainly affecting young women, in which fear of being overweight leads to excessive dieting, and which, in turn, causes chronic anorexia and emaciation. Acupuncture is an effective treatment. See **obesity** and **dietetics**.

ant This insect is a source of formic acid, which Chinese physicians claim to be effective in treating arthritis. See **formic acid**.

antacid A medicine used to neutralize or counter acidity, which is an excess of acid in the stomach. Eggshell, finely ground, which is a natural source of chalk (calcium carbonate), is an antacid in popular use in China.

antagonism In TCM, the relationship between the symptoms of an illness and its treatment is expected to be one of antagonism, or forceful opposition. Thus, illnesses which are yin, cold and empty, are treated with medicines which are yang, hot and full, and vice versa.

ant-eater See **pangolin**.

ante cibum See **a.c.**

antelope *Saiga tatarica* Medicine. Distribution: North China, Mongolia. Parts: horn. Character: cold, salty. Affinity: liver. Effects: antipyretic, antispasmodic, sedative to liver. Symptoms: giddiness, headache, blurred vision, convulsions, spasms, high temperature, swollen eyes, delirium. Treatments: epilepsy, hypertension, apoplexy, illnesses involving liver-yang excess. This is an expensive medicine and one which is not likely to meet with the approval of the people of the West.

antenatal 'Of the period before birth' or 'during pregnancy'.

anthelmintic A medicine to kill or expel parasitic worms in the intestines. Anthelmintics are generally poisonous, so they should be used sparingly, and also in conjunction with cathartics to ensure that the worms and their ova are completely eliminated.

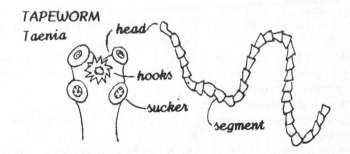

TAPEWORM
Taenia
head — hooks — sucker — segment

Some intestinal parasitic worms are the tapeworm, pin-worm and hookworm. Tapeworms enter the human body in the cyst stage from the flesh of infected pigs, cattle and fish. Over one-third of the human race is infected with roundworms, which include the pin-worm and the hookworm. Some roundworms, such as the vinegar eel, are harmless, and many of those in the soil are beneficial. The pumpkin, *Cucurbita moschata*, and garlic, *Allium sativum*, are effective as anthelmintics, as also are the nuts of the betel palm, *Areca catechu*. A daily dosage of 5 g of a strong decoction of the peel of pomegranate, *Punica granatum*, taken internally for a period of eight days is also considered to be an effective treatment.

anthrax A disease of cattle and sheep which may be transmitted to man, causing skin eruptions, pneumonia or gastro-enteritis. It can be contracted by contact with hides.

antibiotic A medicine which kills disease-causing micro-organisms or inhibits their development. In the West, the most well-known antibiotic is penicillin, and it has been regarded as a breakthrough in modern medical science, though it grows naturally on sheep dung, which has been used in antibiotics since ancient times. Garlic is a selective internal antiseptic which tends to destroy only the harmful flora, and so, on a limited scale, it can be used as an antibiotic. During the Spanish Civil War (1936–9) and the civil war in China, there was an acute shortage of medical supplies, and so garlic was used as an antibiotic. For many centuries, Chinese physicians have treated diseases caused by streptococci with the fermented brine of salted vegetables – a penicillin type of antibiotic.

antibody A substance produced within the body as a defence against foreign substances, including micro-organisms. No doubt, Chinese physicians would regard this as a yin and yang situation, with mutual antagonism being creative of harmony. See **immunity** and **interferon**.

anticoagulant A substance, produced within the body or administered as a medicine, which prevents or reduces the coagulation of blood.

antidiaphoretic Antiperspirant. A medicine to inhibit excessive perspiration. The jujube, *Ziziphus jujuba*, is an effective antidiaphoretic. See **perspiration**.

antidote See **antitoxin**.

antidysenteric A medicine which prevents or alleviates dysentery. See **dysentery**.

antigen A foreign substance which, within the body, stimulates the development of antibodies. See **allergen**.

antihistamine A medicine which counteracts histamines and other allergens. See **histamine** and **allergy**.

antiperspirant See **antidiaphoretic**.

antiphlogistic A medicine to reduce inflammation. Many of the antipyretic medicines (fever-reducers) also function as antiphlogistics.

antipyretic Febrifuge. Refrigerant. A medicine to reduce fevers. All antipyretics are cold or cool yin medicines. Some commonly used antipyretics in TCM are gypsum, *Gypsum fibrosum* (calcium sulphate), self-heal, *Prunella vulgaris*, lotus, *Nulembo nucifera*, dandelion, *Taraxacum officinale*, abalone, *Haliotis gigantea*, and purslane, *Portulaca oleracea*.

antirheumatic A medicine to relieve the painful symptoms of rheumatism and arthritis, or, as the Chinese would say, 'to drive out evil wind-damp excess and facilitate the flow of energy in the meridians'. Some commonly used antirheumatics in TCM are the gentian, *Gentiana macropylla*; Chinese quince, *Chaenomeles lagenaria*; and viper, *Agkistrodon acutus*.

antiseptic A substance which kills or inhibits the growth of harmful micro-organisms. Some commonly used antiseptics in TCM include table salt (sodium chloride); garlic, *Allium sativum*; Chinese spring onion, *Allium fistulosum*; sorrel, *Rumex acetosa*, and vinegar (ethanoic acid). See **disinfectant**.

antiserum A serum with a high content of antibodies which will act against a particular infection, and which will have been taken from an animal which has developed an immunity to that infection. It may be used to protect man or another animal against that same infection.

antispasmodic A medicine to treat abnormal muscular contractions. The chrysanthemum, *Chrysanthemum morifolium*, is mildly antispasmodic. The Borneo camphor tree, *Dryobalanops aromatica*, is used in TCM as a powerful antispasmodic in the treatment of epilepsy.

antitoxin Antidote. A medicine which counteracts a toxin, or organic poison. The chrysanthemum has mildly antitoxic properties. An antitoxin can be an antibody, produced within the body or injected as an antiserum, which neutralizes toxins produced by micro-organisms in the body or, rarely, the bite of a snake. See **antiserum**.

antitussive A medicine to relieve coughs. Antitussives in common use in TCM are the peach, *Prunus persica*; apricot, *Prunus armeniaca*; and beefsteak plant, *Perilla frutescens*.

anus The opening to the exterior at the rectum end of the alimentary canal.

anxiety This is one of the seven emotions of TCM. It is associated with the lungs and the element metal. The lungs control *qi*, or 'vital energy', which is impeded if the lungs are damaged by anxiety. See **lungs**.

anxiety state Phobia. A form of neurosis characterized by persistent and irrational fear, which ranges from vague unease to distinct dread. It can produce physical symptoms: weakness, tiredness, sweating, palpitations, dizziness, muscular tension, nausea, vomiting, diarrhoea, frequent urination, insomnia, and pain in the head, neck, chest, back and abdomen. It is a real illness, and should not be lightly dismissed as being 'all in the mind'. The obvious treatment is to remove the cause of the anxiety – if that is possible, and if there is a cause. Raw carrots and lettuce have a calming effect, as does camomile tea, which is an infusion of the leaves of *Matricaria chamomilla*. Acupuncture and acupressure are often effective treatments. Just as anxiety can produce physical effects, so physical conditions, such as those brought about by changes in the hormone levels, can produce anxiety. Chinese physicians have long recognized that emotional disturbances are psychosomatic, requiring treatment of the body as well as the mind. Apart from the application of herbal remedies, the treatment should involve meditation, breathing exercises, a sound diet, moderate habits and a wise philosophy of living. Chinese physicians believe that emotional disorders, if left untreated, can do severe damage to the vital organs.

aorta The largest artery of the body, issuing from the heart and supplying blood to the arteries. See **circulation**.

aperient A mild laxative. Garlic and onion are mildly aperient, and fibrous vegetables in the diet promote smooth evacuation by the bowel. See **cathartic**.

aphrodisiac A substance which stimulates sexual desire and improves the libido. Many foodstuffs, such as oysters, eggs and beans, and many herbs, such as ginger, cinnamon and black pepper, are reputed to be aphrodisiacs, though their effects as sexual stimulants are negligible. But a person who is in a normal state of health should not require aphrodisiacs, for he will have normal sexual desires. And here, it would be the Chinese view that abnormal sexual desires are unhealthy, if not depraved, and, therefore, they should not be countenanced. But, in the West, where money and sex seem to have become major preoccupations, there will be those people who yearn for sexual potency of a high order. Such people would be well advised to improve their general health, and thereby improve the libido, by adopting a healthier life-style in matters of diet and exercise, and by taking well-tried tonic medicines, such as royal jelly, Asiatic ginseng and the Chinese wolfberry. Those substances which are listed in a pharmacopoeia as being effective as aphrodisiacs, such as damiana, cola, saw palmetto and Spanish fly, or cantharides, are undesirable in so far as they make excessive demands on the body, and Chinese physicians would regard them as being unnatural. Spanish fly, which is the dried and crushed beetle *Lytta vesicatoria*, can be dangerous. Chinese physicians would also condemn the use of those drugs which are not true aphrodisiacs, and which do no more than promote a diminished sense of responsibility in sexual affairs. However, there are three herbs which they would regard as being effective and safe as aphrodisiacs: Asiatic ginseng, *Panax ginseng*; broomrape, *Cistanche salsa*; and horny goat weed, *Epimedium sagittatum*.

apoplexy See **stroke**.

appendicectomy A surgical operation to remove the appendix.

appendicitis Infection and inflammation of the appendix which, if severe, requires removal of the appendix by surgery. But, if the condition is less severe, though often chronic, which is usually described as a 'grumbling appendix', medication is generally sufficient. Chinese physicians consider a decoction of the kernels of the stones of the peach, *Prunus persica*, together with a varied and fibrous diet, to be preventive of appendicitis. Acupuncture is also an effective preventive treatment in that it reduces the tension which may cause constipation and other bowel dysfunctions. See **Glauber's salt**.

appendix An appendage of the caecum, about 7 cm in length and seemingly functionless, but, as is the case with some other bodily structures, such as the sinuses, it was probably bequeathed to us by our ancestors in the process of evolution. See **intestine**.

appetite Chinese meals are appetizing in their colours, textures, flavours and fragrances, which ensures that diners are persuaded to partake of dishes which, though highly nutritious, they might otherwise be inclined to reject. The Chinese cuisine includes a large number of easily digested dishes, such as taro starch jelly and white rice porridge, which are suitable for invalids and elderly people with a poor appetite or an impaired digestion. Chinese physicians have at their disposal a wide range of digestives, which are medicines to stimulate the appetite and assist in the assimilation of nutrients. See **digestive**. Poor digestion and loss of appetite has many different causes: tiredness, stress, lack of exercise, anxiety, constipation, diarrhoea, anaemia, colds, influenza, anorexia nervosa, etc. But loss of appetite may have a serious deep-seated and underlying cause, and so, where the condition persists, medical advice should be sought.

appetizer See **digestive**.

apricot *Prunus armeniaca* Herbal medicine. Distribution: China. Parts: kernels. Character: warm, bitter-sweet. Affinity: large intestine, lungs. Effects: antitussive, cathartic, sedative. Symptoms: coughs, constipation. Treatments: asthma, bronchitis. Dosage: 5–10 g. Mildly toxic.

aqueous solution See **solution**.

aroma See **odour**.

aromatherapy A system of healing in which illnesses are treated with highly scented essential oils that are extracted from plants with medicinal properties. These oils may be inhaled, applied in a compress, added to a bath or rubbed into the skin in massage. They penetrate the skin through the pores and hair follicles. Aromatherapy is not in popular use in China today, but records indicate that, over 4000 years ago, the Chinese were using essential oils medicinally, and they were probably the first people to have knowledge of them. In the West, aromatherapy is mainly used as a massage treatment, but it often incorporates some of the techniques of acupressure and other Chinese-style systems of massage. Each oil has its particular effect and use. Thus, sage oil improves the circulation, and is used as a treatment for rheumatism; and cedarwood oil is sedative, and is used as a treatment for coughs, bronchitis, stress and anxiety. Some essential oils are poisonous, and so they should not be ingested unless they are prescribed by a qualified practitioner. Essential oils have some non-medicinal uses as ingredients in antiseptics, soaps and perfumes. Apart from its medicinal value, aromatherapy is used in beauty treatments. Also, an aromatherapy massage can be very relaxing, and for that purpose alone, it is to be highly recommended. When using an essential oil purchased from a pharmacy or elsewhere, it is important that one should follow the instructions on its container. Essential oils are generally supplied in a diluted form because the pure oils are too strong to be applied directly to the skin. See **massage**.

aromatic An organic compound with a characteristic fragrant and pungent aroma. Essential oils contain aromatic compounds, and being volatile, their particles excite the nerve endings in the nose. See **odour**.

arrhythmia Disturbed heart rhythm. But it is only rarely symptomatic of a heart defect or ill health. See **pulse diagnosis**.

arsenic A brittle and steel-grey metalloid, or semi-metallic element. The so-called arsenic used in medicine is, in fact, the compound arsenic trioxide ($As_2 O_3$), which is a white solid and a violent poison. About 800 years ago, the Chinese were using arsenic, together with calomel and cinnabar, which are compounds of mercury, in the treatment of venereal diseases, but sometimes with disastrous results.

arteriosclerosis Popularly known as 'hardening of the arteries', arteriosclerosis is a condition in which the arteries lose their elasticity, and their walls become thicker and their channels become narrower, thereby causing hypertension, which puts a strain on the heart. It mainly affects elderly people, but it will also affect younger people who are neglectful of their health, particularly in regard to diet and social life. The condition is certainly serious when it affects the coronary artery, which supplies blood to the heart muscles. See **angina**. It can be prevented, or arrested if it has become established, by leading a less stressful life, taking exercise and adopting a healthier diet. Walking, massage and participation in *tai chi chuan*, which is one of the gentler styles of the martial arts, will improve the circulation and maintain the elasticity of the arteries. A low-fat diet will inhibit the formation of cholesterol, whose deposits narrow the channels of the arteries. Red meat, salt, refined sugar and alcohol should be avoided. Obesity and smoking exacerbate the condition, but the former can usually be avoided by adopting a Chinese-style diet, and the latter can be given up by exercising strong will-power for about a fortnight. Nutritionists have suggested that two meals of oily fish – which are rich in polyunsaturated fats – per week would do much to eradicate circulatory and heart complaints altogether. Some helpful Chinese herbal remedies are as follows: garlic, *allium sativum*, vasodilator; onion, *Allium cepa*, vasodilator; tienchi, *Panax pseudoginseng*, vasodilator; ginseng, *Panax ginseng*, vasodilator; hawthorn, *Crataegus pinnatifida*, dissolves cholesterol; dandelion, *Taraxacum officinale*, reduces blood clots; yarrow (milfoil), *Achillea millefolium*, prevents blood clots; chrysanthemum, *Chrysanthemum morifolium*, prevents high levels of cholesterol; ginger, *Zingiber officinale*, reduces cholesterol; earthworm, *Pheretima aspergillum*, relaxes hardened arteries.

arteriole An artery of the smallest size, and not to be confused with a capillary.

artery A blood vessel carrying blood away from the heart to the various organs of the body. With the exception of the pulmonary artery, which carries de-oxygenated blood to the lungs, the arteries contain oxygenated blood, which is bright red in colour.

arthritis Inflammation of a joint. For those who are seriously afflicted with arthritis, it is painful in the extreme, and they do not exaggerate when they say that they are crippled with arthritis. In China, it is not uncommon for very elderly people to be remarkably sprightly, for they are less prone to arthritis and those other illnesses which, in the West, are associated with age. The simple explanation for this state of affairs is that the Chinese of all ages have a healthy diet, take regular exercise and are of moderate habits, and few of them are in sedentary occupations. Chinese physicians regard arthritis as being a wind-damp condition of which there are two main types: wind-cold and wind-heat. With cold arthritis, the joints are particularly painful in cold weather. This conditon is treated with warming medicines, such as ginger root, cinnamon twigs, angelica roots and aconite root. With heat arthritis, the joints are swollen and hot. This condition is treated with gentian root and cork-tree bark, which reduces the swelling. Acupuncture and moxibustion are sometimes effective as treatments. If the joints are not too painful, the exercises of the *tai chi chuan* will help in easing arthritis; but, with rheumatoid arthritis, the joints should be immersed in warm water before they are exercised, which could help to prevent a sudden flare-up of the condition. There are three types of arthritis: osteo-arthritis, rheumatoid arthritis and podagra. Both osteo-arthritis and rheumatoid arthritis affect women more than they do men, probably because of the disturbances in the hormonal balance which are due to menstruation and the menopause. In the West, the methods of alleviation include analgesics to relieve pain – and, in the West, aspirin is still thought to be the best drug for this purpose – a regulated diet, antacids to reduce acids in the stomach and elsewhere in the body, laxatives, diuretics and diaphoretics to eliminate waste, and rubefacients to ease pain and reduce swellings and stiffness. A complete cure is rare where the disease has become severe. Obviously, the function of a badly damaged joint cannot be restored; but, on occasions, a diseased hip may be replaced with an artificial hip made of metal or plastic. For the Chinese physician, the treatment of arthritis is largely a matter of keeping the heart, lungs and liver in a healthy state, for they are the vital organs which maintain the circulation of the blood, so providing nutrients and eliminating waste. An arthritic person should drink copious amounts of water to help in eliminating waste from the blood, and the diet should be essentially vegetarian and alkaline. Fatty, sugary and spicy foods must be excluded from the diet. Royal jelly is considered to be a good dietary supplement, and molluscs, particularly mussels, are thought to have some remedial effect, but not if the person has hypertension. Of the various external treatments that are available, a poultice of comfrey leaves is probably the most efficacious. An infusion of any of the following herbs, using the parts and dry weight indicated, may be taken internally as a daily dosage in treating arthritis, though one should consult a physician before embarking on a course of self-treatment. Angelica, *Angelica archangelia*: root, 5 g. Sage, *Salvia officinalis*: leaves, 6 g. Ginger, *Zingiber officinale*: root, 6 g. Garden nettle, *Urtica urens*: any part, 5 g. Stinging nettle, *Urtica dioica*: any part, 5 g. Dandelion, *Taraxacum officinale*: any part, 15 g. Camomile, *Matricaria chamomilla*: flowers, 6 g. Burdock, *Arctium lappa*: root, 6 g. Chinese cinnamon (cassia), *cinnamomum cassia*: bark, 5 g. Marigold, *Calendula officinalis*: flowers, 6 g. Catmint, *Nepeta cataria*: leaves and buds, 6 g. Coriander, *Coriandrum sativum*: leaves, 4 g. See **joints** and **podogra**.

artificial insemination The introduction of viable semen into a woman's vagina by artificial means. This technique is used where a woman wants to have a baby but is unable to conceive in the normal way. If the husband's semen is viable, even though he cannot ejaculate, it will be used to inseminate his wife artificially. This is called A.I.H., 'artificial insemination by the husband'. But, if the husband's semen is defective, the semen of an anonymous donor will be used. This is called A.I.D., 'artificial insemination by a donor'. This technique produces what are popularly known as 'test-tube babies'. Many Chinese people are likely to have reservations about A.I.D., and Chinese women who are unable to conceive would probably prefer to adopt.

art of living For the Chinese, the art of living is the art of survival and making the best of one's circumstances. To them, this means living as healthily as one can, for as long as one can, and as contentedly as one can. These aims, together with other worthy aspirations, can only be achieved by harmony with nature, within the body and throughout society. Therefore, it is not surprising that the Chinese value health, both physical and mental, above all else, and regard it as the key to success in the art of living. Nor is it surprising that the Chinese have developed the finest system of preventive medicine in the world. See **survival**.

ascending A term ascribed by Chinese physicians to those full and hot illnesses and medications which cause energy to rise and escape as rebellious *qi*. Ascending illnesses are manifested by fever, hotness, sweating, nausea, vomiting, diarrhoea and restlessness. They are treated with descending medicines, which have an opposite effect, and so subjugate rebellious-*qi*. Ascending medicines have a stimulating effect, and will induce the same bodily conditions as are manifested by ascending illnesses: fever, hotness, sweating, etc. See **descending**.

ascorbic acid Vitamin C. Contained in fresh fruits and vegetables, its deficiency in the diet lowers resistance to infection and can be causative of bleeding gums, scurvy, anaemia and weak joints. See **vitamin**.

asepsis Absence of harmful micro-organisms.

Asiatic gingseng *Panax ginseng* Herbal medicine. Distribution: Korea, North-east China. Parts: roots. Character: neutral, sweet. Affinity: lungs, spleen. Effects: *qi* and vital essences, strengthens lungs and spleen, aphrodisiac. Symptoms: lack of energy, loss of appetite, dyspepsia, weak pulse, palpitations, insomnia. Treatments: asthma, hypertension, diabetes, prolapse of the rectum. Dosages: as a general tonic and long-term treatment of debility, and for elderly persons, 4–8 g; for acute and stressful conditions in young persons, 8–20 g, but for no longer than three weeks in any one month. Ginseng must not be consumed with turnips, alcohol or drinks containing caffeine, such as coffee and tea. Ginseng has other benefits which are generally not listed in a pharmacopoeia. It regulates blood sugar and promotes the production of blood. It initiates the secretion of sexual hormones in both men and women, which explains why it is regarded as a safe aphrodisiac. Some of the claims made for the efficacy of ginseng are somewhat exaggerated. Nevertheless, it is one of the most potent and popular medicines in TCM.

Asiatic olive *Canarium album* Herbal medicine. Distribution: South-east China, Vietnam, Laos, Cambodia. Parts: fruits. Character: neutral, sweet-sour. Affinity: stomach, lungs. Effects: antipyretic, antiphlogistic, antitoxic, astringent. Symptoms: pharyngitis, hotness, feverishness. Treatments: bronchitis, coughs, flatulence, nausea. Dosage: 4–10 g. An antidote for seafood poisoning; and, if slowly chewed and swallowed, it will dissolve fish bones lodged in the throat and stomach. The Asiatic olive is also called the Chinese olive.

aspartame An artificial sweetener. See **additives** and **sweetener**.

asphyxia Choking or suffocation.

aspic See **gelatin**.

aspirin The everyday name for acetylsalicylic acid, a white crystalline substance commonly used in the West as an analgesic and antipyretic in the treatment of headaches and rheumatism. Nowadays, it is made synthetically; but, originally, it was extracted from the bark of the willow, a member of the genus *Salix*, from which a part of its name derives. It is considered to be preventive of arteriosclerosis, thrombosis and hypertension if taken regularly in small amounts, say, half a tablet daily. But, in large amounts it can cause nausea, vomiting, indigestion, asthma, allergies and bleeding. It is likely to be safer to take in its natural form as the whole willow bark, and then the other substances in the bark will act as a buffer. See **active ingredient**. Aspirin should NOT be administered to children, nursing mothers and persons suffering from haemophilia or ulcers, and should be administered with great care to pregnant women, elderly persons and those with a history of indigestion, asthma, impaired liver or kidney function and allergy to aspirin. Aspirin must not be used with anticoagulants, steroids and some anti-diabetic medicines and antacids. A wide range of analgesics are commonly available in TCM, but aspirin is not one of them.

asthma Bronchial asthma, as it should be called more accurately to distinguish it from cardiac asthma, which is an entirely different illness, may be briefly defined as contraction of the bronchial tubes and bronchioles due to inflammation, muscular spasms and the secretion of a very sticky mucus, which makes the breathing difficult and wheezy. The causes are allergy and hypersensitivity. Some of the symptoms are coughing, a rapid pulse and panic. A physician must be called when the paroxysms are severe; otherwise the patient could collapse or die from strain, exhaustion or lack of oxygen. Asthma is generally due to inherited factors or such environmental factors as climatic conditions, temperature, infection, stress, anxiety and being allergic to pollen, dust, feathers, hairs, moulds and certain foodstuffs. Where asthma is inherited, it may be associated with hay fever or eczema. Where it is non-hereditary and non-congenital, it may have developed as a consequence of chest infections or heart disorders. In the West, the usual medicines employed in the treatment of asthma are ephedrine and cortisone. By the provisions of the 1968 Medicines

Act, these drugs are available only to qualified medical practitioners; and, in any case, they must not be used where there is severe hypertension, hyperthyroidism, glaucoma or coronary thrombosis. Asthma can be very debilitating, and so the sufferer must take good care of his general health, avoid contact with those substances to which he knows himself to be allergic, and adopt a diet that is more varied and balanced, such as the Chinese diet, for his hypersensitivity may have a dietary cause. Certainly, his diet should contain plenty of fresh fruit and vegetables, garlic, onions and oily fish, and the occasional inclusion of a little wine or cider vinegar would be helpful. He should avoid foods containing synthetic additives, beef and other red meats, refined sugar and flour, dairy products and animal fats. Some sufferers have found that attacks are less frequent after receiving acupressure, acupuncture or massage treatment. The Chinese make

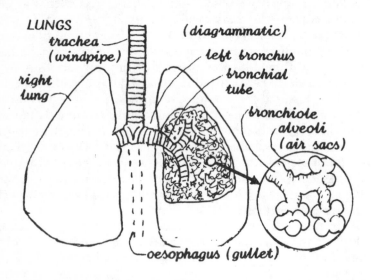

use of breathing exercises – *ch'i kung*, or 'invigorative breathing', and *fang sung kung*, or 'recreative breathing' – to prevent or alleviate asthma. Here, of course, we have one of the fundamental principles of TCM: what cannot be cured or only alleviated with difficulty may often be easily prevented. When one perceives an asthma patient struggling to breathe, one could believe that he is being very energetic. But appearances are sometimes deceptive. He lacks oxygen, so he lacks energy, and he is in a weakened state. Chinese physicians would say that he lacks *qi*, and so they would probably regard asthma as being a wind-cold illness and yin, empty and descending, so requiring a stimulative yang medicine. In Western herbal medicine, there are many asthma remedies, such as thyme, *Thymus vulgare*, coltsfoot, *Tussilago farfara*, and camomile, *Matricaria chamomilla*, but they are relaxants and expectorants, and though they provide some measure of relief, they do not effect a cure. Some of the Chinese herbal remedies for asthma are as follows (although dosages and other details are not given, for do-it-yourself treatment of asthma is not a practice to be encouraged): joint fir, *Ephedra sinica*; ginseng, *Panax ginseng*; Jimson, or loco, weed, *Datura metel*; mandarin orange, *Citrus reticulata*; apricot, *Prunus armeniaca*; beefsteak plant, *Perilla frutescens*; dandelion, *Taraxacum officinale*; Chinese liquorice, *Glycyrrhiza uralensis*. To these, one could add gypsum, *Gypsum fibrosum* (calcium sulphate), which is mineral, and the earthworm, *Pheretima aspergillum*, which is animal. See **cupping** and **smoking**.

astigmatism See **optical defects**.

astragalus See **huang qi**.

astringent Styptic. A medicine which causes contraction of the body tissues, particularly the skin and mucous membranes, so preventing seepage, or fluid loss, as with chronic diarrhoea and dysentery, profuse sweating, nocturnal sweats, severe haemorrhage, spermatorrhoea, premature ejaculation, chronic leucorrhoea, urinary incontinence and chronic coughs. But astringents must not be applied where a fluid loss is desirable in order to remove toxic substances, or evil-*qi*, as with coughs, diarrhoea and other full and external ailments in the earliest stages. Some astringents commonly used in TCM are blackberry, *Rubus coreanus*, rhubarb, *Rheum officinale*, mugwort, *Artemisia vulgaris*, salad burnet, *Sanguisorba officinalis*, opium poppy, *Papaver somniferum*, foxnut, *Euryale ferox*, oyster, *Ostrea rivularis*, cuttlefish, *Sepia esculenta*, praying mantis, *Paratenodera sinensis*, and gypsum, *Gypsum fibrosum*.

astrology The art of estimating the occult influences of the heavenly bodies on human affairs. See **horoscope**. In so far as astrology is used to make predictions, it has some relevance to TCM, for to be forewarned is to be forearmed, and a sick person will surely want to know his prospects in terms of health and longevity. One may suspect that, in past ages, when Chinese physicians dabbled in astrology, gross fabrications guised as predictions were used as placebos, just as placebos – bottles of coloured water – are now used in the West to give patients some self-confidence. And these predictions probably had a moral and dietary content. On the other hand, physicians knew so much about the private life of a patient that they would be able to make reliable predictions based upon known facts. 'Study the past, if you would divine the future,' said Confucius. After all, what is a diagnosis but a prediction based upon observation and a little logical guesswork. The cosmic forces which people are inclined to lightly dismiss as a bit of superstition could be, in fact, gravitational forces and radiation and dust particles from our distant neighbours in outer space. It is as well to remember that some of the discoveries made by astrologers have laid the foundations of modern astronomy.

atherosclerosis A form of arteriosclerosis which is accompanied by fatty degeneration. See **arteriosclerosis**.

athlete's foot A type of ringworm which infects the skin, mainly between the toes and on the soles, and which is caused by the fungus *Tinea pedis*. The condition is contagious and foul smelling, which explains why it is sometimes called 'foot-rot'. It commonly afflicts adolescents and young men, particularly those who engage in athletic pursuits, for it is picked up on the feet in changing-rooms and swimming pools. The skin between the toes becomes itchy and inflamed, and may crack and flake to expose areas of the skin underneath. Spreading of the infection may be curtailed somewhat by going barefoot wherever possible – but certainly not in those public places where the disease can be picked up – and wearing socks made of natural fibres, such as cotton or wool. It is helpful to apply a compress made by dipping cotton-wool into wine or cider vinegar, and leaving it in place overnight. In the West, the usual herbal remedy is tincture of marigold, *Calendula officinalis*, applied externally. A simple and homely but effective treatment in the traditional Chinese style can be achieved by filling a large bowl with hot water, adding 575 ml vinegar and 2 crushed garlic cloves, and immersing the feet in this liquid for 20–30 minutes. This process is repeated until the condition is cured, which may take some considerable time. But if the condition persists or frequently recurs, the sufferer should seek professional medical advice in regard to his general health.

atmosphere The layer of air surrounding the earth, and which the Chinese regard as a source of *qi* or, 'vital energy'. See **air**.

atrophy The wasting away of tissue through disuse or lack of nutriment.

atropine A poisonous alkaloid contained in deadly nightshade, *Atropa belladonna*.

aubergine *Solanum melongena* Also called the egg-plant, the aubergine is classified as a cold food by the Chinese. As an item of diet, it is preventive of diabetes and hypertension.

auditory nerve The eighth cranial nerve, which serves the organs of hearing and balance.

aura A premonition symptomatic of an attack of migraine or epilepsy.

autism See **schizophrenia**.

autoclave A vessel using high-pressure steam to sterilize surgical instruments.

auto-immunity An unusual condition whereby the body reacts abnormally in producing antibodies to counteract the effects of some of its own tissues which are behaving as antigens, or allergens, so causing the tissues to deteriorate. Rheumatoid arthritis and pernicious anaemia are auto-immune diseases.

automatic nervous system Sympathetic nervous system. The part of the nervous system which functions without a person's awareness and regulates involuntary actions, such as peristalsis and the pulse. See **nervous system**.

autopsy A post-mortem examination, involving dissection, of a body to determine the exact cause of death.

auto-suggestion See **self-hypnosis**.

Ayurvedic medicine The traditional Indian system of medicine, in which, as in TCM, the emphasis is on preventive treatment. The patient's life-style is constantly checked by a therapist, who will suggest those adjustments which he deems to be necessary.

B

bacillus See **bacterium**.

backbone Spine. Vertebral column. See **skeleton** and **intervertebral discs**.

back pain This condition has many causes, and so medical advice should be sought to establish whether it is muscular, spinal or nervous in origin or due to a disease of the internal organs. Weak muscles can be treated with herbs, acupuncture, acupressure and massage. The application of soothing ointments and liniments can be very helpful. In TCM, the root of ginseng, *Panax ginseng*, and teasel, *Pipsacus asper*, are commonly used to relieve back pain. A traditional Chinese remedy for cold back pain, is made by steeping 30· g cinnamon, *Cinnamomum cassia*, bark in 1 litre clear spirit, such as gin, for 2 weeks. This preparation is taken orally when the pain arises, but the daily dosage should not exceed about 100 g. A traditional Chinese dietary remedy is a pie or stew made of one pig's kidney and 120 g walnuts which have been soaked until soft and then chopped finely.

bacterium A single-celled plant of microscopic size. Bacteria are widely distributed in the human body and elsewhere. They should not be confused with viruses or single-celled animal organisms. Most bacteria are harmless, but many cause diseases. They multiply by simple fission, that is, by splitting into two. The best conditions for their development are warmth, moisture, darkness and a good supply of nutrients, which important fact should be borne in mind by those people who place their backsides firmly on the seat when using a public convenience. Bacteria are classified according to their shapes: *cocci*, spheres; *bacilli*, rods; *vibrios*, curved; *spirilla*, or *spirochaetes*, spirals. The table shows examples of a few of the diseases caused by bacteria. We owe much of our knowledge of bacteria to the French chemist Louis Pasteur (1822–1895), who noticed the rapid increase in numbers of tiny rod-shaped bodies in fermenting sugar solutions. Prior to Pasteur's discovery, most people and many physicians believed that diseases were due to bad blood or

BACTERIA			
Cocci (coccus)	Bacilli (bacillus)	Vibrios (vibrio)	Spirilla (spirillum)
pneumonia tonsillitis	anthrax tuberculosis	cholera diphtheria (diagrammatic)	syphilis Vincent's angina

the presence of tiny demons within the body. The latter belief was not entirely erroneous in so far as bacteria are alive, as demons are supposed to be. Centuries ago, Chinese physicians were not aware of the existence of bacteria as such, and they probably attributed infections to poisonous substances and evil-*qi*. They would have combated poisons with antidotes, and reduced evil-*qi* with suppressive yin medicines, which is roughly what we, in the West, do today when we use an antibiotic to inhibit the development of disease-causing micro-organisms. Chinese physicians take the view that if a person is in a thoroughly sound state of health, he should be able to throw off most infections. Research in the West has shown that the body has its own immune system which, in general, can cope with invasions by bacteria, even some of those which are pathogenic. See **immune system**.

bad breath See **halitosis**.

ba gang A Chinese medical term meaning 'differential diagnosis'. It is a system of diagnosis in which there are eight principles, or categories, of illness: yin, yang, cold, hot, internal, external, empty and full. An illness will be diagnosed as being yin or yang, cold or hot, internal or external, and empty or full. But this classification is somewhat arbitrary, and so, whilst there is a tendency for yin illnesses to also be cold, internal and empty, and for yang illnesses to be hot, external and full, this will not always be the case, and other combinations of categories are quite common. But, whatever the diagnostic categories indicated by the symptoms, all illnesses fall into the two main categories of yin and yang. If the illness is causing injury to the patient's yin-energy, a yang treatment, herbal or otherwise, will be required.

Conversely, if the illness is causing injury to the patient's yang-energy, a yin-treatment will be required. The table shows the eight categories of *ba gang*, together with the main symptoms and the treatments required:

THE EIGHT CATEGORIES OF BA GANG

Category	Main symptoms	Treatment
yin	paleness, tiredness, shortage of breath, loose stools, clear urine, tender and white-furred tongue, weak and slow pulse	warming, stimulating
yang	flushed, fidgety, heavy and rapid breathing, scanty and dark urine, constipation, bright-red and yellow-furred tongue, heavy and rapid pulse	cooling, sedative
cold	paleness, cold hands and feet, shivering, lack of thirst, loose stools, profuse and clear urine, pale and white-furred tongue, slow pulse	warming, stimulating
hot	flushed, warm hands and feet, great thirst, fidgety, scanty and dark urine, constipation, red and dry yellow-furred tongue, rapid and fluctuating pulse	cooling, sedative
internal	no individual symptoms, changeable tongue, low pulse	indicated by other symptoms
external	chills, hotness, fever, normal tongue with thin white fur, varied pulse	eliminative, diaphoretic
empty	tiredness, weakness, shortage of breath, loss of appetite and weight, tender and thick unfurred tongue, low and slow pulse	warming, stimulating
full	over activity, fidgety, stertorous breathing, scanty and dark urine, abdominal distension, constipation, hard and thick-furred tongue, fluctuating pulse	cathartic, sedative

The treatments will be of an opposite nature to the symptoms. This system of diagnosis may appear to be very complicated; but, in practice, it is quite straightforward if one rigidly abides by the yin-yang principle of complementary opposites: treat a yin illness with a yang medicine, and a yang illness with a yin medicine. See **diagnostic combinations**.

ba gua See **pa kua**.

bai bu *Stemona tuberosa* Herbal medicine. Distribution: China, Taiwan, India. Parts: roots. Character: cool, bitter-sweet. Affinity: lungs. Effects: anthelmintic, antitussive, demulcent to lungs. Symptoms: coughs. Treatments: chronic coughs, whooping cough, tuberculosis, tapeworms. Dosage: 4–10 g. A decoction may be applied externally as a lotion to kill lice.

bai zhi *Angelica anomala* Herbal medicine. Distribution: China, Japan. Parts: roots. Character: warm, bitter, pungent. Affinity: lungs, stomach. Effects: analgesic, antitoxic. Symptoms: headaches, aches and pains. Treatments: colds, abscesses, swellings, leucorrhoea, snake bites. The angelica used in the West is a different species.

balance Harmony. The Chinese regard balance as being the key to success in maintaining a sound state of health, attaining a long life and preventing social friction with all its sad consequences. In the view of Chinese physicians, many illnesses can be attributed to imbalance of the energies within the bodily organs, between the organs, and between the elements. Thus, by fortifying liver-*qi*, the imbalance of the liver may be corrected, and this, in turn, will assist the gall-bladder, and stimulate the heart through the relationship between the elements wood and fire, for wood is supportive of fire. See **harmony** and **element**.

balanced diet The Chinese attach much importance to a balanced diet, which can be briefly defined as one which, in the short term, does not cause indigestion, and which, in the long term, ensures that one does not consume too much of what is beneficial. A balanced diet will contain those health-giving and health-protective substances which prevent infection and dysfunction of the bodily organs. In the West, a balanced diet is achieved by dietetic planning, diet sheets and other paraphernalia. The Chinese have no need of these devices, for their many centuries of rich experience in the culinary arts have provided them with a diet whose in-built components ensure an effective dietary balance, coupled with variety, and thereby a sound state of health. Almost from force of habit, a Chinese cook will effect a judicious and harmonious blending of food ingredients in both their nutritional properties and manner of presentation, that is, in their colours, textures, flavours and fragrances. The *tao* of balanced diet is one of the Eight Pillars of Taoism. In terms of modern chemistry, it is largely a matter of maintaining the correct pH, or acid-alkaline, balance in food. See **acid** and **Eight Pillars of Taoism**.

baldness See **hair loss**.

balloon flower *Platycodon grandiflorum* Herbal medicine. Distribution: China, Japan. Parts: roots. Character: neutral, pungent-bitter. Affinity: lungs. Effects: expectorant, demulcent to lungs, broncho-dilator, pus-eliminator, induces mucus secretions. Symptoms: coughs, sore throat, excess phlegm. Treatments: lungs and throat ulcers. Dosage: 3–4 g.

balm Balsam. A fragrant and medicinal resinous exudation from certain trees, and also a synthetic aromatic oil-based ointment with healing and soothing properties.

balsam See **balm**.

bamboo A giant tropical grass in the genus *Bambusa*. Some species are effective as antipyretics, diuretics and a treatment for arteriosclerosis. Bamboo shoots, which are a popular item of diet in China, are a good source of fibre, which helps to prevent constipation.

banana *Musa sapientum* Easily digested and with a higher energy value than most fruits, the banana is commonly used by the Chinese as an ingredient in diets for invalids and the elderly.

Banti's disease See **splenic anaemia**.

ban zhi lian *Scutellaria barbata* Herbal medicine. Distribution: China, Japan. Parts: entire plant. Character: cold, bitter. Affinity: lungs, heart, gall-bladder, small intestine, large intestine. Effects: antipyretic, diuretic, haemostatic, antidote, reduces swellings. Symptoms: boils, abscesses, fever. Treatments: heat-excess conditions, stomach ulcers, lung ulcers, cancer of lungs, stomach and intestine, poisonous snake bites. Dosage: 8–28 g.

barbiturates Drugs used in the West as sedatives and soporifics. They can be addictive.

'barefoot doctors' A Chinese colloquial name for the travelling one-year-trained paramedical practitioners who, by means of acupuncture and herbal remedies, attend to the health needs of the people in the rural areas of China.

Barefoot Doctor's Manual The official Chinese manual for the guidance of paramedical practitioners. For each of the illnesses listed, both Western and traditional Chinese treatments are given.

barley *Hordeum vulgare* Herbal medicine. Distribution: China, America, Europe. Parts: germinated sprouts. Character: salty, neutral. Affinity: stomach, spleen. Effects: digestive, stomachic, abortifacient, suppressive of lactation. Symptoms: loss of appetite, poor digestion, excessive lactation. Treatments: abdominal distention, weaning, weak spleen and stomach. It eases contractions in childbirth. Dosage: 10–18 g. Barley water is commonly used in the West as a mild diuretic. It is made by pouring boiling water on to pearl barley, and then allowing it to stand overnight. It can be flavoured with sugar and lemon juice.

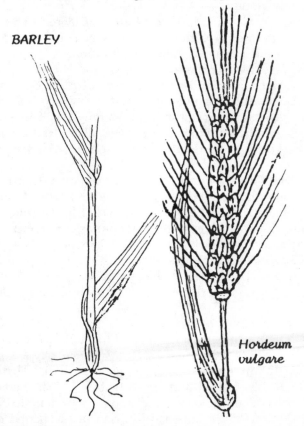

BARLEY

Hordeum vulgare

Bartholin's glands Two small glands, one at each side of the vagina, which secrete lubricants.

base A compound which reacts with an acid to yield a salt and water. Oxides and hydroxides of metals, such as copper oxide and sodium hydroxide (caustic soda), are bases. Water-soluble bases form alkaline solutions. See **acid** and **alkali**.

Basedow's disease See **thyrotoxicosis**.

basic needs See **survival**.

bathing One of the methods used to apply an infusion or decoction to the skin or eyes. A sterile swab is used to apply the liquid to the skin or eyes, but it is usual for the feet to be immersed in a bowl containing the liquid.

bean sprouts A common item of diet in China. They are grown from mung beans and soya beans, but, unlike the dried beans, they contain vitamin C and are easily digested and a good source of dietary fibre. See **soya bean**.

beard See **hairiness**.

bears' paws In China, bears' paws are considered to be a rare delicacy. Traditionally, they are consumed as a remedy for rheumatism and a tonic for a weak constitution.

bed-wetting Nocturnal enuresis. See **enuresis**.

beef With a high content of saturated fatty acid, the consumption of beef leads to the formation of cholesterol, which is a cause of arteriosclerosis. It is not a prominent feature of the Chinese diet. In any case, in the south of China, where all the land is required for growing rice, there is little or no land to spare for grazing cattle.

beefsteak plant *Perilla frustescens* Herbal medicine. Distribution: South China, Japan, India. Parts: leaves, stems. Character: warm, pungent. Affinity: lungs, spleen. Effects: antitussive, stomachic, diuretic, diaphoretic. Symptoms: fever, headaches, Treatments: congestion, colds, chills. Dosage: 6–9 g. Parts: seeds. Character: warm, pungent. Affinity: lungs. Effects: antitussive, expectorant, laxative. Symptoms: coughs, excessive mucus, constipation. Treatments: asthma, bronchitis. Dosage: 4–8 g.

Bell's palsy See **facial paralysis**.

ben cao Chinese words meaning 'herbal medicine'. *Ben cao* has a long history of over 5000 years.

Ben Cao Gang Mu 'Outlines and Branches of Herbal Medicine'. This remarkable work listing nearly 2000 herbal medicines, together with details of their applications, was compiled by Li Shizhen (1517–1593), a famous physician of the period of the Ming dynasty (1368–1644), which was a time when medical science flourished in China. Li Shizhen devoted 27 years to the compilation of this pharmacopoeia, and during that time, he travelled throughout China, conducting his researches. In China, *Ben Cao Gang Mu* is still regarded as the main reference work of medical science, though only about 300 of the medicines it lists are in common use today. It has had some not inconsiderable influence on medical studies in the Western world, and has been translated into a variety of languages, including English, French, German, Russian and Japanese.

benign tumour See **tumour**.

beriberi A disease due to a deficiency of thiamin, and which can cause polyneuritis, oedema and heart failure, its symptoms being paralysis, loss of appetite, atrophy of the muscles and confusion. It was once very prevalent among the Chinese and other Eastern peoples whose staple diet was polished rice, which is rice grains from which the husks, or outer layers, containing thiamin, have been removed. If beriberi is caught in its early stages, it is easily treated with thiamin supplements or merely by adopting a diet that is rich in thiamin. See **Sun Simiao**.

beta-carotene See **carrot**.

betel palm *Areca catechu* Herbal medicine. Distribution: India, Vietnam, Taiwan. Parts: nuts. Character: warm, pungent-bitter. Affinity: stomach, large intestine. Effects: digestive, diuretic, anthelmintic. Symptoms: irregular bowel movements, swollen legs and feet. Treatments: intestinal worms, malaria. Dosage: 4–8 g.

betony *Stachys betonica* Distribution: Europe. Parts: leaves, flowers. Character: warm, bitter. Affinity: lungs, large intestine. Effects: digestive, sedative, anthelmintic. Symptoms: indigestion, breathlessness, irregular bowel movements, headaches. Treatments: sores, ulcers, bronchitis, intestinal worms. Dosage: 3–10 g. The dried leaves are used as an ingredient in herbal tobacco and snuff. See **woundwort**.

bhat gwa mirrors See **mirrors**.

Bian Que Chinese scholars claim that Bian Que (407–310 BC) was the first true physician in China, and that he was the first to practise acupuncture, gynaecology and paediatrics.

bian stones See **acupuncture needles**.

b.i.d. An abbreviation for the Latin words, *bis in die*, meaning 'twice daily', and used in prescriptions.

bile Gall. A viscous, yellow-green liquid and stored in the gallbladder, whence it passes, via the bile-duct, into the duodenum, where it emulsifies fats so that they can be acted upon more readily by the digestive juices in the duodenum and small intestine.

bile-duct See **bile** and **alimentary canal**.

binary numbers Over 5000 years ago, the Chinese were using binary nunbers, and they are often credited with the invention of the binary number system, in which two is the base number. In the denary, or decimal, system, the base number is 10. Binary numbers constitute the principle of the electronic computer, in which a flow of electric current represents one (yang, positive or 'yes') and a non-flow, small flow or opposite flow represents zero (yin, negative or 'no'). It seems that the human brain and nervous system operate in much the same way as a computer. Thoughts are electrochemical impulses, and each thought can be expressed as a question requiring an answer which is either 'yes' (positive, yang) or 'no' (negative, yin). There are degrees of positivity and negativity, it is true, but the principle remains the same. It is, perhaps, in the nature of wild speculation to suggest that the sages of ancient China discovered the manner of operation of the human mind, but if they did, they certainly put the science of psychology on a practical basis. The snippets of wisdom contained in the *I Ching* clearly indicate that they knew much about human nature and ways to attain a sound state of mental health. See **I Ching**.

'biological clock' See **zodiac exercises**.

biorhythms See **zodiac exercises** and **insomnia**.

biotin Vitamin H. See **vitamin**.

bird's nest In China, bird's nest, which is the hard dried saliva of a fish-eating and cave-dwelling species of swift, is steamed with sugar to make a dessert, or stewed with lean pork to make a soup. It is regarded as a great delicacy, but it is also a valuable tonic medicine. The saliva of the birds, which is regurgitated after digestion, and then dried in their nests, which are made of down, contains digestive juices, and one may suppose that, if it is consumed by humans, it will do as much good for their digestion as it does for that of the birds.

birth control The Chinese regard birth control by means of contraceptive devices as being unnatural, and therefore immoral. On the other hand, China is heavily populated, and so, of the two undesirable items – contraceptives and over-population – they have opted for contraceptives. Some of the various types of contraceptive devices used in the West are now freely available in China, and the Chinese government gives encouragement in that direction by providing a money allowance for the first child, but there is no allowance for subsequent children. In fact, if more than one child is born, the allowance for the first child is withdrawn, and so one-child families are encouraged. With the support of the World Health Organization, Chinese biochemists and herbalists are trying to develop an effective and safe herbal medicine to inhibit gestation. The traditional method of contraception in China is sexual intercourse without ejaculation, which must surely indicate that some Chinese males have an iron will and nerves of steel. See **Yellow Emperor** and **safe period**.

birthmark See **naevus**.

bisexual 'Of two sexes'. This term can be used in two contexts: to describe hermaphroditic animals, such as the earthworm, which have male and female sex organs; and to describe a person who, because of his or her glandular make-up, is attracted to both sexes. In China, bisexuality is considered to be inherited and is generally discouraged. See **homosexuality**.

bites The bites from animals can cause problems in several ways. Some animals are able to inject a venom into their victims. This is the case with snakes, which have fangs for this purpose. Some animals which are non-venomous may carry disease-causing micro-organisms in their saliva. An example of this is the anopheles mosquito, which carries the malarial parasite, *Plasmodium*. The rabies, or hydrophobia, virus is transmitted from dogs to humans in the same way. Fortunately for us, many insects do not bite, and those that do bite are generally so small that they can do no real harm. However, there are some notorious exceptions, and the bites of some small insects, such as the rat flea, which carries the bubonic plague, sometimes have dire and even fatal consequences. A simple treatment for a small insect bite is to rub crushed marigold leaves, sage leaves or garlic cloves on the affected part. All spiders are venomous, but most of them are too small or too weak to bite into the skin of a human, and so they do very little harm. Bites from larger spiders and venomous snakes require treatment with sera, which are available at the hospitals in those regions where venomous spiders and snakes feature among the fauna. See **snake bite** and **rabies**.

bitter One of the five tastes in TCM. See **taste**.

bitter almonds These nuts are edible, but they should not be consumed in large quantities, for they contain prussic acid (hydrogen cyanide), which is poisonous.

bitter gourd In China, this gourd is consumed as a health food. 10 g bitter gourd contains as much vitamin C as 170 g apple, which is quite startling. It strengthens the immune system, aids digestion, stimulates the appetite, improves the complexion, removes heat, clears the mind, overcomes tiredness and brightens the eyes. Traditionally, it is a remedy for sore eyes, diarrhoea and diabetes. However, it is of a very cold nature, and it should not be consumed by asthmatics or those with a weak constitution. But the coldness can be counteracted by combining it with ginger or some other warming herb.

blackberry *Rubus coreanus* Herbal medicine. Distribution: China, Europe. Parts: Unripe fruits. Character: sweet, sour, warmish. Affinity: liver, kidneys. Effects: astringent, tonic to kidneys. Symptoms: impotence, premature ejaculation, bed-wetting. Treatments: spermatorrhoea, urinary incontinence, poor vision. Dosage: 4–10 g. There are nearly 400 different species and varieties of blackberry, both wild and cultivated, and all have similar medicinal properties. In China, they are generally administered as medicines by adding the unripe fruits to soups and stews.

blackberry lily See **leopard flower.**

black cardamom *Alpinia oxyphylla* Herbal medicine. Distribution: South China. Affinity: kidneys, spleen. Effects: astringent, stomachic, preventive of diarrhoea and excessive urination, tones kidneys and nurtures bones and connective tissue. Symptoms: impotence, premature ejaculation, diarrhoea, excessive urination and salivation. Treatments: kidney deficiencies, urinary incontinence, abdominal pain and coldness. Dosage: 4–8 g.

black dates See **red dates**.

black eyes See **contusion**.

blackheads See **acne**.

black rice vinegar See **vinegar**.

black soya bean *Glycine max* Herbal medicine. Distribution: China, Japan. Parts: seeds (beans). Character: cold, sweet, slightly bitter. Affinity: stomach, lungs. Effects: antipyretic, carminative, sedative. Symptoms: headaches, insomnia. Treatments: colds, fevers, wind-heat injuries. Dosage: 8–14 g. Black soya beans are fermented before being used medicinally.

blackwater fever A severe but rare complication of one type of malaria. It causes anaemia and damages the kidneys. See **hare's ear**.

bladder One of the sac-like organs which collect and temporarily store a liquid, as with the gall-bladder, which stores bile from the liver. More particularly, this term refers to the urinary bladder, which stores urine from the kidneys. It is one of the hollow organs of TCM. It is yang and its element is water. See **liu fu**.

bladder organ See **liu fu**.

bleeding see **haemorrhage**.

blending of foods The Chinese blend foods most effectively, by methods learned from long experience, to ensure that all the food elements required for proper nutrition are not only available but are also counteractive of ill-effects, so that there is a balance between acid and alkali, irritating and smooth, and so on. This blending also extends to the appetizing qualities of a meal, and there will be an effective blending of textures, colours, flavours and fragrances. Thus, a Chinese meal is as effective in its presentation as it is in the selection of ingredients and preparation.

blepharitis Inflamed eyelid. See **conjunctivitis**.

blister Bulla. An uplifted area of skin containing fluid, which is generally plasma which has escaped from the underlying blood capillaries that have been damaged by heat or friction. A blood blister contains whole blood. If blisters are extensive, treatment for shock is likely to be required. Otherwise, they are self-healing, and require little or no treatment apart from the application of a soothing and antiseptic lotion, such as an infusion of the leaves of sage, *Salvia officinale*, or rosemary. *Rosmarinus officinalis*. If a blister is large, it can be pricked with a sterilized needle to drain the fluid, but the loose skin must not be removed. The blister should then be covered with a sterile dressing to keep out dirt.

block Local anaesthesia. The nerves in a part of the body are rendered insensitive by the injection of an anaesthetizing fluid. In acupuncture, the same effect is produced by inserting a needle into a selected nerve.

blockage A term used in acupuncture, acupressure and reflexology to indicate a condition in which energy is not passing, or is diminished in its passing, along a meridian.

blood A red fluid tissue circulating in the arteries and veins of higher animals, and which contains a number of constituents – plasma, erythrocytes leucocytes and thrombocytes – each having its particular function. The blood is the transport system of the body, taking nutrients and oxygen to the tissues and removing waste. It provides chemical communication between the tissues and organs by means of hormones and other secretions. The average adult person has about 7 litres of blood, which makes up about 10 per cent of his body by weight. In Chinese, blood is called *xue*, which is one of the four humours of traditional medicine. See **humour** and **circulation**.

blood blister See **blister**.

blood circulation See **circulation**.

blood cleanser Strictly, this is not a medical term, but it is one which effectively describes many of the wide range of medicines and health foods which improve the quality of blood by eliminating toxic waste, counteracting allergens and destroying harmful micro-organisms, either directly, acting within the blood itself, or indirectly, in the small intestine, stomach and other organs which supply the blood with nutrients and other essentials. Garlic, *Allium sativum*, sage, *Salvia officinalis*, stinging nettle, *Urtica dioica*, chervil, *Anthriscus cerefolium*, burdock, *Arctium lappa*, and dandelion, *Taraxacum officinale*, are quite effective in this regard. Nettle tea, which is an infusion of nettle shoots in a dosage of 2–4 g, is renowned for its powers as a spring tonic. See **brimstone and treacle**.

blood clot Blood clots, or coagulates, on exposure to air. If this were not so, a person sustaining a nosebleed or the slightest cut would bleed to death. However, blood clots sometimes form in inconvenient places, and so hinder the normal functions of the body. An infusion of the dandelion, *Taraxacum officinale*, using the whole plant, is a treatment for clots in the lungs. See **coagulation** and **thrombosis**.

blood-excess One of the theories of TCM is that an excess of blood in the system, or blood-excess, causes anger. And it is true that a person who is angry may have a flushed face. But, being self-perpetuating, anger is likely to develop into violent rages. This could damage the liver, which is the organ that controls the quality and quantity of blood. See **emotion**.

blood-letting In this treatment, a sharp needle, which is first sterilized, is inserted into the damaged area of an external disease or a vital acupoint for an internal disease, so releasing a small amount of blood, together with excess evil-*qi* and heat energy. Leeches are not used for this purpose, as they were once used in the West. Blood-letting is a treatment for swellings, fevers, heat stroke, apoplexy, vomiting, colic and diarrhoea. See **leech**.

blood poisoning This is the everyday name for what, more correctly, should be called septicaemia.

blood pressure Blood pressure may be high, which is called hypertension, or low, which is called hypotension. See **hypertension** and **hypotension**.

bloodshot eyes See **eyesight**

blood sugar Glucose ($C_6 H_{12} O_6$). This food, which is formed by the digestion of starches and more complex sugars, such as sucrose, is present in the blood plasma, and is a source of energy for the tissues. Lack of blood sugar leads to lack of energy, as will be manifested by tiredness. An excess of blood sugar, some of which passes into the urine, is often a symptom of diabetes. See **diabetes mellitus**.

blood system See **circulation**.

blood tonic This is a medicine which cleanses or enriches the blood or makes it more effective in its functions. See **blood cleanser**. The blood may be enriched by being provided with nutrients, including vitamins and minerals, which it will pass on to the tissues where they are required, or which it will utilize to increase its oxygen-carrying capacity. This is generally achieved by a more varied and wholesome diet and tonic medicines which contain minerals, particularly iron, calcium and phosphorus. Of course, medicines which tone the heart, lungs and liver will also indirectly benefit the blood, and so they could be regarded as blood tonics also. A medicine or health food containing iron, and administered as a treatment for anaemia, which is an iron-deficiency disease in its commonest form, could also be regarded as a blood tonic. Infusions of dandelion, *Taraxacum officinale*, root in a dosage of 10–18 g and stinging nettle, *Urtica dioica*, leaves in a dosage of 2–4 g are effective as blood tonics. Other blood tonics include: *shu di huang*, *Rehmannia glutinosa*, roots, 10–20 g; angelica, *Angelica sinensis*, roots, 10–12 g; longan fruit, *Euphoria longan*, dried fruit, 10–12 g; cornbind, *Polygonum multiflorum*, all

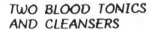

TWO BLOOD TONICS
AND CLEANSERS

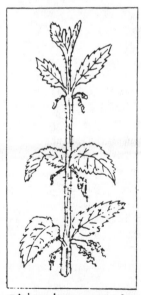

stinging nettle
Urtica dioica

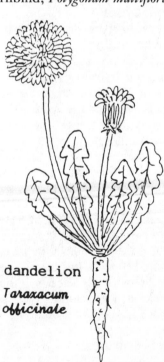

dandelion
Taraxacum officinale

parts, 7–10 g ; tienchi, *Panax pseudo-ginseng*, to be taken as directed by the instructions on the container in which it was purchased.

bodily fluid In Western medicine, it is accepted that the main body fluid other than blood is lymph, which is a colourless alkaline fluid similar to blood but without erythrocytes. In TCM, this bodily fluid is called *jin ye*, and it is considered to have two components, which are *jin*, a thin fluid, and *ye*, a dense fluid. *Jin ye* derives from water and substances in food, and is converted by the vital organs into various forms which have different functions. This is the Chinese physician's seemingly over-simplistic interpretation based upon superficial observations, but it is essentially accurate and, as far as TCM is concerned, it works in practice. See **lymph** and **jin ye**.

'body clock' See **insomnia** and **zodiac exercises**.

body odour This condition is due to the action of bacteria on accumulated perspiration, sebum and dirt, the parts of the body most affected being the armpits, groin and feet. Apart from being clean in one's personal habits, an effective treatment is to add 500 ml lemon juice or tomato juice to the bath water. See **athlete's foot**.

body temperature See **temperature**.

boil See **furuncle**.

bones There are a few serious diseases of bones; but, in general, apart from fractures and defects of the joints, as with arthritis, bones do not seem to give much trouble, but they can become weakened or brittle with age. A traditional Chinese dietary remedy to strengthen the bones is as follows: add 500 g pig's trotters, pig's houghs or mutton bones and 60 g vinegar to 2 litres water, simmer for 2 hours, and then consume as a soup. Otherwise, the bones can be strengthened by providing tonics for the kidneys. In TCM, it is assumed that the bones are dependent upon the kidneys for nourishment, and so they are associated with the element water.

boneset See **comfrey**

Book of Odes *Shijing*. One of the greater literary classics of the period of the Zhou dynasty (1100–221 BC). Its many references to medicinal herbs clearly indicate that TCM was beginning to flourish at least 3000 years ago, but there is archaeological evidence to show that it had its origins in a much earlier period in history.

borage See **eczema**.

botany The scientific study of plants, involving their anatomy, physiology, classification and distribution. Chinese physicians and scholars have studied plants, particularly those which are medicinal herbs, for thousands of years. In a Chinese pharmacopoeia in the style of TCM, the emphasis is on a classification based more upon medicinal properties than anatomical structures. In the southern provinces of China, and also in Sichuan, in Central China, herbs are cultivated extensively, and various techniques are employed: grafting, induced pollination and fertilization, seed selection, irrigation, crop rotation, etc. In China, the cultivation of herbs, requiring a great deal of botanical knowledge, is a major industry, which supplies its products to all parts of the world. In one way or another, the Chinese contribution to the health of mankind must be enormous. However, some of the more potent wild plants cannot be cultivated, and so the Chinese government is taking the appropriate measures to ensure that these valuable plants do not become extinct. It is important that the medically useful parts of the plants should be collected, and that they should be collected in a clean and healthy condition at the time of year when they are most medicinally active: roots and rhizomes in early spring and late autumn, flowers in the spring and summer, and so on. And they must be correctly sorted, dried and stored so that they are not damaged by micro-organisms, moulds, heat, frost, etc.

botulism The most deadly of all forms of food poisoning, causing weakness, double vision, paralysis and respiratory or heart failure. Closely related to tetanus, botulism bacteria thrive in airtight containers, such as cans of food. The Chinese have fewer problems in this regard because they insist on food ingredients being really fresh, and generally do not consume canned and processed foods. See **food poisoning**.

bovine spongiform encephalopathy 'Mad-cow disease'. Staggers. A disease affecting the brain and spinal cord of cattle, horses and sheep, resulting in giddiness, paralysis and death. In cattle, it is probably due to feeding them on infected sheep offals. This disease causes no problems in China, for the Chinese do not feed their cattle on sheep offals or any other form of unnatural diet. In any case, apart from those few small areas in the north of China where the land is suitable for grazing, few cattle are reared. What is more, the Chinese do not regard beef as being a particularly healthy item of diet.

bowel Intestines. The state of the bowel – constipation, hard stools, diarrhoea, foul-smelling faeces, etc. – provides the Chinese physician with many helpful symptoms.

boxthorn See **wolfberry**.

BP The abbreviation for *British Pharmacopoeia*.

brain This organ has three main parts, which are the cerebrum, cerebellum and medulla oblongata. The cerebrum, which has a convoluted surface, or cortex, to give it a large area, is the thinking part of the brain. It also controls the sense organs and limbs and records impressions. The cerebellum co-ordinates the voluntary activities of the body, maintains balance and controls many of those actions which are regarded as being instinctive. The medulla oblongata, which is commonly known as the brain stem, connects the cerebrum and cerebellum, through the base of the skull, with the spinal cord. The bones which enclose the brain are called the cranium. But, although the brain is regarded as the seat of the intellect, it is not the seat of the emotions, or, at least, not entirely so, for modern research has shown that some emotional reactions are initiated by hormones, which are secretions from the endocrine glands in various parts of the body.

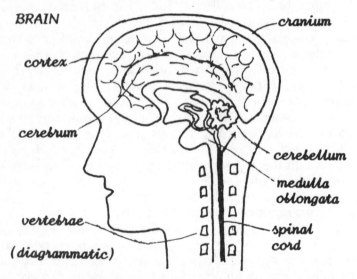

BRAIN — cranium — cortex — cerebrum — cerebellum — medulla oblongata — vertebrae — spinal cord — (diagrammatic)

But the brain will register and perhaps modify these reactions. It seems that the physicians of ancient China displayed great perspicacity when they decided that the emotions are associated with the vital organs. Perhaps we are nearer the truth than we realize when we describe a bad-tempered person as being liverish, a cowardly person as being 'yellow-livered', and a happy person as having joy in his heart. Anxiety states and nervous breakdowns, which are regarded as mental illnesses, are often due more to bodily conditions than any serious defect of the brain. It is largely a matter of body chemistry. The menopause, which is a devastating experience for some women, is a good example of a breakdown in the chemical control system of the corporeal frame.

brandy These days, this spirit, especially French cognac, is favoured by Chinese physicians for making spring wine, which is the most potent form of medicinal wine. See **spring wine**.

bread Those people who value their health will prefer wholemeal bread to white bread, for the former contains 100 per cent wholemeal flour, which is made from grains from which the outer layers have not been removed, and so is rich in vitamins, minerals and dietary fibre. However, it is becoming the well-established practice for white flour to be fortified by the addition of thiamin, niacin, calcium and iron in amounts which are comparable with those in wholemeal flour. In the Western world and the north of China, where bread is made mainly from wheat flour, yeast is used as a raising agent. It feeds on the sugars in the dough and produces carbon dioxide gas, which causes the dough to rise and acquire a spongy texture. But yeast is rich in vitamins and minerals, and so it adds to the nutritive qualities of bread, though some of its vitamins are destroyed by the heat produced during baking. See **yeast**.

breasts See **mammary glands**.

breast-feeding Chinese women prefer to breast-feed their babies, on the not unreasonable principle that nature intended cow's milk for baby cows. Chinese women behave wisely in this respect, for research in the West has shown that dairy products contain allergens, and that babies fed on cow's milk are susceptible to eczema.

breathing This term describes the process by which air is taken in and given out by the lungs. In more scientific terms, breathing-in is described as inspiration or inhalation, and breathing-out as expiration or exhalation. These processes should not be confused with respiration, which is the process of oxidation and gaseous exchange that occurs within the tissues. The full process of breathing and respiration in mammals, including humans, which is closely linked with their blood circulation, may be briefly described as follows. Air enters the lungs, where its oxygen dissolves in the moisture in the spongy tissue, and is then absorbed into the blood capillaries. It combines with the haemoglobin in the erythrocytes to form oxyhaemoglobin. The haemoglobin, which is a protein compound containing iron, is carried by the pulmonary vein to the arteries, and thence to the tissues, where it oxidizes carbonaceous substances, releasing heat and energy and producing carbon dioxide gas, which is carried by the pulmonary artery to the lungs. The moisture in the lungs could be said to be a small ocean providing the medium by which oxygen passes into the capillaries. It is a legacy from our fish-like ancestors, which breathed the oyxgen dissolved in sea water. This explains why people whose lungs become dry, as with asthma and pneumonia, have difficulty in breathing. Respiration and breathing are influenced by external factors, such as temperature, pollution and the moisture, oxygen and carbon dioxide content of air, and by internal factors, such as the condition of the heart, lungs and blood vessels. Long ago, the Chinese realized the importance of breathing and blood circulation, which is why they have always advocated breathing exercises as being one way of promoting the general health. One may wonder if *qi*, or 'primordial vital energy', which is one of the fundamental concepts of TCM, is really the oxygen in the atmosphere, together with the energy released when it combines with carbon and other elements. This is more than just an interesting speculation, for the physicians of ancient China must have concluded that, since man cannot live without air, or whatever it is that one feels on a windy day, it must contain something that is vital to his existence. See **circulation** and **air**.

breathing exercises The Chinese consider that *qi*, or 'vital energy', is best produced by breathing correctly. This would certainly be the case if *qi* were oxygen. See **oxygen**. Physical activity combined with breathing exercises improves the circulation and ensures that the organs and tissues receive an adequate supply of oxygen and nutrients, encourages relaxation and improves the quality of meditation by providing the brain with an adequate supply of oxygenated blood. Breathing exercises also ensure oxidation of toxic waste, so preventing headaches, liverishness, stuffiness, and so forth. In so far as the lungs and heart are involved in breathing and respiration, breathing exercises will help to tone their connective tissue. It is important that one should breathe clean air. But clean air is simply not available in many of the industrial regions of the West. It is also important that one should breathe through the nose, and not the mouth, and then the inhaled air will be filtered, and so some of the impurities will be removed. To promote a sound state of health and prevent many ailments, the Chinese government has issued an exercise manual which covers a wide range of exercises of all kinds – meditation, breathing, relaxing, bathing, walking, massage and the martial arts – and it seems that those who are suffering from chronic conditions, such as asthma, arteriosclerosis, hypertension and haemorhoids, can reap substantial benefits from these exercises. Taoist philosophy teaches that the seven glands of the body may be invigorated and life prolonged by a set of exercises which are aptly described as 'immortal breathing'. An awareness of the benefits of breathing exercises has spread to the West, where there is now a vogue for a combined system of exercises, involving breathing and physical activity, called aerobics, which increase stamina, improve the circulation, emotional state and sleeping habits, relieve depression and increase resistance to disease. See **qi gong**.

Bright's disease See **nephritis**.

brimstone and treacle In Victorian times in Britain, children were regularly dosed with a mixture of brimstone and treacle to cleanse the blood and eliminate waste from the bowel. Brimstone is an archaic name for sulphur, and treacle is a sweetener which, being viscous, could hold together the finely powdered sulphur, or flowers of sulphur, as it is called by pharmacists. It was an effective but drastic treatment, but the same results could have been achieved in a gentler and more natural way by adopting the Chinese practice, and feeding them on garlic, *Allium sativum*, which is rich in sulphur compounds. The other constituents of garlic function as a buffer. See **buffer**.

British Pharmacopoeia In Britain, it is a legal requirement that proprietary medicines should be of the standard of purity indicated by the British Pharmacopoeia. Chemical substances that are likely to be required for medicinal use are generally marked with the abbreviation BP. Chemical substances of commercial standard, such as those used in industrial processes, often contain impurities.

brittle bones See **bones**.

bronchus One of the two bronchi, branching from the trachea, or windpipe, into the lungs.

bronchial asthma See **asthma**.

bronchiole One of the smallest of the bronchial tubes contained within the lungs.

bronchitis Inflammation of the bronchial tubes. In TCM, there is a wide range of remedies for this condition, which include the following, taken internally, using the parts and daily dosages indicated: garlic, *Allium sativum*, 3 cloves, eaten uncooked; gypsum, *Gypsum fibrosum* (calcium sulphate), aqueous suspension,

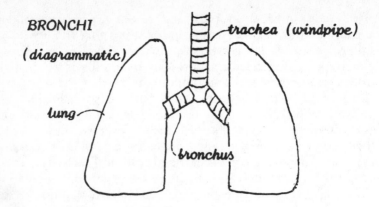

BRONCHI
(diagrammatic)
trachea (windpipe)
lung
bronchus

10–30 g; apricot, *Prunus armeniaca*, decoction of ground stones, 5–10 g; plantain, *Plantago asiatica*, infusion of seeds, 5–9 g; agrimony, *Agrimonia pilosa*, infusion of leaves and flowers, 10–15 g; comfrey, *Symphytum asperum*, infusion or decoction of leaves and roots, 3–12 g. Honey is effective as a demulcent and emollient.

broomrape *Cistanche salsa* Herbal medicine. Distribution: China, Mongolia, Siberia. Parts: stems. Character: warm, salty-sweet. Affinity: large intestine, kidneys. Effects: demulcent, cathartic, tonic to kidneys, aphrodisiac. Symptoms: impotence, premature ejaculation, constipation. Treatments: spermatorrhoea, lumbago, weak bones and connective tissues, hypertension. Dosage: 8–15 g.

broth In China, a broth is the commonest, as well as the oldest, technique for administering a medicine. Its main advantage is that a liquid is assimilated more easily than a solid, and so it takes effect more quickly. Simmering for a long time ensures that all the medicinal ingredients are extracted from the herb. The time taken to boil or simmer the herb, which is generally done in an earthenware pot, is determined by the texture of the parts used. Mineral substances usually need to be boiled at an intense heat for a long period. A broth usually needs to be strained to remove the debris. See **decoction**.

brucellosis A disease caused by bacteria of the genus *Brucella*. In cattle and goats, it is called contagious abortion; in humans, it is called undulant fever because it can recur every few weeks. Caught through contact with infected cattle and goats or their milk, its symptoms are fever, aching limbs, severe sweating and prostration. This disease presents few problems for the Chinese because they do not raise cattle or goats on a large scale.

bruise See **contusion**.

bruisewort See **comfrey**.

BSE The abbreviation for *bovine spongiform encephalopathy* ('mad-cow disease').

bubonic plague See **flea**.

Buddhism The third largest religion in China, but many Chinese view it with suspicion, partly because it has a celibate priesthood, which they regard as being unnatural, and partly because of the Buddhist belief that the human soul passes from one animal to another in a series of reincarnations, which they consider to be nonsensical. On the other hand, Buddhists are peace-loving people, which makes them a good influence; and, since they are opposed to the slaughter of animals, they have evolved a wide range of delectable and health-giving vegetarian dishes, some of which have medicinal properties, and which have been a great boon to the Chinese, and done much to improve their health. It was the Buddhist monks who popularized the tea-drinking habit; and tea, in the Chinese view, is beneficial to the health in a variety of ways. They also devised some forms of kungfu, or martial arts, as a means of self-defence, but which now provide opportunities for keep-fit exercises, and which have meditative overtones that are conducive to a sound state of mental health.

Buerger's disease See **thrombo-anginitis obliterans**.

buffer A term used by pharmacists for a substance which maintains the constant acidity of a solution or renders a medicinal substance less potent. A buffer is sometimes added to a medicine to reduce the risk of toxicity or other side-effects. One of the advantages of herbal medicines is that the whole herbs are less likely to produce side-effects than are the active ingredients when isolated. See **active ingredients**.

bulimia Closely related to anorexia, bulimia is an eating disorder of a psychological origin. It is characterized by excessive dieting, an overwhelming desire to be thin and sudden cravings for food, bouts of overeating, taking laxatives and attempts at vomiting. It can cause hypertension, menstrual problems, anxiety, stress, kidney disorders, urinary problems, dehydration and poor circulation. Acupuncture or acupressure may be helpful, but professional medical advice should be sought. See **obesity**.

bulla See **blister**.

burdock *Arctium lappa* Herbal medicine. Distribution: China, Europe. Parts: seeds, root. Character: cold, pungent-bitter. Affinity: lungs, stomach. Effects: diuretic, expectorant, anti-pyretic, antiphlogistic, diaphoretic, antitoxic. Symptoms: fever, headaches, wind-heat conditions. Treatments: pneumonia, abscesses, throat infections, psoriasis, acne, eczema, dandruff, boils. Dosage: 3–12 g. Burdock is an effective blood cleanser. The young leaf stalks can be boiled as a vegetable or eaten raw in salads. It is sometimes called the greater burdock to distinguish it from the lesser burdock, *Arctium minus*, which is a smaller species but with similar properties.

bulrush See **reedmace**.

bunion See **bursitis**.

burns This condition can be caused by heat, chemicals, electricity or radiation. Tissue is destroyed and plasma seeps from damaged blood vessels and accumulates as blisters. Severe burns cause shock and may become infected. Treatments: rhubarb, *Rheum officinale*, powdered rhizome applied externally; marigold, *Calendula officinalis*, flowers applied as a wet compress; salad burnet, *Sanguisorba officinalis*, powdered root mixed with sesame oil and applied as a lotion; gypsum, *Gypsum fibrosum* (calcium sulphate), powdered crystals applied externally.

burnt See **odour**.

bursa Anatomically, a bursa is a sac of fibrous tissue containing a little fluid, and which serves as a cushion, reducing friction where ligaments move against joints. A bursa may develop where there is abnormal pressure.

bursitis An inflamed bursa, as with housemaid's knee, tennis elbow and a bunion (usually on the big toe). The condition may be aggravated by gout, arthritis or an infection. Treatments: acupressure; massage; comfrey, *Symphytum asperum*, hot poultice of leaves; cayenne pepper, *Capsicum frutescens*, hot compress of powder; camomile, *Matricaria chamomilla*, infusion of flowers taken internally or applied externally as a lotion, 4–6 g. See **meridian massage**.

bu yuan qi A Chinese term meaning 'stimulating the primordial vital energies', which involves diet, herbal medicines, acupuncture, massage, breathing exercises and kungfu. It is one of the fundamental purposes of TCM. See **yuan qi**.

C

caffeine An alkaloid stimulant with a diuretic effect which occurs in tea, cocoa, coffee and the cola nut. It can be addictive, and if taken to excess, say, more than 200 mg per day, which is equivalent to about 4 cups of tea or coffee, it can cause nervousness, depression, delirium and sleeplessness. Some herbal medicines, such as ginseng, cannot be safely taken with drinks containing caffeine.

cai The meat, fish and spicy dishes in the Chinese diet. They are balanced by *fan*, which consists of vegetables and cereals. See **fan**.

Caladium sequinium This herb causes impotence in men. It is potentially a safe and natural contraceptive drug. Japanese scientists have been conducting research in that direction.

calcium This mineral is required for the growth and maintenance of healthy bones and teeth, and so pregnant women and nursing mothers should be provided with a calcium-rich diet. Calcium deficiency may cause osteomalacia in adults and rickets in children, but this condition is rare where the diet is balanced and varied, as is the Chinese diet. Bones are an important component of the Chinese diet, and are chopped small and added to soups and stews, in which, after being simmered for a long time, their nutrients and minerals are extracted. See **mineral**.

calculus Stone. A concretion, or hard deposit, formed in a hollow organ. The commonest calculi are gallstones and kidney stones, but they also occur in the urinary bladder, prostrate gland and salivary glands. They may cause bleeding and severe pain if they block a duct. When large, they need to be removed surgically or dissolved by means of drugs. Chinese physicians insist that, to a large extent, they can be prevented by a sound diet and healthy living. See **gallstone** and **urinary stone**.

callisthenics Gymnastic exercises to achieve both physical and mental health, together with elegance of movement. The Chinese government has issued a manual of exercises devoted entirely to this purpose.

callus See **corn**.

'calm the spirit' See **sedative**.

calomel Mercurous chloride. A poisonous compound of mercury which, about 1000 years ago, the Chinese began to use as a purgative and a treatment for venereal diseases. In the West, it came into use for the same purpose about 400 years later. See **mercury**.

Calorie Large calorie, or kilocalorie. Spelt with a capital C, it is equivalent to 1000 small calories, spelt with a small c. See **calorie**.

calorie A unit of heat, which is defined as the amount of heat required to raise the temperature of 1 g water through 1° Celsius. 1000 calories = 1 kilocalorie = 1 Calorie. The calorie is too small for use in dietetics, and so the energy values of foods are measured in kilocalories, Calories or kilojoules. 1 kilocalorie = 4.18 kilojoules. See **Calorie**, **joule** and **temperature**.

calorific value of food The energy, or calorific, value of foods is measured in kilocalories or kilojoules per stated weight of a solid or stated volume of a liquid. Kilocalories per 100 grams, abbreviated as kcal/100 g, for solids, and kilocalories per 100 millilitres, abbreviated as kcal/100 ml, for liquids, are convenient units for most purposes in dietetics. These measures are useful, and so they will be employed by Chinese physicians and pharmacists, even those practising TCM.

caltrop *Tribulus terrestris* Herbal medicine. Distribution: China, Africa, South America, Australia. Parts: mature fruits. Character: warm, sweet. Affinity: liver, kidneys. Effects: nutrients for bones and connective tissue, stimulates kidneys and liver, improves vision. Symptoms: impotence, premature ejaculation, profuse urination, blurred vision, backache. Treatments: tinnitus, spermatorrhoea, lumbago, leucorrhoea, kidney-yang deficiency. Assists labour contractions in childbirth. Dosage: 10–14 g.

camomile *Matricaria chamomilla* Herbal medicine. Distribution: Europe, Asia, North America. Parts: flowers, leaves. Character: warm, bitter. Affinity: stomach, spleen. Effects: stomachic, antipyretic, antiphlogistic, sedative. Symptoms: indigestion, fever, headaches, insomnia. Treatments: dysmenorrhoea, tension, menopausal conditions, catarrh, skin complaints. Very effective in reducing allergies. Dosage: 1–4 g.

cancer A malignant growth, or tumour, which is one that is likely to spread, as opposed to a benign tumour, which does not spread and generally does no harm unless it happens to be inconveniently positioned, so interfering with the function of an organ. A cancer may be a carcinoma, which is one that occurs in the epithelia, that is, the skin and membranes, such as those of the intestinal tract, or it may be a sarcoma, which is one that occurs in bone, muscle and other connective tissue. Cancer is a condition which is more easily prevented than cured, and for this purpose, the Chinese have a wide range of preventive medicines and health foods, including garlic, red-tea fungus, mandarin orange, Chinese wolfberry, Chinese angelica and Chinese yam, most of which do no more than strengthen the body's immune system. Chinese physicians consider that the immune system, or what they would regard as a sufficiency of pure- or protective-*qi*, is strengthened by acupuncture and acupressure, which reduce stress, anxiety and debility, conditions that exacerbate any deficiencies in the immune system. They also consider that a sound diet, exercise, moderate habits and natural living can do much to prevent cancer, just as an unsound diet, sedentary habits and unnatural living can be causative of cancer. In this connection, it is interesting to note that in countries such as Italy, Spain and the south of China, where garlic, olive oil or cereal oil, fresh fruits and vegetables, fish and cereals feature prominently in the diet, there is a lower incidence of cancer than elsewhere. But, no doubt, other factors are involved in this state of affairs. The Italians and the Spanish have an abundance of sunshine, drink a great deal of coffee, and do not have an overwhelming weakness for dairy products; and the Chinese, being a Mongoloid race, are possessed of an inherent stamina. On the other hand, some Italians, Spaniards and Chinese do succumb to cancer, and so the role played by diet in its prevention is, to some extent, a matter of conjecture. There are many theories about the causes of cancer, but the contention that it is a lawless, and perhaps non-genetic, growth of cells, brought about by unnatural, and generally man-made, influences does seem to be an adequate explanation. There is certainly no shortage of unnatural influences, which include chemical and mechanical irritants and radioactivity: damaging drugs, certain contraceptive devices and sex stimulants, synthetic additives in food, alcohol, tobacco, pesticides, fertilizers, fumes from motor-car exhausts, pollutants from industrial processes, over-use of detergents, and so on. Knowing, as we do, what a microwave oven will do to an item of food, we may wonder just how much damage is being done to human-body cells by the high frequency radiations from the electronic devices with which we are surrounded, and by which we are being constantly bombarded. It would seem that cancer is a by-product of modern civilization, and that tobacco has been selected to be the scapegoat, which is rather surprising since motor-car exhausts probably constitute one of the gravest menaces to the health of urban man. Exhaust fumes, together with industrial waste, contain carbonaceous substances, and many of these are suspected of causing cancer. See **carbon** and **free radical**. In the West, the usual treatments for cancer are surgery, chemotherapy and radiotherapy, but these are generally more alleviative than curative. With Chinese physicians, the emphasis is on prevention and the kind of healthy life-style which does not invite disaster; and their well-founded opinions in this regard are supported by the simple fact that there is a low incidence of cancer in China. It is important to note that the person who has a cancer, or merely suspects that he has a cancer, would be indeed foolish to pin his faith on traditional or preventive remedies, for they are usually of little avail once a cancer has become established. To quote from *Huang Di Nei Jing*, 'The Internal Book of Huang Di': 'To administer medicines for illnesses which have already developed is akin to the conduct of a man who begins to dig a well after he has become thirsty.' Medical advice must be sought immediately, for a cure can often be effected if the disease is caught in its earliest stages. See **ban zi lian** and **fungi**.

Candida albicans Monilia. Yeast. Its excessive reproduction in the intestinal tract, where it is normally present, causes an infection of the large intestine, vagina or mouth, which is known medically as *candidiasis*, and more commonly as thrush. Its symptoms include diarrhoea, flatulence, headaches and migraine. It may be caused by a sugary diet, on which it feeds, or by antibiotics or other drugs which interfere with the normal balance of the micro-organisms in the intestine. In the West, the usual treatment is a sugar-free diet. But this cannot be applied to the Chinese, for the Chinese diet is virtually sugar-free. Chinese physicians would recommend tonic medicines to counteract the lowering of vitality which is often associated with this condition. For a vaginal infection, a douche of a solution of 40 ml vinegar in 1 litre water is usually effective. Fresh garlic, consumed regularly, helps to prevent this condition. See **thrush**.

cantharides See **aphrodisiac**.

capillary One of the smallest blood-vessels, which form a network between arteries and veins, so ensuring that the tissues receive oxygen and nutrients, and waste matter is removed.

caraway *Carum carvi* Herbal medicine. Distribution: Europe,

Central Asia, North America. Parts: seeds. Character: warm, sweet. Affinity: lungs, stomach, liver. Effects: expectorant, carminative, antispasmodic. Symptoms: flatulence, chestiness, bad breath. Treatments: colds, congestion, bronchitis, indigestion, colic, hysterics. Dosage: 1–2 g. A decoction may be used as a mouthwash and gargle to sweeten the breath and soothe a sore throat, and the seeds may also be chewed as a remedy for flatulence and bad breath. A poultice of the crushed seeds may be applied to relieve earache, a sprain or a painful bruise. An infusion drunk as a tea will increase lactation. The roots serve the same purpose if cooked and eaten as a vegetable.

CARAWAY

Carum carvi

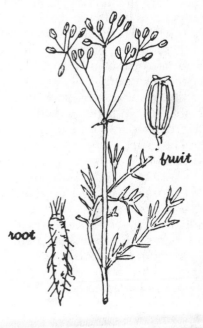

fruit

root

carbohydrate One of a group of carbon compounds which includes sugars, starches and cellulose. Sugars and starches are a source of energy, and cellulose is the main constituent of the walls of plant cells. See **food** and **cellulose**.

carbon An element which, together with hydrogen, is contained in all organic substances, which are those of plant or animal origin. Carbon is quadrivalent, or tetravalent, which means that it has a valency of four, and so an atom of carbon is able to combine with or displace one, two, three or four atoms of another element. Thus, carbon is able to form a large number of compounds, and chemists have succeeded in synthesizing many carbon compounds which do not occur in nature. These have many useful applications, and some are used in medicines. Unfortunately, the readiness of carbon to unite with other substances could be one of the causes of changes in the nuclei of animal cells, which, in turn, could lead to a lawless growth of cells, and so give rise to a cancerous condition. It could also be a cause of ageing. Carbon is a fundamental constituent of all living matter, and when oxidized, it is a source of energy, which could be the 'primordial vital energy' that Chinese physicians designated as *qi*. See **free radical** and **qi**.

carbon compounds Some carbon compounds, such as sugars and starches, are of natural origin, but many, such as those contained in plastics and synthetic dyes, flavourings and medicines, are man made. Many of the carbon compounds, particularly those that are synthetic, which are listed in a chemical supplier's catalogue are marked with an asterisk to indicate that they should be treated with caution because they could be carcinogens. This is one of several reasons why, in general, herbal medicines are preferable to synthetic medicines. It is alarming to think that coal-tar derivatives were once freely used, with little or no medical research, in antiseptics and medicines. See **carbon**.

carbon dioxide A colourless, odourless gas which, chemically, is fairly unreactive, and which constitutes less than 1 per cent of air. When fuels and other organic compounds burn, the carbon they contain combines with the oxygen in air to form carbon dioxide and produce heat energy. In respiration, the carbon in the nutrients in the tissues combines with oxygen from the bloodstream to form carbon dioxide, together with the production of energy. This carbon dioxide is eliminated from the body, via the lungs, as a waste product. In the presence of sunlight, by a

PHOTOSYNTHESIS

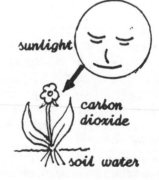

carbon dioxide + water
= sugar + oxygen

$$6CO_2 + 6H_2O$$
$$= C_6H_{12}O_6 + 6O_2$$

sunlight

carbon dioxide

soil water

process called photosynthesis, green plants synthesize sugars and starches from carbon dioxide and water. Some of the energy of sunlight is stored in the sugars and starches, and oxygen is evolved. This oxygen will be respired in animal tissues. Thus, the waste products of animals become the food of plants, and plants become the food of animals. This is a good example of the balance of nature, and shows that nature, by 'biological recycling', allows nothing to go to waste. This reinforces the traditional Chinese view that vital energy, which they call *qi*, is contained in plants, animals and the atmosphere. The inter-dependence of plants and animals clearly indicates that Chinese physicians have never been unreasonable in thinking that plants contain substances which can be beneficial to the health of man. See **air** and **qi**.

carbon monoxide A colourless, odourless gas produced by the incomplete combustion of carbon compounds. It is said to be extremely toxic, though its effect on the human body is more in the nature of tissue suffocation than poison. It combines with haemoglobin, which it does about 250 times more readily than oxygen, to form carboxyhaemoglobin, so the haemoglobin is no longer able to take up oxygen. Thus, the tissues become starved of oxygen, and death soon follows. Carbon monoxide is present in the exhaust gases of petrol and diesel engines. However, there are few motor cars in China. The Chinese have a preference for bicycles, both as a system of transport and a means of taking exercise. This makes a great deal of sense.

carbuncle A severe abscess due to the spreading of a boil. See **furuncle**.

carcinogen A substance which causes cancer. See **carbon**.

carcinoma See **cancer**.

cardamon *Elettaria cardamomum* Herbal medicine. Distribution: South China, India, Thailand, Vietnam, Sri Lanka. Parts: seeds. Character: warm, pungent. Affinity: heart, stomach. Effects: digestive, carminative, stimulant to the circulation. Symptoms: dyspepsia, flatulence. Treatments: cold-excess conditions, constipation, colic. Dosage: 1.5–6 g.

cardiac Of the heart.

cardiac asthma A severe congestion of the lungs due to acute heart failure. It has no relationship to bronchial asthma. See **asthma**.

cardiogram A chart on which heart movements are recorded, and which is obtained with an instrument called a cardiograph.

cardiology The study of the heart and its defects and diseases.

cardiotonic A medicine to stimulate the heart. Cardiotonics commonly used in TCM include: wheat, *triticum aestivum*; Chinese jujube, *Ziziphus jujuba*; aconite, *Aconitum carmichaeli*; musk, *Moschus moschiferus*; and pig's gall-bladder.

care with medicines See **medicines, Medicines Act 1968** and **dangers with medicines**.

caries Decay, particularly of the bones and teeth.

carminative A medicine to relieve flatulence by expelling gas from the stomach and intestines. See **flatulence**.

carotene See **carrot**.

carrier A person who carries infectious micro-organisms in his body with no harm to himself but which he unwittingly passes on to people who will succumb to them. The carrier of a disease is a far greater menace to the health of the community than the person who has succumbed to the disease, for the former is unaware of his condition, and so he will infect many, whereas the latter, being under treatment, will be isolated from the rest of the community. A carrier is generally a strong and healthy person whose immune system is operating efficiently, so preventing the infection from taking its toll. This bears out the validity of the opinion of Chinese physicians that, if one takes good care of one's general health, and the vital organs especially, one should be able to throw off most infections, and so one will have no need of specific remedies for particular diseases.

carrot This vegetable has a prominent place in the Chinese diet, and it is generally added to soups, stews and tonic medicinal broths as well as being consumed in salads. In scientific terms, the explanation for the popularity of the carrot as a dietary item is that carrots, along with dark-green leafy vegetables, apricots and pumpkins, are a good source of carotene, which exists in several forms, alpha-, beta- and gamma-, and which is converted by the body into retinol, or vitamin A. Reninol is needed for growth and healthy skin and mucous membranes. It is also essential for distinguishing colours and to good vision at night.

cartilage Gristle. A white fibrous tissue which provides smooth surfaces in joints and at the ends of bones, and cushion-like pads, called intervertebral discs, between the bones in the vertebral column. Cartilage is a low-grade protein and a source of gelatin.

cassia *Cinnamomum cassia* Also called Chinese cinnamon. Herbal medicine. Distribution: South China, Vietnam, Laos. Parts: young stems. Character: warm, pungent-sweet. Affinity: heart, bladder, lungs. Effects: carminative, diaphoretic, antiseptic, emmenagogue. Symptoms: chills, fever, diarrhoea, nausea. Treatments: colds, menstrual disorders. Dosage: 2–5 g. Parts:

unscraped bark. Character: hot, sweet, pungent. Affinity: liver, spleen, kidneys. Effects: stimulant, analgesic. Symptoms: coldness, especially of hands and feet, loss of appetite, diarrhoea, tiredness. Treatments: yang-deficiency in kidneys and spleen, debility, poor blood, anaemia, dysmenorrhoea. Dosage: 2–5 g.

casual sex See **sex**.

catabolism See **metabolism**.

catalepsy Sleep-like hypnotic state in which the body becomes rigid and immobile. The cause is emotional – extreme fear, extreme ecstasy, etc. A rare condition, perhaps partly due to hereditary factors, for which Chinese physicians would recommend acupuncture and massage. Tonic medicines, such as ginseng, royal jelly and Chinese wolfberry, might be helpful.

catalyst A substance which is involved in a chemical reaction, inducing it to proceed more quickly or at a lower temperature but which, in itself, remains unchanged at the end of the reaction. See **enzyme**.

cataract A condition in which the whole or a part of the lens of an eye becomes opaque, so impairing vision. Chinese physicians regard this condition as being due to weakness of the liver and kidneys and lack of nourishment for the blood. The development of the cataract may be slowed down or even arrested by infusions of the following taken internally, using the parts in the dosages indicated: Chrysanthemum, *Chrysanthemum morifolium*, flowers, 5–10 g; Chinese wolfberry, *Lycium chinense*, fruits, 5–10 g; abalone, *Haliotis gigantea*, powdered shell, 15–30 g; cicada, *Cryptotympana pustulata*, exuviae, 2–5 g. Abalone is considered to be particularly effective, but the powdered shell should be stirred in water to make a suspension. A solution, though recommended in Chinese herbals, would be of an ineffective potency. The infusion of cicada exuviae, or moultings, would be more effective if mixed with that of chrysanthemum flowers. *Chrysanthemum morifolium*, the species of chrysanthemum indicated here, is indigenous only to China, and so may not be readily available in the West, but other species which have similar medicinal properties are available in the West.

catarrh Inflammation of a mucous membrane with an excessive discharge of mucus, although the term is commonly and more specifically applied to inflammation of the nose, nasal sinuses, throat and bronchial tubes. Nasal catarrh is referred to as rhinitis, and that of the sinuses as sinusitis. Catarrh in the nose, nasal sinuses, throat or bronchial tubes is caused or aggravated by a cold or some other infection, smoke and other airborne irritants, alcohol, confectionery, starchy food and milk products. Needless to say, one should try to avoid those things which aggravate the condition. Relief may be provided by expectorants, and also by mild sedatives where there is distress. The usual treatments in TCM are infusions of the following, using the parts and dosages indicated, taken internally, and to be sipped slowly: coltsfoot, *Tussilago farfara*, flowers and floral buds, 3–10 g; honeysuckle, *Lonicera japonica*, leaves and flowers, 10–16 g; fennel, *Foeniculum vulgare*, fruits and leaves, 1–2 g; magnolia, *Magnolia liliflora*, floral buds, 4–8 g; angelica, *Angelica anomala*, roots, 3–7 g. As a treatment for catarrh of the nasal sinuses, the Chinese would favour a hot and spicy stew of lean meat, vegetables, barley, dried orange peel, coriander and pepper. The immune system will be strengthened by including eggs, liver, lean pork, fish, shellfish, wholegrain cereals, nuts, beans and peas in the diet.

caterpillar fungus *Cordyceps sinensis*. This is a plant, not an animal. It owes its animal-like name to the fact that it begins its life by growing parasitically in the body of a caterpillar. It is a tonic food held in high esteem in China. It is steamed or boiled with meat, and has an extremely appetizing flavour. It is sedative and soporific, a remedy for deteriorating eyesight and memory, and strengthening for those in a poor state of health.

cathartic A medicine which induces a positive evacuation from the bowel. Those of gentle action are called aperients, those of medium strength are called laxatives, and those of powerful action are called purgatives. See **aperient**, **laxative** and **purgative**.

cathartic treatment This is one of the eight methods of herbal treatment in TCM. Its purpose is to lubricate the small intestine and encourage the formation of loose, hot stools, which will bring out the accumulated heat. Purgatives are suitable for patients who are young and strong. Laxatives, which are not so strong, are suitable for weak and elderly persons with a chronic illness. See **cathartic**.

catmint *Nepeta cataria* Also called catnep or catnip. There are many species of mints, and most have similar medicinal properties. But Chinese physicians seem to have a preference for field mint, *Mentha arvensis*, which is also called corn mint in the West. See **mint**.

catnep, catnip See **catmint**.

cat's tail See **reedmace**.

cause and effect There is a difference between Western and

Chinese conceptions of cause and effect. Acceptance of predestination is a feature of Chinese philosophy, in contrast to the Western notion of free will, or self-determination. According to the Chinese conception of predestination, the decisions that a person takes are conditioned by a host of factors indiscernible to the individual, including past experience, emotional characteristics and environmental factors. When a person makes a decision he is confronted with a set of alternatives of which only one is possible, and that is not the end-product but only a stage in many long series of events which have been in progress since the beginning of time. In this sense they have been preordained. Although the outcome of a series of events may be unforeseen by the individual, it is still a certainty. This important philosophical difference has a bearing on medical practice. Western medicine, at least until recently, emphasised curative techniques on the implicit assumption that these can alter the course of events. Chinese medicine, on the other hand, is mainly preventive, and aims to anticipate destiny and take action before it is too late. See **AIDS, causes of illness** and **universe**.

causes of illness Of the various differences between Western medicine and TCM, one of the most revealing is the attitude towards the causes of illness. The physicians of the West will say, quite categorically, that pneumonia is caused by a bacterium, dysentery is caused by a type of amoeba, ringworm is caused by a fungus, influenza by a virus, and so on. But Chinese physicians will say that the body is largely self-healing and self-regulating, and that the cause of illness is the inability of the body, and the vital organs in particular, to cope with the malign influences which enter the body. Similarly, Western physicians will say that a fracture is due to an excessive force being exerted on a bone. But Chinese physicians will say that it is due to a bone being too weak to resist a strong force. These two different points of view show a difference of emphasis. In Western medicine, it is on the curative, with a specific cause requiring a specific treatment. In TCM, the emphasis is on the preventive, with medicines of a less specialized nature but which will stimulate or tone the vital organs. This explains why a Chinese pharmacopoeia includes many tonic medicines, and they will be described as being a yang tonic (for yang conditions), a tonic for kidney-*qi*, a tonic for liver-*qi*, and so on. To accurately prescribe a medicine for the treatment of a particular organ requires accurate diagnosis, but Chinese physicians are very adept in diagnosis. It is important that symptoms should not be confused with the causes of illness. Causes must not be mistaken for effects and vice versa. The Chinese physician trained in both Western medicine and TCM will adopt both approaches, and he will play for safety by eradicating the micro-organisms which have entered the body, and by toning the organs which have been affected by the invaders. He will both cure the condition and take steps to prevent its recurrence. See **cause and effect**.

celery *Apium graveolens* Herbal medicine. Distribution: warm and temperate regions of the Northern Hemisphere. Part: seeds. Character: cool, salty. Affinity: kidneys, stomach. Effects: sedative, refrigerant, diuretic, urinary antiseptic, digestive, carminative, galactogogue. Symptoms: flatulence, arthritic conditions. Treatments: arthritis, gout, hypertension, calculi, urinary infections. Dosage: 3–9 g. This medicine must NOT be taken during pregnancy.

celibacy See **sex**.

cell The cell, which is of microscopic size, is the basic component of all plants and animals, and the smallest unit capable of life. See **virus**. The higher organisms consist of millions of cells which are interdependent in their functions, whereas the simplest organisms, such as bacteria and the amoeba, are single cells and can lead a separate existence. Plant and animal cells have the same basic functions: they respire, assimilate nutrients, expel waste, grow and reproduce themselves by binary fission, that is, by splitting into two. But there are some important differences between them. An animal cell has a thin cell-wall, whereas a plant cell has a thick cell-wall that is made of a dead substance called cellulose. Unlike an animal cell, a plant cell has a large space, called a vacuole, containing sap. A plant cell also has chloroplasts containing chlorophyll, which is a green pigment that, in the presence of sunlight, enables it to manufacture sugars and starches from carbon dioxide and water. An animal cell contains no chlorophyll and feeds on organic food. The similarity of all cells in both structure and function and the gradual increase in complexity from the simplest unicellular organisms to the highest mammals and flowering plants suggests that all living things have a common ancestry, perhaps in a virus-like organism which, by some freak of chemistry, developed within the murkiness of primeval slime. No explanation other than the theory of evolution could account for this state of affairs. See **evolution**. It is humbling to realize that man is distantly related to all the other living things. A cell has a nucleus, which could be regarded as a primitive nervous system that controls its

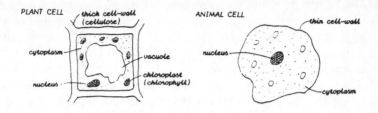

functions. The nucleus also controls its destiny, for the genes within the nucleus, which has been described as a 'genetic blueprint', ensure that the inherited characteristics of the cell are transmitted to the next generation of cells; and, in theory, this process should carry on indefinitely, the characteristics being passed on from generation to generation. But, occasionally, things go awry, and changes in the genes, called mutations, occur, so producing a different set of heritable characteristics. It is more than likely that it is the damage done to the genes by radiation or mechanical or chemical irritants which causes the patternless and unhealthy growth of cells that we describe as cancer. See **cancer**. It is hardly likely that the physicians and philosophers of ancient China were aware of the cell structure of plants and animals. Nor is it likely that they had any clear-cut ideas about the evolution of man. Some of the Chinese emperors regarded themselves as demigods, and the peasants, like their counterparts in the West, had some curious notions about the origin of mankind. The popular view was that the human body is a miniature version of the universe. See **universe**. However, belief in the existence of *qi*, or 'vital energy', which can be transmitted along meridians on the surface of the body, indicates that the sages of ancient China were aware that the body tissues consist of energy-seeking and energy-giving material, and that the energy processes of the body are not confined to the muscles and vital organs. Also, they knew that some illnesses could be treated without medicine by regulating the bodily functions by means of diet and exercises, just as we, in the West, are beginning to realize that some illnesses could be eradicated by genetic control, that is, by manipulating the genes. It is certain that the educated Chinese have never had any illusions about the quality of man. The Taoists perceive man as a child of nature, whose future will largely depend on the manner in which he co-operates with the natural forces around him. In the Taoist view, much illness and misery is due to man's precocious rebellion against nature. See **genetics**.

cell nutrition It could be said that the term *nutrition* would be more accurately defined as cell nutrition, for the cells are the basic units of the body, and each type of cell has its own particular nutritive requirements, and it is only by satisfying the particular nutritive requirements of each and every cell of the body that one can satisfy the nutritive requirements of the body as a whole. For example, the cells of bones have a special need of calcium, and the erythrocytes, or red blood cells, have a special need of iron. However, Chinese physicians trained in TCM will not think in terms of minerals and vitamins, but will be inclined to think in terms of medicines and health foods that will stimulate, tone or nutrify specific organs, and which will be variously described as 'stimulating of the heart', 'toning of the kidneys', 'nutrifying of the liver', and so forth. Fortunately for the Chinese, their diet is so correctly balanced and varied that they have no great need of mineral and vitamin supplements. See **mineral** and **vitamin**.

cellular tissue A connective tissue of loose texture, particularly that beneath the skin.

cellulite Unsightly pockets of fat protruding from the cellular tissue beneath the skin. It is best treated by adopting a diet that contains no dairy products, fatty meat and refined sugar, and by regular exercise and deep breathing to provide oxygen, which will oxidize, and so reduce, the unwanted fat.

cellulitis Inflammation of the cellular tissue. Treatments: a fat-free diet, exercise and deep breathing, as for cellulite; external application of an infusion of sage, *Salvia officinalis*, leaves in a dosage of 2–8 g, or ginger, *Zingiber officinale*, root in a dosage of 2–4 g. These infusions must NOT be taken orally.

cellulose A complex carbohydrate, called a polysaccharide, which plants manufacture from glucose, and which strengthens their cell-walls. It is a source of dietary fibre, but it cannot be broken down by digestive juices. However, it is decomposed into assimilable forms by fermentation in the caecum of a rabbit or a similar animal.

Celsius The official temperature scale, also called centigrade, abbreviated as C, on which water freezes at 0° and boils at 100° under normal conditions of pressure. *Celsius*, not *centigrade*, is the more acceptable term. See **temperature**.

centigrade See **Celsius**.

centipede *Scolopendra subspinipes* Medicine. Distribution: global. Parts: whole animal. Character: warm, pungent. Affinity: liver. Effects: sedative to liver, antitoxic, antispasmodic. Symptoms:

fright, traumatic shock, abscesses. Treatments: tetanus and other serious infections, snake bites, cancer. Poisonous, and so it must not be taken during pregnancy or without medical supervision.

central nervous system The brain and spinal cord.

centre See **direction**.

cereal One of the various species of grass with edible seeds, including wheat, oat, barley, rye, maize, rice and millet. They are staple foods in all parts of the world, and are good sources of starch, sugar, protein, dietary fibre, minerals and vitamins. Wheat, barley and maize have mild medicinal properties. A diet high in cereal, such as the Chinese diet, is healthy.

cerebellum See **brain**.

cerebral haemorrhage See **stroke**.

cerebral palsy See **spastic**.

cerebro-spinal fever See **meningitis**.

cerebrum See **brain**.

cervical Of the neck, as in 'cervical vertebrae', or of the cervix, which is the narrow entrance to the womb.

cervical cancer This condition can be successfully treated if caught in time. The test for this condition is carried out using a smear, and the usual treatment in the initial stages is radiotherapy. But with cervical cancer, as with other forms of cancer, preventive methods, when people bother to apply them, are generally more effective than curative methods, as Chinese physicians well know. There are several possible causes of cervical cancer, including friction. See **cancer** and **sex**.

cervical mucus The purpose of this sticky fluid, secreted around the cervix, is to prevent infective micro-organisms from entering the womb. But it sometimes acts as a barrier to the spermatozoa, which is one of the rarer causes of infertility in women.

cervix See **cervical**.

Ceylon cinnamon See **cinnamon**.

cha See **tea**.

Cha Ching Also written as *Cha Jing*, 'Book of Tea'. This classical treatise, written in AD 780 by Lu Yu, enthuses about the refreshing and medicinal properties of tea. He comments: 'Tea improves the spirit, and soothes and balances the mind. It stimulates thought and disposes of lethargy, elevates and invigorates the body and clarifies perception.'

chafing See **cuts**.

Cha Jing See **Cha Ching**.

chancre See **venereal disease**.

chancroid See **venereal disease**.

chang The Chinese name for wines fermented directly from medicinal herbs. See **medicinal wine**.

change of life See **menopause**.

Chang San-feng According to Chinese legend, the gentle sport of *tai chi chuan* owes its existence to Chang San-feng, an eleventh-century philosopher, who was so concerned about the violent and aggressive nature of the martial arts that he sought a gentler form which would aid meditation and develop spiritual values.

channel One of the bodily channels along which *qi*, or 'vital energy', flows. See **meridian**.

Ch'ao Yuen Fan See **diabetes mellitus**.

character of herbs See **medicinal properties of herbs**.

cheese Some medicines, both herbal and synthetic, cannot be safely consumed with cheese. But a warning to this effect is usually displayed on the containers in which such medicines are purchased.

chemicals In the West, chemicals are widely used as ingredients in detergents, cosmetics, toiletries, pesticides and fertilizers. They are often injurious in so far as they are irritants, and so cause rashes, eye and nose irritations, allergies and throat and breathing problems. Some hair dyes, for example, are suspected of causing dermatitis and skin cancer. Some insecticides are poisonous if inhaled, and the sniffing of glue or solvents can become a dangerous addiction. There is a tendency for people to use cleaning agents which do more harm than the micro-organisms they are intended to eradicate. One should be wary of washing and scouring powders, bleaches, polishes, air-fresheners, cosmetics, soaps and other toiletries, insecticides, fungicides, glue, wood preservatives, varnishes, paints, paint strippers, fillers, sealants and weedkillers. One should employ those 'green' products which are now available at most supermarkets and stores. Of course, the use of chemicals for the purposes described above would be sheer anathema to the Chinese, who have a preference for natural products, and would opt for a little 'clean dirt' rather than dangerous chemicals.

chemistry The physicians of ancient China had some considerable knowledge of chemistry. They were using sulphur, iodine, mercury and gold as medicinal ingredients, but not always to good effect. They understood the principles of fermentation, and were using alcohol as a solvent and in making tinctures. And, many centuries later, both the Chinese alchemists and their Arab counterparts made important discoveries which helped to lay the foundations of modern chemistry. See **alchemy**. But modern chemistry has proved to be a bane as well as a boon, for it is the irresponsible use of chemicals which is the main cause of pollution of the environment. Maybe the greatest blessing of chemistry is our knowledge of biochemistry, wherein lies a fuller understanding of the structures and functions of plants and animals, and which has led to improvements in the applications of the healing arts. Most assuredly, it is chemistry which holds the secret of life.

chemotherapy This is the branch of Western medical science that is concerned with the treatment of illnesses by means of drugs, which are generally synthetic. Some of these drugs are drastic in their effects, but it must be admitted that desperate situations usually call for desperate remedies, for there are sometimes no alternatives. Be that as it may, Chinese physicians practising within the established framework of TCM will prefer to administer herbal medicines, whose actions are much less powerful and without unpleasant side-effects, but quite effective if taken over a long period. See **active ingredient**.

chen chiu The Chinese name for moxibustion, which is a form of acupuncture in which heat is applied. See **moxibustion**.

chervil *Anthricus cerefolium* Herbal medicine. Distribution: Europe and Western Asia. Parts: leaves. Character: warm, sweet-pungent. Affinity: kidneys, liver. Effects: diaphoretic, antipyretic, diuretic, stomachic. Symptoms: fever, indigestion, lack of appetite. Treatments: skin blemishes, jaundice, gout, bruises, swellings, blood clots. Chervil is used as a seasoning and in soups, which settle an upset stomach and improve the appetite. Dosage: 6–10 g.

chi See **qi**.

ch'iang chuang kung A system of invigorative breathing exercises which is less demanding than some of the other forms. It is a treatment for hypertension, heart diseases, anxiety, depression and emphysema. One may perform these exercises in sitting comfortably on a chair. Details of these exercises are to be found in the *Chinese Exercise Manual*.

Chiao Yi-tang See **Chinese Doctors' Day**.

chicken *Gallus gallus domesticus* Medicine. Distribution: global. Parts: gizzard. Character: neutral, sweet. Affinity: stomach, intestines, spleen, bladder. Effects: stomachic, digestive. Symptoms: fullness of stomach and abdomen, nausea, vomiting. Treatments: accumulation of undigested and unassimilated food, gastro-enteritis, urinary incontinence, spermatorrhoea. Dosage: 5–8 g.

chicken-pox See **varicella**.

chicken's feet A popular dietary item in China, and a good source of interferon. See **connective tissue**.

chicken soup A person who has a cold or influenza is advised to take plenty of liquid in order to offset dehydration and eliminate toxic waste. The Chinese regard chicken soup as being one of the best liquids for this purpose because it is nutritious and easily digested.

chickweed *Stellaria media* Also called starweed. All parts of this herb may be applied externally as a compress to relieve inflamed, eruptive and itchy skin conditions.

chi kung See **qi gong**.

chilblains A condition in which excessive coldness causes severe constriction of the blood vessels in the extremities, that is, the feet, hands, nose and ears, and which is characterized by swelling, redness, itching and burning sensations. It affects women more than men, and is partly due to poor circulation. It is not unlike frost-bite, though it is much milder. It is helpful to wear woollen socks and gloves and to avoid sitting or working in low-temperature conditions. Chinese physicians regard chilblains as a condition due to yang-*qi* deficiency. For the circulation, they would recommend infusions of the following herbs, using the parts and dosages indicated, and taken internally: ginger, *Zingiber officinale*, rhizome, 4–8 g; cassia *Cinnamomum cassia*, unscraped bark, 2–5 g; angelica, *Angelica sinensis*, roots, 8–14 g; red sage, *Salvia miltiorrhiza*, roots, 4–6 g. But, for people who live in the West, an effective and readily available treatment is an infusion of 3–12 g of the flowers of marigold, *Calendula officinalis*, to be taken internally.

childbirth Acupuncture is effective in assisting labour contractions and reducing labour pains. An infusion of the mature fruits of caltrop, *Tribulus terrestris*, taken internally also assists labour contractions, and the appropriate herbs can be used to arrest bleeding. See **haemorrhage**. One should note that, in the United Kingdom, it is illegal for a person other than a registered nurse or certified midwife to attend a childbirth without proper medical supervision. However, there have been many cases where women have safely entered into labour or given birth without assistance from people other than medical experts. After all, childbirth is a natural process, as Chinese physicians would readily declare. Hasty elimination of the placenta and stimulation of involution may be effected by an infusion of the leaves of the raspberry, *Rubus idaeus*, taken internally in a dosage of 6–20 g.

Postnatal abdominal pain may be alleviated by an infusion of the fruits of the hawthorn, *Crataegus pinnatifida*, taken internally in a dosage of 5–15 g. This species of hawthorn is indigenous to East China and Japan, but there are many species native to Europe which have similar medicinal properties.

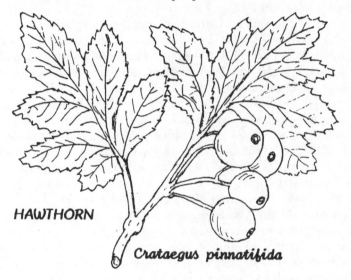

HAWTHORN

Crataegus pinnatifida

childhood The Chinese liken a child to a bush which needs to be pruned occasionally if it is to grow in the right direction and without ugliness. Chinese families are close-knit, being held together by strong ties of loyalty and affection, but the Chinese would contend that, even so, one does not demonstrate true love for children by allowing them to develop precociously, selfishly and totally without restraint, for that is not freedom but licence. Children are the most recent stage in a long lineage, and if its worthiness is to be maintained, they must be disciplined so that they will develop in a way that is not self-destructive but beneficial both to themselves and to society as a whole. For the Chinese, childhood is a period of inspired learning, when a healthy outlook and healthy habits are acquired, and which will ensure a long and healthy life of youthful vigour, together with the self-satisfaction and other rewards which derive from moral responsibility and communal harmony. The Chinese teach their children by precept and example. Every day, in the early morning, in the cities and towns throughout China, the parks and other open spaces are thronged with people, including the

131

elderly and the very young. They will be doing the invigorative and relaxing exercises of the *tai chi chuan* and some of the other gentler forms of kungfu, and so maintaining themselves in a sound state of health. These exercises have meditative aspects, and so the children will develop mentally as well as physically, and with self-discipline and self-respect.

chill A sudden lowering of the body temperature which is often accompanied by feverishness. The usual Chinese home remedy is equal parts of ginger and spring onion boiled together, with a little honey or brown sugar added, and drunk as a tea. An infusion of chillies, *Capsicum frutescens*, dried or whole, taken internally is also a popular treatment. See **chills and fever**.

chilli *Capsicum frutescens* This spice is indigenous to Mexico, but it is now cultivated in most of the spice-producing countries, and is used throughout the world as a flavouring for sauces and a garnish for various dishes. Chillies stimulate the appetite and have a warming effect, and so they are of some medicinal value.

chills and fever Taken together, chills and fever are symptoms which provide the Chinese physician with information which will assist him in making an accurate diagnosis of a patient's condition. A chill without fever indicates a yang-deficiency, and fever without a chill indicates an excess of yang-energy. Fever and thirst without a chill indicate an internal ailment, and spasmodic alternations of chills and fever generally indicate an ailment which is affecting both the internal and the external organs.

Chinese Almanac This remarkable work, which is revised and reissued each year, is probably the oldest continuous publication in the world, dating from about 2200 BC. The original was compiled by the best of China's astrologers and philosophers, and on the command of Emperor Yao. In Taiwan, it is called the 'Farmers' Almanac', and in Hong Kong, it is called *Tong Sing*, which means 'Know Everything Book'. It is crammed with information about astrology, the festivals, traditional beliefs, and so forth. Although the Chinese officially use the Western-style calendar, which is based on solar movements, they still use the lunar calendar for astrology and agricultural purposes, for the times for sowing and harvesting are better decided by the influences of the moon than those of the sun. The lunar year begins on a variable day which, in the Western calendar, is in late January or early February. The Chinese Almanac is essentially folklorish in content, but beneath the myths and traditional beliefs, there is a great deal of common-sense thinking, as there is with all Chinese beliefs, and the information given in regard to agricultural arrangements, health and suchlike is quite reliable. There are sections on the interpretation of dreams, feast days, baby care, love-making, diet, cookery recipes, wine-making, herbal medicines, palm-reading, physiognomy, numerology, the teachings of Taoism and Confucianism, proverbs, horoscopes and divination generally. Divination in China is not a bit of superstition, for the predictions are not based on blind guesswork as is often the case of the West, but on known facts, intelligent observations and logical inferences, and they are sometimes more in the nature of those proverbs which are universal truths and snippets of profound wisdom. The needs of the modern world are not overlooked, and there are sections on postal information, official statistics, etc.

Chinese anemone *Pulsatilla chinensis* Closely related to the pasque flower, *Pulsatilla vulgaris*. Herbal medicine. Distribution: North China, Korea, Japan. Parts: roots. Character: cold, bitter. Affinity: stomach, large intestine. Effects: antipyretic, antitoxic, antidysenteric. Symptoms: severe diarrhoea. Treatment: amoebic dysentery. Dosage: 6–10 g. This herb is considered to be one of the most effective for the treatment of amoebic dysentery.

Chinese angelica See **angelica**.

Chinese cinnamon See **cassia**.

Chinese diet See **diet**.

Chinese Doctors' Day After the establishment of the Republic of China, in 1911, Western medicine was introduced into China, and soon began to act in opposition to TCM. However, in 1929, a meeting of physicians from all parts of China was held in Shanghai; and, on 17 March, its elected delegation petitioned the Nationalist government in Nanjing to support TCM. The petition was successful; and, as a happy outcome, 17 March has since been celebrated as Chinese Doctors' Day. The TCM physicians consolidated their victory four years later, when the Central Chinese Hospital was opened in Nanjing, and Chiao Yi-tang, a chief justice of the Supreme Court, was appointed to oversee the promotion and systemization of TCM.

Chinese Exercise Manual This is an official publication issued by the Chinese government to provide a complete guide to those physical and breathing exercises which may be used to promote health and prevent or treat a wide variety of ailments. It is remarkable in that it shows how so many ailments, some serious and some chronic, can be effectively treated without recourse to medicines, herbal or otherwise. See **Tsa Fu Pei**.

Chinese gentian *Gentiana scabra* Herbal medicine. Distribution: China. Parts: roots. Character: cold, bitter. Affinity: liver, gallbladder. Effects: antipyretic, astringent, stomachic. Symptoms: headaches, sore eyes, pains in chest, swollen and painful scrotum, dark leucorrhoea. Treatments: damp-heat ailments, jaundice. Dosage: 4–8 g. Taken before meals, this medicine promotes digestion; taken after, it impedes digestion.

Chinese history China could claim to have the oldest civilization in the world, and archaeological finds have indicated that its long history began more than 7000 years ago in the fertile valleys of the Huanghe, or 'Yellow River'. But little is known about its early history, for most of the written records were destroyed when the first emperor, Qin Shi Huang Di, ordered that all books should be burnt, for he feared that freedom of speech might lead to opposition to his rule. Perhaps he was the first ruler to introduce 'censorship of the press'. During the legendary period, prior to the Xia dynasty (*c.* 2100–1600 BC), the arts of weaving, pottery, agriculture and tool-making were developed. But the emperors of this period have always been regarded as legendary figures, though there is now evidence to show that they were real people. The period of the Zhou dynasty (*c.* 1100–221 BC) was one of great cultural development, to which Lao Zi, Confucius and Mencius made valuable contributions, and which has been described as the Golden Age of Chinese Philosophy, when Chinese society took on the form that it still retains today. Students of Chinese culture will perceive that throughout the history of China, there has always been a long and continuous and ever-present thread of practical philosophy, which has enabled China to become economically and politically self-sufficient. Although the Chinese have had little need or desire to look far beyond their own borders, China has had need to withstand many invasions. In modern Chinese history, the most significant turning points have been the collapse of the Manchu dynasty (1644–1911) and the establishment, in 1912, of the Republic of China under the presidency of Dr Sun Yatsen (1866–1925), and, in 1949, the establishment of the People's Republic of China under the leadership of Mao Zedong (1893–1976). At present, China seems poised to become one of the foremost world powers.

Chinese jujube See **jujube**.
Chinese liquorice See **liquorice**.
Chinese medicine See **herbal medicine**.
Chinese olive *Canarium album* Herbal medicine. Distribution:

South China. Parts: fruits. Character: neutral, sweet-sour. Affinity: stomach, lungs. Effects: antipyretic, antiphlogistic, astringent, antidote. Symptoms: sore throat, overheated stomach. Treatments: pharyngitis, allergic reactions, seafood poisoning, fish bones caught in throat. Dosage: 6–10 g. The Chinese olive should not be confused with the European olive, *Oleo europea*, which is an entirely different species; and, in fact, it belongs to a different genus. See **fish bones**.

Chinese plum *Prunus japonica* Herbal medicine. Distribution: Central China. Parts: seed kernels. Character: neutral, bitter-sweet, pungent. Affinity: intestines, spleen. Effects: laxative, diuretic, emollient. Symptoms: constipation, headaches. Treatments: water-retention, dropsy. Dosage: 3–7 g.

Chinese quince *Chaenomeles lagenaria* Herbal medicine. Distribution: North China, Taiwan, India. Parts: fruits. Character: warm, sour. Affinity: liver, spleen. Effects: analgesic, stomachic, astringent, antirheumatic, antispasmodic. Symptoms: swollen legs and feet, stomach cramps, weak and painful legs and knees, vomiting. Treatments: rheumatism, arthritis, gout, diarrhoea, spasms. Dosage: 4–9 g.

'Chinese restaurant syndrome' See **monosodium glutamate**.

Chinese spring onion See **cong bai**.

Chinese violet *Viola yedoensis* Herbal medicine. Distribution: China, Japan, India. Parts: entire plant. Character: cold, bitter, pungent. Affinity: liver, heart. Effects; antipyretic, antiphlogistic, antidote. Symptoms: abscesses, boils. Treatments: carbuncles, ulcers. Dosage: 5–9 g. The juice may be applied externally to abscesses, and that of the entire plant to snake bites.

Chinese wolfberry See **wolfberry**.

Chinese years Chinese astrology is based on a cycle of 12 years, each being named after an animal. An old legend says that, just before Buddha departed from the earth, he summoned all the animals to appear before him. But only 12 obeyed his call. As a reward, he named each of the 12 years after one of the animals in the order in which they had arrived: rat, ox (buffalo), tiger, rabbit (hare), dragon, snake, horse, goat (sheep), monkey, rooster, dog and pig (boar). According to Chinese astrology, a person's character and life are determined by the animal which governs the year in which he was born. Thus, a person who is born in the Year of the Rooster will be vain, moody and talkative; and a person who is born in the Year of the Ox will be strong, reliable and calm. It is interesting to note that, in China, one of the most respected animals is the rat. This is because he is a great

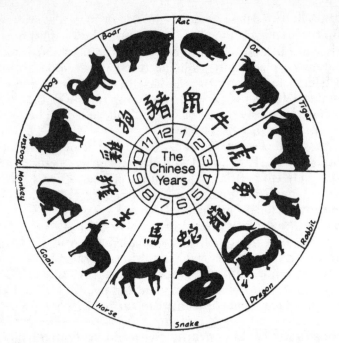

survivor. But the dog is despised – except as an item of diet. Of course, these animal-named Chinese years could be regarded as a bit of superstition, but they do at least show that the sages of ancient China were beginning to make a study of human emotions and conduct, and were categorizing people as being aggressive, timid, taciturn, talkative, introvert, extrovert, and so on; and these qualities do tell a physician much about a patient's state of health. They would have noticed that a person's behaviour and outlook can be changed by an intake of alcohol or herbs, some having a soothing effect, some having a soporific effect, and so on. This, surely, is how the science of psychology began. Psychiatry, which is an offshoot of psychology, is the study and treatment of mental illnesses. See **Chinese Almanac** and **horoscope**.

ching lo See **qing lo**.

chiropractic A Western system of massage and manipulation of the bones, especially the vertebrae, based on the principle that some ailments are due to pressure on the nerves caused by bones being displaced. It is similar to osteopathy but the emphasis is more on the spine, and it makes use of modern scientific devices, such as X-rays. It is not unlike some of the massage and manipulative techniques employed in TCM.

chlorophyll See **cell**.

chocolate The Chinese do not regard chocolate as being a particularly healthy item of diet. It has a high content of sugar and saturated fat. In large quantities, this increases the risk of coronary heart disease. The Aztecs, who lived in what is now Mexico, were of the opinion that chocolate does much for the libido. It certainly has a high energy value. For milk chocolate, this is about 530 kcal/100 g. It contains theobromine, which is a stimulant similar to caffeine.

cholagogue A medicine to stimulate the production of bile.

choler Bile. One of the four humours of traditional Western medicine. See **humour**.

cholera A serious disease, often fatal, that results from contact with food or water contaminated by faeces infected by the bacterium *vibrio cholerae*, which multiplies rapidly in the intestine. The symptoms are watery diarrhoea, severe dehydration, painful cramps and complete prostration. It is prevented by satisfactory methods of sanitation.

cholesterol A hard and fatty substance which occurs in all animal tissues, and which the liver makes from saturated fatty acids. An accumulation of cholesterol in the blood vessels is causative of arteriosclerosis, hypertension, thrombosis and coronary heart disease. To some extent, it can be reduced by excluding animal fats, cream and butter from the diet, and consuming foods which are high in polyunsaturated fatty acids, such as fish and vegetable oils. It is significant that the Chinese diet is low in red meat and dairy products. Chinese physicians regard garlic and ginseng as being preventive of the conditions which arise from an excess of cholesterol in the bloodstream. See **fat**.

chopping See **percussion**.

chopsticks See **eating utensils**.

chorea See **St Vitus' dance**.

Chou An older Anglicized form of *Zhou*. See **Zhou dynasty**.

chronic A term which describes an illness, whether minor or serious, of long duration, as opposed to one which is acute.

chrysanthemum *Chrysanthemum morifolium* Herbal medicine. Distribution: China, Japan. Parts: flowers. Character: cool, bitter-sweet. Affinity: liver, lungs. Effects: antipyretic, refrigerant, antitoxic, sedative, lowers hypertension, improves eyesight. Symptoms: headaches, giddiness, sore eyes, fever. Treatments: cirrhosis, wind-heat injuries. Dosage: 5–10 g. An infusion may be used both internally and externally to treat abscesses, and as an eyewash to treat conjunctivitis. Cultivated varieties of the chrysanthemum will be available in the West. There are a number of herbs native to Europe which are closely related to the chrysanthemum, and which have similar medicinal properties. Examples: feverfew, *Chrysanthemum parthenium*; tansy, *Chrysanthemum vulgare*; corn marigold, *Chrysanthemum segetum*.

chrysanthemum wine The flowers of the chrysanthemum are said to inhibit the ageing process and prevent hypertension and arteriosclerosis. For these purposes, the Chinese take chrysanthemum wine. Here is a simple recipe. Ingredients: 60 g dried chrysanthemum flowers, 575 ml rice wine, 90 g refined sugar. Detach the stems flowers and put all the ingredients into a large clean jar. Cover, seal and store in a cool, dry, dark and undisturbed place. After 12 months, strain the wine, discarding the flowers, and store for another 12 months before drinking. The Chinese sometimes take this wine as a nightcap. See **medicinal wine**.

Chu Ping Yuan Hou Lun See **diabetes mellitus**.

chyme Semi-liquid, partly digested food which passes from the stomach into the small intestine.

cicada *Cryptotympana pustulata* Medicine. Distribution: China, Taiwan, Japan. Parts: exuviae (moultings). Character: cold, sweet. Affinity: liver, lungs. Effects: antipyretic, antispasmodic. Symptoms: weak eyesight, convulsions. Treatments: cataracts, wind-heat injuries. Dosage; 2–5 g. See **cataract**.

cider vinegar See **vinegar**.

cinnabar Red mercuric sulphide. This is a poisonous compound, and it is certainly NOT used in Western medicine. But, in TCM, it is used as a sedative, antispasmodic and antidote. In small doses, it is a treatment for hypertension, abscesses on the body and in the mouth, and a wide range of nervous disorders, including excitement, anxiety, traumatic shock, hysteria and nightmares. The Chinese alchemists ascribed great powers to this substance, and the Taoists included it as one of the main ingredients in their 'elixir of life', which was supposed to confer a youthful immortality on its users.

cinnamon There are two types of cinnamon, but they have similar medicinal properties: Chinese cinnamon, or cassia, *Cinnamomum cassia*, which is native to South China; and Ceylon cinnamon, *Cinnamomum zeylanicum*, which is native to Sri Lanka. It is the former type that is used in TCM, but both types are cultivated in South-east Asia, and both are used for culinary purposes in the West. See **cassia**.

'cinnamon-sap soup' In his *Shang Han Lun*, or 'Discussions on

CASSIA

Cinnamomum cassia

Cinnamon is usually supplied as a powder or sticks of rolled bark.

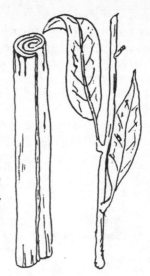

Fevers', the celebrated physician Zhang Zhongjing records an all-purpose prescription for the treatment of chills, fevers and other ailments, and which he describes as 'cinnamon-sap soup'. It is a mixture of cinnamon sap, ginger root, jujubes, liquorice root and Chinese peony root.

cinnamon twigs In TCM, cinnamon twigs are commonly used in the treatment of diseases of the heart and circulation. See **heart**.

circadian rhythm The natural daily cycle of the body, which is partly due to established habits, and partly due to physiological factors. Such terms as 'body clock' and 'biological clock' are used to describe this pattern. See **insomnia, jet lag** and **zodiac exercises**.

circulation In the West, the English physician William Harvey (1578–1657) is credited with the discovery of the circulation of the blood; but, in fact, it had already been discovered by the Chinese many centuries earlier during the time of the Han dynasty (206 BC – AD 220). The illustration shows, in diagrammatic form, the heart and main arteries and veins, together with the organs and tissues which they serve. The blood, under the pumping action of the heart, is in continuous motion, carrying oxygen from the lungs, and nutrients from the small intestine, to the tissues, and also carrying carbon dioxide from the tissues to the lungs, and other waste products, which are mainly nitrogen compounds, to the kidneys. The general rule is that the arteries carry oxygenated blood away from the heart, and the veins carry de-oxygenated blood towards the heart; but, exceptionally, the pulmonary artery carries de-oxygenated blood away from the heart to the lungs, and the pulmonary vein carries oxygenated blood from the lungs to the heart. The oxygen and nutrients are transferred by the lymph, a colourless fluid, from the capillaries to the tissues; and, in reverse, the lymph transfers waste products from the tissues to the capillaries. The functions of the vital organs and the blood vessels which serve them are described under separate entries. See **heart**.

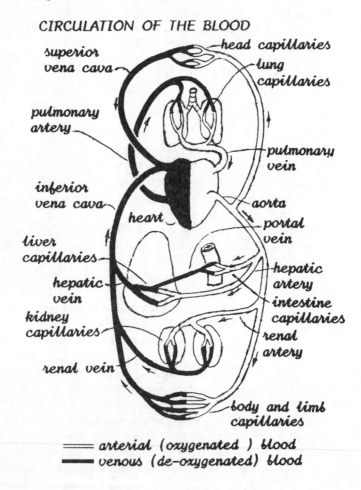

CIRCULATION OF THE BLOOD

circulatory defects The circulatory system sometimes becomes defective as the outcome of disease, accidents, ageing or some other damaging agency. Arteriosclerosis, or hardening of the arteries, hypertension, or high blood pressure, hypotension, or low blood pressure, thrombosis, coronary thrombosis, angina pectoris and varicose veins are defects of the circulatory system which commonly occur in the Western world, and which can be largely prevented by regular exercise and a healthy diet. Chinese physicians recommend a diet that is low in animal fats, sugar and salt, but rich in fish, vegetables and cereals. A regular intake of garlic, ginger, sage and rosemary are helpful. There is now some evidence to show that Siberian ginseng, *Eleutherococcus senticosus*, is also helpful.

circumcision Removal by surgery of a part of the foreskin, which covers the tip of the penis. This is not a common practice in China, and such an operation would be performed only for a strictly medical reason.

cirrhosis A condition of the liver where inflamed and damaged tissue is replaced by scar tissue. Its causes include alcoholism, hepatitis and gallstones. The liver has many functions, and so there are many things which can go wrong. Preventive procedures in matters of diet and exercise should be followed. See **liver**.

citric acid A mild acid contained in many fruits, especially citrus fruits, and which is involved in metabolism in the release of energy from food.

citrus fruit A fruit, such as the lemon, orange or lime, which is rich in citric acid and ascorbic acid, or vitamin C. Citrus fruits are one of the major items in the Chinese diet, and the mandarin orange is employed as a medicine. See **citric acid**.

classification of foods Many foods, especially those herbs and spices which are used more for flavouring than for their nutritive effects, have medicinal properties, and when the Chinese physician uses them in treatments, he will classify them by their therapeutic effects, the symptoms to which they appear to be related, and the organs to which they have an affinity. See **classification of medicines**. The Chinese cook, however, has a somewhat simpler system of classification of foods, and it is one which works well in practice. It is the Chinese view that foods not only affect a person's general state of health but will also influence his temperament. Thus, the person who consumes too much animal fat will become irritable; and there is medical evidence to show that people with hypertension, which is sometimes the consequence of a fatty and sugary diet, do easily become agitated. The cook's main classification will be on the basis of yin and yang, the former being cooling and the latter being heating. It follows that a person who has a fever will be given cooling foods, and a person who is cold will be given a heating food. Similarly, a person who has an impaired digestion will not be given foods which are irritating or too nutritive. Of particular value to the Chinese cook are those foods which are classified as neutral, for they do not upset the yin-yang balance of the body, and so they can be used in almost any situation. This table shows the main classes of foods, together with a few examples. Seemingly, this classification does contain some contradictions. For instance, pork and onions, which have energy values of 390 kcal/100 g and 233 kcal/100 g respectively, are regarded as being very heating, whereas duck and bamboo shoots, which have energy values of 340 kcal/100 g and 18 kcal/100 g, are regarded as being cooling. One explanation is that the energy value of a food as determined by laboratory experiments may be different from the actual energy released when the food has entered the body. But, in China, the fat is removed from duck before it is roasted, which reduces its energy value from 340 kcal/100 g to 190 kcal/100 g. A food that is nourishing, such as ginseng tea, may also be irritating, which creates a few problems for the inexperienced cook. Obviously, the type of food which suits one person may not suit another, and so, in preparing meals for a particular person, it is important that the cook should know as much about the person as he does about the ingredients. Certainly, there is a relationship between a person's eating habits and his temperament. 'Tell me what you eat, and I will tell you what you are,' said J. A. Brillat-Savarin in his *The Philosopher in the Kitchen*. It is a part of a Chinese physician's diagnostic technique to ask his patients about the nature of their diet. Needless to say, if the cook is to prepare a meal which is fully appetizing, he will need to consider the tastes of the ingredients. See **taste**.

VERY HEATING beef, fatty pork, dog meat, lamb, smoked fish, onions.

HEATING chicken's liver, brown sugar, eggs, leeks, walnuts, wine.

COOLING bamboo shoots, apples, barley, duck, fish, mushrooms.

VERY COOLING bean sprouts, cucumber, shellfish, green tea, bananas, soya bean milk.

NEUTRAL carrots, cauliflowers, lean chicken, dates, plums, steamed white rice.

VERY NOURISHING pigeon, pig's liver, ginseng tea, bird's nest soup.

NOURISHING lean chicken, duck, fish roe, quail's eggs, dog meat, eels.

MODERATELY NOURISHING garlic, honey, spinach, carrots, abalone, rice wine.

VERY IRRITATING vinegar, shellfish, smoked fish, spirits.

MILDLY IRRITATING beef, ginseng, garlic, carrots, onions, wine.

classification of herbs In **Shen Ben Cao Jing**, or 'The Pharmacopoeia of Shen Nong', scholars of the early part of the period of the Han dynasty (206 BC–AD 220) recorded all knowledge of herbal medicines which had existed from the time of the legendary emperor Shen Nong. In this book, all herbal plants have been put into three classes: those which support life, those which merely provide energy, and those which are poisonous but which could be used, within certain limits, to combat the most virulent diseases. In the last category, one could include those herbs which could be fatal if taken internally, but which are efficacious in treating external conditions. Since then, Chinese physicians have tended to classify medicines by their many various effects: analgesics, which reduce pain; antiseptics, which inhibit the development of micro-organisms; carminatives, which reduce flatulence, emetics, which induce vomiting; and so forth. See **herbal treatments**.

classification of medicines In TCM, the classification of medicines, no matter whether they are whole herbs, parts of herbs, herbal extracts, minerals or of animal origin, is based upon the fundamental principle that there must be inverse correspondence between the symptoms of an illness and the effects of the medications used in its treatment. Thus, yang symptoms, which are hot, full and external, will call for treatment with yin medicines, which are cooling, sedative and suppressive. Conversely, yin symptoms, which are cold, empty and internal, will require treatment with yang medicines, which are heating, toning and elevating. See **yin-yang illnesses**. Hotness, warmth, coldness and coolness are called *si qi* or 'four energies'. Medicines are also classified according to *wu wei*, or 'five tastes', which are hot, sweet, sour, bitter and salty, and the five elements, which are metal, earth, wood, fire and water. See **taste, element** and **herbal medicines**.

classification of plants See **botany**.

clean air One of the fundamental principles of TCM is that air is a source of *qi*, or 'vital energy', and that an intake of *qi* is facilitated by breathing exercises. Therefore, it is understandable that the Chinese should attach much importance to air being clean. Those mountain recluses who, during the time of the Zhou dynasty (*c.* 1100–221 BC), made a study of herbal medicines considered the air in the mountains to be a source of pure-*qi*. Perhaps a simpler explanation is that, since carbon dioxide gas is slightly denser than air, there is a little more oxygen and a little less carbon dioxide at the higher levels than at the lower levels of the atmosphere. Furthermore, the mountain mists have a moistening effect on the lungs, which would make breathing easier. See **breathing** and **xian**. It is surely highly desirable that we, in the West, should take steps to deal with the industrial waste which is largely responsible for the pollution of the environment. See **chemicals**.

cleaning agents See **chemicals**.

cleft palate A congenital defect in which a fissure in the palate joins the cavities of the nose to those in the mouth. In the West, it is rectified by plastic surgery.

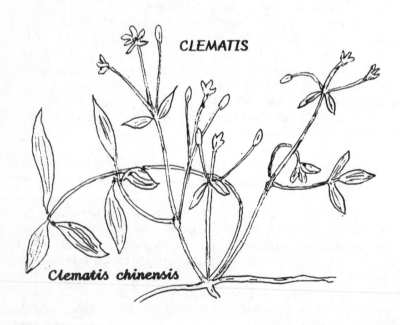

CLEMATIS

Clematis chinensis

clematis *Clematis chinensis* Herbal medicine. Distribution: China, Taiwan, Vietnam, Laos. Parts: roots. Character: warm, pungent.

Affinity: bladder. Effects: analgesic, diuretic, antipyretic, anti-rheumatic. Symptoms: aching limbs and painful joints, slight fever. Treatments: arthritis, gout, rheumatism. Dosage: 4–10 g. This medicine must NOT be taken with tea. Chinese clematis is related to traveller's joy, *Clematis vitalba*, a European species of clematis. See **fish bones**.

climacteric The period, between 45 and 60, when a person's energy begins to decline. See **menopause**.

climate In ancient times, the Chinese regarded the human body as a world in miniature; and, as such, it was influenced by climatic conditions which, when deficient or in excess, would tend to have an adverse effect on the body. The truth of this is borne out by modern medical science in the West, which has shown that most germs will flourish only under certain conditions of humidity and temperature, and that the organs of the body do not function well in conditions where it is excessively hot or cold. Anyone who has sat near an open window or doorway for several hours on a bright summer's day, when it is warm and dry and the air appears to be still, and yet has been troubled with a stiff neck on the following day, will know that these climatic conditions, however slight, do exist, and can be very treacherous. Basically, there are five climates, and each is associated with the vital organ which it most affects: windy for the liver, damp for the spleen, hot for the heart, dry for the lungs, and cold for the kidneys. But these climates can exist in various combinations, such as wind-dry, wind-hot, wind-cold, cold-damp and hot-damp. Very excessive, or tropical heat, which TCM describes as fire, as opposed to summer heat, is sometimes added to these climates, and then they are known as the six excesses. See **six excesses**.

climax See **orgasm**.

cloud ears See **silver wood ears**.

coagulation Clotting. This is brought about by threads of a protein called fibrin which is formed when chemicals and the platelets in the blood interreact. This occurs on blood being exposed to air, as when a blood vessel is damaged. See **blood clot** and **thrombocyte**.

coal tar A viscid and dark flammable liquid which is obtained by the dry distillation of wood or coal. It is a source of naphtha, paraffin, benzene, creosote, aniline dyes and many other derivatives, some of which are almost certain to be carcinogenic. Amazingly enough, coal-tar derivatives were once commonly used in the preparation of soap and other toiletries. The Chinese do not use coal-tar derivatives or any other kinds of synthetic substances as dyes and flavourings for food. See **cancer** and **chemicals**.

cobalamin Vitamin B. This vitamin is essential for the formation of red blood cells. Liver is a good source, which explains why Chinese physicians recommend chopped raw liver as a remedy for some forms of anaemia. See **vitamin**.

cobweb Many years ago in China, and also in the West, a cobweb would be placed on an open wound in order to induce the blood to coagulate. The explanation is that the fluid ejected from the spinnerets of a spider coagulates immediately on exposure to air, and the coagulant which it contains has the same effect on blood. This may appear to be a most unhygienic practice; but, seemingly, cobwebs contain natural penicillin. The manufacture of rayon and nylon fibres from plastic substances, such as viscose, which is derived from cellulose, is similar to the way in which the spider makes silk for its web. One may conclude that modern scientific discoveries are not always very original, and that we have much to learn from nature. See **penicillin** and **antibiotic**.

coccus See **bacterium**.

coconut milk A pleasant drink for those people who, for reasons of health, prefer not to consume cow's milk. See **milk and milk products**.

coelic disease See **gluten**.

coffee Very little coffee is drunk in China, but this situation is likely to change now that worldwide studies by the International Agency for Research into Cancer have revealed that coffee-drinking wards off cancer, particularly that of the colon, for the Chinese are generally quick to adopt any dietary practice which is likely to be beneficial to the health. See **caffeine**.

cola See **kola**.

cold In TCM, cold is one of the four energies. Dominant in winter and governed by the element metal, it is also one of the six excesses. It is an evil-yin and destructive to yang energy. Externally, it causes fevers, chills, headaches and bodily pains; and, if in contact with a meridian, it causes pains in the bones and joints. Internally, when it is called inner-cold, it causes nausea, vomiting, flatulence, diarrhoea, abdominal pains, sensations of coldness in the limbs and a pale complexion. Over-consumption of cold foods can cause inner-cold. See **six excesses** and **cold food**.

cold-dryness See **six excesses** and **excess combinations**.

cold food It is not always possible to translate Chinese words into

English without any loss of exactitude, and so some of the terms used in TCM can be misleading. Thus, a cold food is not necessarily one which is at a low temperature, but one which has a low energy value. For example, ice-cream is at a low temperature but is high in energy, for it is made of vegetable oil, whereas a cup of tea is at a high temperature but is low in energy, for it contains very little nutrient. Likewise, a hot food is not necessarily one which is at a high temperature, but one which has a high energy value. And so, in TCM, ice-cream is regarded as a hot food. See **classification of foods** and **temperature**.

cold illness A cold illness is generally internal, empty, descending and suppressive, and its symptoms will indicate this. See **cold** and **ba gang**.

colds A cold is due to a virus infection, and may be accompanied by feverishness and a rise in temperature. The word *cold* as defined in Western medicine is different in meaning from the word *cold* as defined in TCM, and so a cold must not be confused with a cold illness, for the latter term covers a wide range of conditions. See **cold** and **common cold**.

cold sores An infection which is characterized by small blisters around the nose or lips. It is caused by a virus, *Herpes simplex*, and may follow or be associated with a common cold, though it is not the same condition. It is very infectious, and may be transmitted by kissing. Normally, the virus remains dormant in the body for many years, but it appears on the skin, and sometimes the genitalia, when the resistance of the body is lowered by illness, stress, cold weather or hormone imbalances during menstruation or pregnancy. It can be prevented by a diet which omits sugar and other refined foods, chocolate, beer and nuts, and which includes honey, fruit and vegetables. It is helpful to paint the affected parts with lemon juice. Chinese physicians would advise a wholesome diet, a healthy life-style and a regular intake of garlic, occasionally supplemented with royal jelly or Asiatic ginseng.

cold-summer-heat See **excess combinations**.

'cold turkey' See **withdrawal symptoms**.

colic Cramping pains, fluctuating in intensity, which are due to inflammation or a blockage in one of the hollow organs, particularly the intestines, and which is accompanied by distension and contraction of the involuntary muscles of the organ. A simple but effective remedy is an infusion of one of the following taken internally, using the parts and dosages indicated: ginger, *Zingiber officinale*, root, 3–8 g; thyme, *Thymus vulgare*,

147

leaves, 2–12 g; peppermint, *Mentha piperita*, leaves, 2–4 g; catnip, *Nepeta cataria*, leaves, 3–12 g. Tarragon, *Artemisia dracunculus*, is helpful if consumed as a seasoning. Chinese physicians sometimes recommend blood-letting as a treatment. If the condition persists, medical advice should be sought, for it could be indicative of a more serious condition, such as appendicitis, lead poisoning, strangulated hernia, gallstones and cancer. Colic is a common condition in infants, causing them much distress. The best remedy is probably a gripe water made as an infusion of the leaves of dill, *Anethum graveolens*. It is also important that a baby with colic should be kept warm and comfortable, for this creates reassurance, and the diet be kept free of irritating foods, such as coffee, strawberries, oranges, bananas, chocolate and spicy foods.

colitis In its milder form, which is called mucus colitis, or nervous bowel, colitis can be described as inflammation and over-activity of the large intestine accompanied by diarrhoea and a discharge of mucus. It can be treated with relaxants and carminatives which will allow the bowel to re-establish its natural rhythm.

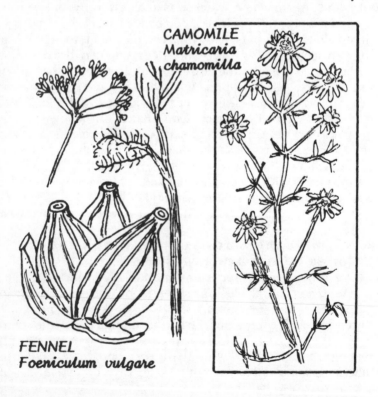

CAMOMILE
Matricaria chamomilla

FENNEL
Foeniculum vulgare

These could include infusions of the following herbs taken internally, using the parts and dosages indicated: camomile, *Matricaria chamomilla*, flowers, 4–12 g; hop, *Humulus lupulus*, strobiles (cones), 1.5–3 g; fennel, *Foeniculum vulgare*, leaves, 1 g, seeds, 3 g; dill, *Anethum graveolens*, fruit, 4–12 g. In its severest form, which is called ulcerative colitis, the condition is chronic, and there is severe diarrhoea, pain and blood in the stools, which are also the symptoms of dysentery. The causes are complex, and so medical advice should be sought, for expert attention, with the possibility of surgery, will certainly be required.

collagen See **connective tissue**.

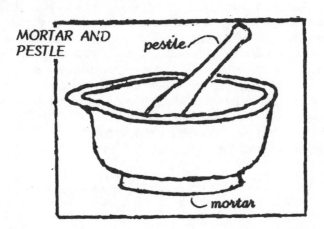

MORTAR AND PESTLE — pestle — mortar

collecting herbs In collecting medicinal herbs from the field or garden, one should pick those which are dry, clean and growing in unpolluted places, but bearing in mind that some species are protected, which means that it is illegal to pick them. The roots must be washed, but the other parts must NOT be washed. A few herbs can be used immediately in the fresh state, but most will need to be dried so they can be conveniently stored for later use. To do this, one should place them on clean cloth or paper, and keep in a dry, airy and dark or shaded place until they become dry and brittle. They can be stored whole or ground, but the hard parts – seeds, roots and bark – will generally need to be ground. This can be done with a mortar and pestle (which may be purchased from a pharmacy). The herbs should be stored in cardboard boxes, paper bags and dark-glass jars so that they will be unaffected by sunlight, but not in cans and plastic bags, in which they would be liable to ferment. They should keep in a good condition for 6–8 months. Fresh herbs can be stored in a deep-freeze. See **preparation of herbs** and **culinary herbs and spices**.

colon See **large intestine**.

colour Colour has a certain significance in Chinese mythology. Red, for example, is associated with the heart, the planet Mars, the element fire and the emotion of joy. Green is associated with the liver, the planet Jupiter, and so on. Each of the five solid vital organs has its associated colour: *heart* red, *liver* green, *spleen* yellow, *lungs* white, *kidneys* black. These associations should not be lightly dismissed as superstition, for they have their uses in TCM. On the charts and models which are used by acupuncturists, each meridian line is shown in the colour symbolizing the organ to which it relates, and this makes for ease in identification. Colour also has a fair degree of psychological significance, as painters, Chinese or otherwise, have always known. Red is exciting, yellow is cheerful, green is restful and blue is depressing. A painting in which there is a preponderance of shades of red, yellow, orange, brown and green creates an impression of warmth and comfort.

colour-blindness See **hereditary defects**.

colourings See **additives** and **food colours**.

COLTSFOOT

Tussilago farfara

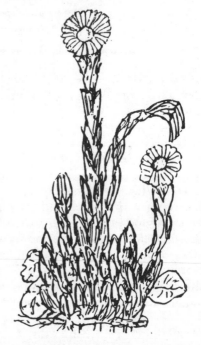

coltsfoot *Tussilago farfara* Herbal medicine. Distribution: North China, Europe, Africa. Parts: flowers, buds. Character: warm, bitter. Affinity: lungs. Effects: expectorant, antitussive. Symptoms: coughing, wheezing. Treatments: asthma, bronchitis. Dosage: 2–6 g. The dried leaves of coltsfoot are sometimes made into herbal cigarettes, which are occasionally recommended as a treatment for asthma.

coma Deep and prolonged unconsciousness.

comedo Comedone. Blackhead. See **acne**.

comfrey *Symphytum officinale* Herbal medicine. Distribution: Europe, Asia, North America. Parts: leaves, roots. Character: warm, sweet. Affinity: stomach, lungs. Effects: stimulant, emollient, astringent, expectorant. Symptoms: coughing, colic, cuts, grazes, sprains. Treatments: ulcerative colitis, fractures, internal wounds, bronchitis. Dosage 3–12 g. Comfrey was once used in the West for treating fractures and sprains, which explains why four of its everyday names are knitbone, knitback, boneset and bruisewort.

commensal An animal or plant living harmlessly, and not parasitically, and sometimes with mutual benefit with or in another animal or plant. Some of the bacteria in the intestines of humans are commensals.

comminuted fracture See **fracture**.

common cat's tail See **reedmace**.

common cold A virus infection causing acute inflammation of the mucous membrane of the nose and throat. The common cold viruses circulate in the atmosphere, and so it is difficult to avoid them. But one can increase one's immunity to viral infections of all kinds by keeping in a sound state of health. A regular intake of garlic as an item of diet is helpful, for it has antiseptic properties. A traditional Chinese remedy is to gently sip a tea made by boiling 20 g each of ginger root, spring onion and cinnamon in 575 ml water for 5 minutes, and then adding 20 g honey, and stirring. The common cold should not be confused with a chill. The former is an infection, and can be contracted in hot weather, whereas the latter is a mere lowering of temperature as a consequence of cold weather or for some other reasons, which are sometimes obscure. See **chill**.

common plaintain *Plantago major* Also called the greater plaintain. Distribution: global. Parts: leaves, seeds. Character: cold, sweet. Affinity: liver, kidneys, lungs, small intestine. Effects: diuretic, expectorant, demulcent, astringent. Symptoms: difficult urination, coughs, diarrhoea, painful and swollen eyes, excess mucus.

Treatments: dysentery, infections of the urinary tract, hypertension. Dosage: 4–12 g. This herb has some value as an aphrodisiac, and a compress of its fresh leaves may be applied locally as a treatment for haemorrhoids.

compatibility of medicines See **dangers with medicines** and **synergy**.

complementary medicine See **alternative medicine**.

complex A term used in psychology and psychiatry to describe a set of fixed beliefs or ideas which arise subconsciously from past experiences, forgotten or repressed, but which strongly affect and direct behaviour. Complexes develop mainly in childhood – the period of the formative years – and can remain with people, influencing their conduct for good or for ill, for the rest of their lives. There is no doubt that the political opinions, religious beliefs and social attitudes of many people stem more from their complexes than from any attempt at logical thought or accurate observation. The Chinese live in a thoroughly integrated society, and they have long recognized that social disharmony can create unsocial attitudes, or what we would describe as complexes of guilt and inferiority. These can lead to mental disorders, which, in turn, may lead to physical disorders. The Chinese would contend that, if the minds of young people are properly influenced, they will develop attitudes which are inhibitive of violence, greed, dishonesty and impropriety, but it is all-important that the influences brought to bear must be flawless in their reliability and sincerity. Here, it must be said that it would be difficult indeed to find any serious defects in the teachings of Confucius and the *I Ching*, or 'Book of Changes', a classical work of great antiquity, which have influenced the Chinese for many centuries and done so much to mould their character. In the Chinese view, the illnesses of society, as with the illnesses of the body, are more easily prevented than cured. Similarly, in dealing with crime and other forms of antisocial behaviour, training to condition the mind, which is a preventive technique, is more effective than crude punishments, which are a curative technique, but it must be accepted that the threat of punishment, even though rarely carried out, may be a necessary part of this preventive training. It is the Chinese policy in this regard, which a psychologist in the West might describe as 'conditioning to produce desirable complexes', that has created a society in which antisocial behaviour and mental illness are not commonplace. See **childhood, Confucius** and **I Ching**.

complexion 'All is not gold that glitters', says a Latin proverb, and it is true that one cannot always judge by appearances, and it must sometimes be the case that a person with a youthful complexion will not feel youthful or be healthy. But, in general, the condition of the skin is an indication of the condition of the body. It is in the eyes, mouth and skin that the physician finds many of the symptoms of illness – and signs of health. Chinese physicians contend that the health of the skin is largely determined by the health of the body, and the bloodstream in particular, for therein lie the vital essences which control many of the activities of the body. The blood also contains those toxic wastes which cause skin eruptions, painful joints and aching muscles. Certainly, regular elimination of waste from the bowel by a diet high in fibre, and from the blood by a diet high in medicinal herbs, will do more for the health and youthful complexion of the skin than will those cosmetic preparations which clog the pores and destroy the natural protective oils, and which do nothing for the health of the blood and internal organs. An eminent chemist in his capacity as a public analyst has said that the use of perfume is largely a matter of using one smell to cover up another. Some diseases and defects of the skin, such as warts and dermatitis, have external causes, and they may be spread by contact. But many, such as acne, eczema, psoriasis, wrinkles and baldness, have internal causes, such as inadequate diet, food allergies, constipation, nervous tension and the changes in hormone levels at the time of puberty and middle age. Taking care of the skin, and so eliminating the tell-tale signs of age, need be no problem if one adopts the Chinese diet, for it has in-built components which are beneficial to the health of the skin, and thereby provide a youthful complexion. The skin will benefit considerably if the diet includes dandelions, *Taraxacum officinale*, garlic, *Allium sativum*, ramsons, *Allium ursinum*, nettles, *Urtica dioica*, jujubes, *Ziziphus jujuba*, and plenty of leguminous vegetables. Ramsons are wild garlic. The leaves and stems of the dandelions and all parts of the garlic and ramsons should be washed, finely chopped and eaten raw in a salad, but the nettles and jujubes should be taken as a tea – 10 g in 1 litre boiling water. Small pimples will generally disappear if they are rubbed with the cut end of a garlic clove. Age spots, or senile keratosis, can be treated by applying the juice (extracted with a blender) of the marigold, *Calendula officinalis*, and the leek, *Allium porrum*. See **pimples** and **spots**.

compress A folded sterilized cloth, such as lint, or a pad which is heated or soaked in a hot or cold herbal infusion or decoction or some other liquid and applied to bruises or other affected parts to relieve pain or improve the circulation.

compression A term used in massage to describe the pressure movements, of which there are two main kinds – petrissage and friction. Petrissage is the slow, gentle and rhythmic kneading of the muscles, which increases the circulation and removes waste, and thereby reduces fatigue, and might even eliminate some of the excess fat. Friction is firm rubbing in circles, done with the palms of the hands, the bases of the thumbs or one or more fingers, the skin moving with the hand, so gliding over the underlying tissues. This technique stimulates the circulation, removes excess fluid and sometimes reduces fat and fibrous thickenings and nodules. See **reflexology** and **massage**.

compromise For the Chinese, compromise is one of the major components of the art of survival. It is their capacity for compromise and their avoidance of violent extremes, which is an extension of the yin-yang principle that few things are either completely yin or completely yang, that enables them to make the best of a bad situation and achieve some measure of success by a realignment of their thinking and behaviour. They believe that harmony in all things, including the bodily functions, is not a matter of aiming for what is ideal, for that may be impossible to achieve, or aiming for what is undesirable, for that could be disastrous, but a matter of finding a balance between the ideal and the unideal. Perhaps this compromise, or the middle way, is sometimes the true ideal, the apparent ideal being unattainable because it is a product of self-deception. Two eyes are better than one. By this reasoning, it could be said that three eyes are better than two. But, as three eyes are impossible, we must make do with two eyes, for that is the most that can be achieved. The Chinese attitude in this respect is best expressed by a quotation from the literature of India: 'I complained because I had no shoes; but I ceased to complain when I met a man who had no feet.' See **moderation**.

computer Over 5000 years ago, the Chinese invented binary numbers, which were used in devising the 64 hexagrams of the *I Ching*, and which constitute the principle of the electronic computer. But the human brain functions in much the same way as a computer, and so it could be said the Chinese paved the way for the science of psychology and psychiatry. See **I Ching** and **psychology**.

concentrated A term used by chemists to describe a solution in which there is a very high proportion of the dissolved substance, or solute. See **solution**.

concentration One of the seven emotions of TCM, and related to the spleen. Over-concentration, as with an obsessive fixation, can harm the mind and interfere with the functions of the spleen and stomach, so impairing digestion and producing abdominal pains. Anyone who has suffered from nervous indigestion will know that this can be the case. People who need to concentrate heavily in their work should take a break occasionally, preferably by participating in a physical activity which requires no mental effort. See **seven emotions**.

conception Fertilization in mammals. See **fertilization**.

conception-vessel A Chinese medical term which aptly describes the genitalia.

concoction A medicine which is a mixture of ingredients.

concussion A condition of immediate unconsciousness caused by a blow to the head, so giving a shock to the brain. Generally, complete recovery occurs within less than 24 hours provided there is no actual injury to the brain.

condiment Seasoning. Most seasonings, such as salt, pepper and mustard, have medicinal properties. See **culinary herbs**.

conditioned reflex See **involuntary movement**.

condom A thin rubber or plastic sheath which is used to cover the penis during intercourse, and so prevent conception and infection. This is the officially preferred method of contraception in China.

confectionery The Chinese do not consume large amounts of confectionery, for they consider refined sugar to be detrimental to the health.

Confucian classics Among the earliest literary works of China are the five Confucian classics: the *Shijing, Yijing, Shujing, Liji* and *Chunqui*. They are authoritative works, and they are often consulted by Chinese scholars. Parts of these classics are sometimes attributed to Confucius, though no one knows what kind of contribution, if any, he made to their compilation. However, it is known that his students made notes of what he said, and it could well be that some of the information in the Confucian classics was derived from these notes. The *Shijing* is a collection of lyrics from the period of the Zhou (or Chou) dynasty (*c.* 1100–221 BC), the *Yijing* is a book of divinations, the *Shujing* is a collection of historical documents and speeches made by Zhou rulers, the *Liji* provides descriptions of the classical rites, and the *Chunqui* is a historical chronicle which describes the state of Lu, where Confucius lived, at Qufu, which is now a large city, during the time of the Zhou dynasty. Of these works, the

Yijing is the one that is the best known in the West, where it is more likely to be called the *I Ching*. This is an alternative spelling that is more familiar to Western people, and it is the one which is used elsewhere in this book. Perhaps the main significance of these works to students of history is that they give a clear indication of the condition of the Chinese civilization at the time of the Zhou dynasty. There are many references to herbal medicines and physical and breathing exercises, and so it is clear that the Chinese developed a tremendous interest in health and the healing arts at an early stage in their history. But, at that time, the Chinese also made great advances in other directions. See **Zhou dynasty**.

Confucianism One of the principal religions of China, though it is really a moral philosophy, or way of life, and not a religion in our sense of the term. Mysticism and superstition are anathema to Confucians, who consider that virtue brings its own rewards – as does vice. They look askance at Christianity with its promises of eternal bliss and threats of eternal damnation. The main aim of Confucianism is to produce the *zhunzi* (*chun-tzu*), or true gentleman, who will behave correctly in all situations, and it places great emphasis on the five virtues of wisdom, justice, sincerity, charity and propriety. Confucianism is the greatest moral force in China, and it has been the main instrument in producing a stable society based on a stable family life; and this, in turn, has produced stable individuals. It could be said that the low incidence of mental and nervous disorders in China is largely due to the Confucian influence.

Confucius Although he is China's greatest sage and the founder of Confucianism, very little is known about the personal life of Confucius. His name, as we know it, is a Latinized version of *Kong Fuzi*, his Chinese name, which was contrived for him by the Jesuit missionaries who came to China many centuries after his death. He was a person of profound wisdom, immense benevolence and incisive logic. He contended that man must constantly strive to make his presence felt in the eternal cycle of good and evil. There is no doubt that his teachings, which are totally rational and free of superstition, have given the Chinese a sound set of unassailable moral values, and thereby a strong lead, health-wise as well as socio-politically, over the rest of the world.

cong bai *Allium fistulosum* Herbal medicine. Distribution: North China, Mongolia, Siberia. Parts: fresh rootlets and white stems. Character: warm, bitter. Affinity: stomach, lungs. Effects: antiseptic, diaphoretic, stomachic. Symptoms: shivering, feverishness, stomach ache. Treatments: wind-injury, colds and chills, stomach upsets. Dosage: 4–10 g. For external use, the fresh herb, finely chopped, is mixed with honey to make an ointment which is effective in treating abscesses and skin infections. For treating colds and chills, it may be decocted with ginger root and honey or brown sugar, and taken internally. Although *cong bai* is native to Asia, it is cultivated in the West, where it is generally eaten uncooked in salads. In Britain, it is called the onion green, Welsh onion or Chinese spring onion.

congener A substance formed in fermentation, and which, especially in such drinks as lager and brandy, irritates the lining of the stomach, and so heightens the effect of a hangover. See **hangover**.

congenital A defect or other condition which is present or occurs at the time of birth, but which is not necessarily hereditary. See **hereditary defects**.

congestion An abnormal condition where there is an excessive accumulation of blood in an organ. The term is also applied to the condition whereby there is an excess of mucus in the lungs and nasal passages. The latter condition may be effectively treated with an infusion, taken internally, of any of the following, using the parts and dosages indicated: angelica, *Angelica sinensis*, roots or seeds, 3–6 g; magnolia, *Magnolia liliflora*, buds, 4–8 g; stinging nettle, *Urtica dioica*, shoots, 2–4 g. Garden angelica, *Angelica officinalis*, may be used as an alternative to the Chinese angelica listed above. An external treatment for congestion is a poultice of the crushed seeds of black mustard, *Brassica nigra*, applied to the chest.

conjunctiva The thin membrane covering the eyeball and the internal surfaces of the eyelids.

conjunctivitis 'Red eye' or 'pink eye'. Inflammation of the conjunctiva, which TCM physicians ascribe to wind-heat in the liver. A suitable treatment for this condition, and also for blepharitis, provided there are no serious associated conditions, is an eyewash of an infusion or decoction of any of the following, using the parts and dosages indicated: marigold, *Calendula officinalis*, flowers, 3–12 g; chrysanthemum, *Chrysanthemum morifolium*, flowers, 4–10 g; jasmine, *Jasminum officinale*, flowers, leaves, 3–6 g; fennel, *Foeniculum vulgare*, leaves, 1 g, seeds, 3 g; raspberry, *Rubus idaeus*, leaves, 5–10 g; camomile, *Matricaria chamomilla*, leaves, flowers, 4–6 g; eyebright, *Euphrasia officinalis*, leaves, flowers, 4–6 g. An infusion of eyebright can also be taken internally, as can infusions of the following: tea, *Camellia sinensis* (green or black), 2–4 g; self-heal, *Prunella vulgaris*, leaves, seeds, 5–7 g. Both fresh eyebright and parsley, *Petroselinum crispum*, may be used as a compress.

connective tissue A somewhat loose term which describes the less specialized tissues which bind together and support nerve, muscle and skin tissues and the various organs, glands and systems. Much of it is fibrous and fatty, and the rest consists of bone, cartilage, blood, lymph and collagen, which is a low-grade protein. See **interferon**.

constipation Difficult, irregular or infrequent evacuation of the bowels, which is characterized by small, hard stools. Bowel action varies from person to person, and it is largely determined by diet and personal habits. Its main causes are lack of fibre, fluids and exercise, an excess of meat or dairy products, food allergies, the side-effects of some medicines, pregnancy, anxiety and stress. If the condition persists, medical advice should be sought. Otherwise, delayed bowel action generally does little harm, though stagnant food waste can have a deleterious effect on the bodily organs, and chronic constipation can lead to bowel disorders and haemorrhoids. As gentle laxatives, Chinese physicians would recommend infusions of the following, using the parts and dosages indicated, and to be taken internally: stinging nettle, *Urtica dioica*, leaves, 2–4 g; yarrow, *Achillea millefolium*, leaves, 4–5 g; dandelion, *Taraxacum officinale*, leaves and root, 10–30 g; apricot, *Prunus armeniaca*, fruits, 5–10 g. Some Chinese dietary remedies are fig wine, white rice porridge, stewed pears and bananas with honey and eaten cold, and 30 g powdered walnuts mixed with 15 g honey and eaten with boiled rice. Glauber's salt (sodium sulphate) and senna, *Cassia tora*, are strong purgatives. However, strong purgatives should not be administered to frail or elderly people or anyone with a heart condition. Regular exercise helps to prevent constipation. For therapeutic exercises, Chinese physicians would recommend *nei yang kung*, or 'internally nourishing exercises'. Information about these is to be found in the exercise manual issued by the Chinese government. Taoist philosophy has provided a set of 12 exercises, one of which is effective in preventing constipation provided that it is performed between 5 and 7 o'clock in the morning. See **zodiac exercises, fig wine, white rice porridge** and **Chinese Exercise Manual**.

constituents of herbs See **herbal constituents**.

consultation The treatment of a patient is almost always preceded by a consultation in which the physician takes note of the physical indicators of disease, such as the complexion, skin temperature, pulse, colour and texture of the tongue, diet and personal habits. In TCM, neither the diagnosis nor the treatment is completely fixed from the outset. The physician is prepared to reconsider his original diagnosis, and so, as the symptoms change, he will alter the procedure of the treatment. In a consultation, the Chinese physician uses four basic methods of diagnosis: discussion, observation, listening and touch. These methods of diagnosis yield information about chills and fever, stools, urine, perspiration, temperature, food, drink, taste, sleep, sexual habits, menstruation and pregnancy. See **diagnosis**.

consultative discussion An important aspect of a consultation with a physician is the information obtained by discussion, and which, generally, could not be obtained in any other way. This discussion elicits from the patient details of the more obvious symptoms of his illness, the history of the illness from its commencement until the time he visits the physician, changes in symptoms, the circumstances in which the illness first arose, various manifestations in regard to aches and pains, food, drink, taste, perspiration, urine, stools, sleep, sexual habits, menstruation, pregnancy, childbirths, past history and illnesses, personal habits, environmental factors and the family history. The patient's family may be required to provide information, particularly if the patient is a child or is incapable of speaking for himself, as would be the case if he were deaf or dumb or had been afflicted by a stroke.

consumption An archaic name for a wasting disease, especially pulmonary tuberculosis.

contact dermatitis Severe dermatitis due to the patient being in contact with a substance, such as paint or oil, to which he is allergic. See **eczema**.

contagious disease A disease which is transmitted only by direct contact with an infected person or the things with which he has been in contact – his stools, spittle, urine, perspiration and personal possessions. See **infectious diseases**.

contagious abortion See **brucellosis**.

contaminated food Food is contaminated mainly by contact with chemicals, such as detergents and pesticides, and micro-organisms, such as salmonella and listeria. Contaminated food gives rise to a wide range of illnesses, some of which may prove to be fatal. Therefore, it is imperative that food should be stored and prepared in hygienic conditions and away from possible contact with toxic and corrosive substances. The Chinese attitude in this regard is simple but effective. All foodstuffs must be fresh, and chemical substances, including food additives, must not be brought into contact with food. See **chemicals, food hygiene** and **fresh food**.

contraception See **birth control** and **condom**.

contusion Bruise or other injury without any break in the skin. Black eyes are bruises in a particularly sensitive area. A helpful treatment is a wet compress of any of the following, using the parts indicated: marigold, *Calendula officinalis*, flowers; comfrey, *Symphitum officinale*, leaves; chervil, *Anthriscus cerefolium*, leaves. Marigold flowers may also be mixed with lard or petroleum jelly and applied as an ointment. A poultice of the capsules of the corn poppy, *Papaver rhoeas*, is another treatment. See **cupping**.

convenience food See **junk food**.

conventional medicine Orthodox medicine. This is the system of medicine that is favoured and mainly practised in the West, though it is now being realized that it has certain limitations, and that other systems of medicine, as are practised traditionally in such countries as India and China, and which are called alternative medicine, have certain advantages. See **traditional medicine**.

convulsion See **fit**.

cooking See **classification of foods**.

cooking oil See **vegetable oil**.

cookery recipes These days, there is a great abundance of Chinese cookery books on the market, and so the wise person who decides to adopt the Chinese diet as a means to health will have no difficulty in obtaining recipes for Chinese dishes.

cool See **four energies**.

copper See **mineral**.

copulation Sexual intercourse.

cordial An infusion or decoction of medicinal herbs flavoured and sweetened by the addition of fruit and sugar, with alcohol occasionally added, and used as a pleasant and warming drink and sometimes as a stimulant for the heart.

coriander *Coriandrum sativum* Herbal medicine. Distribution: Middle East. Parts: leaves, seeds. Character: warm, sweet. Affinity: stomach, spleen. Effects: analgesic, stomachic, carminative, aphrodisiac, emmenagogue. Symptoms: loss of appetite, aches and pains. Treatments: indigestion, flatulence, arthritis. Dosage: 10–12 g. An infusion of crushed coriander seeds, called coriander water, makes a refreshing drink, and it is helpful to women if taken at the time of the menstrual flow. Crushed coriander seeds or leaves can be applied as a wet compress to relieve the pain in arthritic joints. As an item of diet, coriander is regarded as an aid to long life. Coriander is sometimes called Chinese parsley, though it is not indigenous to China.

cork tree *Phellodendron amurense* Herbal medicine. Distribution: North China, Siberia, Japan. Parts: bark. Character: cold, bitter. Affinity: bladder, kidneys, large intestine. Effects: antipyretic, antidote. Symptoms: diarrhoea, painful urination, vaginal pain and swelling, dark leucorrhoea, painful joints, aching limbs. Treatments: jaundice, arthritis, rheumatism, skin diseases, dysentery, cystitis, enteritis, urethritis, hypertension, nocturnal emissions, ailments due to yin-deficiency and damp-heat excess. Dosage: 4–5 g.

corn Callus. A small region of hard and thickened skin, generally on the feet and toes, and caused by rubbing or pressure. One simple treatment is to wear shoes which do not fit too tightly. See **keratosis**.

cornea The transparent skin on the front of the eye.

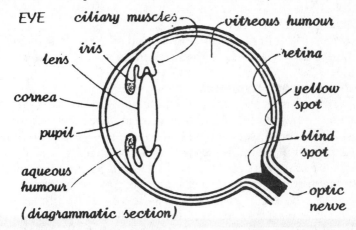

EYE ciliary muscles — vitreous humour
lens, iris — retina
cornea — yellow spot
pupil — blind spot
aqueous humour — optic nerve
(diagrammatic section)

corn marigold *Chrysanthemum segetum*. Related to the Chinese chrysanthemum, *Chrysanthemum morifolium*. See **chrysanthemum**.

corn mint *Mentha arvensis* Herbal medicine. Distribution: China, Vietnam, Europe. Parts: leaves and stems. Character: cool, pungent. Affinity: liver, lungs. Effects: diaphoretic, stomachic, digestive, carminative. Symptoms: colds, headaches, sore throat, feverishness. Treatments: colds, chills, some wind-heat conditions. Dosage: 2–4 g.

corn oil Maize oil. See **fatty acid** and **oil**.

corn poppy See **poppy**.

coronary arteries The arteries which supply blood to the muscles of the heart.

coronary heart disease See **coronary thrombosis**.

coronary thrombosis Coronary occlusion. The blockage of a coronary artery by a blood clot, or thrombus, and which can cause intense pain, shock and heart failure. See **thrombosis** and **qi gong**.

cortex Outer part of the brain or a kidney.

corticosteroids The collective name for the hormones secreted by the adrenal glands. The name is also used for similar chemicals which are made synthetically. They are commonly known as steroids. See **steroids**.

cortisone One of the corticosteroids. In the West, it is used to treat inflammation and allergies.

coryza The common cold, particularly where there is a severe nasal discharge. See **common cold**.

cosmetics See **chemicals** and **complexion**.

costal Of the ribs.

costive Constipated.

cotton-seed oil In the West, cotton-seed oil is used for frying, but Chinese physicians are of the opinion that it causes infertility in men.

Coúeism See **self-hypnosis**.

cough There is no shortage of Chinese remedies for a cough. They include infusions of the following, using the parts and dosages indicated, and sipped slowly: coltsfoot, *Tussilago farfara*, flowers, buds, 3–10 g; Chinese plantain, *Plantago asiatica*, seeds, 5–9 g; fennel, *Foeniculum vulgare*, leaves 1 g, seeds 3 g; angelica, *Angelica officinalis*, stems, roots, 3–6 g; liquorice, *Glycyrrhiza glabra*, roots, 3–10 g; thyme, *Thymus vulgare*, leaves 2–12 g; agrimony, *Agrimonia eupatoria*, leaves, flowers, 10–15 g; stinging nettle, *Urtica dioica*, young shoots, 2–4 g; gypsum (calcium sulphate), 10–30 g. A decoction of 10–15 g of the skin of the roots of the Chinese wolfberry, *Lycium chinense*, taken internally is helpful, as is ginger rhizome if cooked in with a soup or stew, and in a dosage of 3–8 g.

counter-irritant A treatment such as a poultice or liniment which is applied to the skin to increase the local blood supply and so relieve pains in the underlying tissues and organs.

cowpox See **immunology**.

cramp Spasms. A painful involuntary muscle contraction. Among its causes are coldness, as with swimming in cold water, a poor circulation of blood to the muscles and a deficiency of salt and other minerals as a consequence of diarrhoea and heavy perspiration. A person who is susceptible to cramp should learn how to relax, for tension can make this condition more painful. Massage by gliding and kneading movements will stretch the contracted muscle, and thereby bring relief. Effleurage will stimulate circulation to the affected muscle. A decoction of 3–8 g ginger root taken internally is helpful.

cranium See **brain**.

creeping lily turf See **lily turf**.

cretin See **hypochyroidism**.

Creutzfeldt-Jakob disease A most virulent disease in man, and the equivalent of bovine spongiform encephalopathy in cattle. There was a high incidence of this disease among the natives of New Guinea until they gave up cannibalism, which meant that they ceased to consume human brains infected with the disease. See **bovine spongiform encephalopathy**.

crime and illness See **complex** and **mental health**.

critical dosage With Western medicines, which are usually synthetic, dosages are generally critical, and, if the medicines are not taken within the prescribed limits, they are likely to be ineffective, and perhaps give rise to unpleasant side-effects or even fatal consequences. This is also true of some Chinese herbal medicines, but, in general, herbal medicines can be administered in non-critical dosages. This, of course, is one of the several advantages of herbal medicines. See **dosages**.

cross-linkage One of the theories of recent Western medical research into ageing is that highly active atoms or groups of atoms, called free radicals, which result from wear and tear on the body, or enter the body in drugs and pollutants and by radiation, react chemically with others, and thereby damage body cells and fibres of collagen, which is a protein. The fibres become 'cross-linked', or tangled, and so the skin loses its suppleness, and wrinkles develop, arteries and veins harden, muscles become soft and joints become stiff. This is one of the causes of ageing. It could also be one of the causes of cancer. See **ageing, cancer** and **free radicals**.

crustaceans A class of aquatic animals, closely related to the insects, which have hard exoskeletons (external skeletons). Crayfish, lobsters, crabs, woodlice, prawns, shrimps, waterfleas (*Daphneae*) and barnacles are crustaceans. The woodlouse is a terrestrial creature, and the water-flea is of microscopic size. Those crustaceans which are edible are called shellfish, though

EDIBLE CRUSTACEANS

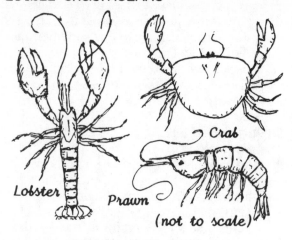

Lobster · Crab · Prawn *(not to scale)*

they are not true fish. See **shellfish**.

culinary arts The healing arts, especially in the realm of herbal medicine, are offshoots of the culinary arts, and came into being when it was first noticed that certain items of diet have health-giving and curative effects. But, as the Chinese have excelled and led the world in their mastery of the culinary arts, it must surely follow that they have excelled and led the world in their mastery of the healing arts; and that is indeed the case. See **herbal medicines**.

culinary herbs and spices Most of the common culinary herbs and spices which are almost always available in the kitchen, whether in China or the Western world, have useful medicinal properties and, together with the herbs and spices available in the field and garden, they provide a wide selection of simples, as they would be called in the West, which are inexpensive, readily available and safe to use, and which may be employed to treat quite a large number of minor and chronic ailments.

cupping This technique involves the use of a suction cup, made of bamboo or glass, in the treatment of boils, abscesses, bruises, swellings, infected wounds, asthma, some forms of arthritis and rheumatism, colds and chills. The Chinese theory underlying this technique is that it removes poisons and withdraws and disperses evil-*qi*. A piece of combustible material, such as cotton-wool or paper, is dipped into spirit, ignited and then held inside an inverted cup. The oxygen in the air inside the cup is used up by the burning material, which is then extinguished. This air has become less dense, so creating a difference in pressure between the inside and the outside of the cup. The cup is then placed at the point where treatment is required, and the resulting suction extracts pus, lymph, fat, leaked blood and foreign bodies. The author of this book once saw an elderly Chinese woman treating herself by means of this technique. She used an ordinary earthenware cup and a small candle, which she rested on her chest. What would have happened if the candle had been accidentally knocked over need hardly be a matter for conjecture. The use of a suction cup could be described as 'knifeless surgery'. The same technique was used by the physicians of the West until the end of the nineteenth century.

curative medicine The Chinese have a preference for preventive medicine, which makes sound sense, for it is often the case that conditions which can be easily prevented can be cured only with great difficulty, if at all. Therefore, in China, curative medicine is used only when preventive medicine has failed or been neglected. It is also used to treat those conditions, such as virulent infectious diseases, serious wounds and injuries and other conditions which, by their nature, cannot be treated by preventive medicine. Obviously, preventive medicine can delay or inhibit hardening of the arteries, but it cannot prevent a ruptured artery due to a stab wound or an accident. Curative techniques attempt to correct imbalances within the body and tone weak organs which have allowed diseases to develop. In addition to taking the prescribed medicines, the patient must adjust his life-style so that it fits in with the requirements of the medicines prescribed. A Chinese herbal cure is slow to take effect but, once established, it is generally permanent. Some chronic ailments require months or even years of treatment before a cure is permanently effected. See **preventive medicine**.

cuts In TCM, there are several herbal medicines for the treatment of cuts, scratches, abrasions and other small wounds. The following are effective: a wet compress of sage, *Salvia officinalis*; a poultice of sorrel, *Rumex acetosa*, leaves; a lotion of an infusion of 2–12 g thyme, *Thymus vulgare*, leaves; a wet compress or ointment of marigold, *Calendula officinalis*, flowers.

cuttlefish *Sepia esculenta* Medicine. Distribution: global. Parts: bone. Character: warm, salty. Affinity: liver, kidneys. Effects: astringent, haemostatic, antacid. Symptoms: dyspepsia, nausea, itchy skin. Treatments: stomach ulcers, biliousness, pruritis, menorrhagia, leucorrhoea, spermatorrhoea, abscesses, sores, open wounds. Dosage: 4–10 g.

cyanocobalamin Vitamin B_{12}. See **vitamin**.

cyanosis A blueness of the skin, especially around the lips and on the nose and ears, and due to a lack of oxygen in the blood.

cyst An abnormal, sac-like and fluid-filled swelling.

cystitis Inflammation of the bladder, which is generally due to an infection. See **urinary disorders**.

D

Da Costa's syndrome A state of anxiety, accompanied by palpitations and vague chest symptoms, which derives from a person's erroneous belief that his heart is diseased.

dairy products Milk, cream, butter, yoghurt and cheese do not feature prominently in the Chinese diet, for they are not regarded as being particularly healthy items of diet. All dairy products are sources of saturated fatty acids, which the body converts into cholesterol. They also contain allergens which can be causative of asthma, eczema, hay fever and other conditions. See **breast-feeding, milk and milk products** and **bovine spongiform encephalopathy**.

daltonism Colour-blindness. See **hereditary defects**.

damiana *Turnera diffusa* A plant indigenous to Mexico, Central America and Texas, and which is used in the West as an aphrodisiac and restorative for the nerves. See **aphrodisiac**.

damp-heat Also stated as 'hot-damp'. See **climate**.

dampness One of the six excesses, and which is associated with the element water, being most active in late summer and early autumn. Damp-excess conditions derive from sudden exposure to mists, fog and rain, immersion in water and dwelling in a damp place or climate. The symptoms are aching joints and limbs, sluggishness and a feeling of fullness in the chest. The dampness turns inwards if spirits, melons and greasy and sugary foods are consumed to excess, so affecting the spleen, the symptoms being vomiting, diarrhoea and a distended stomach.

dancing Various artifacts unearthed by archaeologists in Changsha, in China, indicate that, about 2300 BC, the Chinese were using dancing as a treatment for arthritis. See **healing exercises**.

dandelion *Taraxacum officinale* Herbal medicine. Distribution: temperate regions worldwide. Parts: all. Character: cold, bitter-sweet. Affinity: liver, stomach. Effects: antipyretic, antidote, reduces swellings, mildly diuretic and aperient. Symptoms: fever, headaches. Treatments: influenza, abscesses, breast tumours, blood clots in lungs, constipation. Dosage: 10–30 g.

The juice from the stems may be applied to warts, so causing them to shrivel. It may also be applied to bites from venomous snakes. In Europe, a delicious wine with health-giving properties is made from the flowers. The dandelion is rich in vitamin C, carotene, iron, potassium and manganese. It is much relished as a salad vegetable in China, whereas in the West it is regarded as a troublesome weed. Its preventive and curative properties as described above are as they would occur in a Chinese herbal, but herbalists in the West would say that it can also be used as a digestive and hepatic tonic and in the treatment of urinary problems in general, hepatic and post-hepatic jaundice, gallstones and chronic joint and skin inflammations.

dandruff There is some doubt about the causes of dandruff, of which the symptom is an excessive shedding of flakes of dead skin cells; but, in its severest state, it could be a form of seborrhoeic eczema, and involving a dry scalp, over-production of skin cells, debilitation in general health and bacterial infection of the sebum, which is a natural oil secreted by the hair follicles. Suitable treatments are lotions made as infusions of 2–12 g thyme, *Thymus vulgare*, leaves and 4–10 g burdock, *Arctium lappa*, leaves, and a poultice of the crushed fresh leaves and stems of watercress, *Nasturtium officinale*. Additionally, the sufferer should avoid using shampoos, wearing a hat and using a sharp comb or brush, and he should keep his scalp clean with surgical spirit or gin! The diet should be low in fats and carbohydrates, and high in fruits and vegetables.

dangers with medicines There are some dangers involved with the taking of medicines, herbal or otherwise. Therefore, the following instructions should be read very carefully – they could prevent a few mishaps:

1. Do NOT take medicine when it is unnecessary, and on the misleading principle that one cannot have too much of a good thing.
2. Do NOT rely too much on medicines. For many ailments, there are other forms of treatment, such as diet, exercise, massage and acupuncture, which are more effective than medicines. A mistaken belief in medicines and a total dependence on them will lead to hypochondria, which is a form of mental illness. However, this advice does not apply to those preventive medicines which are regularly taken by the Chinese, and which are not intended to be curative.
3. Do-it-yourself medicine may be satisfactory for the treatment of many minor and chronic ailments, but with more complex

illnesses, especially where the cause has not been accurately diagnosed, as with persistent headaches, anxiety and circulatory and menstrual defects, and there are manifestations of complications and a serious condition, professional medical advice should be sought.

4. Medicines generally operate at their most effective level only when they are taken within the prescribed limits. Therefore, stated doses must NOT be misread, and so, perhaps, exceeded. Overdoses of medicines of any kind, including those proprietary brands regarded as safe and which may be obtained without a doctor's prescription from a grocery store, may lead to a disaster, and even be fatal.

5. Mineral substances, such as Glauber's salt, must be obtained from a pharmacy to ensure that they are of the standard required by the *British Pharmacopoeia Codex*. Commercial forms usually contain impurities.

6. Certain medicines must NOT be administered to pregnant women. These medicines include medicinal wines, mugwort, sage, penny royal, thyme, basil and marjoram.

7. Certain medicines must NOT be administered where there is a heart condition or treatment for cancer is being undergone. A powerful cathartic could lead to disaster in these situations.

8. Medicines which are beneficial in one situation may be harmful in another. Aspirin may be good for a headache, but it can severely irritate the membranes of the stomach. Therefore, in using a medicine, it is important to make sure that it is appropriate for the condition being treated.

9. Some medicines are mutually negating in their effects, or even dangerous, when taken together. Such combinations must be avoided.

10. Many medicines cannot be safely taken with alcohol or certain foods, such as cheese, eggs or fish.

11. Some medicines give rise to allergies. Unfortunately, an awareness of the ill-effects of these is generally produced only by experience.

12. Medicines for external use may be unsafe for internal use, and vice versa.

13. The correct part of a herb must be used. For example, the stems of rhubarb, *Rheum raponticum*, can be consumed quite safely, but its leaves are poisonous.

14. There are two broad guidelines to be offered in dealing with medicines of any kind. BE VERY CAREFUL and TAKE NOTHING FOR GRANTED.

dan shen *Salvia miltiorrhiza* Herbal medicine. Distribution: North China, Manchuria, Japan. Parts: roots. Character: cool, bitter. Affinity: heart, pericardium. Effects: sedative, anticoagulant, refrigerant, tonic, improves blood circulation. Symptoms: abdominal pains, bodily pains, chest pains, palpitation, insomnia. Treatments: amenorrhoea, metrorrhagia, mastitis, thrombosis. Dosage: 4–6 g. This herb is in the sage family of plants. It must NOT be confused with *dang shen, Codonopsis tangshen*.

dang shen *Codonopsis tangshen* Herbal medicine. Distribution: North China. Parts: roots. Character: warm, sweet. Affinity: lungs, spleen. Effects: stomachic, tones lungs and spleen. Symptoms: shallow and stertorous breathing, tiredness, loss of appetite, dyspepsia, insomnia. Treatments: exhaustion, prolapse of rectum. This herb is similar to ginseng in its medicinal properties, but it is less potent – and less expensive. It is sometimes called the 'poor man's ginseng'. It must NOT be confused with *dan shen, Salvia multiorrhiza*.

dan medicines These medicines, which are usually in the form of pills or powders, contain very potent mineral substances, some of which are toxic, and which were originally used, thousands of years ago, in making an elixir of life, which would confer immortality on its users. The Chinese word *dan* means 'elixir'.

dao yin A system of psycho-physiological exercises which was introduced during the era of the Warring Kingdoms (476–221 BC) by the Taoists as a means of preventing and treating certain illnesses. See **healing exercises**.

Dao Yin Tin This work, published in 168 BC, depicts exercises in unusual healing skills as they were first practised in China. Physical exertion is combined with mental control. See **healing exercises**.

'dead man's fingers' The finger-like sections of the gills of lobsters and crabs, and which must be removed before consumption.

deaf-mutism See **hereditary defects**.

deafness Loss of hearing has a variety of causes, which include blockage by wax, a damaged eardrum, infection, inflammation, abnormal bone formation in the ossicles and a damaged auditory nerve. Deafness due to infection and some types of inherited deafness can be cured by acupuncture. Wax and mucus following an infection can be treated with warm lotions of infusions of 2–4 g peppermint, *Mentha piperita*, leaves, 4–10 g chrysanthemum, *Chrysanthemum morifolium*, flowers, 5–9 g plantain, *Plantago asiatica*, seeds and 5–7 g self-heal, *Prunella* *vulgaris*, flowers or seeds. Deafness due to old age can be treated with infusions, taken internally, of 10–12 g *han lian cao*, *Eclipta prostrata*, leaves and 10–12 g eucommia, *Eucommia ulmoides*, bark.

death Among the older generation of peasants, there are a few people who believe that their ancestors exist in spirit form, and, if not placated, will haunt and molest their descendants. But the educated Chinese take the Confucian view that earthly affairs are of much more significance, and are certainly better understood, than some imaginary residence in the sky. They also take the view that a long and healthy life of vigorous youthfulness is as near as they will ever get to a state of immortality, and that, though the individual will cease to exist at death, he will take on the role of a worthy ancestor if he has lived worthily, and this will help to ensure the worthiness and the continuance of the Chinese race. According to TCM, death occurs when the whole of *yuan qi*, or 'primordial vital energy', has been dissipated. See **air** and **yuan qi**.

debility Feebleness of health. It has a wide range of symptoms, including lassitude, nervousness, loss of appetite and sleeplessness, some of which can be misleading. An infusion of 10–12 g angelica, *Angelica sinensis*, roots taken internally is considered to be an effective treatment, but the Chinese have a wide range of tonic medicines, all of which are helpful in treating this condition, though a sound diet, exercise, sleep and peace of mind constitute the best remedy. See **tonic**.

decoction This is much stronger than an infusion, and is prepared by adding the stated dosage of the herb to ½ litre water in an earthenware cooking pot, bringing to the boil and then simmering until the liquid has about half of the volume of the original water. The degree of concentration is determined by the heat applied and the amount of plant material used and the length of time for which it is simmered. This method is preferable to an infusion when preparing extracts from seeds, bark and other hard parts. Flowers and other delicate parts will need to be simmered gently over low heat for only a short time, perhaps for no more than a few minutes, whereas minerals will need to be boiled over high heat for a long time, which could be as much as a whole day. Tonic herbs will generally need to be gently simmered for a long time. See **broth**.

decongestant A medicine to reduce swelling or congestion. In TCM, some decongestants are infusions or decoctions of the following taken internally, using the parts and dosages indicated: grains of paradise, *Amomum xanthoides*, seeds, 2–4 g; mandarin orange, *Citrus reticulata*, rind of fruit, 3–7 g; trifoliate orange, *Poncirus trifoliata*, unripe fruits, 5–8 g; balloon flower, *Platycodon grandiflorum*, roots, 3–5 g; yellow starwort, *Inula britannica*, flowers, 3–8 g; coltsfoot, *Tussilago farfara*, flowers and floral buds, 3–8 g; gulf seaweed, *Sargassum fusiforme*, all parts, 6–10 g; Job's tears, *Coix lacryma-jobi*, seeds, 12–28 g.

defaecation Evacuation of the bowel.

defence See **survival**.

deficiency disease A disease or defect due to the lack of certain vitamins or minerals in the diet. See **vitamin** and **mineral**.

deficient-qi See **qi**.

deflection treatment This is one of the eight methods of treatment by herbs in TCM. Medicines are used to correct imbalances within the body by reorientating energy and dispelling congestion, accumulations of stagnant food and sputum and other forms of unwanted liquid. There are five types of deflection treatment: improving energy, purifying blood, stimulating digestion, transferring moisture and liquifying sputum.

defloration 'Loss of virginity'. Rupture of the hymen.

dehydration An abnormal reduction of the water in the body as a consequence of severe perspiration, vomiting or diarrhoea. Excessive urination, as when imbibing alcoholic drinks, can cause dehydration. Obviously, one needs to take in more water in hot weather than in cold weather in order to offset that lost as perspiration. A decoction of 15–30 crushed grains of wheat, *Triticum aestivum*, taken internally will help to prevent dehydration by perspiration. See **perspiration**, **salt** and **diaphoretic treatment**.

delirium A condition of mental confusion characterized by excitement and restlessness. It is often accompanied by hallucinations.

delirium tremens A condition of delirium accompanying severe alcoholism. This is one of those many instances where a Chinese physician would be inclined to say, 'Why bother to search for a cure for a condition which can be easily prevented?'

delivery Giving birth to a baby.

delusion A fixed and irrational belief. See **illusion**.

dementia A condition of chronic mental deterioration, usually with loss of memory and intellectual ability.

dementia paralytica See **general paralysis of the insane**.

dementia praecox See **schizophrenia**.

demulcent Emollient. A medicine which soothes inflamed or irritated mucous membranes. An infusion of honey is an effective demulcent in the treatment of inflamed membranes in the mouth and throat. Some demulcents in TCM are infusions or decoctions of the following taken internally, using the parts and dosages indicated: coltsfoot, *Tussilago farfara*, flowers and floral buds, 3–8 g; plantain, *Plantago asiatica*, seeds, 5–8 g; mandarin orange, *Citrus reticulata*, rind of fruit, 3–7 g; balloon flower, *Platycodon grandiflorum*, roots, 3–5 g.

dense-fluid See **jin ye**.

dental caries See **caries**.

dentifrice A paste or powder for cleaning the teeth. Some Chinese manage very well with a dentifrice which is a mixture of equal parts of salt (sodium chloride) and powdered eggshells, the former being antiseptic and the latter being abrasive.

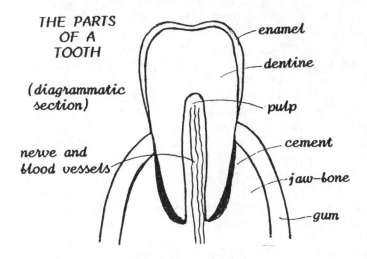

THE PARTS OF A TOOTH

(diagrammatic section)

enamel

dentine

pulp

cement

nerve and blood vessels

jaw-bone

gum

dentine A very hard substance of which the main part of the tooth is composed.

dentistry In the West, teeth are extracted on the principle that an extracted tooth is preferable to an aching tooth. In China, the traditional and common-sense view is that teeth are intended for a very important purpose, and so it must be more advantageous to have bad teeth than no teeth at all. After all, pain can be managed. But, in any case, in so far as decayed teeth are a consequence of poor diet, there is sure to be a lower incidence of dental caries in China than in the West. To some extent, dental treatment of the kind carried out in the West is a cosmetic exercise. See **toothache**.

depression An abnormal condition of deep and long-lasting melancholy. It may arise from debility or changes in the hormone levels, which the Chinese would regard as imbalances of energy and the presence of evil-*qi* or stagnation of liver-*qi*. It is sometimes due to an event which gives cause for extreme sadness, but which affects the sufferer with a severity which is irrational and out of all proportion to what would be regarded as its normal impact. However, there is no easy solution in this regard. Some people have delusions, illusions and complexes, and some are more strong-minded than others, and so what is a mere trifle for one person could be a calamity for another. TCM treatments include an infusion or decoction of the following taken internally, using the parts and dosages indicated: scullcap, *Scutellaria baicalensis*, roots, 5–7 g; angelica, *Angelica sinensis*, roots, 8–14 g; longan, *Euphoria longan*, flesh of fruits, 8–14 g; eucommia, *Eucommia ulmoides*, bark, 8–14 g. Note that Chinese scullcap, *Scutellaria baicalensis*, must not be confused with the scullcap, *Scutellaria laterifolia*, used in the West, and which is indigenous to North America, though they have similar properties. Also beneficial are basil, *Ocimum basilicum*, leaves, 3–5 g, thyme, *Thymus vulgare*, leaves, 2–12 g, and peppermint, *Mentha piperata*, leaves and stems, 2–4 g. A traditional treatment among the Chinese peasantry is a tea made by infusing a mixture of 25 g crushed grains of wheat, *Triticum aestivum*, and 10 g roots of Chinese liquorice, *Glycyrrhiza uralensis*, and adding 10 g honey or brown sugar. Acupuncture is often helpful, as also are the *qi gong* exercises. But a sound diet, regular elimination from the bowel, adequate exercise, sleep, laughter and association with normal, friendly and understanding people is probably the most effective remedy of all.

Dercum's disease See **adiposis dolorosa**.

dermatitis Inflammation of the skin which is generally regarded as a less chronic form of eczema. See **eczema**.

dermis The deeper layer of skin, just below the epidermis, which contains the blood vessels, nerve endings, hair follicles and sebaceous glands.

descending A term used in Chinese medicine to describe those illnesses which have a depressive, or lowering effect, and which appear to enter deeply into the body, so affecting the internal organs. Descending illnesses need to be treated with ascending medicines, which will elevate and scatter vital energy, as with perspiring or vomiting. Descending illnesses are yin, empty and cold or cool, and descending medicines are suppressive or sedative, downward moving or inward moving, and have a concentrative effect. See **ascending**.

desquamation The flaking and shedding of dead skin. This is a normal process but it can be excessive with some conditions, such as dandruff.

detergent See **chemicals**.

detoxification The removal of poison. But this should not be confused with the counteraction of poison, as is done with an antitoxin or antidote. See **antitoxin**.

dextrose See **sugar**.

dhobie itch A fungal infection of the skin of the groin. The medicinal treatment can be the same as for athlete's foot; but, of course, it is to the groin that the compress and liquid are applied, not the feet. See **athlete's foot**. One chopped and crushed fresh garlic clove consumed daily is also helpful.

diabetes insipidus A rare condition in which abnormally large amounts of urine are passed, and which is caused by the pituitary gland failing to secrete the appropriate hormone to regulate the function of the kidneys. This condition is not related to diabetes mellitus, a much more common and entirely different condition.

diabetes mellitus Known commonly as sugar diabetes or more simply as diabetes, this condition must not be confused with diabetes insipidus, a rare and totally different condition, though their symptoms are similar in their initial stages – unquenchable thirst and passing abnormally large amounts of urine. The cause is the failure of the pancreas to produce sufficient insulin, which is the hormone that controls the level of blood sugar. The condition may be hereditary or due to a virus infection. Its symptoms include swelling, redness, bruises, cracks, cuts and infections of the feet, together with drowsiness and extreme emaciation in severe cases. Do-it-yourself treatment is not advisable for diabetes, and professional medical advice should be sought. In the West, severe cases are treated with regular injections of insulin, and less severe cases are treated with insulin tablets, and so, provided that the patient is careful and does not neglect his medication, he can live a full life despite his condition. The mildest cases can usually be treated with diet alone. The diet of the diabetic should contain little or no alcohol or caffeine, and plenty of green and red vegetables, such as lettuce, brassicas and carrots, and his meals should be smaller. The Chinese have a wide range of herbal medicines which act by reducing the level of blood sugar or toning the kidneys or pancreas. Complete cures have been effected in some of those cases where patients have been insulin-dependent. These medicines include the bean, *Phaseolus vulgaris*, plantain, *Plantago asiatica*, dogwood, *Cornus officinalis*, wolfberry, *Lycium chinense*, knotty yam, *Dioscorea opposita*, ginseng, *Panax ginseng*, gentian, *Gentiana macrophylla*, water plantain, *Alisma plantago-aquatica*, cork tree, *Phellodendron amurense*, lotus, *Nelembo nucifera*, and greater burdock, *Arctium lappa*. Ch'ao Yuen Fan, a physician of the time of the Sui dynasty, explained in his medical classic *Chu Ping Yuan Hou Lun*, or 'About the Causes of Diseases', how exercise could be used to reduce the ill-effects of diabetes-related ailments. He suggested that the sufferer should take 120 paces or more, but not more than 1000 paces, before taking a meal, and then take 200 paces. Wang Shou, a physician of the period of the Tang dynasty, gave similar advice, but he went further by suggesting that exercise could be used to prevent diabetes and not merely mitigate some of its ill-effects. The explanation is that exercise utilizes the excess sugar in the bloodstream. For mild diabetes, Chinese physicians would recommend *qi gong* and *tai chi chuan*. However, these exercises should not be taken without medical advice, for, if overdone, the level of blood sugar may fall too low, so inducing a coma.

diagnosis Two of the main weaknesses of any system of medicine in any part of the world are inaccurate diagnosis and the temptation to treat symptoms rather than the actual illnesses. But, since some totally unrelated illnesses, minor or severe, have similar symptoms, it is easy enough for a physician to make an error of judgement. But even the layman would perceive that, though sedatives and soporific medicines have their value, especially as a temporary measure, sleeping tablets are not the ideal way to treat a condition of which insomnia is only a symptom, nor are tranquillizers the best way to treat a state of anxiety which has a fundamental emotional or physical cause. Chinese physicians are very much aware of the perils involved in merely suppressing symptoms, particularly aches and pains. The nervous system is, among its various functions, the body's alarm system, and the aches and pains which it manifests are nature's way of proclaiming that something is amiss. To treat backache with a mild diuretic, such as barley water, from the wide range of medicines that are available, instead of treating the disease or dysfunction of which it is a symptom, is just about as sensible as trying to extinguish a fire by switching off the fire-alarm. However, it must be conceded that there are some extremely painful and distressing conditions for which there is no cure, and then the alleviation of pain is as much as the physician can hope to achieve. But the complete conquest of pain is a tremendous medical advance in itself. Who would deny terminally-ill patients the right to 'shuffle off this mortal coil' without pain and with dignity? See **pain** and **symptom**. Over the centuries, Chinese physicians have evolved a wide range of techniques by which they are able to make accurate diagnoses, and in so doing, they are sometimes as much concerned with the signs of health as with the symptoms of illness, for they need to be assured that the remedies they are applying are operating to good effect, which is not likely to be the case if they have made a wrong diagnosis. The diagnostic techniques employed by a Chinese physician are basically the same as those used by his counterpart in the West, the essential difference being that he uses them more extensively, and probably more skilfully, for Chinese medicine is much older than Western medicine, and the TCM practitioner generally has no X-rays, cardiograms and the like to aid him. With so much care and complication in diagnosis, it follows that a medical examination in China is always thorough, never cursory. In TCM, diagnosis has three main stages, the first being *si zhen*, or consultation, at which the physician obtains all the information he can about the patient's condition by the four basic methods of discussion, observation, hearing and touch. See **consultation**. The second is *ba gang*, or differential diagnosis, by which an illness is classified according to its symptoms and nature within a broad framework of eight principles. The third is an extension or modification of the original diagnosis, and is based upon the effects produced by the treatment. Thus, a herbal remedy not only prevents, alleviates or cures but may also provide some additional information about the patient's condition. This is a safeguard against errors in diagnosis. The physician may need to revise the treatment. See **yin-yang diagnosis** and **ba gang**.

diagnostic combinations The symptoms, causes and nature of an illness do not exist in isolation, and they need to be considered as a whole if a treatment is to be truly effective. Thus, a condition which is regarded as external may be either hot and yang or cold and yin, though it is more likely to be hot and yang. Similarly, a condition which is regarded as internal may be either full and yang or empty and yin, though it is more likely to be empty and yin. Here, of course, there is an example of the Taoist yin-yang principle that nothing can be either completely positive or completely negative – external or internal, hot or cold, full or empty, and so on. Thus, the Chinese physician is sometimes on the horns of a dilemma in trying to decide whether in

177

suppressing rebellious-*qi* in one direction he might be encouraging it in another. To the Western mind, this may seem to be a senseless approach, yet TCM practitioners are often successful in situations where Western physicians fail. But, unlike the physicians of the West, Chinese physicians do not take the view that there is a cut-and-dried solution – or no solution at all – for each and every illness. For example, a medicine which is effective in the treatment of a certain condition in one patient would not necessarily be effective in the treatment of the same condition in another patient. A medicine for an external-cold ailment would not be suitable for an external-hot ailment. In this respect, there are a number of factors to be considered. Safety is one of them. A medicinal wine may be excellent as a tonic for a young man who is basically healthy, but it could be disastrous for an elderly person with a heart condition. This table shows some examples of simple diagnostic combinations:

SOME DIAGNOSTIC COMBINATIONS

Principles	Symptoms
external-hot	feverishness, headaches, aversion to draughts, occasional perspiration, rapid and fluctuating pulse, red tongue with white or pale-yellow fur
external-cold	fever, chills, headaches, body aches, dry skin, heavy pulse, normal tongue with thin white fur
internal-hot	feverishness, fidgety, bloodshot eyes, great thirst, rapid pulse, red tongue with yellow fur
internal-cold	aversion to coldness, cold hands and feet, loose stools, low and jumpy pulse, white and smooth fur on tongue
external-full	headaches, body aches, dry skin, jumpy pulse, normal tongue with white fur
external-empty	aversion to draughts, perspiration, slow and fluctuating pulse, pale tongue
internal-full	heavy breathing, perspiration on hands and feet, abdominal fullness, strong pulse, hard tongue with thick yellow fur

internal-empty	weakness, shortness of breath, diarrhoea, weak pulse, pale-red tongue with pale and thin fur

One notices that the symptoms for each combination are a mixture of the symptoms associated with each of its two principles when they stand alone. A combination such as external-hot is obviously yang, and one such as internal-cold is obviously yin. But what of a combination such as external-cold? It could be a little more yin than yang, or a little more yang than yin. But which? A Chinese physician of long experience would be able to answer this question. He would consider both the symptoms and the ailment, and then decide whether the effects on the vital organs were more suppressive than stimulating, or more stimulating than suppressive. See **symptoms** and **yin-yang diagnosis**. The combinations shown in the table are no more than simple examples, but other, more elaborate, combinations are possible – external-hot-damp, internal-cold-windy, etc.

diaphoresis Perspiration, especially when excessive. See **hyperhidrosis**.

diaphoretic Sudorific. A medicine which induces or increases perspiration. Some commonly used diaphoretics in TCM are as follows, taken internally as infusions or decoctions, using the parts and dosages indicated: ginger, *Zingiber officinale*, root, 3–8 g; *cong bai* (Chinese spring onion), *Allium fistulum*, roots and stems, 4–10 g; joint fir, *Ephedra sinica*, stems, 4–10 g; cassia (Chinese cinnamon), *Cinnamomum cassia*, young stems, 2–5 g; corn mint, *Mentha arvensis*, leaves and stems, 2–4 g.

diaphoretic treatment This is one of the eight methods of treatment by herbs in TCM. Diaphoretics, which induce perspiration, are used to counteract the effects of ailments due to external exposure. Diaphoretics are of two types: warm, which are used to treat wind-cold ailments, and cold, which are used to treat wind-heat ailments.

diaphragm See **hiatus hernia**.

diarrhoea A condition in which loose and fluid stools are frequently passed. Its causes include improperly cooked or contaminated food, impure water, infections by micro-organisms, such as bacteria and viruses, lactose intolerance and medications taken for other conditions. Generally, it should not be viewed with alarm, for it is one of the body's defence mechanisms in so far as it eliminates unwanted or harmful substances. On the other hand, if excessive, it can cause dehydration and debility. Dietary treatment can be effected by avoiding dairy products, carminative (gas-producing) foods, such as Brussels sprouts, cabbage, peas and baked beans, foods which can contribuite to dehydration, such as bread, cereal products, apples, pears, peaches, plums, prunes and potatoes, and antacids and other medications which are likely to be causative of diarrhoea. The bowel should be given a rest by following a liquid diet of clear, thin soup, such as chicken broth. Dehydration can be offset with a drink, taken often, of 4 pinches salt and 2 teaspoons honey to 1 litre water. When back on solid food, the intake should consist of non-irritant foods, such as toast, bananas, hard-boiled eggs and boiled carrots. TCM remedies include infusions or decoctions of the following, taken internally, using the parts and dosages indicated: garlic, *Allium sativum*, 3 cloves; hawthorn, *Crataegus pinnatifida*, fruits, 5–15 g; plantain, *Plantago asiatica*, seeds, 5–9 g; cassia (Chinese cinnamon), *Cinnamomum cassia*, bark, 1–3 g; water plantain, *Alisma plantago-acquatica*, tubers, 4–14 g; comfrey, *Symphitum officinale*, leaves or roots, 3–12 g. Also helpful are suspensions of talc (magnesium silicate), powder, 4–10 g, and oyster, *Ostrea rivularis*, crushed shells, 4–10 g. Scullcap, *Scutellaria baicalensis*, roots, 5–7 g, and cork tree, *Phellodendron amurense*, bark, 4–5 g, are considered to be very effective. A homely and traditional remedy much favoured by Chinese peasants is an infusion of 2 tablespoons each of ginger powder and green tea in ½ litre boiling water, and drunk as a tea. Chinese physicians sometimes recommend blood-letting as a treatment for diarrhoea, especially if it is of the full-hot type. See **white rice porridge**.

diastase See **maltose**.

diet The Chinese certainly do not underestimate the importance of food as a means of keeping healthy. Over 2000 years ago, the eminent sage Confucius (551–479 BC), pointed out that food and sex are vital to man's existence, and to treat them as if they were otherwise would be an unnatural act, and also one of immense folly. They are two of man's most fundamental needs; and his other needs, if not superfluous, are only ancillary to food and sex. Here, the term *food* is meant to be inclusive of water, air, warmth and light, which are components of the nutritional process. Food of the right kind ensures the health and longevity of the individual, and sex ensures the continuance of the race. As far as the Chinese are concerned, diet is not just a matter of nutriment. It is the basis of preventive medicine, of which herbal remedies are an offshoot. If a person has a wholesome diet, he is less likely to succumb to disease, and also, if disease does strike, it is likely to be less debilitating. It is their preoccupation with diet which has given the Chinese a complete mastery of the art of living. They have always recognized that the diet must be regulated, and in this, it is as much a matter of ethics as nutrition and health. And to the Chinese mind, ethics means social harmony, and health means bodily harmony. It must indeed be the case that a country which allows its citizens to be ill fed and unhealthy cannot be said to have ethical standards. With diet, as with all else, the Chinese pursue the middle way, which is the way of harmony, and so they avoid the extremes of gluttony and fasting, just as they avoid the extremes of promiscuity and celibacy, which they regard as being unhealthy. In China, many medications are administered as items of diet, and the principles which govern herbal therapy also govern the intake of food. Cold foods, which are yin, are consumed to prevent heat-excess conditions, which are yang, whereas hot foods are consumed to offset cold conditions. In this respect, the legendary emperor Shen Nong gave the Chinese some good advice: 'Treat hot illnesses with cooling medicines, and treat cold illnesses with warming medicines.' One can be sure that, in this, he did not differentiate strictly between what is a medicine and what is a food. Foods are classified in the same way as medicines, that is, by the four energies and the five tastes, or as stimulating or suppressive, toning or sedative, yin or yang, and so on. In TCM, food is the first stage in defence. Sun Simiao, one of the great physicians of the period of the Tang dynasty (618–907) advised people to resort to medicine only when food fails to effect a cure or an alleviation. See **dietetics**, **food**, **longevity** and **sex**.

dietary fibre Roughage. This is the collective term for those indigestible substances of plant origin, mainly cellulose, which absorb water and so add moisture and bulk to the stools, so encouraging a regular and easy evacuation of the bowel. A diet that is high in fibre and accompanied by a high intake of liquid is generally the most effective way of preventing constipation. The best sources of dietary fibre are cereals and cereal products, pulses, fruits and vegetables. Dietary fibre does not occur in substances of animal origin, which is one of the several reasons why the Chinese regard a meat-rich diet as being unhealthy.

dietary treatment The treatment of many ailments, either as a whole or in part, can often be effected by dietary methods, particularly if they are accompanied by physical and breathing exercises. Many Chinese medicines can be administered as items of diet, and most culinary herbs and spices can also be employed as medicines. Anyone who takes the trouble to study a Chinese cookbook of the more authoritative kind will find many recipes for dishes which are specifically designed to prevent, alleviate or cure certain undesirable bodily conditions. Furthermore, the Chinese diet is balanced and varied, and so those people who adhere to a Chinese diet are not likely to fall victim to deficiency diseases. See **diet** and **vitamin**.

dietetics The study of nutrition, and which, in both China and the West, involves the prescribing of certain diets or specific foods for the treatment of various ailments and other bodily conditions. In the West, the scientific study of food has been pursued for no more than about 200 years, but, in addition to its many benefits, it seems to have produced a wide range of fears and phobias; and, with some people, dieting and the use of drugs and 'natural foods', deceptively advertised in glowing terms, to reduce weight and 'defeat cellulite' has become a fetish, which is sometimes associated with bulimia and anorexia nervosa. Some people have an inherited predisposition to obesity, it is true, and others put on weight as a consequence of lack of exercise and a surfeit of fatty, sugary and starchy foods; but, in general, these conditions can be treated in a common-sense and non-drastic way by a judicious regulation of the diet in terms of balance and variety. The Chinese have fever problems and no fetishes in this regard, for their diet, based on over 5000 years of culinary experience, is balanced and varied and has in-built components which are conducive to both sound nutrition and health protection, and they certainly have no need of diet sheets, crash courses to induce weight loss and other similar devices. Here, the Chinese principle, which is simple but effective, is that if one's diet is balanced and varied, one cannot have too much of what is harmful, nor too little of what is beneficial. One of the most significant aspects of dietetics as studied in the West is the realization that the health and proper functioning of the body is largely determined by vitamins, enzymes and hormones. For example, men who have a high level of testerone, the male sex hormone, in the blood, have total immunity to some diseases and a high resistance to others. Thus, recent scientific research in the West has confirmed what the Chinese have known for thousands of years: diet is as much a matter of health as one of nutrition, and that foodstuffs, whether plant or animal in origin, contain energies, or essences, some of which are similar to those already contained in the body, and which are essential to its general functioning, and also tone or stimulate the vital organs and promote longevity and resistance to disease. See **vitamin, enzyme, hormone** and **humour**.

dieting For the treatment of certain conditions, such as those due to mineral or vitamin deficiencies, dieting can be a valuable treatment, but it must be carried out under proper medical supervision, for an excess of minerals or vitamins can sometimes be as damaging as a deficiency. But the term *dieting* is generally used in reference to those weight-reducing regimens which some people choose to follow in an attempt to achieve a youthful appearance. The benefits of this kind of dieting are sometimes more aesthetic than clinical, and sometimes not even that, though a weight reduction, provided it is not too drastic, is generally of benefit to the heart. But obesity is sometimes associated with other conditions, and so medical advice should be sought before embarking upon a programme of dieting. For most people in a normal state of health, a Chinese-style diet consisting, by weight, of 40 per cent cereal, 30 per cent vegetables, 20 per cent miscellaneous – fish, shellfish, eggs, vegetable oil, etc. – and 10 per cent meat is adequate, and does away with all the complications of dietary planning. See **diet, dietetics, food** and **obesity**.

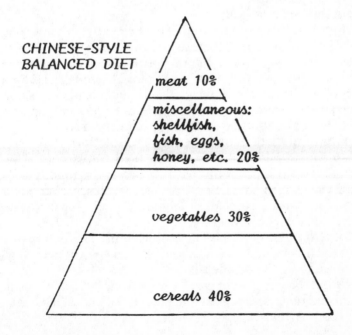

CHINESE-STYLE BALANCED DIET

meat 10%

miscellaneous: shellfish, fish, eggs, honey, etc. 20%

vegetables 30%

cereals 40%

differential diagnosis See **ba gang**.

digestion The chemical processes, occurring in the mouth, stomach and duodenum, which convert foods into simpler forms so that they can be readily assimilated by the wall of the small intestine. See **ingestion, food** and **indigestion**.

digestive Appetizer. A medicine to stimulate or aid the digestion, and which must not be confused with a medicine to cure indigestion. In TCM, there is a wide range of digestive stimulants, including infusions of the following taken internally, using the parts and dosages indicated: hawthorn, *Crataegus pinnatifida*, fruits, 5–15 g; barley, *Hordeum vulgare*, germinating grains, 10–20 g; hop, *Humulus lupulus*, strobiles (cones), 1.5–3 g; fennel, *Foeniculum vulgare*, leaves 1 g, seeds 3 g; mugwort, *Artemisia vulgaris*, flower buds, 2–6 g. The Chinese much favour green tea and ginseng tea as digestives. See **white rice porridge, taro starch jelly** and **stomachic**.

digestive ailments These are shown as separate entries: **indigestion, flatulence, heartburn**, etc.

digestive tract See **alimentary canal**.

digitalis See **herbal medicines**.

dilute A term used by chemists to describe a solution in which there is a very low proportion of the dissolved substance, or solute. See **solution**.

dipsomania See **alcoholism**.

direction Traditionally, in Chinese medicine, the five vital organs have directional relationships as follows: *heart* south, *liver* east, *spleen* centre, *lungs* west, *kidneys* north. These descriptions are symbolic and have very little geographical significance. Similar symbolism is employed when describing medicines as being ascending and stimulating if yang, and descending and suppressive if yin. See **ascending, descending** and **universe**.

disciplining-qi medicines See **energy regulation**.

disease An unhealthy condition of the body, or part of the body, the mind or a plant. But this term should not be applied to those conditions which have defects or inconveniences but are not unhealthy, such as colour-blindness, a cleft palate or an amputated leg. See **illness**.

disinfectant A chemical substance which is used to destroy micro-organisms, but, unlike an antiseptic, it is too potent to be applied to human flesh. See **antiseptic**.

dislocation The displacement of a bone from its correct position. The condition is cured by manipulation, at which Chinese physicians are most adept.

dissection See **anatomy**.

disseminated sclerosis See **multiple sclerosis**.

distribution This term as used in this book refers to the natural distribution of plants and animals. It should be understood that some of the plants and animals living wild in a region are not truly indigenous, or native, to that region, but have been introduced by man or other agencies, as, for example, the Chinese wolfberry, *Lyceum chinense*, which grows wild in the hedgerows in Britain, and has escaped from gardens, and the rabbit, which has flourished in Australia, where it was introduced from Europe.

diuretic A medicine which stimulates or increases urination. Some commonly used diuretics in TCM are infusions or decoctions of the following taken internally, using the parts and dosages indicated: barley, *Hordeum vulgare*, sprouts, 10–20 g; Indian bread, *Poria cocos*, whole plant, 6–10 g; parsley, *Petroselinum crispum*, leaves and stems, 5–10 g; dandelion, *Taraxcum officinale*, all parts, 10–30 g; self-heal, *Prunella vulgaris*, seeds, flowers, 5–7 g; plantain, *Plantago asiatica*, seeds, 5–9 g; fennel, *Foeniculum vulgare*, leaves 1 g, seeds 3 g; water plantain, *Alisma plantago aquatica*, tubers, 4–15 g; burdock, *Arctium lappa*, seeds and roots, 4–10 g. Other TCM diuretics are a suspension of 4–10 g talc (magnesium silicate) powder and an extract from the gall-bladder of a pig.

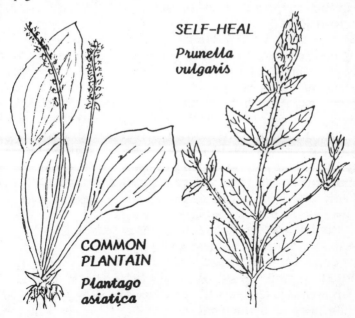

SELF-HEAL
Prunella vulgaris

COMMON PLANTAIN
Plantago asiatica

diverticulosis Inflammation of the small pouches, or diverticulli, which occur in the wall of the large intestine usually as a consequence of a long period of constipation and continual passing of hard stools. The best treatment is a diet high in fibre, such as cereals and pulses, but without fruits containing seeds which could exacerbate the condition. Infusions of 3–12 g comfrey, *Symphytum officinale*, leaves or root, and 2 crushed garlic, *Allium sativum*, cloves are helpful.

divination It would be helpful to know what the future has in store for us, particularly in matters of health, for to be forewarned is to be forearmed. The events of the past are often a guide to the future, and so it is sometimes possible to make accurate predictions. For thousands of years, the learned men of China have practised the art of divination, making predictions which are coupled with wise advice. See **I Ching** and **prediction**.

dizziness Giddiness. This condition is due to a slight change in blood pressure or a sudden change of position. An attack generally lasts for no longer than 30 seconds, but if an attack lasts longer and is accompanied by headaches and nausea, medical advice should be sought, for the cause could be serious. Chinese physicians sometimes recommend acupuncture as a treatment for dizziness. See **fainting** and **vertigo**.

dock *Rumex crispus*. This plant contains antihistamines, which explains why there is instant relief if one of its leaves are rubbed on a nettle sting.

dodder *Cuscuta japonica* Herbal medicine. Distribution: China, Japan. Parts: seeds. Character: neutral, pungent-sweet. Affinity: liver, kidneys. Effects: tonic to kidneys and liver, nourishes bones and connective tissue, improves eyesight. Symptoms: impotence, premature ejaculation, frequent and excessive urination, blurred vision. Treatments: spermatorrhoea, tinnitus, urinary incontinence, leucorrhoea, lumbago, kidney and liver deficiency. Dosage: 9–14 g.

dog meat A very warming food which is administered as a broth in those conditions where there is a yang deficiency, as with cold hands and feet, cold sweats and a weak pulse. However, it can have a toxic effect if consumed to excess.

dominant characteristic See **hereditary defects**.

dongku See **winter mushrooms**.

donggua See **winter melon**.

Dong Zhongshu A neo-Confucian scholar who, at the time of the Han dynasty (206 BC–AD 220), had so modified the Taoist philosophy of harmonious relationships that the Chinese had come to regard man as a miniature version of the universe. See **universe** and **Pangu**.

dosages These days, in TCM, dosages are measured by weight in grams, and indicate the prescribed daily intake of the dried herb, and not the infusion or decoction prepared from it. Where the fresh herb is prescribed, the quantity must be doubled. For example, 10 g fresh herb is equivalent to 5 g dried herb. If a prescription says '8 g sage leaves', the herbalist or pharmacist will prepare 8 g dried sage leaves or 16 g fresh sage leaves if no other instructions are given. The prepared infusion or decoction is usually divided into three equal parts so that it may be taken three times daily. Of course, if a large quantity of an infusion or decoction is prepared in advance, the quantity of herb will need to be adjusted accordingly. Thus, if the dosage of a herb is stated as 12 g, a week's supply of its infusion will require 84 (12 × 7) g of the dried herb or 168 (24 × 7) g of the fresh herb. The amount of water used is optional, but for most infusions, ½ litre water is satisfactory and convenient. In TCM, many dosages are non-critical, but, as a matter of safety, it is best to administer medicines within the prescribed limits. See **critical dosage**. It is also important to understand that a medicine intended for external use may be harmful if taken internally. In the pharmaceutical industry of the West, liquid medicines are prepared to such an accurately standardized degree of concentration that 1 ml of an infusion, decoction or other form of liquid extract is medicinally equivalent to 1 g fresh herb.

douche A jet of water or other liquid which is used to reach and wash inaccessible parts of the body, such as the vagina and the anus.

dragon We, in the West, regard the dragon as a legendary creature, but the Chinese believe that it was a real creature, which is not surprising since the fossilized bones of giant reptiles, now extinct, that lived millions of years ago, have been commonly found in China. These bones are powdered and used as medicines which are believed to be of great potency as aphrodisiacs. They are also expensive, for such has been the demand for these medicines that the supplies of these bones have been greatly depleted. See **White Tiger**.

dreams 'We are such stuff as dreams are made on . . .' wrote Shakespeare; and, indeed, humans do have a great capacity for imaginative thought. With a few talented people, such as inventors and novelists, this leads to immense creativity, but for most people, day-dreaming is a temporary escape from the harsh or tedious realities of life. However, fantasizing is not always harmless, for it can produce delusions, illusions, dishonest deceptions, beliefs which are remote from the truth and even insanity. It is not uncommon for a person who sets out to deceive others to end up by deceiving himself. From time to time, there emerges the odd character who declares himself to be a Messiah, and there are many people who manage to be on conversational terms with the Almighty, which is surely a supreme act of self-deception. Just as a computer can recall some of the data stored in its memory bank, so the brain can recall past events and the thoughts and sensations associated with them. If this recall occurs during sleep, when the mind is not in full operation, it is rapid and mixed-up and strange, and sometimes of the nature of fantasy, and very commonplace, very pleasant, or very frightening, as with a nightmare. Dreams occur during light sleep, when the mind is not deeply resting, and they are prompted in a wide variety of ways, such as a cold bedroom, a warm bed, a cold draught from a window, an uneven pillow, one's mood before retiring and one's current anxieties or successes. A cool draught could lead to arctic scenes, a warm bed to sexual fantasies, anxieties to nightmares, and so on. Dreams are sometimes very vivid and impressive. It was such dreams that encouraged our superstitious ancestors to believe that a human had a soul-life which could exist separately from his body. Until recent times, it was the belief of some of the Chinese peasantry that, during a dream, the soul had escaped from the body, and was able to travel to all parts of the world; and, if it did not return, the body would be without direction, and so death of the body, but not the soul, would ensue. Sadly, there are people who live in a kind of 'waking sleep', in which a dreamlike fantasy has taken over control of the mind, and so they believe quite totally in what, initially, they had regarded as a pleasant escape from reality. In the study of dreams, psychiatrists have found the keys to a better understanding of fixations, complexes and the like. Chinese physicians have long regarded dreams as being symptomatic of mental conditions. The astute physician can sometimes learn something of a person's character and state of mental health by studying his dreams, though this technique is hampered by the fact that dreams are soon forgotten. Chinese physicians are humane as well as practical, and so they recognise that day-dreaming, faith in beliefs that are remote from reality and other forms of self-deception sometimes have a therapeutic value in that they are an anodyne for the simple-minded, and providing they do not give rise to violence and other forms of outrageously antisocial behaviour, there is little harm done. In so far as dreams are concerned with past events, they may sometimes be used in making divinations. 'If you would divine the future, study the past,' said Confucius. See **nervous disorders**.

dressing A covering to protect a wound or a similar condition.

dried herbs Most of the herbs used as medicines will keep best if they are dried. The herbal enthusiast who requires only a few medicinal herbs for his own use can achieve this by storing the herbs in a dry, airy and dark or shaded place. See **collecting herbs**. But, in China, where the collecting, storage and distribution of herbs are aspects of a vast industry, the drying of herbs is done in a variety of ways as are determined by the nature of the herbs, where and when they are collected and the parts used. Impurities must be removed by washing, though some, such as plantain, must not be washed. Drying methods include exposure to direct sunlight, storage in well-ventilated shade, warming by a fire indoors and exposure to the wind.

dropsy See **oedema**.

drug A term which, strictly speaking, describes all kinds of medicinal substances, but *drugs* is more commonly used as a collective description of narcotics, hallucinogens and stimulants. A narcotic is a substance which induces drowsiness, sleep, stupor or insensibility. A hallucinogen, as its name suggests, is a substance which induces hallucinations. Some narcotics are cocaine, marijuana and opium, from which morphine and codeine are derived. Mescaline is a hallucinogen obtained from mescal buttons, which are the dried tops of peyote, a species of cactus indigenous to Mexico. See **drug effects** and **medicine**.

drug addiction This is a blight on modern society in all parts of the world, and vast profits are being made by those unscrupulous people who deal in drugs. It is only in those countries such as China and Thailand, where the law imposes severe penalties, that drug dealing is effectivelly controlled. 'Once a guy gets hooked on a drug, he can't kick the habit' is how a popular magazine has described the situation so succinctly. Chinese physicians would contend, with no little justification, that drug addiction is a self-inflicted injury, and one of those many instances where preventive methods, which are largely a matter of health education and will-power, are more effective than curative methods. Acupuncture of the ear, with a success rate of over 80 per cent, is effective as a treatment for drug addiction. But, unfortunately, the relapse rate is also very high. See

addiction, **withdrawal symptoms** and **ear acupuncture**.

drug effects Many drugs of synthetic origin have unpleasant side-effects. This is also the case with drugs of herbal origin which contain only the active ingredients. For this reason, Chinese physicians have a preference for medicines in which the whole plant is used. See **active ingredient**. It is important that, as far as is possible, drugs should be correctly prescribed for a particular condition, for a drug which will cure or alleviate one condition may exacerbate another. The taking of drugs has become a fetish among the people of the West, which is unfortunate, for better treatments are sometimes effected by diet, physical and breathing exercises, acupuncture and massage. The Canadian physician Sir William Osler (1849–1919), in his *The Principles and Practice of Medicine*, wrote: 'One of the first duties of a physician is to educate the masses not to take medicine.' However, the situation is somewhat different in China, where many medicines are taken as items of diet, and more for their preventive than for their curative effects. There are some drugs, such as narcotics and stimulants, which have harmful effects. See **drug** and **withdrawal**.

drumming See **percussion**.

dry dressing A dressing in which no liquid substances are used.

dryness This is one of the six excesses of TCM. It is governed by the element metal and is dominant in the autumn season. There are two types: hot-dryness and cold-dryness. Hot-dryness is characterized by a dry skin, which may become wrinkled and scaly, dry hair, a dry scalp, a dry mouth, cracked lips and hard, dry stools. It is harmful to the lungs, nose, throat and fluid balance of the body. Internal, or cold-, dryness is caused by vomiting, diarrhoea, haemorrhages or excessive perspiration, which conditions may be induced by certain medicines, such as cathartics and diuretics. See **dry skin**.

dry skin A condition caused by moisture being removed from the skin by over-dry air in a dry environment. The simplest treatment is to sit in a bath of warm, but not hot, water for about 20 minutes, and then apply a vegetable oil as a moisturizer to seal in the moisture in the skin. This process should be repeated several times daily.

d.t., d.t.s. Abbreviations for **delirium tremens**.

duct A tube which carries secretions from a gland.

ductless glands See **endocrine glands**.

du huo *Angelica pubescens* Herbal medicine. Distribution: Sichuan and Hubei provinces of China. Parts: roots. Character: warm, bitter-pungent. Affinity: kidneys, bladder. Effects: analgesic, antirheumatic. Symptoms: pain and stiffness of back and limbs. Treatments: rheumatism, lumbago, arthritis. Dosage: 4–9 g.

Duke of Argyll's Tea-tree See **wolfberry**.

duodenal ulcer See **ulcer**.

duodenum Situated between the stomach and the jejunum, the duodenum is the first part of the small intestine. See **alimentary canal** and **intestine**.

dye See **additives** and **food colours**.

dysentery Infection and inflammation of the large intestine. There are two types: bacterial, which is the more common, and amoebic, which occurs only in tropical and subtropical countries. See **amoebic dysentery**. But both types have the same causes: infected food, contaminated water and poor hygiene. They also have similar symptoms: abdominal pains, flatulence, vomiting and severe diarrhoea. But amoebic dysentery is the severe condition, and it should be treated by a physician. Bacterial dysentery can be treated by acupuncture. TCM treatments include infusions or decoctions of the following, taken internally, using the parts indicated: garlic, *Allium sativum*, 3 cloves; Job's tears, *Coix lacryma-jobi*, seeds 8–28 g; plantain, *Plantago asiatica*, seeds, 5–9 g; salad burnet, *Sanguisorba officinalis*, roots, 4–10 g; purslane, *Portulacea oleracea*, leaves and stems, 15–30 g; baical scullcap, *Scutellaria baicalensis*, roots, 5–8 g.

dysfunction A malfunction of an organ.

dysmenorrhoea Difficult and/or painful menstruation. TCM treatments include infusions or decoctions of the following, taken internally, using the parts and dosages indicated: peach, *Prunus persica*, kernels of the stones, 4–10 g; nut grass, *Cyperus rotundus*, roots and tubercles, 4–10 g; mugwort, *Artemisia vulgaris*, leaves, 2–6 g; wild turmeric, *Curcuma aromatica*, roots, 4–8 g. Acupressure is sometimes helpful.

dyspepsia See **indigestion**.

E

ear The diagram shows the main parts of the ear. The ear-drum, which is a thin membrane, is made to vibrate by the sound waves that enter the outer ear and travel along the auditory canal. The ossicles, which are three small bones – the malleus, incus and stapes – carry these vibrations across the middle ear to the base of the cochlea, which is a spiral-shaped sound-box that magnifies the vibrations. A fluid in the cochlea transfers the vibrations to nerve endings, and they are then transmitted as sound impulses along the auditory nerve to the brain. The three semi-circular canals, each in a different dimensional plane, have nothing to do with hearing. The movements of the fluid which they contain enables the brain to register the position and movement of the head, and so the balance of the body as a whole. See **vertigo**. The Eustachian tube connects the middle ear to the throat, which explains why infections of the nose, throat and mouth can easily affect the ears. Those who value their appearance will

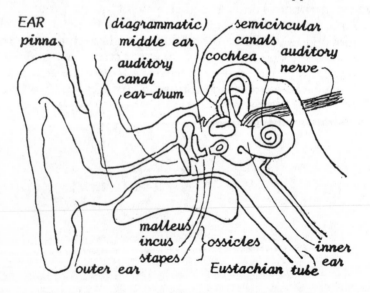

know that clean ears, together with a clean nose and clean eyes and finger-nails, are among the hallmarks of pride in one's personal hygiene. Wax in the ears is unsightly, but apart from that, it can cause defective hearing. See **tinnitus**. Do not attempt to remove wax with an instrument, for this could damage the eardrum. Instead, put a few drops of vegetable oil into the ear to soften the wax, and then, after a few days, gently squirt warm water into the ear. If this fails, consult a physician. Ear infections are generally uncommon in adults, and only occur when the sinuses become infected. Deafness has several causes. See **deafness** and **earache**.

earache A condition which has a variety of causes: blocked Eustachian tubes, colds, infected sinuses, the presence of foreign bodies, changes in atmospheric pressure, as when ascending or descending in an aircraft, allergies and infections of the nose and throat. Persistent earache may be symptomatic of a more serious condition, and so a physician should be consulted. Yawning and chewing will often open a blocked Eustachian tube. If earache occurs when in flight, hold your nose, take a mouthful of air and use your cheek muscles to force it back into the throat so that some of it will enter the Eustachian tube and the middle ear, and thereby equalize the pressure. Pain may be relieved by putting a few drops of garlic, marigold or almond oil into the ear. A sedative will relieve pain and ensure sleep at night.

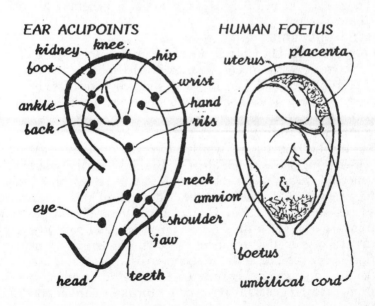

EAR ACUPOINTS

kidney, knee, hip, foot, wrist, ankle, hand, back, ribs, neck, eye, shoulder, jaw, head, teeth

HUMAN FOETUS

uterus, placenta, amnion, foetus, umbilical cord

ear acupuncture This technique, which has been in use for many centuries, is based on the principle that there are points in the outer ear which correspond to the organs of the body, and that by stimulating certain selected points, the corresponding organs will be strengthened so that the conditions associated with them will be alleviated or cured. The shape of the outer ear has some resemblance to the human foetus in its amnion. This is purely coincidental; but, many centuries ago, it may have influenced the development of this technique, with the undoubted efficacy of ear acupuncture being sufficient justification for any beliefs in this direction. Ear acupuncture is now being used, and quite successfully, in the treatment of tobacco addiction, obesity, alcoholism and drug addiction.

earth One of the five symbolic elements of Chinese philosophy and medicine, and not to be confused with *earth*, meaning 'ground', 'soil' or 'world'. It is yang and is associated with the spleen, the mind and dampness. See **element**.

earthworm *Pheritima aspergillum* Medicine. Distribution: global. Parts: whole animal. Character: cold, salty. Affinity: liver, stomach, kidneys, spleen. Effects: antipyretic, diuretic, sedative to liver, relaxant to bronchi, unblocks the meridians. Symptoms: convulsions, wind-damp pains, paralysis, difficult and/or painful urination. Treatments: stroke, asthma, swellings, hypertension, arteriosclerosis. There are hundreds of species of earthworms. The species named here is the one that is generally listed in a Chinese herbal.

east See **direction**.

eating utensils The Chinese are of the opinion that food is tainted by contact with metals, and so their spoons are made of porcelain, their ladles are of wood, their chopsticks are of wood, ivory or some other non-metallic substance, and their cooking pots are of earthenware.

ecdysis See **moulting**.

eczema This skin disease, which can cruelly undermine a person's self-esteem, causes much distress. In the West, this condition is generally regarded as being quite intractable, but Chinese physicians could claim to have had a considerable measure of success in this direction. The eczema sufferer should take heart from the attitude of the Chinese physician, and patiently accept that success in the treatment of eczema is largely a matter of time, perseverance and a trial-and-error approach. There is no definite distinction between eczema and dermatitis, but the former term is generally reserved for the more chronic condition.

Dermatitis may be defined as inflammation of the skin, and eczema as inflammation of the skin accompanied by itchiness, redness, rashes, spots, a discharge from vesicles, and exfoliation. It is popularly known as 'dry eczema' when the skin becomes thick and dry, and as 'weeping eczema' when the skin erupts and discharges. Eczema is often confused with acne, or blackheads, though they are quite different ailments. Eczema is also often associated with hay fever, asthma and a wide variety of skin complaints, such as psoriasis, pruritis, impetigo and dandruff, which is not surprising since all of these complaints may be triggered off by an allergic reaction or nervous condition, though there are some causal differences. In the Western world, medical opinion is that eczema is the adverse reaction of skin tissue to an internal or external irritant, though there could be some other causes. But this opinion is not entirely shared by Chinese physicians, who are inclined to regard eczema as being more of a symptom than an illness in itself. The suggested causes of eczema include hyperaesthesia (excessive sensitivity), hyperactivity (excessive physical activity), ageing, fatigue, sleeplessness, stress, irregular or difficult menstruation, premenstrual tension, constipation, renal problems, hormonal imbalance, radiation, viral infections, zinc deficiency, poor diet, toxins in the blood, alcoholism, the hydrogenated oils in some margarines, and many allergies. Of course, one must consider these conditions when treating eczema, though one may wonder if some of these items are the effects rather than the causes of eczema. No doubt, worrying about having eczema only serves to exacerbate the condition. The physicians of the West seem to have settled for a classification of eczema into five main types, each with its set of causes: seborrhoeic, contact, detergent, pompholyx and discoid. Seborrhoeic eczema, which is the commonest form, is inherited, and contact eczema and detergent eczema (industrial dermatitis) are caused by allergic reactions to a wide variety of substances, such as zinc, detergents, paint, textiles, pollen grains and cow's milk. Pompholyx eczema, which is due to stress, and which causes itchy and discharging vesicles to form on the palms and soles, is quite uncommon and usually clears up without treatment after a few weeks. Discoid eczema, whose cause is unknown, is also uncommon, and is characterized by reddened itchy patches which flake, discharge and become blistered and encrusted, and which last for several months. Recent research in the West has shown that the evening primrose, *Oenochera biennis*, and borage, *Borage officinalis*, are effective in the treatment of eczema because, apart from human breast-milk and the body itself, they are the only known sources of GLA (gamma-linolenic acid), an essential fatty acid which assists in the regulation of the cell activity of the body. The Chinese physician regards eczema as an external manifestation of one or more internal conditions associated with the heart, lungs, stomach and blood, and classifies them as three main types: that due to damp heat, where the skin is hot, itchy and weeping; that due to dryness-heat, where the skin is red, dry and itchy; that due to wind-heat, where the skin erupts to form scabs. As far as the general health is concerned, the eczema sufferer should take regular exercise, drink copious quantities of water, consume one clove of garlic per day, and adopt a diet that is in the Chinese style, or, failing that, to avoid beef, shellfish, eggs, refined foods, confectionery, fats and fried foods, junk food, dairy products and drinks containing stimulants. The diet should include an abundance of wholemeal cereal foods and fresh fruit and vegetables. Where eczema is accompanied by stress, ginseng, royal jelly and acupuncture are helpful. In China, the standard treatment for eczema is an infusion, taken internally, of 6 g dried root of *fang feng*, *Ledebouriella seseloides*, or stems, leaves and buds of Japanese catnip, *Schizonepeta tenuifolia*. But these herbs are indigenous only to China and Japan, and so they will have to be purchased from a Chinese herbalist, who might offer some sound advice into the bargain. The following herbs, in the dosages and for the purposes indicated, have been found to be effective in the treatment of eczema. Stinging nettle, *Urtica dioica*: as a blood cleanser, take internally as an infusion of 10 g dried herb, all parts, in 1 litre water. Drink two small cups, sipping slowly, daily for about 4 weeks. Garden nettle, *Urtica urens*: as for stinging nettle. Burdock, *Arctium lappa*: as a blood cleanser and internal antiseptic, take internally and as an infusion of 6 g dried root. Apply externally as a lotion. Dandelion, *Taraxacum officinale*: as a blood cleanser and mild aperient, and to reduce inflammation, take internally as an infusion of 15 g dried herb, all parts. Sage, *Salvia officinalis*: as a blood cleanser and mild sedative, take internally as an infusion of 6 g dried leaves. Apply externally as a decoction of 12 g fresh leaves in a compress. Comfrey, *Symphitum officinale*: to relieve pruritis, add an infusion to the bath water or apply as a lotion in a dosage of 15 g dried leaves or roots or 30 g fresh leaves or roots. Hop, *Humulus lupulus*: as a tranquilliser and to relieve insomnia, take internally as an infusion of 3 g dried strobiles (cones). Watercress,

Nasturtium officinale: to relieve itchiness and reduce inflammation, apply crushed stems and leaves as a poultice. Green cabbage and camomile, *Matricaria chamomilla*, may be used similarly. Speed-well, *Veronica officinalis*: as for stinging nettle.

eel *Anguilla anguilla*. A good source of interferon. See **interferon**.

EFFLEURAGE

←———————————————————————

light stroke away from the heart

———————————————————→

deep stroke towards the heart

effleurage A stroking technique used in massage, and which may be light or deep. In light stroking, the palms and fingers are used, and the rhythm is slow and even. In deep stroking, the whole of the hand is used and greater pressure is applied, the movement always being towards the heart in order to encourage venous flow and the elimination of toxins. Light stroking may be used either singly or in combination with deep stroking, when the two types of stroking must be in opposite directions. This form of massage also assists lymphatic circulation, and it is soothing and relaxing. See **massage** and **reflexology**.

egg-plant See **aubergine**.

eggs A rich source of protein, minerals and vitamins, but they must be fully cooked in order to destroy harmful micro-organisms, such as salmonella. Because of their association with the sexual process, they are sometimes regarded as an aphrodisiac, but this is a superstition. Eggs cannot be safely consumed with certain medicines. See **fertilization**.

ego A term used by psychologists in the West to denote the conscious mind or personality, as opposed to the *id*, which is the most primitive part of the personality, and concerned only with the basic instincts. See **super-ego**.

eight herbal treatments See **herbal treatments**.

Eight Pillars of Taoism These are the eight branches of Taoist thought and practice, which are symbolized by the eight trigrams of the Pa Kua (also written as *Ba Gua*), the symbol of Taoism, and which are supported and explained by the *Tao Te Ching*, a philosophical and political treatise written by Lao Zi,

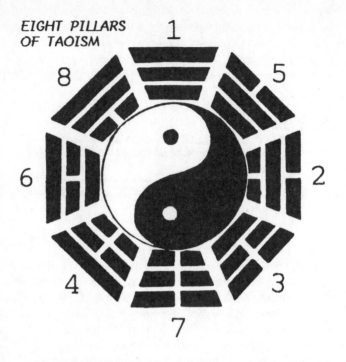

who is generally regarded as the founder of Taoism. *Tao* means 'the Way'. The Eight Pillars, which have always strongly influenced the healing arts in China, may be briefly summarized as follows:

1. The *tao* of philosophy.
2. The *tao* of revitalization.
3. The *tao* of balanced diet.
4. The *tao* of the diet of forgotten food.
5. The *tao* of healing.
6. The *tao* of sex wisdom.
7. The *tao* of supremacy.
8. The *tao* of achievement.

The numbers of the items in this summary correspond with the numbers on the symbol shown below. The central part of this symbol is the Tai Chi (also written as *T'ai Chi* or *Tai Ji*), or yin-yang, symbol. In a study of the Eight Pillars of Taoism, one becomes aware of the immense depth and complexity, but also immense practicality, of Chinese philosophy. To be successful in the art of living, say the Taoists, it is not enough to have altruistic thoughts. One must also have a healthy body and a healthy mind, together with a practical approach in matters of survival and everyday living, or as we in the West might say, 'Wise actions speak louder than empty words.' See **Tai Chi** and **I Ching**.

eight principles of differential diagnosis See **ba gang**.

ejaculation The sudden and forceful discharge of semen from the penis during sexual intercourse. See **premature ejaculation**.

élan vital 'Life-force'. The French philosopher Henri Bergson (1859–1941) postulated the concept that all living things, both plant and animal, contain a 'life-force' which is vital to their existence. When the life-force ceases to be, the physical structure ceases to function, and so assumes the condition that we know as death. This life-force conveniently provides a somewhat naïve explanation of the functioning of plants and animals, but it cannot be equated with the soul, which, according to some religious teachings, can have a separate existence from the body after the death of the body. However, these days, most scientists are extremely sceptical about Bergson's theory or any other theories about spiritual existence. See **qi**.

electro-acupuncture One of the more important advances in Chinese medicine has been the introduction of electro-acupuncture, whereby a photo-electric cell coupled to a meter indicates the areas of reduced skin resistance over the acupoints. These objective diagnostic readings enable the practitioner to proceed with greater accuracy, and he can test the patient before and after each treatment. Electro-acupuncture has confounded some of the medical experts in the West by providing conclusive evidence that the meridians and acupoints do exist, and are not a mere philosophical concept or conjecture.

element In modern chemistry, an element is defined as a substance which cannot be changed into simpler substances by a chemical process. There are about 100 natural elements: oxygen, hydrogen. sulphur, carbon, etc. But some elements exist in different forms as isotopes. An example is deuterium, an isotope of hydrogen, which combines with oxygen to form deuterium oxide, which is commonly known as 'heavy water'. And so, whilst the above definition holds good for most practical purposes, it does not tell the completely true story. The wise men of ancient Greece pondered about the structure of matter, and they came to the conclusion that all substances are composed of two or more of four elements: air, earth, fire and water. Their facts were wrong,

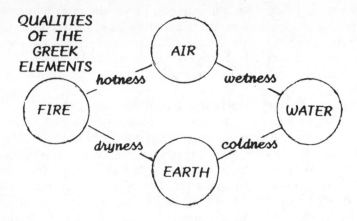

QUALITIES OF THE GREEK ELEMENTS

but their reasoning was not unsound. After all, water oozes out of the ends of a damp log when it is burning, and it produces fire, smoky vapours – or 'air' – and a residue of ash – or 'earth'. They also concluded that qualities are due to a mixing of the elements. Here, there was some degree of accuracy. Air is humid when it contains water, as with steam or water vapour. Air rising from a fire is hot. Waterlogged ground, or earth, is cold. The residue of ash, or 'earth', from a fire is dry. The Taoist sages of ancient China also gave some thought to the structure of matter, and they devised a system of five elements – fire, earth, metal, water and wood – which became well established as a component of Chinese philosophy and medicine. But these elements are not concerned with real fire, earth, metal, water and wood, but only with attributes and influences as exhibited by objects, plants, animals and humans. They are convenient labels for philos-

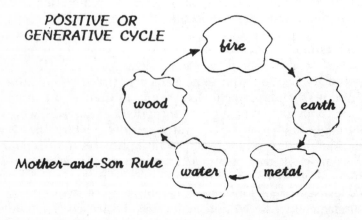

POSITIVE OR GENERATIVE CYCLE

Mother-and-Son Rule

ophical concepts, and are used in much the same way as the scientists of the West use α, β and γ (alpha, beta and gamma) – letters of the Greek alphabet – or A, B and C – letters of the Roman alphabet – to represent unknown or theoretical quantities and qualities. These five elements, together with yin and yang, encompass all the phenomena of nature, and interact in two cycles – the positive, or generative, and the negative, or suppressive. In the positive cycle, each element generates the succeeding element. Fire generates earth, earth generates metal, metal generates water, and so on, as the diagram shows. But, here, there is some association with real things. Fire does generate ash, or 'earth', earth yields metals in its ores, wood generates fire when it burns, water encourages the growth of those plants which yield wood, and metal becomes liquid, like water, when it is molten. In the negative cycle, each element suppresses the succeeding element. Thus, fire melts metal, metal cuts wood, trees and other woody plants break up earth, earth absorbs water, and water extinguishes fire. The relationships between elements in the generative cycle is described as the

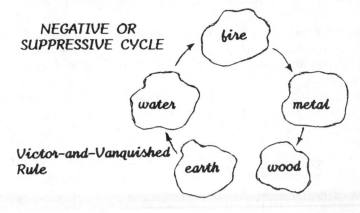

NEGATIVE OR SUPPRESSIVE CYCLE

fire
metal
wood
earth
water

Victor-and-Vanquished Rule

mother-and-son rule. Fire is mother to earth, which it generates; but fire is son to wood, which generates it; when water is son, its mother is metal; and so on. The relationships between elements in the suppressive cycle are described as the victor-and-vanquished rule. Water vanquishes fire by extinguishing it, fire vanquishes metal by melting it, metal vanquishes wood by cutting it, and so on. The generative and suppressive cycles can be shown as a single diagram, which is an aid to the memory. The qualities and functions of the vital organs and viscera are linked with the elements, as this table shows:

ELEMENTS, ORGANS AND VISCERA

Fire: heart, small intestine, triple-warmer, heart-constrictor, blood, endocrine glands
Earth: spleen, stomach, muscles
Metal: lungs, large intestine, skin
Water: kidneys, bladder, bones
Wood: liver, gall-bladder, nerves

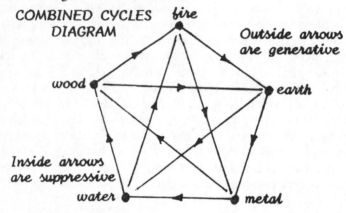

COMBINED CYCLES DIAGRAM

fire

Outside arrows are generative

wood

earth

Inside arrows are suppressive

water

metal

See **vital organs** and **viscera**. The elements also have relationships with the emotions, tastes, planets, colours and other items. It is important to understand that these relationships are not based on guesswork but are derived from long experience, with the elements being a convenient shorthand way of expressing them. For example, the planet Mars does appear to be red when viewed through a telescope, and so it should be obvious why it is said to be related to the element *fire*, the colour *red*, the climate *hot*, the organ *heart*, the emotion *joy*, the sound *laugh*, and so on. Earth and metal are yang, and fire, wood, and water are yin.

RELATIONSHIPS OF THE ELEMENTS

Fire	*Earth*	*Metal*	*Water*	*Wood*
heart	spleen	lungs	kidneys	liver
Mars	Saturn	Venus	Mercury	Jupiter
red	yellow	white	black	green
hot	damp	dry	cool	windy
joy	desire	anxiety	fear	anger
laugh	sing	weep	moan	shout
bitter	sweet	pungent	salty	sour
horse	cow	dog	pig	chicken
seven	five	nine	six	eight

elephantiasis A condition in which the skin and its underlying tissues thicken and swell because of blockage of the lymphatic vessels. It is sometimes confused with acromegaly. See **filariasis**.

elevating A term used in TCM to describe a medicine which causes energy to rise and scatter, as with perspiration or vomiting. Elevating medicines are yang, and are used to treat yin or yang-deficiency conditions.

eliminative A medicine which stimulates one or more of the eliminatory functions, which remove toxic wastes and whose full functioning is highly desirable where diseases produce chronic inflammation, as with eczema, arthritis and cancer, or where there is a high ingestion of additives and other chemicals. Eliminatives include cathartics, expectorants, diuretics, lymphatics, emetics, diaphoretics and antiseptics.

elixir An aromatic liquid medicine that is sweetened and of pleasant flavour. This term is used more specifically to denote a preparation to prolong life indefinitely – the so-called 'elixir of life' pursued by the alchemists.

emaciation A very severe loss of weight, making a person look unhealthily thin, and which is brought about by excessive dieting and certain diseases, such as anorexia nervosa, diabetes mellitus and cancer. Where the cause is dietary, a full and balanced diet, together with sedatives to reduce stress, is the treatment. Otherwise, the causative disease must be treated.

embolism The sudden blockage of an artery by an embolus. See **pulmonary embolism** and **thrombosis**.

embolus Material in the bloodstream which blocks an artery. It may be a clot, fat or an air bubble. See **thrombosis**.

embrocation See **liniment**.

embryo A developing baby from the time of conception until the beginning of the third month of pregnancy. See **foetus**.

emetic A medicine to induce vomiting, and which is of particular value where poisonous or contaminated substances have been swallowed. Induced vomiting can be very exhausting, so emetics should be administered only under proper medical supervision. But, in an emergency, a strong saline solution may be used as an emetic.

emetic treatment This is one of the eight methods of treatment by herbs in TCM. Emetic herbs, which induce vomiting, are administered to treat acute or full ailments which affect the stomach and the upper parts of the body. These herbs eliminate toxic and pathogenic matter from the stomach and small intestine. They are sometimes of benefit to the lungs.

emmenagogue A medicine to stimulate the menstrual flow. Some of the emmenagogues used in TCM are infusions or decoctions of the following taken internally, using the parts and dosages indicated: angelica, *Angelica sinensis*, roots, 10–12 g; safflower, *Carthamus tinctorius*, flowers, 3–5 g; pangolin, or scaly ant-eater, *Manis pentadactyl*, scales, 5–8 g; peach, *Prunus persica*, kernels of the stones, 5–8 g.

emollient See **demulcent**.

emotion Emotion has much clinical significance in TCM. Each of the five solid vital organs is associated with one of the emotions: heart, joy; liver, anger; spleen, desire; lungs, anxiety; kidneys, fear. In the West, the lungs are thought to be associated with anxiety, for a person's breathing is shallow, heavy or irregular when he is anxious. Also, a person who is angry is said to be liverish. The emotions also have other associations, such as the elements, planets and colours. See **element** and **seven emotions**.

emphysema A condition in which there is an abnormal accumulation of air in organs and tissues. In pulmonary emphysema, there is a permanent distension of the alveoli, or air sacs, in the lungs and their bronchioles, causing the patient to be short of breath. Pneumonia, tobacco smoke, pollutants in the atmosphere and allergies are common causes of emphysema, and chronic bronchitis and asthma cause further complications. There is no cure for this condition, but it can be alleviated by avoiding smoke-laden atmospheres, allergens, heavy metals and tight clothing on the chest, and by taking regular exercise, reducing weight and living in a humid atmosphere. Some of the exercises in the *Chinese Exercise Manual* are helpful provided that they are correctly regulated. A person in a very weakened condition must not be expected to perform very strenuous exercises. See **ch'iang chuang kung**.

empty illness A term used in TCM to describe those illnesses which are yin and tend to be internal and descending and are due to a deficiency of *qi*, and whose symptoms are weakness of voice, shallow respiration, a feeble cough, a white tongue and a weak or slow pulse. Such illnesses are treated with yang medicines which are toning. Breathing exercises are also helpful. See **ch'iang chuang kung**.

empty kidney-glands A term used in TCM to describe a deficiency of *qi* in the kidneys, and which causes nervousness and a decrease in the action of the heart, blood pressure and the rate of breathing, resulting in a lowered resistance to disease and a shortened life-span. An infusion of 4–8 g fruits of the Chinese wolfberry, *Lycium chinense*, taken internally is an effective treatment for this condition. The kidney-glands are the adrenal glands, and *qi* in this regard is probably adrenalin and the other hormones they secrete. Of course, the physicians of ancient China did not know the chemical composition of adrenalin, or even of its existence as such, but they were aware of the effects produced by the kidney-glands. See **adrenal glands** and **adrenalin**.

empty symptoms These symptoms are indicative of a yin condition. See **ba gang**.

emulsifier A substance, occurring naturally in the alimentary canal or added to foodstuffs, which converts fats and oil into emulsions.

emulsion A suspension of tiny droplets of one liquid in another, usually oil in water, which will not separate out after shaking. See **bile**.

enamel A hard substance providing a thin protective layer on the outside of a tooth. See **dentine**.

endocrine glands These are ductless glands that secrete hormones, which are the 'chemical messengers' that regulate the bodily activities, including the emotions, and which, in TCM, are known collectively as *jing*, one of the four humours. It seems that the existence of these glands was known to physicians in ancient China, and that they regarded them as energy centres, or houses, which produce the energies that regulate the body, and that disease could occur where these energies are weak or depleted. There are seven glands, each with its particular functions, which are listed below. In this respect, the opinions of the Taoists of ancient times are not altogether different from those of the Western medical scientists of the present day.

1. Pineal, or house of spirit. In Western medicine, its function is regarded as being uncertain; and, in fact, it may not even be an endocrine gland. According to Taoism, it controls the other glands and is the spiritual centre of the body, being associated with conscience and intuition. Only humans have this gland, for only humans have spiritual values and indulge in worship. But, perhaps, it would be nearer the truth to say that only humans are capable of unbridled imagination which sometimes undermines their intelligence.

2. Pituitary, or house of intelligence. In Western medicine, it is thought to be a regulator of growth and an influence on the sexual glands. According to Taoism, it controls the intelligence, wisdom and the memory.

3. Thyroid, or house of growth. It controls metabolism and growth.
4. Thymus, or house of the heart. In Western medicine, its function is regarded as being uncertain. According to Taoism, it governs the heart and circulation.
5. Pancreas, or house of transcendence. It controls the digestive system, body temperature and levels of blood sugar. With a weak pancreas, there is hypoglycaemia, or low levels of blood sugar, which leads to a craving for sugary foods and confectionery, so causing hyperglycaemia, or high levels of blood sugar. See **diabetes mellitus**.
6. Adrenal, or house of water. See **empty kidney-glands**.
7. Sexual, or house of essence – testes and prostate in the male, and ovaries and breasts in the female – which controls the sexual activities. Understandably, in TCM, the sexual glands and their associated organs are called the conception vessel. See **hormone**, **humour** and **qi**.

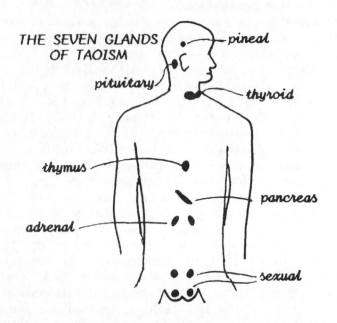

THE SEVEN GLANDS OF TAOISM

pineal
pituitary
thyroid
thymus
pancreas
adrenal
sexual

endorphin, enkephalin Morphine-like neuropeptides which relieve pain, and which are released by the brain when certain acupoints are stimulated.

enema The injection of a liquid medication into the rectum to treat inflammation or an infection of the bowel, to promote a bowel movement or to bypass the liver in providing internal medication. This technique is also useful in administering medicines which cannot be safely or helpfully taken orally. It is very much a feature of Western medicine. See **lavage**.

energy This term is an English translation of a Chinese word which could also be translated as 'essence' or 'spirit'. It may be representative of *qi*, or 'vital energy', but it is also indicative of lesser forms of energy. In TCM, hot, warm, cold and cool are called *si qi*, or 'four energies'. The difference between hot and warm, and cold and cool, is only one of degree. Common sense would dictate that young and robust patients be given the potent and quick-acting hot or cold medicines, and elderly and frail patients be given the mild and slow-acting warm or cool medicines. Hot and warm ailments and medicines are yang, and cold and cool ailments and medicines are yin. Cold or cool yin ailments are treated with hot or warm yang medicines, and vice versa. This principle of complementary opposites is stated in the *Pharmacopoeia of Shen Nong*: 'Treat hot illnesses with cooling medicines, and treat cold illnesses with warming medicines.' We, in the West, observe the same principle when we say, 'Starve a fever but feed a cold.' But it is imperative that this principle be strictly observed. If a yang hot-energy illness, characterized by a high temperature, extreme thirst, and so on, were treated with a yang hot-energy medicine, the condition would be intensified and the yin-yang balance so disturbed that death might ensue. See **energy value of food**.

energy and taste combinations It is important that foods and/or medicines administered to a patient should be alike in energy and taste. For instance, a medicine of bitter taste has an astringent effect, and so to administer it together with a medicine of cold energy would produce no benefit, the former nullifying the benefit of the latter. Some herbs of the same taste have different energies, and some of the same energy have different tastes, as this table shows:

MEDICATION	ENERGY	TASTE
Ginger, *Zingiber officinale*	warm	hot
Magnolia, *Magnolia officinalis*	warm	sour
Longan, *Euphoria longan*	warm	sweet
Plantain, *Plantago asiatica*	cold	sweet
Viper, *Agkistrodon acutus*	warm	sweet
Cassia, *Cinnamomum cassia*	hot	sweet

Sometimes, ingredients are added to a concoction to offset any ill effects which might arise where the other ingredients are of an opposite character in taste and energy. See **active ingredient** and **taste**.

energy centre See **endocrine glands**.

energy regulation This is the process by which medicines are used to calm the nerves, relax the body and ease the mind. Such medicines, which are called sedatives, or tranquillizers, are of two kinds: those which treat over-stimulation and excessive excitement caused by full ailments, and those which tone the heart and liver when the symptoms indicate empty ailments. These medicines need to be combined with other medicines which will cure or alleviate the specific ailments which have given rise to the need for sedation. For example, insomnia and hysteria may be reduced by sedation, but it is likely that they will have specific causes, such as a heart condition or an excess of liver-yang. See **sedative**.

energy value of food Not only medicines but foods also have an energy value – very hot, hot, warm, cool, cold, very cold – and so, with foods as with medicines, it is important that a hot ailment should be treated with a cooling food, and vice versa. The Chinese physician knows from long experience how to arrange both medicines and diet so they are best suited to the needs of the patient; but, in the West, the energy values of food are measured and expressed in kilocalories or kilojoules. See **calorific value of food**.

enfleurage See **essential oil**.

enkephalin See **endorphin**.

enteritis Inflammation of the intestine. Provided that there are no complications, the standard treatment in TCM for this condition is an infusion or decoction taken internally of 5 g bark of the cork tree, *Phellodendron amurense*. See **gastro-enteritis**.

enuresis Bed-wetting, which is more common among children than adults. In older children, nocturnal enuresis, or bed-wetting at night, is likely to be due to anxiety or some other psychological cause, and the treatment should be based on this assumption. In TCM, a helpful treatment is an infusion or decoction taken internally of 5–8 g unripe fruits of the blackberry, *Rubus coreanus*, or 10–25 g leaves and stems of agrimony, *Agrimonia pilosa*.

environment A person's state of health is determined in some measure by the state of the environment in which he lives. A person living in a warm, dry region will be less likely to succumb to bronchitis and rheumatism than a person living in a cold, damp region; and a person living in a cold region will generally not be infected with insect-borne diseases, such as malaria and sleeping sickness. A person cannot expect to be totally healthy if he lives in an unhealthy environment. Nothing is done for the good of our health by the pollution of the atmosphere, seas, rivers and soil by industrial effluence, which includes radioactive waste, and the contamination of crops by artificial fertilizers and pesticides, together with the inferior food products which result from intensive farming and food-processing methods. What is more, our technologically and commercially biased way of life produces hazards, such as leaded petrol and synthetic food additives, and encourages nervous and mental disorders, which set the odds against us attaining a ripe old age. Some people are accident-prone by temperament, and some are congenitally ill, and the hazards in our environment aggravate their weaknesses. A reckless driver is very vulnerable to accidents on a busy road, and an asthmatic person is at a great disadvantage in a polluted atmosphere. Many health hazards are by-products of a material-istic society. The Chinese have far fewer problems in this regard, for they abide by the teachings of Taoism, which advocate harmony with nature. They fully realize that, if they do not take care of their natural environment, including the plants and animals contained therein, their natural environment will not take care of them, and they will not have adequate supplies of clean air, pure water and uncontaminated food. See **chemicals** and **environmental health**.

environmental health Care of the environment has always been one of the main features of the Chinese approach to health. Many centuries ago, at the time of the Zhou dynasty, medicine men were aware that one could fully benefit from breathing exercises only in an atmosphere of clean air. In the West, preoccupation with environmental health, which is popularly known as the 'green revolution', is quite a recent development, and one which should be welcomed, and is long overdue.

enzyme Bio-catalyst. A complex protein produced by living cells and which activates some of the essential chemical changes within the body of a plant or animal. For example, ptyalin, the enzyme in saliva, converts starch into maltose. See **catalyst**, **maltose** and **qi**.

ephedra See **ephedrine**.

ephedrine An alkaloid derived from the roots and stems of *ma huang*, or joint fir, *Ephedra sinica*, and which is considered to be the most effective of all the medicines for the treatment of asthma. It is widely used in the West as well as in China, but Chinese physicians prefer to use the whole herb rather than simply the ephedrine. See **active ingredient**.

epidermis The outer layer of the skin of animals. It has a single layer of living cells, above which is a layer of dry dead cells which are constantly being shed.

epiglottis A projection of cartilage in the larynx which prevents food from entering the trachea, or windpipe, during swallowing.

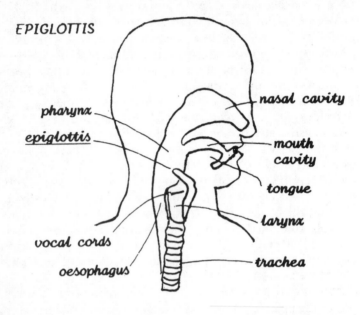

EPIGLOTTIS

pharynx
epiglottis
vocal cords
oesophagus
nasal cavity
mouth cavity
tongue
larynx
trachea

epilepsy A condition in which a person suffers convulsions, or fits, and loses consciousness for a period lasting from a few seconds to several minutes. The two main types are *grand mal* and *petit mal*. The former is the more serious form, and it generally only affects adults, who sometimes foam at the mouth and may swallow the tongue. *Petit mal* affects only children and teenagers, and attacks are so brief, with loss of consciousness lasting for no more than a few seconds, that they may barely be noticed. There is some doubt about the causes of epilepsy; but, in the West, it is generally accepted that some of the causes are excessive electrical discharges among the brain cells and brain damage due to head injuries and tumours. Also, it seems that, with some people, the condition is inherited. However, Chinese physicians take a somewhat different view, and they would contend that epilepsy is caused by blood– or *qi*-stagnation and internal dampness, and so they treat the heart, spleen and liver. However, the treatment is complicated, and involves a carefully planned diet and a number of herbal remedies, which include the Chinese quince, *Chaenomeles lagenaria*, sweet flag, *Acorus calamus*, and various species of bamboo in the genus *Phyllostachys*. Epileptics must NOT take evening primrose oil. See **hereditary defects**.

epinephrine See **adrenalin**.

erection See **impotence**.

erectile insufficiency See **impotence**.

erysipelas Local inflammation due to infection by streptococci. The TCM treatment is external application of an infusion of 10–16 g flowers of Japanese honeysuckle, *Lonicera japonica*, or 4–9 g fruits of golden bell, *Forsythia suspensa*.

eructation Belching.

eruption Rash.

erythrocyte A red blood cell, or corpuscle, which contains a pigment called haemoglobin that combines with oxygen to form oxyhaemoglobin, and so carries oxygen to the tissues. See **blood**.

essence 'Jing'. A Chinese term, also given as vital essence, which denotes the special form of *qi*, or 'energy', which is associated with the semen and sexual organs. In Taoist philosophy, the sexual glands are described as the 'house of essence', and it is the Taoist view that conservation of the semen and a regulated sex life preserves the vital essence, and so promotes longevity. In the *Principles of Longevity*, a treatise written during the seventeenth century by Liu Ching, there is some advice about regulated sex: 'In the spring, a man may ejaculate every three days. In the summer and autumn, he may ejaculate no more than twice a month. In the winter, when it is cold, he must not ejaculate at all, and so conserve his semen and amass yang-essence, which is the way to heaven and the attainment of longevity. An ejaculation in winter is a hundred times more harmful than an ejaculation in the spring.' It is a fact that debility and nervous disorders among men – but not women – are sometimes caused by sexual excess. Chinese physicians prescribe herbal tonics which thicken the semen, and so increase the vital essence. The horny goat weed, *Epimedium sagittatum*, and broomrape, *Cistanche salsa*, are very effective in this respect. See **jing**, **endocrine glands**, **Yellow Emperor** and **nervous disorders**.

essential oil One of a wide range of fragrant volatile oils extracted from plants and used in medicines and as flavourings for foods.

They are extracted in three ways: hand expression, enfleurage and maceration. With hand expression, which is an old-fashioned technique and confined to citrus fruits, the peels of the fruits are squeezed by hand until the oil glands burst. The oil is collected in a sponge which, when saturated, is transferred to a container. With enfleurage, the flower-heads are immersed in purified fat, and, when their oils have been absorbed by the fat, the fat is mixed with warm alcohol. The fat is insoluble in alcohol, but the essential oil dissolves in it quite readily, and is then extracted from the alcohol by distillation. With maceration, leaves and flowers are crushed and added to warm oil, and the resultant liquid can be used directly as a herbal cream or lotion, or the essential oil can be removed by distillation. See **aromatherapy**.

ethanoic acid An organic acid (CH_3 COOH) which occurs in vinegar, and which was known as acetic acid in an older system of chemical nomenclature. See **vinegar**.

ethanol See **alcohol**.

ethyl alcohol See **alcohol**.

eucommia *Eucommia ulmoides* Herbal medicine. Distribution: Central China. Parts: bark. Character: warm, sweet. Affinity: kidneys, liver. Effects: nutrient to bones and connective tissue, tonic to kidneys and liver, sedative to restless foetus. Symptoms: headaches, dizziness, tiredness, weakness, backache, impotence, bed-wetting, restless foetus in women. Treatments: lumbago, kidney deficiency, liver deficiency, hypertension. Dosage: 8–15 g. This medicine is effective in preventing a miscarriage.

eugenics This science, founded by Sir Francis Galton (1822–1911), makes a study of how the human race might be improved by selective breeding. It has few practical applications, for we cannot breed humans as we breed animals. Who is to decide just what are the most desirable qualities in humans? However, eugenics can be practised successfully on a limited scale. People who have some hereditary defect could be advised against having children or even be compulsorily sterilized. Arranged marriages, as are still commonly practised in China, are an attempt to produce worthy descendants who, eventually, will become worthy ancestors. See **hereditary defects** and **inbreeding**.

Eustachian tube See **ear**.

euthanasia The Chinese seek to attain longevity and a good state of health, which interest stems from their ancestors' attempts to achieve immortality. Their respect for their ancestors borders on reverence, and so they are not likely to be willing to assist in an act of euthanasia, particularly in regard to those elderly persons who are destined to become their ancestors. However, it seems that in past ages certain privileged persons who had committed a crime or were terminally ill were allowed to dispose of themselves – to commit honourable felo de se, so to speak – and were thus spared the indignity of public punishment or a lingering death. For this purpose, they were provided with the poisonous comb of a certain species of crane; and, when the time was propitious, they would take the fatal bite. This species of crane is remarkable in that it can consume all manner of poisonous plants and animals without any harm to itself, the poisons being stored in its comb.

evacuation The removal of waste from the bowel. See **eliminative**.

evening primrose *Oenothera biennis* This herb is helpful in the treatment of premenstrual tension, breast tenderness, alcoholism, inflammation and eczema, and it reduces cholesterol and regulates the female reproductive system. But it must NOT be taken by epileptics. It is not extensively used in Chinese medicine. See **eczema**.

evil-qi See **qi**.

evil-qi excess A term used in TCM to describe a condition where there is an excess of stimulation or toning or what in the West would be described as over-stimulation, as is caused by certain medicines. Some poisons have this effect, as is the case with strychnine and some of the other substances used in tonic medicines. See **qi**.

evil-yang See **qi**.

evil-yin See **qi**.

evolution The Taoists have always regarded man as being very much an animal with close links with nature; but, in Chinese literature, there is no evidence to suggest that the Chinese have ever given serious consideration to theories of evolution of the kind initiated by Charles Darwin. However, the *Ben Cao Gang Mu*, or 'Outlines and Branches of Herbal Medicine', a classic herbal prepared by Li Shizhen, is thought to have influenced Darwin in his study of evolution and natural selection. Li Shizhen was struck, as was Darwin, by the close similarity between the anatomical and physiological features of both plants and animals. See **Ben Cao Gang Mu**.

excess combinations The six excesses, which are wind, cold, summer-heat, dampness, dryness and fire, can exist in various combinations, such as wind-cold, wind-heat, cold-dryness and hot-dryness. The inner forms of the excesses occur in the internal organs and are not caused by climatic conditions. Thus, inner-cold is caused by a deficiency of yang-energy in the spleen and stomach, and inner-wind originates in the heart, kidneys and liver. Cold drinks taken during the summer will produce the combination cold-summer-heat, which produces abdominal pains, chills and perspiration. Of course, a healthy person will be less affected by the excesses than an unhealthy person. It is the purpose of preventive medicine to ensure that the body maintains its resistance to the conditions induced by the excesses and their combinations. A disease due to one of the six excesses is more likely to occur when the weather conditions are abnormal, for it is then that the body must counter a condition for which it is unprepared. For example, a sudden cold spell in the summer may cause colds, coughs and influenza. People who visit a country where the climate is different from that at home are more likely to fall victim to a climatic excess than are the inhabitants, who will have developed an immunity to the local conditions. See **climate** and **six excesses**.

excess flavour See **excess taste**.

excess food and drink According to TCM, most of the causes of disease are climatic and emotional. The other causes include an excess of food and drink and an improper diet, which can bring about indigestion, constipation, diarrhoea, dysentery, halitosis, loss of appetite, and so on. Stomach-ache, vomiting and diarrhoea are often caused by too much cold food. See **diet** and **food**.

excess-qi See **qi**.

excess taste Over-indulgence in food that is strong in one of the five tastes is harmful to the solid organ associated with the taste. Thus, too much bitter-tasting food can be injurious to the heart, too much sour food can be injurious to the liver, too much salty food can be injurious to the kidneys, and so on. Those in the Western world who are sceptical of the merits of TCM would be quick to regard this as superstition, but medical research in the West has shown that the taste of food is often a reliable guide to its quality – or its harmful properties. An excess of sour food does aggravate the liver, and an excess of salty food does cause renal dysfunction. Those who study their domestic animals will know that animals fight shy of foods that are excessively hot, bitter, sour, sweet or salty. It is only the apes and monkeys – man's nearest relatives – which will consume confectionery. It seems that, in matters of taste, Chinese physicians have discovered by long experience what we, in the West, have only recently discovered by laboratory experiments. See **taste**.

excision A term used in surgery to indicate the cutting away of an organ, tumour or some other unwanted tissue.

excretion The expulsion of waste from the body. This term refers particularly to the evacuation of the bowel, but it is also inclusive of other forms of elimination: urination, perspiration and breathing. See **eliminative**.

exercise In TCM, exercise, together with diet, breathing, regulated sex, herbal medicines and moderate habits, is a fundamental component of preventive treatment. People who are engaged in laborious work are generally much fitter than those in sedentary occupations – and few Chinese are in sedentary occupations. Regular exercise helps to ensure that muscles do not become soft and flabby, joints do not become stiff, and the most benefit is derived from the intake of food. Oxygen enters the body via the lungs, but the actual process of respiration occurs in the tissues, and a good circulation of the blood, which is prompted by regular exercise, conveys oxygen and nutrients to the tissues where they are required. It also conveys the waste products of respiration to the kidneys and lungs, where they are excreted. Exercise is also an aid to the digestion, for the bodily movements assist peristalsis, which is the involuntary contractions and relaxations of the wall of the alimentary canal, and so the chyme, which is the food that has undergone gastric digestion, is kept in motion, thereby aiding assimilation and preventing constipation. A little exercise often relieves flatulence, or 'shifts the wind', as this process may be described in colloquial terms. However, it is inadvisable to take violent exercise after a meal, for this puts too much strain on the heart. Exercise should not be too strenuous. Those sporting activities in which some of the young people of the West indulge themselves, such as the fortnightly game of football or hockey, or the occasional game of tennis, are too infrequent and too exertive to be of any positive value. What is gained is negated by long periods of sedentary living. There is much to be said for the twice-daily walk as a safe and healthy form of exercise, and it is an activity in which the young and old alike can freely indulge. But, for those to whom a steady walk might seem to be totally unexciting, following the Chinese example by taking an interest in kungfu, or the martial arts, would seem to be the sensible alternative. Chinese physicians would say that lack of exercise causes ill health by making the blood and energy sluggish, which leads to deterioration of the vital organs, muscles and *qi*. They would also say that excessive labour or exercise causes weakness and fatigue and deterioration of *qi*. Some Chinese keep fit by performing the 12 zodiac exercises, each of which is influenced by one of the two-hourly periods of the day. These exercises derive from ancient Taoist philosophy. But most Chinese keep fit by performing callisthenics, which are gymnastic exercises to improve both the body and the mind. These are components of the *tai chi chuan*, which is based on one of the systems of martial arts. See **martial arts**, **games**, **zodiac exercises** and **tai chi chuan**.

exercise therapy The Chinese perform callisthenic exercises not only to keep fit by improving the body and mind and energy but also as a form of therapy for a wide range of ailments, which include myopia, hypertension, asthma, emphysema, pleurisy, tuberculosis, constipation, haemorrhoids, insomnia, hepatitis, paraplegia, arthritis and cystitis. Since these exercises generally involve co-ordination of the mind and body, they are particularly effective in treating diseases which are closely associated with the emotions, such as depression, hypertension, insomnia and colitis. The exercises have been developed from the psychological and breathing exercises which were first introduced by the Taoists, and which have close links with the martial arts. Further information about these exercises is to be found in the *Chinese Exercise Manual*, which derives much of its data from two ancient works – *Nei Ching*, or 'Classic of Internal Medicine', and *Xien Chin Fang*, or 'The Thousand Prescriptions'. See **Chinese Exercise Manual** and **tai chi chuan**.

exfoliation The shedding of skin scales, as in eczema and dandruff.

exhalation See **breathing**.

exhaustion This may be due to a period of unusually difficult or intensive work, either physical or mental, and then there is no cause for alarm. But if the condition persists, it is likely to be due to a *qi* or blood deficiency, such as anaemia. Asiatic ginseng, royal jelly, wolfberries and *huang qi* are helpful. See **tiredness**.

expectorant A medicine that initiates or eases the coughing up of sputum. TCM has a wide range of medicines for this purpose, which include infusions or decoctions of the following herbs taken internally, using the parts and dosages indicated. Common plantain, *Plantago asiaticus*, seeds, 6–10 g; mandarin orange, *Citrus reticulata*, peel, 4–8 g; balloon flower, *Platycodon grandiflorum*, roots, 2–5 g; loguat, *Eriobotrya japonica*, leaves, 10–14 g; coltsfoot, *Tussilago farfara*, flowers and floral buds, 4–10 g; liquorice, *Glycyrrhiza glabra*, root, 3–12 g; garlic, *Allium sativum*, 3 cloves.

Liquorice must not be used where there is hypertension.

'expel-worms medicine' See **anthelmintic**.

experience Chinese physicians attach much importance to experience, and they do not regard themselves as being fully qualified
until they have had many years of experience, as opposed to
mere book knowledge. In the past, when chemistry was not as
advanced as it is today, there were many instances where
Chinese physicians produced an effective cure by treating an
illness whose cause was unknown with a herbal medicine whose
functioning was not understood. They relied upon the experience
gained from previous treatments. To the Western mind, this
would seem to be a most unscientific approach. But it is a
humane approach, and so it is the right approach if the recovery
and welfare of the patient is the physician's first priority. It is no
consolation to a very sick person to be told that some clever
doctor knows all about the cause of his illness but is unable to
effect a cure. Of course, it is not unreasonable to assume that
knowing the cause of an illness could lead to finding a cure, but
that is not always the case. See **patience**.

expiration See **breathing**.

external A term used in TCM diagnosis to indicate the location,
extent and direction of a disease. It is one of the eight principles
of differential diagnosis. If a disease moves towards the outside of
the body, the symptoms become external, which means that the
treatment is probably taking effect. External symptoms and
ailments are regarded as being yang, but they must be considered
together with the other principles of diagnosis. See **ba gang**.

'external-release medicine' This is the Chinese description of a
diaphoretic, which is a medicine to induce perspiration in order
to release evil-*qi* in external ailments, such as those brought about
by excessive exposure to heat, dampness and wind. See
diaphoretic treatment.

external symptoms and treatments The external symptoms of
illness may be briefly listed as follows: chills, hotness, fever,
normal tongue with thin white fur, fluctuating pulse. The
treatments are the administering of diaphoretic and other
eliminative medicines. See **external** and **ba gang**.

external therapy TCM lays great emphasis on external therapy,
which is those treatments that are applied to the outside of the
body, though their effects can be either external or internal.
These treatments include acupuncture, acupressure, moxibustion,
massage, blood-letting, skin-scraping, suction cups, compresses,
poultices, ointments, lotions and liniments. For external diseases

and injuries, external treatments are applied directly to the areas affected. For internal ailments, external treatments are applied to the acupoints and meridians which are associated with diseased or defective organs. External treatments are often combined with internal treatments, and so it is sometimes a case of what cannot be achieved by one technique may be achieved by another. Thus, eczema will require both external and internal therapy. See **internal therapy**.

extraction of medicines The medicinal substances in herbs are extracted by a variety of methods, which include infusion, decoction, hand expression, enfleurage and maceration. See **infusion**, **decoction** and **essential oil**.

extremities As a medical term, this word means 'hands and feet'.

extrovert A term used in psychology to describe a person who is socially active, impetuous and outgoing, and whose interests and activities are directed away from himself. The Chinese would say that he has a yang personality. See **yang** and **nervous disorders**.

exuviae See **moulting**.

eye In both structure and function, the eye is similar to a camera. With a camera, light rays enter through the aperture and are focused by the lens on to a light-sensitive film from which a picture is obtained by the chemical processes of developing and printing. With the eye, light rays enter through the pupil and are focused by the lens on to the retina, which contains light-sensitive nerve endings. The impressions formed on the retina are carried to the brain by the optic nerve. The membrane on the front of the eye, called the cornea, is transparent and is kept clean by the wiper action of the upper eyelid. See **cornea**. The size of the pupil is altered by the iris, so controlling the amount of light which enters the eye. Humans and all other vertebrate animals have binocular vision, that is, they have two eyes which, in giving slightly different views of the same object, enables them to judge distance. Objects seen with only one eye appear to lack depth, and seem to be 'flat', or two-dimensional. The physician examines the eyes to find symptoms of disease – and signs of health. Listless eyes, taken with other symptoms, may indicate exhaustion, anaemia, a nervous disorder, drug addiction or a serious stage in a wide variety of ailments. A yellow iris could be symptomatic of jaundice. There is a Chinese proverb, often attributed to Li Shizhen: 'The eyes are the windows of the body, and the skin is its mirror.' According to TCM theory, the liver converts *jin ye*, one of the four humours, into tears. See **jin ye**.

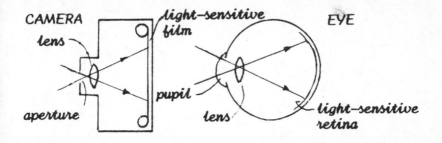

CAMERA
lens
aperture
light-sensitive film
pupil
lens
EYE
light-sensitive retina

eyesight Good eyesight is an asset that we cannot afford to lose, and so it is important that we should take care of our eyes. Common diseases and defects of the eye are blepharitis, conjunctivitis, myopia, hypermetropia, eyestrain, bloodshot eyes and tired eyes. Bloodshot eyes are caused by a slight infection or dehydration, as occurs after a bout of heavy drinking. The best treatment is a good sleep of about eight hours duration, which allows rehydration to occur naturally. See **optical defects**.

eyestrain This condition is due to loss of focusing power, which is usually caused by ageing, but it can also be caused by bad habits in using the eyes, such as constant reading in light that is too weak or too strong, or simply by overworking the eyes, as often occurs with people engaged in clerical or computer work. An eye test and, if necessary, the provision of spectacles are to be recommended. The eyes should be rested as often as is possible, and a strong but non-glare light should be used for reading. Chinese physicians advise a gently daily massage of the area around the eyes in order to defer the onset of eyestrain due to age. Treatments for tired and sore eyes are royal jelly, green tea and infusions of the following taken internally, using the parts and dosages indicated: wolfberry, *Lycium chinense*, fruits, 5–10 g; chrysanthemum, *Chrysanthemum morifolium*, flowers, 5–10 g; plantain, *Plantago asiatica*, seeds, 4–10 g; fennel, *Foeniculum vulgare*, leaves 1 g, seeds 3 g. It is also helpful to apply a compress of fresh parsley, *Petroselinum crispum*, to the closed eyes, or to bathe them with cold tea.

F

facai Hairweed. A hairlike alga which grows in Inner Mongolia, the Gobi Desert and the semi-desert regions of the north-west of China. Greenish brown when wet, and black when dried, it is a highly valued item of diet, for it has medicinal properties, and is used as a diuretic, antitoxin, expectorant, antitussive and tonic. If it is consumed regularly, generally in a soup or stew, it prevents hypertension and malnutrition. By tradition, it is always served on New Year's Eve.

facial paralysis Bell's palsy. This condition is due to damage to the nerve controlling one side of the face. With immediate treatment, recovery is generally complete, though some weakness may persist in elderly people. A Chinese physician would recommend acupuncture and remedial exercises from the *Chinese Exercise Manual*. An infusion of 4–10 g fruit of the Chinese quince, *Chaenomeles lagenaria*, taken internally is also helpful.

faeces See **stools**.

fainting Known medically as syncope, this brief loss of consciousness is due to lack of oxygen to the brain. The usual cause is standing too long, when the blood, which carries oxygen, is not circulated to the brain. Other causes of poor circulation are pain,

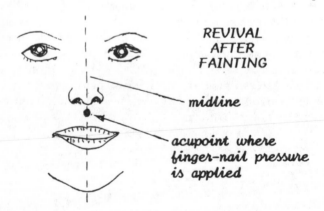

REVIVAL
AFTER
FAINTING

— *midline*

*acupoint where
finger-nail pressure
is applied*

hunger, fatigue, weakness after an illness, shock, diabetes and drugs, which lower the heartbeat. But fainting can occur when the heartbeat is rapid and the blood well circulated if, for some reason, it is deficient in oxygen. This is the case with anaemia. Treatment is simple. Tight clothing at the neck must be loosened so that the circulation is not restricted. The patient must be made to lie down or sit down with the head held forward so that the brain is supplied with blood. Immediately after recovery, he should get into the fresh air. Whereas we might use smelling salts to revive a person who has fainted, the Chinese would use acupressure. The finger-nail is applied to stimulate the acupoint on the midline two-thirds of the way up between the patient's upper lip and nose. A person who faints frequently for no apparent reason should seek medical advice. See **dizziness**.

fallopian tubes See **reproductive systems**.

family history In making a diagnosis, the Chinese physician will ask the patient about his family history, for he will need to know about the patient's private life and if there are any hereditary defects which might have some bearing on the patient's condition and the type of treatment that might be necessary. See **consultative discussion**.

fan This refers to the cereals and vegetables in the Chinese diet, of which rice is the usual mainstay. *Fan*, which literally means 'cooked grain', provides bulk and is filling and satisfying, and it is easily digested, protective, smooth and not irritating to the alimentary canal. It absorbs the excess grease and acids in the richly spiced meat and fish dishes. See **cai**.

fang Canine tooth of a mammal or the venom-filled tooth of a snake. See **bites**.

fang feng *Ledebouriella seseloides* Herbal medicine. Distribution: North China, Japan. Parts: roots. Character: fairly warm, hot and sweet. Affinity: liver, spleen, bladder. Effects: analgesic, antipyretic, expectorant, astringent, haemostatic. Symptoms: aches and pains in muscles, joints and limbs. Treatments: windmoist ailments, chills, fevers. Dosage: 3–7 g.

fang sung kung This is a relaxation breathing exercise which is used to treat a wide variety of ailments, including bronchitis and bronchial asthma. In this, the technique of *ju ching* is used. It involves special words and poetry which induce quietness into the relaxation. *Fang sung kung* is described and explained in the *Chinese Exercise Manual*.

Farmers' Almanac See **Chinese Almanac**.

fasting In general, the Chinese do not approve of fasting, and they would regard it as the height of folly to enter into voluntary starvation for the sake of some religious principle. Why do people fast? Perhaps their thinking is that, as gluttony is a sin, fasting, which is the antithesis of gluttony, must be a virtue. But it is naïve thinking, and it is not good for the health. On the other hand, the Chinese do see the need for frugality, which is a sensible compromise, for it is an established fact that more people die from overeating that from under-eating. Some Chinese physicians recommend an occasional reduction in the food intake to give the alimentary canal a rest and to assist the processes of elimination. But they insist that this should be done

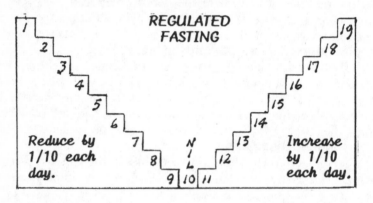

REGULATED FASTING

Reduce by 1/10 each day.

Increase by 1/10 each day.

gradually over a period of, say, 20 days, so that there is no severe shock to the system. On the first day, the normal food intake is reduced by one tenth, on the second day by two tenths, and so on, until, on the tenth day, it will be nil. Then, on the eleventh day, the intake is increased by one tenth, on the twelfth day, by two tenths, and so on, until, on the twentieth day, it will be back to normal. The gentle shock provided by this 'regulated fasting' is sometimes effective where blood-cleansing is required, as with arthritis, gout and eczema. But this could be a risky undertaking for a pregnant woman or a person with a weak heart, and so medical advice should be sought before this procedure is attempted. See **frugality**.

fat An organic compound which is insoluble in water, and which occurs in both animals and plants. Fats consist of fatty acids, triglycerides and compounds of glycerol. A fat has an energy value which is about twice that of the same weight of a carbohydrate. The body can make fats from carbohydrates and protein, requiring only fatty acids to be present in the diet.

Foods with a high fat content include dairy products, bacon, lamb and vegetable oils. A high intake of fat can lead to obesity, and those containing saturated fatty acids can produce cholesterol, and so may be causative of coronary heart disease, atherosclerosis (a form of arteriosclerosis) and cancer of the breast. An oil is a fat which is liquid at ordinary temperatures. See **food**, **glycerol**, **oil** and **fatty acid**.

fatigue Exhaustion. Breathing exercises help to remove toxic waste products, which cause drowsiness. Tienchi and ginseng are helpful where this condition is due to a *qi* or blood deficiency, but a medical examination is advisable if it persists. See **exhaustion**.

fatty acid This is the main component of fat. Fatty acids are classified as saturated, unsaturated and polyunsaturated. Some of the polyunsaturated acids, described as essential fatty acids, or EFA, are important as components of all cell membranes. Good sources of these are corn (maize) oil, sunflower oil and evening primrose oil. Polyunsaturated acids, which are contained in vegetable and fish oils, maintain correct cholesterol levels, and so reduce the risk of thrombosis, strokes and atherosclerosis, which is a form of arteriosclerosis associated with fatty degeneration. The Chinese have few problems here, for their diet is low in animal fats, and they do their cooking in vegetable oil. See **fat** and **oil**.

fauna The animals of a region or an epoch. In China, some animals are used in medicines, and so the Chinese physician needs to study the fauna of the region where he practises. See **flora**.

fear One of the seven emotions of TCM, fear is associated with the kidneys. Chinese physicians would say that a person is fearful because the *qi* of his kidneys is weak. When one's will-power is weak, one gives in to fear, and this, in turn, weakens the kidneys, and the weakened kidneys produce even more fear. And so excessive fear and physical injury go together, creating a psychosomatic cycle which may be difficult to break. There is evidence to support this view. Involuntary urination and even defaecation may occur during a period of intense fear, and medical research in the West has shown that the adrenal glands, situated at the upper ends of the kidneys, secrete a hormone – adrenalin, which is, perhaps, kidney-*qi* – that helps in over-coming fear. Too much fear can deplete these glands, which leads to weakness, as occurs when people shake with fright. Fear, like pain, is a part of the body's alarm system, and indicates that one must take action to avoid danger. The usual reaction to fear is either to fight or to take flight. In Western culture, running away from danger, particularly in regard to military situations, is regarded as cowardly and totally dishonourable, and yet it is a natural defence mechanism and the obvious thing to do. Heroes may be awarded medals but cowards tend to live longer. There is a difference between being brave and being foolhardy. Women in childbirth and mentally-ill people with an anxiety state are sometimes compelled to behave with a high degree of courage for which no medals are awarded. One suspects that heroes are sometimes motivated by the fear of being thought to be afraid. Sometimes a person may continue to be afraid even though the cause of his initial fear has ceased to be. This is one form of anxiety neurosis. See **panic**, **adrenalin** and **seven emotions**.

febrifuge See **antipyretic**.

febrile Caused by or causing a fever.

feeling See **touch** and **tactile diagnosis**.

female semen-essence See **jing**.

femininity According to Taoist ideas, as indicated by the Tai Chi, yang represents the masculine principle, which is positive, and yin represents the feminine principle, which is negative. But this is not intended to mean that men are superior to women. On the contrary, women are superior to men in many respects, and their gentleness and patience should not be regarded as weakness. The Confucian view is that the opposite natures of women and men – yin and yang – create harmony within the family. A woman should be respected for being a woman and not as a pale imitation of a man, and any attempt to alter the natural status quo is unhealthy and undesirable. Those women who say that they want to be equal with men do a great disservice to womankind, for such an attitude implies that they are envious of the status of the male, which they believe to be superior to their own. To be more constructive, and so more convincing, they should be saying that they want men to be equal to them. The Chinese have no problems here. After many centuries of Taoism and Confucianism, they regard men and women as being opposite but complementary, and the immense joy and self-fulfilment derived thereby is good for the health of the mind and the stable fabric of society, and infinitely preferable to the rather pointless inter-gender warfare which is now all the fashion in the West. See **masculinity**.

femur Thigh-bone.

feng shui See **fung shui**.

fennel *Foeniculum vulgare* Herbal medicine. Distribution: Europe,

Asia, North Africa. Parts: leaves, fruits, seeds. Character: warm, hot. Affinity: kidneys, liver, stomach, spleen. Effects: analgesic, stomachic, digestive, soporific, carminative, controls *qi*. Symptoms: nausea, vomiting, pains in groin and abdomen, prolapsed testicle, sleeplessness. Treatments: hernia, insomnia, ailments due to coldness. Dosage: leaves 4–7 g, seeds or fruits 2–5 g. This medicine may induce flatulence and eructation.

fenugreek *Trigonella foenum-graecum* This herb is indigenous to the Mediterranean lands and the Middle East, and is not used extensively in TCM. An infusion of 3–18 g seeds taken internally is a treatment for debility, poor digestion and gastritis. It promotes lactation and can be applied externally as a remedy for infections and inflammation of the skin.

fermentation This term describes the process by which wine and beer are made. In wine-making, fruit or vegetables, sugar and yeast are added to warm water. The yeast, which is a mass of tiny single-celled fungal plants, feeds on the sugar and gives off alcohol as an excretory product. The fruits and vegetables give wines the distinctive flavours. In brewing, malt, hops and yeast are added to warm water. The yeast feeds on the sugar contained in the malt, which is germinating barley grains, and yields alcohol. The hops serve as a flavouring and a preservative. Spirits are made by distilling wine and beer. Brandy is distilled from wine, and gin is distilled from beer. The term *fermentation* also describes a Chinese process for making medications. Powdered herbs, flour and water are kneaded together, shaped into balls and then put aside to ferment. These medications have a natural affinity for the stomach and spleen, and so they are used to promote digestion and treat diseases of those organs. See **alcohol, yeast** and **wine**.

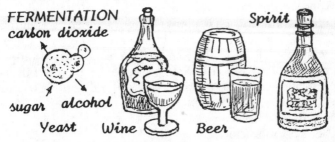

FERMENTATION
carbon dioxide
sugar   alcohol
Yeast   Wine   Beer   Spirit

fermented vegetables See **antibiotic**.

fertilization In humans, this may be described as conception. It is the beginning of pregnancy, when a spermatozoon, or male sex cell, unites with an ovum, or female sex cell, which is then known as an egg. The same process occurs in mammals. In flowering plants, a pollen grain, or male sex cell, unites with an ovule, or female sex cell, which is then known as a seed.

FERTILIZATION

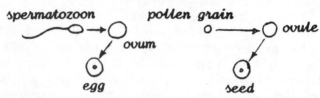

fertilizer A chemical or a mixture of chemicals which is applied to the soil as a source of nutrients for plants. Nitrates from fertilizers sometimes seep into the water supplies, where they can be harmful to humans. See **chemicals**.

feverfew *Chrysanthemum parthenium* Also known as bachelor's buttons, feverfew and midsummer daisy, this herb is distributed globally, but it is not used extensively in TCM. One fresh leaf taken three times daily is a treatment for arthritis, migraine, vertigo, tinnitus, dysmenorrhoea and amenorrhoea. After labour, it cleans and tones the womb, but it must NOT be taken during pregnancy.

fevers Abnormal rises in the body temperature which are generally due to infections, but which can also be caused by other conditions, such as brain damage and heat stroke. Fevers are common among children, for they are susceptible to a large number of diseases which generally do not affect adults. They include diphtheria, rubella (German measles), morbilla (measles), scarlatina (scarlet fever) and pertussis (whooping cough). Fevers are yang and external and usually associated with hot and full ailments, and are characterized by a flushed complexion, restlessness and a great thirst. They need to be treated with yin medicines which are cooling and suppressive, such as antipyretics and diaphoretics. Blood-letting is sometimes helpful but it must be performed by a TCM physician, and only on his recommendation. See **chills and fever**.

fibre See **dietary fibre**.

fibrin See **coagulation**.

fibroblast One of the cells contained in fibrous connective tissue. Fibroblasts form the scar tissues on wounds. See **interferon**.

fibroid See **uterine disorders**.

fibrositis Inflammation of fibrous tissue, especially that covering the sheaths of muscles. The treatment is as for rheumatism.

fibula The smaller of the two bones in the lower leg.

field mint See **corn mint**.

fig *Ficus carica* As an item of diet, and consumed regularly, the fruits of the fig prevent constipation, piles, halitosis and bloodshot eyes. They are also regarded as a dietary remedy for hypertension, anaemia (but not pernicious anaemia) and exhaustion. They have a tonic effect on the stomach and intestines. In the Western world, a syrup made from figs has a good reputation as a gentle laxative. Chinese white figs stewed with pork and consumed as a soup are beneficial to a poor liver condition.

fig wine Figs have medicinal properties. See **fig**. Here is a simple recipe for fig wine. Ingredients: 175 g dried figs, 575 ml rice wine, peel of a large lemon, 45 g refined sugar. Finely chop the lemon peel and enclose it in a piece of muslin. Put all the ingredients – do not wash the figs – together with the lemon peel in muslin, into a large clean jar, cover, seal and store where cool, dry, dark and undisturbed. After a month, dispose of the lemon peel. Reseal and store again. After 5 months, dispose of the figs. Store for 12 months before drinking. Two small glasses a day is the maximum dosage. There may be certain risks involved with consuming medicinal wines. See **medicinal wine**.

filariasis A tropical disease in which there is infestation by worms introduced as larvae by the bite of an insect. The worms may block the vessels of the lymphatic system, so causing elephantitis.

finger-nails See **personal hygiene**.

fingerprints The Taoists in ancient China were aware of the significance of fingerprints, which is quite remarkable since their use by the police in the West for identifying criminals is a recent development. They were first used in Britain in 1901 at New Scotland Yard. The *tao* of supremacy, or mastery, which is one of the Eight Pillars of Taoism, informs us that a person's fingerprints are indicators of his personal character and career potential, and provide warning signs of his inherited weaknesses, which he must conquer if he is to be sound in health and master of his situation.

fire One of the five elements of Chinese philosophy and medicine. It is yin, and is associated with the heart, the emotions and hotness. It is also one of the six excesses, and it is the form taken on by any of the other excesses if they should become too extreme. Thus, if coolness becomes more extreme, its symptoms of muscle cramps and pains in the limbs will be more intense, and there will also be symptoms of violent heat-excess. Too much food, alcohol and sex may cause inner-fire, which is manifested as violent anger. Grief or passion causes fire to collect in the lungs. Violent anger is associated with fire in the liver. See **six excesses** and **element**.

fire-energy See **huo qi**.

'fire-organ' As fire is the element associated with the heart, it is understandable that Chinese physicians describe the heart as the 'fire-organ'. But this association is not the outcome of an arbitrary decision, and it is based upon a real relationship in nature. A person who has a fiery complexion may have an over-active heart. Also, the heart is sedated when the kidneys are toned, which is because water is the element associated with the kidneys, and water extinguishes fire. Here, of course, Chinese physicians use the elements to express symbolically what is occurring in reality. See **joy** and **heart**.

'fire-sound' In TCM, fire is associated with the heart, and so laughter, which has the crackling sound of a wood fire, is called 'fire-sound'. Too much high spirits, as manifested by uncontrolled laughter or even hysterics, may injure the heart. Even in the West, it has been noticed that the person who laughs a great deal often has an over-active heart. See **joy** and **laughter**.

first aid This is the first assistance that a sick or injured person receives before a more responsible person, such as a doctor, nurse or ambulance man, takes charge of the situation. Whatever other treatments are applied, the order of priorities is: 1. breathing, 2. bleeding and 3. shock. The airway must be kept clear, loosening the clothing at the neck, chest and waist if necessary, the severe bleeding must be arrested, and the patient covered with a blanket to prevent loss of heat, which increases shock. The Chinese have the same order of priorities in first-aid treatment, but a Chinese physician would use a different mode of expression. He might say, 'Keep the airway clear so that the patient is not deprived of *qi* ("vital energy"), arrest the flow of *xue* ("blood") so that there is no loss of *xue-qi* ("blood-qi"), and keep him warm so that his condition does not become internal, empty and yang-deficient.' This makes a great deal of sense if one can accept that the *qi* in air is oxygen, which is certainly essential to the production of energy. See **qi**.

fish Two of the main sources of protein in the Chinese diet are fish and shellfish, the latter being crustaceans and molluscs, which are not true fish. Fish is also a good source of fat, minerals and vitamins, and it is easily digested and easily cooked. Marine fish are a source of salt in its most natural form, and this salt contains iodine, which is essential to the proper functioning of the thyroid glands. Nervous disorders and pellagra, a disease that may lead to insanity, are partly caused by deficiencies of thiamin and niacin, two vitamins contained abundantly in fish, and so the popular belief that fish is good for the brain is not an old wives' tale. Edible fish may be put into two main categories: white fish, such as plaice and whiting, which contain less than 3 per cent fat; and oily fish, such as herrings and mackerel, which have a high fat content. All fish contain many minerals, including sulphur, phosphorous and calcium, and a wide variety of B-complex vitamins, but oily fish also contains vitamins A and D. Unlike the fat in meat, the fat in fish is mainly polyunsaturated, and so helps considerably in reducing the cholesterol level in the bloodstream. This does much to prevent cancer, strokes, coronary heart disease, arteriosclerosis and other circulatory complaints. It has been suggested by some nutritionists that two or three helpings of oily fish per week might prevent coronary heart disease altogether. The Chinese have few problems in this regard, for fish features prominently in their diet. However, as a dietary item, fish has two disadvantages. It cannot be safely consumed with certain medicines, and it 'goes off' very quickly. Food poisoning of any kind is unpleasant, but it is more so, and sometimes fatal, where fish is the culprit. Therefore, it is important that fish should be perfectly fresh when purchased and consumed. See **fresh food**.

fish bones All bones contain calcium, and so herrings, sardines, sprats and other fish which are eaten whole, including the bones, are a good source of calcium. But fish bones which become accidentally lodged in the throat can cause great discomfort. The usual remedy is to slowly chew and swallow Chinese olives (*Canarium album*), which will dissolve the bones. Another remedy is to sip a decoction of 8 g roots of clematis, *Clematis chinensis*, in 150 g vinegar. This decoction must NOT be consumed with tea.

fish liver This contains, among other things, a number of unsaturated fatty acids, including eicosapentaenoic and docosahexanoic acids, which are known collectively as Omega 3. For many years in the West, proprietary brands of cod-liver oil, flavoured with orange juice and malt, have been used to provide energy and resistance to illness, but salmon oil, now available in capsule form, is becoming popular as a source of polysaturated oils and vitamins A and D, which reinforces the Chinese view that fish, including fish liver, is a valuable item of diet. See **oil**.

fish oil See **fish liver** and **oil**.

fissure As a medical term, a fissure is a crack or split in the skin or a mucous membrane. Fissures commonly occur in the anus and at the corners of the mouth. If fissures at the anus persist, they could be indicative of a more serious condition, and medical advice should be sought. Generally, this condition is of short duration if one adopts a high fibre and liquid diet, avoids acid foods and uses an emollient. Chinese physicians would recommend the application of talc (magnesium silicate) to reduce perspiration in the affected areas.

fistula See **ulcer**.

fit A sudden and transitory or recurring bout of an illness, such as epilepsy, apoplexy, hysteria, fainting and paralysis. Strictly, it is a non-medical term, *convulsion* being more correct. A convulsion may be defined as an involuntary relaxation and contraction of muscles, often accompanied by unconsciousness. Chinese physicians would regard this as a condition where there might be some rebellious-*qi*. See **epilepsy**.

fitness The Chinese techniques for the achievement of fitness could be briefly summarized as a sound diet, regular exercise, correct breathing, regulated sex, moderate habits, peace of mind, preventive medicines and the wisdom to cope with the unforeseen, such as accidents and the other vicissitudes of life.

five elements In Chinese philosophy and medicine, there are five elements: wood, fire, earth, metal and water. Together with yin and yang, they account for all the causes and effects in nature and explain all the motivations of mankind. But these elements are symbolic, and are sometimes used to express great truths which cannot be explained in simple terms. The system of five elements, together with the characteristics of taste and odour, is used as a guide to the determination of the affinities of herbs, as the table below shows. See **element**.

Element	Taste	Odour	Yin Organ	Yang Organ
wood	sour	acid	liver	gall-bladder
fire	bitter	burnt	heart	small intestine
earth	sweet/plain	fragrant	spleen	stomach
metal	hot/plain	raw	lungs	large intestine
water	salty	rotten	kidneys	bladder

fixation Obsession. A term used in psychology for a person's concentration on a single idea or aim. It can be characteristic of determination and a worthwhile ambition, but if it is unreasonable, too prolonged or the subject of an unattainable desire, it can lead to frustration, anxiety, a complex or even nervous or mental illness. The *Analects* of Confucius contain many wise sayings which advise people against taking up foolish beliefs and so becoming the victims of fixations. Examples: 'Thought without learning is labour lost; learning without thought is dangerous. The superior man is distressed by his want of ability. Fine words and a flattering appearance are seldom associated with true virtue.' See **complex** and **mental health**.

fizzy drinks See **flatulence**.

flat feet Fallen arches. A condition in which the natural arches of the feet become flattened, and which affects young people and elderly persons whose ligaments have become slack. In the West, shoes with built-in supports may be worn if the feet ache. In China, the usual treatments are massage and remedial exercises.

flatulence 'Wind'. An excessive accumulation of gas in the stomach and intestine, and which may cause considerable discomfort and no little embarrassment when making an audible and odorous escape. Gas in the stomach is generally air which has been unconsciously swallowed or carbon dioxide from fizzy drinks, and that in the intestine is due to the fermentation of certain foods which have been incompletely digested. The main culprits are pulses, green vegetables, cucumber, nuts, onions and prunes. Flatulence can be prevented by regular exercise, a plain diet, avoiding those foods which are known to cause the condition, and seasoning foods with ginger, thyme, sage, rosemary and marjoram. Otherwise, a carminative can be used. An infusion, taken internally, of 2–4 g leaves and stems of corn mint, *Mentha arvensis*, or 2–5 g leaves and flowers of camomile, *Matricaria chamomilla*, makes an effective carminative. It is helpful to chew the seeds of the mandarin orange, *Citrus reticulata*, or fennel, *Foeniculum vulgare*. If the condition persists, medical advice should be sought, for its cause may be serious. See **white rice porridge**.

flatus Also called a fart, which is a vulgarism. Gas or 'wind' escaping from the intestine via the rectum and anus.

flavour See **taste**.

flea A wingless jumping insect, the commonest species being *Pulex irritans*. Fleas feed on the blood of humans and some other animals, and so transmit the micro-organisms which cause diseases, such as typhus fever and bubonic plague. Fleas carried by rats were responsible for the bubonic plague or Black Death, which, during the fourteenth century, killed 60 million people in Europe, Asia and Africa. Fennel, *Foeniculum vulgare*, will deter fleas if placed in bedding. See **vector**.

flora The plants of a region or epoch. In China, many plants are used in medicines, and so the Chinese physician needs to study the flora of the region where he practises. This term is also used as a collective description of the bacteria which are naturally present in the intestine and other organs. See **fauna** and **yeast**.

flour-paste pills See **paste pills**.

flowers of sulphur A powdered and pure form of sulphur used in medicine and obtained by sublimation, that is, by being changed from a solid to a vapour, and vice versa, without an intermediate liquid stage. See **brimstone and treacle**.

flower tea A herbal tea in which only flowers or floral buds are used, and which is an infusion that is made in the same way as many other herbal medicines. The Chinese have a wide range of flower teas, such as chrysanthemum, jasmine and honeysuckle, which they value both as refreshing drinks and for their medicinal properties. See **herbal tea**.

flu See **influenza**.

fluke One of the several species of parasitic worms which infect humans and other animals. A fluke has a complicated life history and undergoes a metamorphosis, or change of bodily form, in which there are several stages. Centuries ago, the Chinese probably knew nothing about the life history of the fluke, but they were aware that meat which is uncooked or insufficiently cooked could be a source of illness. See **parasite**.

flutter A regular but abnormally rapid heartbeat. See **pulse**.

foetus A developing baby from the beginning of the third month of pregnancy until birth. See **embryo** and **restless foetus**.

folk remedies These are the traditional remedies, mainly herbal, which are a component of the folklore of a culture. They were once used on a large scale in rural areas for treating common and minor ailments for which professional medical help was not thought to be needed – or was too expensive. Some of these so-called remedies are not very effective or are totally ineffective, and some are no more than bits of superstition, but they do provide a little comfort for those who live by faith. The folk remedies of the Chinese, which are now being vigorously tested, are being shown to be generally thoroughly reliable. However, there are a few exceptions. For example, the belief that ginseng,

Panax ginseng, is effective as an aphrodisiac is based on the fact that the forked root of ginseng has a shape that is similar to that of the Chinese written character for *ren*, which means 'man'.

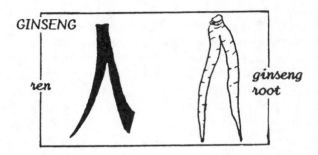

GINSENG

ren

ginseng root

follicle A small sac or gland in the body. A hair follicle is an example.

fomentation A warm dressing, poultice or lotion applied as a stimulant or to alleviate a condition.

food Food is one of man's basic needs, which are air, water, food, warmth, light and some means of defence. To these, Confucians would certainly add sex, which ensures the survival of the race. Of course, satisfying these needs will only ensure mere survival, and life would be very bleak indeed if man were not able to also satisfy his cultural needs and his social, moral and intellectual aspirations. Foods are body-building, energy-giving and health-protective, and may be placed into seven distinct categories: proteins, carbohydrates, fats, dietary fibre, minerals, vitamins and trace elements. Proteins are compounds of hydrogen, oxygen, carbon and nitrogen, which the body requires for growth and the replacement of tissue damaged by illness or injury. Their sources are meat, fish, eggs, cheese, milk, pulses and cereals. Carbohydrates are starches and sugars, which are compounds of hydrogen, oxygen and carbon, and which supply energy. Their sources are cereals, pulses, fruits, vegetables and honey. Enzymes in the alimentary canal convert starches into simple sugars so that they can be assimilated by the wall of the alimentary canal. Fats are stored energy foods because, unlike carbohydrates, their energy is not always immediately available, and they are stored in the tissues as a reserve. The body can synthesize fats from carbohydrates and proteins, which explains why a person who consumes a great deal of starchy and sugary foods may become obese. Dietary fibre is mainly cellulose,

233

which is an insoluble form of carbohydrate that cannot be broken down by digestive juices. It does not provide nutrients, but it does aid the digestive and assimilatory processes and assists elimination from the bowel, and so it is not unreasonable to regard it as a food. There are a number of items of diet which have little or no nutritive value, and so, strictly speaking, should not be regarded as foods. Some of the items sold in health-food shops are vitamin or mineral supplements, and, in themselves, have no nutritional value. Minerals, vitamins and trace elements are substances which have little or no nutritive value but which assist the bodily functions in a variety of ways including the digestion, assimilation and tissue absorption of food. Lack of these causes a wide variety of diseases and defects, which are called deficiency diseases. But if one's diet is varied, the body should receive adequate amounts of all its food requirements. The Chinese have always attached considerable importance to food, but this has not always been the case in the West, where it is now being realised that a balanced and varied diet, free of additives and other contaminants, and with fresh ingredients, will do much to eradicate certain diseases. Chinese physicians are ever ready to point out that a sound diet does much to create a healthy body, functioning harmoniously, which will effectively resist attack by external agencies. See **diet**, **mineral**, **vitamin** and **survival**.

food additive See **additives**.

food allergy Western medicine informs us that people with a true allergy, as opposed to those who are merely hypersensitive, have a defect in their blood system which is due to an abnormally large amount of a blood protein called immunoglobulin. Foods are by far the most numerous of the environmental items causing allergic reactions, for the obvious reason that food cannot be avoided because everyone needs to eat. Foods causing allergic reactions include sugar, milk and other dairy products, coffee, tea, chocolate, eggs and wheat. It seems that young children are particularly allergic to lactose, or milk sugar. The sensible person who has a condition due to an allergy will avoid those foods which he knows to be inducive of the condition, but this is not always easy, for allergens cannot always be easily detected. Some physicians take the view that conditions which appear to be due to allergens are more likely to be due to stress and anxiety or some other form of neurosis, and it is a fact that those conditions which are attributed to allergens are generally accompanied by the symptoms of a mild nervous disorder. One is tempted to think that an allergy provides an all too convenient explanation when the cause of an ailment cannot be accurately diagnosed. One is also tempted to think that some so-called allergic reactions are really natural reactions. Food additives, dust, pollen and mites are irritants when they come into contact with the delicate membranes of the eyes, nose, throat or lungs, and any copious flow of tears, mucus, etc., is surely no more than the body's normal defensive response to a foreign body, which is hardly an illness, though it may be unpleasant if the membranes happen to be extra-sensitive. The 'allergy theory' of illness would have no great appeal for Chinese physicians, who take the view that a healthy body is self-healing and self-regulatory, and so should be able to cope with minor conditions. However, they would think in terms of a *qi*-deficiency or rebellious-*qi* being caused by the wrong kind of food or contact with strange substances. See **allergy** and **hypersensitivity**.

food and health According to Taoist philosophy, food should not be taken just for pleasure or sustenance and survival but as a means to regulate and improve the health, both physical and mental. In China, therefore, food is consumed for its therapeutic effects as well as its other effects, and it is categorized accordingly: warm foods to counter cold ailments, cold foods to counter hot ailments, non-irritating foods for an upset stomach, and so on. To correct any imbalance between the yin and yang influences within the body, food is the first treatment, and medicines are prescribed only when all else has failed. See **diet** and **health foods**.

food and medicine The Chinese do not make a sharp distinction between what is a food and what is a medicine, for some medicines are administered as items of diet, and many of the culinary herbs also have medicinal properties. Foods may be classified according to their medicinal properties: heating, cooling, non-irritating, etc. The manner of cooking also plays a part in the classification of foods. For instance, a duck egg is classified as a cool food, but it is classified as a warm food when it is cooked in an omelette. Some of the food remedies used in Chinese folk medicine are remarkably effective. For example, the treatment for recurrent but non-acute cystitis is to fill a pig's bladder with a handful of peppercorns, boil it for an hour and then drink the juice. Pork offals, such as the heart, gall-bladder and trotters, yield a number of effective remedies. See **classification of foods**, **diet** and **health foods**.

food and sex Confucius recognized that food and sex are two of man's fundamental needs, the former being necessary for the survival of the individual, and the latter for the survival of the race. The Tang physician Sun Simiao, in his 'Precious Prescriptions', points out the benefits of a sound diet, adequate exercise and regulated sex: 'A man may have a long and healthy life if he regularly takes wholesome food and proper exercise and effects an emission twice monthly or 24 times yearly.' See **diet** and **dietetics**.

food balance See **balanced diet**, **cai** and **fan**.

food classification See **classification of foods**.

food colours The Chinese are very much averse to using synthetic additives in food, and so they use natural food colours, which are the juices of herbs, fruits and vegetables: tea for yellow or brown, soy sauce for brown, beetroot for crimson, tomato for scarlet, spinach for green, caramel for dark red or brown, and so on. See **additives**.

food concentrates See **health foods**.

food contamination See **contaminated food**.

food, drink and taste In making a diagnosis, the Chinese physician obtains information about a patient's state of health by asking him questions about his diet and eating habits generally. A desire for cold food and drinks indicates a hot condition, such as a fever. A desire for hot food and drinks indicates a cold condition, such as a chill or fatigue. The taste of a food – bitter, sour, sweet, plain, etc. – especially if different from the taste normally associated with it, indicates some other condition. For example, an insipid taste could indicate coryza or pharyngitis. A strong desire to eat spicy food or some unusual item of diet might indicate that parasites are present in the intestine. Pregnant women sometimes crave for strange foods. See **consultative discussion**.

food hygiene The attention given to food hygiene in China is basically the same as it is in the West. The cook takes steps to ensure that food ingredients are fresh and uncontaminated by contact with animals and poisonous and corrosive substances, or by defects in his own personal hygiene. The difference is that food hygiene in China is a matter of common sense and tradition, whereas, in the West, it is implemented by using a formal system of regulation and inspection. The sources of food contamination are many, and they include dirty hands and finger-nails, coughing, sneezing, a runny nose, dust, grease, grime, rusty utensils, cracked crockery, litter and other waste materials, cats, dogs, rats, mice, decaying food, detergents, paint, cleaning materials, cigarette ends, unboiled water, preserved foodstuffs which have beeen kept too long, stale left-overs, reheated food, human hairs, broken glass, additives and adulterants. Fruit and vegetables to be eaten uncooked should be washed thoroughly. One should not attempt to freshen stale food by cooking it. See **contaminated food**, **frozen food** and **personal hygiene**.

food ingredients There is much more variety among the food ingredients available to the Chinese than there is among those available to the people of the West, though this situation has been modified somewhat by improved methods of refrigeration and transport. Fruits, vegetables and rice grow in abundance in the warm, wet climate of South China and the equable climate of East China. Also, China has a long coastline, and so there is no shortage of fish and shellfish, which thrive in the warm waters of the South Pacific Ocean. This state of affairs gives the Chinese cook two main advantages. He has more scope for preparing meals which are varied and highly nutritious and appetizing, and he has more resources for preparing dishes with health-giving or medicinal properties. See **fresh food**.

food poisoning Ptomaine poisoning. The symptoms of food poisoning are vomiting, nausea, diarrhoea, feverishness and heavy perspiration. The main cause is micro-organisms which inflame the membranes of the stomach and intestine, and when the condition is severe, it can be fatal. *Salmonella* and *Staphylococcus* bacteria occur in half-cooked food which has been reheated, *Lysteria* in soft cheeses and pâtés, and *Campylobacter* in poultry, infected fish and unpasteurized milk. The condition can also be caused by direct contact with vomit or diarrhoea containing rota-viruses. There is probably a higher incidence of food poisoning in the West than in China, where there is a distinct preference for fresh foods, and there are fewer frozen, canned and processed foods to create opportunities for bacteria to develop. The main danger of food poisoning is dehydration, and so, if afflicted, one should drink plenty of water. Chinese liquorice, *Glycyrrhiza uralensis*, is effective as an antidote for poisoning by fungi, and ginger, *Zingiber officinale*, reed grass, *Phragmites communis*, and the Chinese olive, *Canarium album*, for seafood poisoning. Mishmi bitter, *Coptis sinensis*, is effective in suppressing a wide range of micro-organisms and toxins. However, food poisoning can generally be prevented by observing a few simple rules.

1. Use fresh foods rather than preserved or processed foods.
2. Take care to avoid contamination.

3. Make sure that food is sufficiently and correctly cooked.
4. Do not consume left-overs and stale and reheated food.
5. Thoroughly wash foods which are to be eaten uncooked.
6. Avoid foods which are known to have ill effects.

See **food hygiene**.

foods to avoid There are many dietary items consumed in the West which, in China, would be kept at a bare minimum or excluded altogether because they have poisonous or deleterious effects, or because they are damaging to the health if consumed over a long period. They include unboiled water, synthetic additives, refined sugar, dairy products, animal fats, red meat, hung pheasants, eggs that are not well cooked, bitter almonds, ginkgo nuts, chocolate and other confectionery, unwashed fruits and vegetables, the 'dead man's fingers' in crabs, stock cubes, stale and tainted food, reheated food, preserved foods and junk food. See **food hygiene**.

foods to include The Chinese set great store by a varied diet because they realize that there are very few foods which are seriously damaging to the health providing that they are not consumed to excess. On the other hand, there are some dietary items which are of so much benefit to the health that they should be included in the diet of anyone who perceives the value of good food as a means to a sound state of health. They include garlic, honey, royal jelly, oily fish, shellfish, peanuts, soya bean products, pork offals, edible fungi, cereals, abalone, aubergines, celery, figs, spring onions and green tea.

foot aches See **painful feet**.

foot odour See **body odour**.

forgetfulness See **amnesia**.

forgotten food The *tao* of forgotten food is one of the Eight Pillars of Taoism, and it refers to those herbal foods which are required to supplement the ordinary items of diet, particularly when a person is in a debilitated condition. These are foods which are taken for reasons of health and nutrition rather than mere pleasure. Royal jelly, garlic, figs, abalone and pig's trotters are within this category. Some thousands of years ago, Taoist surgeons were using herbs as anaesthetics in performing surgical operations, but these practices were largely discontinued when it was realized that many illnesses could be prevented by herbal medicine and an improved life-style, and that surgery may temporarily alleviate a condition, such as a tumour, but not prevent its recurrence. See **foods to include** and **health foods**.

formication A sensation as if ants are crawling over the skin.

formic acid See **methanoic acid**.

fortune sticks One of the several devices used by the Chinese for making predictions, and which they take very seriously because they believe that all events are preordained, and nothing happens by chance. A stick is drawn at random – as we would say in the West – from a bundle of numbered sticks. Each of the numbers has a corresponding text which is interpreted by a medium in a way which best suits the needs of the prediction seeker. See **divination** and **predictions**.

fortune-telling See **prediction**.

fossil bones Called 'dragon bones' by the Chinese. Medicine. Distribution: global. Parts: crushed bones. Character: neutral, sour-sweet. Affinity: heart, kidneys, liver. Effects: sedative, astringent, suppresses excess liver-yang. Symptoms: fright, panic, hysteria, shock, dizziness, insomnia. Treatments: hypertension, spermatorrhoea, leucorrhoea, diarrhoea, external styptic on abscesses. Dosage: 9–20 g. See **dragon**.

four energies In TCM, there are four energies: hot, cold, warm and cool. Where there appears to be an absence of energy, as with fossil bones, the term *neutral* is used. See **energy**.

four humours See **humour**.

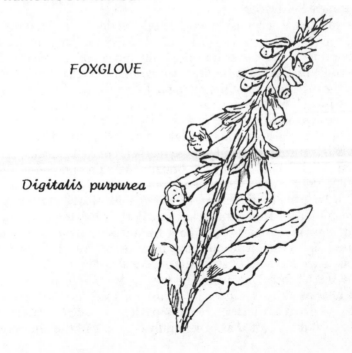

FOXGLOVE

Digitalis purpurea

foxglove *Digitalis purpurea* Source of digitalis, a drug used as a heart stimulant, but which must only be administered under proper medical supervision. It also yields digitalin, which is a steroid poison.

foxnut *Euryae ferox* Herbal medicine. Distribution: China, Japan, India. Parts: seeds. Character: neutral, sour and sweet. Affinity: kidneys, spleen. Effects: analgesic, astringent, stimulant to kidneys and spleen. Symptoms: impotence, premature ejaculation, nocturnal emissions, dyspepsia. Treatments: spermatorrhoea, urinary incontinence, leucorrhoea, chronic diarrhoea, spleen and kidney deficiencies. Dosage: 12–30 g.

fracture A break in a bone. In a simple fracture or a green-stick fracture, the treatment is largely a matter of keeping the bone immobile until the broken ends knit together. The Chinese have a number of herbs which they use to assist in this process. At one time, in the West, comfrey, *Symphytum asperum*, was used for this purpose, which explains why its everyday names are knitbone, boneset and bruisewort. But in a comminuted fracture, where the bone is broken into several pieces, or a compound fracture, where the break is exposed by a skin wound, the treatment is more difficult and may require surgery. See **green-stick fracture**.

fragrance See **odour**.

free radical A chemist might loosely define a free radical as a molecule which is deficient of an electron, and so behaves abnormally and destructively, influencing other molecules to become free radicals. Some medical scientists regard free radicals as one of the causes of the ageing of living tissues. See **ageing**.

fresh food The Chinese have a distinct preference for fresh food because its health-giving properties will not have been destroyed by decay or preservation methods, and it is not likely to give rise to food poisoning. In a Chinese market, chickens, ducks, rabbits and other small animals are bought live. The purchaser selects the item he requires and the vendor slaughters it there and then. Fish are usually on display in a large tank of water, from which the purchaser makes his selection. Pork is not frozen or chilled but comes from pigs which have been freshly slaughtered on the same day. One could not have meat or fish much fresher than this. Such methods of slaughtering are illegal in most countries in the West, where they would be regarded as inhumane.

fresh herbs When fresh herbs are used in medicines, the dosage is always given as the dried-herb equivalent. A weight of fresh herb is generally accepted as being equivalent to half the same weight of the dried herb. Thus, 2 g fresh herb = 1 g dried herb. See **dosages**.

friction See **compression**.

fright See **panic**.

fringe medicine A term used to describe unorthodox methods of treatment, such as acupuncture and osteopathy, which have not been fully accepted into the conventional medicine of the West, but which may be very successful. Most forms of alternative medicine fall into this category.

frog's legs A popular item of diet in the south of China, and which is valued dietetically as a source of protein that is cooling and non-irritating.

frost-bite A condition caused by freezing of the skin and underlying tissue of the nose, cheeks, hands and feet, and characterized by numbness due to a reduction in blood circulation. The immediate treatment, though painful, is to immerse the affected parts in warm water at a temperature between 40°C and 42°C, and then keep the extremities covered with insulating materials, such as woollens, until medical assistance can be obtained. Frost-bite could occur in North China and Manchuria, where the conditions are near-arctic during the winter, but experience and health-awareness has taught the Chinese and Manchurians to avoid exposure to extremes of coldness.

frozen food The Chinese have no great enthusiasm for preserved food, frozen or otherwise, but where freezers are used, they will adopt the same practices as obtain in the West. Food is not improved by freezing, but only preserved in the condition that it was in when it was put into the freezer, and that for only a limited period of time, for even frozen food will slowly deteriorate. Each item should be contained in a sealed bag to prevent contamination by absorption of unwanted flavours from other foodstuffs. The temperature of the frozen food should be kept below −5°C. Items taken from a freezer should be allowed to thaw out completely before use, and they should not be returned to the freezer in the hope that they will be restored to a good condition. Hot items should not be put into a freezer. They should be allowed to cool down first.

frozen shoulder A colloquial term which describes arthritis, or stiffness, of the shoulder due to the inflamed state of the membranes enclosing the shoulder joint. The Chinese treatment is the same as that for arthritis in any other part of the body, together with remedial exercises of the kind described in the *Chinese Exercise Manual*. See **arthritis**.

fructose See **sugar**.

frugality The climate and other geographical features of China are such that, for many centuries, the Chinese have suffered from famine and other privations, which have encouraged them to develop habits of frugality. As a consequence, they are not overfed, which is very much to their advantage, for they are not susceptible to obesity and its associated conditions, such as heart and circulatory diseases. See **fasting**.

fruits A wide range of fruits are employed in Chinese medicine, but it is as well to remember that, in general, it is only the kernels of the fruit stones which have the desired medicinal properties; and when the flesh of the fruit is used, it is generally that of the unripe fruit, not that of the mature fruit. The Taoist thinking here is that an unripe fruit or a fruit stone is yang, developing, energetic, full of *qi*, a 'concentration of the future', and without decay, whereas a ripe fruit is yin, in decline, tired, deficient of *qi*, without a future and well on the way to decay. In the West, the simple conclusion would be that, whatever the chemical substances in the whole plant may be, they are likely to be contained in a greater concentration in the seeds, with all their potential as the future plants.

fu kay Automatic, or spirit, writing is one of the several devices used by the Chinese for making divinations. It is similar in its function to a technique used at spiritualist seances in the West. See **prediction**.

full illness A term used in TCM to describe those illnesses which are yang and tend to be external and ascending and are due to excess of *qi*, and whose symptoms are restlessness, hyperactivity, noisiness, coarse breathing, constipation, distension of the abdomen, dark and scanty urine, a hard tongue with thick fur and a 'jumpy' pulse. Such illnesses are treated with yin medicines which are sedative or purging. See **ba gang**.

fumigation Disinfecting a room by means of fumes which are destructive to micro-organisms. The Chinese use joss-sticks as fumigants. See **joss-sticks**.

fungi These plants, of which there are hundreds of different species, grow very easily and in great profusion in the hot, wet regions of south China, and so they are consumed in much larger quantities and in far greater variety in China than in the West. They are an immense boon to the Chinese, for many have valuable medicinal properties, though a few are poisonous. Some fungi are preventive of coronary thrombosis because they arrest the build-up of cholesterol in the blood, and some are thought to

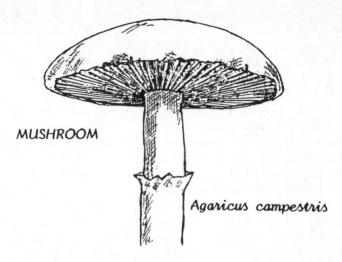

MUSHROOM

Agaricus campestris

be preventive of cancer if consumed as a regular item of diet. Cancer has many causes, and so it would be naïve to assume that fungi could give complete immunity, but if they are consumed as a component of a diet which is essentially healthy in other directions, the chances of developing cancer will be considerably less. Most British people have never tasted any fungus other than the common mushroom, *Agaricus campestris*, and its several varieties. However, it has its merits. Although it contains no nutrients apart from a tiny amount of protein, it provides dietary fibre, and it is flavoursome and easily digested, and it contains substantial amounts of niacin and riboflavin.

fung shui This term, also spelt as *feng shui*, which literally means 'wind and water', is concerned with the influence, for good or ill, of material things, particularly property, on human affairs. The *fung shui* concept arises from the Chinese belief that nature is not inanimate and without emotion and movement, but is alive and possessed of spirituality, and that man is a component of this natural system and is strongly influenced by it. Critics in the West might argue that this is superstition, but it is certain that man is influenced by the forces of nature, such as wind, rain, lightning, thunder, sunshine and other items of which he may have no direct knowledge, and so it is important that a person should arrange his position in relation to the environment in such a way that it will be favourable to him, or bring him good *fung shui*, as the Chinese would say. According to the scholars of the Song dynasty (960–1279), the cause of all that exists is one abstract principle, or the Supreme Absolute, which produces

243

yang, the male principle, and yin, the female principle, which are activated by *qi*, or 'primordial energy'. *Qi* permeates all things, and so, if a man and his family wish to live without harm to themselves, he must site his buildings so that they have good *fung shui*. Thus, a house that is in a village in a valley which is well watered by streams and rivers and surrounded by hills which act as a barrier against strong winds is likely to have good *fung shui*, whereas a house built on the top of a mountain, where it is exposed to the elements, is almost sure to have bad *fung shui*. But do we not adopt the same approach in the West when, given the opportunity, we prefer to live in a cottage in the country rather than a tenement in an industrial town, or choose to live in a house whose living-room windows face towards the sun? And we heed the blurbs in travel agents' brochures: 'with a pleasing aspect', 'a pleasant view of the sea', 'bedrooms facing south', etc. Really, the selection of a favourable position, or a good *fung shui*, is a step towards a sound state of health, both physical and mental. See **radiation**.

fur The condition of the fur on a patient's tongue provides some indication of his state of health. See **tongue diagnosis**.

furuncle Boil. A skin abscess which has developed from within a hair follicle or sebaceous gland. A group of furnuncles forms a carbuncle. The treatment is the same as for most other skin abscesses. See **carbuncle**, **abscess** and **cupping**.

Fuxi A legendary sage who is said to have lived over 7000 years ago, and who devised the mystic symbols, or trigrams, of the *Pa Kua*. See **Pa Kua**.

G

galactagogue A medicine to induce lactation. Galactagogues in common use in TCM include lily turf, *Liriope spicata*, snake gourd, *Trichosanthes kirilowii*, akebia, *Akebia quinata*, and farmer's tobacco, *Malva verticilla*. Pig's feet cooked in black rice vinegar are a helpful item of diet in this respect. See **lactation**.

gall See **bile**.

gall-bladder Its associated element is wood, and its associated emotions are anger and depression. Traditional Western medicine also associates depression – or melancholy – with this organ. Its function is to provide temporary storage for bile, which is a digestive fluid secreted by the liver. If the bile duct, which is the tube leading from the gall-bladder, becomes clogged by a gallstone or a quantity of mucus, bile enters the bloodstream, so causing a yellowing of the skin and eyes. This condition is known as jaundice. See **bile**, **liver**, **tin fu** and **liu fu**.

gallop rhythm A bounding heartbeat with three distinct sounds which are suggestive of the sounds made by a galloping horse. See **pulse diagnosis**.

gallstone One of the functions of the gall-bladder is to concentrate bile by the removal of some of its water. Sometimes, too much water is removed, and then the concentrates may accumulate as solid structures, which are called gallstones. Blockage of the bile duct by a gallstone causes jaundice, and there is likely to be an accompaniment of pain and fever. An infusion or decoction of 10–30 g stems, leaves or roots of the dandelion, *Taraxacum officinale*, taken internally and regularly helps to prevent or relieve this condition. See **calculus**, **gall-bladder** and **bile**.

gambling See **social evils**.

games Chinese physicians regard such games as chess and draughts as being good for the mental health. They provide pleasant involvement and companionship for those who are frustrated or beset with anxiety. They are a restful form of occupational therapy. See **sports**.

gangrene The death of a tissue, usually in the lower extremities, which is due to a decreased blood supply. Where there is illness or injury, it is important that the blood circulation be maintained. The condition is known as gas gangrene where the dead tissue becomes infected with bacteria called clostridia, which thrive in dead muscle in the absence of air, producing gas in the affected region.

gan ho A Chinese phrase which is used to describe impetuous and irrational actions due to stagnant liver-*qi*. See **liver-stagnation**.

Gansu books Relics of the Han dynasty, including books, discovered in the Gansu province indicate that, two thousand years ago, medical treatment in China was well established and sophisticated, though it was, perhaps, available only to the wealthy or the influential. The medical books used in the time of the Han dynasty were not the same as the books in use today. They consisted of about 35 strips of bamboo or wood held together with silk, each strip bearing a prescription and the recommended dosage. See **Han dynasty**.

garden burnet See **salad burnet**.

gardenia *Gardenia jasminoides* Herbal medicine. Distribution: China, Japan, Taiwan. Parts: ripe fruits. Character: cold, bitter. Affinity: heart, liver, stomach, lungs. Effects: antipyretic, antiphlogistic, refrigerant, antidote, haemostatic. Symptoms: fever, restlessness, irritation, sore and swollen eyes, nosebleeds, abscesses. Treatments: ailments due to heat excess, blood in the urine and sputum. Dosage: 4–10 g. A paste made by mixing this

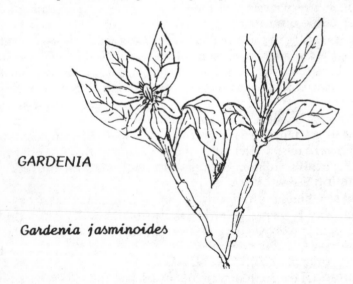

GARDENIA

Gardenia jasminoides

herb with flour and wine is effective as a poultice in the treatment of sprains, bruises, abscesses and injuries to muscles, joints, tendons and ligaments.

garlic *Allium sativum* Herbal medicine. Distribution: global. Parts: cloves. Character: warm, pungent. Affinity: stomach, large intestine. Effects: antiseptic, stomachic, antidote, anthelmintic, tonic, blood cleanser, cathartic, vasodilator. Symptoms: diarrhoea, convulsions, coughing fits, colds. Treatments: constipation, dysentry, parasitic worms, especially pin-worms and hook-worms, abscesses, tuberculosis, ringworm, influenza, anaemia, bronchitis, whooping cough, asthma, hay fever, rheumatism, thrombosis, hypertension. Dosage: 3–6 cloves, preferably fresh. Garlic is indeed a wonder-working panacea, and so deserving of special mention. It can be used as a treatment for many conditions, including those listed above. It is used internally, and most effectively, as a blood cleanser, expectorant and antiseptic, and, since it does not destroy the beneficial flora in the bowel, also as a selective antibiotic. Being a vasodilator, that is, a dilator of blood vessels, it is preventive of arteriosclerosis (hardening of the arteries). It is also considered to be preventive of cancer, for it has been noticed that there is a lower incidence of cancer in those countries where large amounts of garlic are consumed, such as China, Spain and Italy. But there may be other factors involved. The Chinese, Spanish and Italians consume large amounts of vegetables, fruit and shellfish, and do their frying in vegetable oils, which are rich in polyunsaturated fatty acids. In Spain and Italy, olive oil is the popular cooking oil. In China, peanut oil is the usual medium for stir-frying. Externally, garlic is a treatment for insect bites and stings, ringworm and skin infections generally. Steeped in oil, it makes an effective liniment for rheumatism and sprains, and may also be used as drops for earache. Everyone would benefit by a regular intake of garlic. The recommended amount, except where it is used specifically as a medicine, is one clove per day, crushed and infused in boiling water, and drunk as a tea, or chopped and added to a salad. Apart from many other benefits, it would reduce the cholesterol level, and so also minimize the risk of circulatory complaints. Garlic has one great disadvantage, which is the unpleasant odour it produces – 'Your best friends won't tell you' – but it would be the acme of folly to omit garlic from the diet for reasons of vanity. See **brimstone and treacle**.

gas gangrene See **gangrene**.

gastric Of or related to the stomach.

gastric ulcer See **ulcer**.

gastritis Inflammation or infection of the stomach. If the condition is acute and chronic, a medical check is necessary, for the cause could be ulcers or something worse. But, if it is not chronic, a plain and wholesome diet, including white rice porridge, and without alcohol, caffeine and tobacco, is required, together with a decoction, taken internally, of 4 g bark of Chinese cinnamon, *Cinnamomum cassia*, 8 g roots of liquorice, *Glycyrrhiza glabra*, or 10 g flowers of marigold, *Calendula officinalis*.

gastro-enteritis A combination of gastritis and enteritis. The treatment is the same as for gastritis.

gastropod See **mollusc**.

gate control theory This theory, which has been tested experimentally, explains how acupuncture or acupressure may be used to control pain; although, with acupressure, deep pressure must be applied if the technique is to be effective. A nerve consists of bundles of fibres, of which some are thick and some are thin. The thick ones transmit the sensation of touch, and the thin ones transmit the sensation of pain. An increase in the intensity of an impulse in the thick fibres closes a 'gate', which consists of certain nerve cells in the spinal cord, and so blocks the transmission of the sensation of pain in the thin fibres. Thus, the pain in an injured joint may be relieved if strong pressure is applied, which is contrary to what one would expect.

gelatin A low-grade type of protein derived from skins, bones and connective tissue. It is soluble in water; but, if the solution is concentrated, it solidifies to form a jelly on cooling. It is mixed with fish or meat stock to make aspic, which is a savoury jelly used as a mould for cold dishes. In China, it is used on a large scale for making jelly-type confectionery, which is considered to be healthier than that made entirely of sugar.

gene A tiny body attached to a chromosome in a cell, and which carries an inheritable characteristic, such as blue eyes, haemophilia and night-blindness. See **hereditary defects**.

general paralysis of the insane Dementia paralytica. Generally, a manifestation of untreated or ineffectively treated syphilis which occurs many years after the original infection. The nervous system is extensively damaged, which causes emotional instability, loss of intellect, fits, paralysis, insanity, delusions of grandeur and religious mania.

generative cycle See **element**.

genetics The scientific study of heredity, which is the manner in which the inheritable characteristics of humans, animals and plants are transmitted from one generation to the next. This is not a simple study, for the process of inheritance is not as straightforward as it might appear to be. For example, a tall man and a short woman may generate a tall son, but why is he tall, and not short? The explanation could be that he has inherited the characteristic of tallness, which is dominant, from his father, and that of shortness, which is recessive, from his mother, but the characteristic of tallness masks that of shortness. But the son could have a number of children, some short and some tall. Taking all the very many inheritable characteristics into account, the number of possible combinations is almost infinite, which explains why it is almost impossible to find two people who are exactly alike. It is important to distinguish between acquired characteristics and inherited characteristics. A man with a wooden leg, which he may have acquired as the result of an accident, will not have children with wooden legs; but a man with brown eyes, which is a dominant inherited characteristic, could have children whose eyes are brown. But there are exceptions. Now and again, an acquired characteristic may so influence the structure of the sex cells that it becomes an inherited characteristic. This process is called a mutation, and many scientists believe that it is one of the ways in which new varieties and even new species of animals and plants have been evolved. One can be sure that, thousands of years ago, the Chinese did not have a full understanding of the laws of inheritance, but they did see the need for some form of selective breeding so that desirable characteristics could be perpetuated, and undesirable characteristics eradicated. To this end, they would have favoured arranged marriages. See **hereditary defects**, **eugenics**, **ancestor worship** and **inbreeding**.

Genghis Khan See **Mongols**.

genitalia External organs of reproduction, which are sometimes called secondary sex characteristics, for a person's sexual nature is determined by the glands, and not by the external organs. It sometimes happens that a person with male genitalia has the sexual desires of a female, and vice versa, which can create problems – medical, social, moral and legal.

genital herpes See **herpes**.

genital thrush The many possible causes of this condition include sex with an infected partner, bubble baths, tight-fitting trousers or tights, antibiotics, emotional disturbances, contraceptive pills, lack of sleep, debility, diabetes, menstruation, pregnancy and the menopause. Wine, tea, coffee and fruit juices can exacerbate this condition. See **Candida albicans**.

gentian *Gentiana macrophylla* Herbal medicine. Distribution: China. Parts: roots. Character: neutral, pungent-bitter. Affinity: stomach, liver, gall-bladder. Effects: antipyretic, analgesic. Symptoms: painful and stiff extremities, muscles and joints. Treatments: arthritis, rheumatism, jaundice due to excess of damp-heat, yin-deficiency. Dosage: 5–10 g. Gentian is considered to be a good remedy for genital herpes. It is sometimes called Chinese gentian to distinguish it from the European species, *Gentiana lutea*.

genu The medical name for the knee.

geomancy Fortune-telling by signs exhibited by the earth, as with the positions of natural features, the shape of the terrain and markings in sand. It is related to *fung shui*, or 'earth magic', which was once commonly practised in China. See **prediction**.

geriatrics The medical study and treatment of the ailments of elderly people. In China, geriatric treatment is based upon physical and breathing exercises of the kind contained in the *Chinese Exercise Manual*.

German measles See **rubella**.

germicide A preparation designed to destroy bacteria and some other micro-organisms.

gestation Pregnancy. In humans, the period of gestation, or pregnancy, is about nine months or 283 days. It is interesting to compare the gestation period of humans with those of other mammals: opossum, 12 days; rabbit, 31 days; dog, 61 days; horse, 340 days; elephant, 645 days. One should note that it is quite common for human babies to be born prematurely, and, occasionally, after only seven months; but, with proper care, such babies develop normally and healthily.

Gest Oriental Library One of the finest collections of Chinese medical books in the world is contained in the Gest Oriental Library at Princeton University in the United States. It was established by G.M. Gest, an American businessman, as a token of his gratitude to a Chinese physician who had cured him of an eye disease which, hitherto, had been thought to be incurable. Gest himself collected about 75,000 volumes which became the basis for the collection in the library.

giddiness See **dizziness**.

gigantism An abnormal enlargement of the body which is due to an excessive secretion by the pituitary gland of the hormone which regulates growth and bone formation. This condition must not be confused with acromegaly, which affects only the hands, feet and head.

gin Distilled from beer and flavoured with juniper berries, gin is regarded as one of the purest of the potable spirits, and it makes a good substitute for medicinal alcohol, and also for rice wine when preparing Chinese-style medicinal wines.

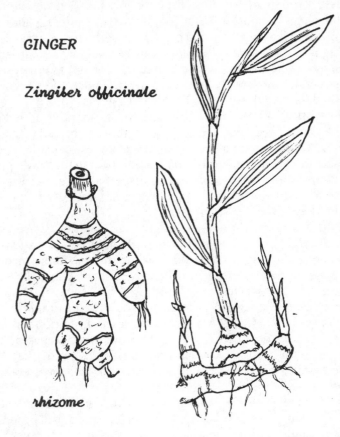

GINGER

Zingiber officinale

rhizome

ginger *Zingiber officinale* Herbal medicine. Distribution: tropical countries. Parts: dried rhizomes. Character: warm, pungent. Affinity: heart, lungs, stomach, spleen, kidneys. Effects: warming, particularly to the lungs, expectorant, loosens phlegm, stomachic, antiemetic, stimulating to yang-*qi*. Symptoms: nausea, vomiting, diarrhoea, coldness in hands, feet and abdomen, weak pulse, coughing, profuse sputum. Treatments: cold-excess in stomach and spleen, painful abdomen, cold-excess in lungs, travel sickness. Dosage: 3–8 g. One should note that the so-called ginger root is actually a rhizome. The fresh root – or rhizome – is a remedy for colds, nausea and seafood poisoning. Fresh or dried, it may be used as a remedy for chills, coughs, colic, flatulence and visceral spasms, when it is best administered in a soup or a stew. It is very versatile in its culinary uses. It is added to fish dishes in order to destroy any unpleasant fishy odour.

gingivitis Inflamed or infected gums. An infusion of one of the following as a mouthwash, using the parts and dosage indicated, is an effective treatment: sage, *Salvia officinalis*, leaves, 2–6 g; marigold, *Calendula officinalis*, flowers, 3–12 g; cardamom, *Elettaria cardamomum*, crushed seeds, 2–6 g. Chewing fresh watercress, *Nasturtium officinale*, which must be thoroughly washed, is a good treatment for bleeding gums.

gingko nuts These nuts are the fruits of the gingko, or maidenhair, tree, which has a very ancient ancestry but now survives only in China and Japan. The Chinese consider them to be a delicacy, but they shell and blanch them before adding them to soups and meat and sweet dishes. However, they are poisonous if consumed in large quantities, and so they are best omitted from the diet altogether.

ginseng There are three types of ginseng: Asiatic, *Panax ginseng*, American, *Panax quinquefolium*, and Siberian, *Eleutherococcus senticosus*. They are similar but not identical in their medicinal properties. Asiatic ginseng, which is said to retard the ageing process, is the species commonly used in China, though large quantities of American ginseng are now being imported into China via Hong Kong. Many substitutes and inferior specimens of ginseng are being sold, and so the would-be purchaser should proceed with caution. Among these substitutes are pfaffia, which is sometimes called Brazilian ginseng, and *dang shen*, *Codonopsis tangshen*, which is similar to ginseng in its properties but is less potent. Tienchi, *Radix pseudo-ginseng*, which grows abundantly in the Yunnan province, has many valuable medicinal properties, and it could outdo ginseng in its popularity. Women with menstrual irregularities should not take ginseng. It is available at health-food stores as a root to be chewed, in powdered form in tablets and capsules, and as loose powder or extracts to be made into herbal teas. See **Asiatic ginseng**.

ginseng syndrome This term describes the popular belief that ginseng is a wonder-working panacea, and that a regular intake is certain to keep one in a sound state of health. But ginseng does have its limitations, and, though it is generally safe, it does have side-effects, which include headaches and irritability, and so it should not be taken as a single course for more than three weeks.

ginseng tea This is an infusion of ginseng leaves or flowers with sugar added. It is a refreshing and tonic drink, but it is less potent than the root. However, it is safe and effective if taken regularly over a long period. Commercially, it is obtained as a mixture containing ingredients which, by weight, are usually in the proportions of 90 per cent sugar and 10 per cent ginseng extract.

GLA The abbreviation for gamma-linolenic acid. See **eczema**.

gland An organ which secretes a chemical substance with a specific function. Those glands which have ducts, such as the sweat glands, are called exocrine glands. Those whose secretions are transmitted via the bloodstream are called endocrine glands. A lymph node of the lymphatic system is also described as a gland.

glandular fever See **infectious mononucleosis**.

Glauber's salt Mirabilite. Sodium sulphate. Medicine. Distribution: global. Parts: crystals (decahydrate). Character: very cold, bitter, salty. Affinity: stomach, large intestine, triple-warmer. Effects: purgative, antiseptic. Symptoms: constipation, sore mouth and gums. Treatments: heat-excess conditions, abscesses, appendicitis. Dosage: 9–10 g. If this salt is used as a mild cathartic, the dosage is reduced. It is combined with rhubarb when used as a purgative. Externally, a solution is applied to abscesses or used as an eyewash or gargle. Being of a bitter taste, it may be applied to the nipples to wean children off breast-feeding. In China, a poultice of a mixture of Glauber's salt crystals, chopped rhubarb rhizomes and crushed fresh garlic cloves is applied to the abdomen as a treatment for acute appendicitis. But this treatment is not to be recommended for the people of the West. A physician should be called if appendicitis is suspected.

glaucoma A condition in which an abnormally large amount of fluid within the eyeball exerts a pressure on the retina and optic nerve. See **eye**.

globus hystericus A 'lump' in the throat'. This sensation is caused by anxiety or tension.

glossitis Inflammation of the tongue. The treatment is the same as that for gingivitis.

glottis The region of the vocal cords in the larynx, which is situated just below the epiglottis. See **epiglottis**.

glucose See **sugar**.

gluten A protein found in wheat and rye. The other cereals – barley, maize, oats, millet and rice – contain little or no gluten. Intolerance to gluten causes coeliac disease, which is more common in children than in adults, and is characterized by severe diarrhoea, foul-smelling and pale stools, a distended abdomen, poor growth, loss of weight, anaemia and rickets. The gluten causes the formation of lesions in the small intestine, which results in poor absorption of fats, iron and certain vitamins. The treatment is to provide the patient with a gluten-free diet. There is a low incidence of this disease in South China, where rice is the staple item of diet.

glycerine See **glycerol**.

glycerol A dense and sweetish syrupy alcohol, which was called glycerine in an older system of chemical nomenclature, and which is a constituent of fats. It is a by-product of soap manufacture, which is made by adding a strong alkali, such as caustic soda (sodium hydroxide) or caustic potash (potassium hydroxide), to fat or an oil. Glycerol is used as a solvent in tinctures.

glycogen Animal starch. A type of carbohydrate which is stored in the liver and muscles, but which breaks down into glucose when required to maintain the constant concentration of glucose in the blood.

gnat bite See **mosquito**.

goatish See **odour**.

goats It seems that goats have played a part in the development of Chinese medicine, for there is a story, which could well be true, that a long time ago, in ancient China, a goat-herd noticed that his billy-goats were always sexually active for several hours after they had eaten a certain weed. It was found that this herb is just as effective with human males as it is with male goats. Chinese herbalists named it *yin yang huo*, which means 'horny goat weed'. Even today, this herb is regarded as being one of the best and safest of all aphrodisiacs. See **horny goat weed**.

goitre A morbid enlargement of the thyroid gland due to iodine deficiency, and which often occurs as a pendulous swelling of the neck. In ancient China, this condition was treated by administering the iodine-rich black ash from burnt seaweed. Sun Simiao, one of the great physicians of the period of the Tang dynasty, prescribed extracts from the thyroid glands of deer and lambs. The situation has been very different in the West. Until recent times, a goitre was thought to necessitate an operation, which had certain risks. Nowadays, the treatment is tablets containing thyroid extracts from the dried thyroid glands of sheep. Preventive measures include the addition of iodine compounds to table salt and the water supply, using sea salt as a condiment and having a diet containing foods that are rich in iodine, such as fish and seaweed products. It is noticeable that there is a lower incidence of goitre among people who live in coastal regions than among those who live in mountainous areas, where the soil is deficient in iodine. See **hyperthyroidism**.

gold The alchemists of both China and the West included gold in their elixirs. No doubt, they believed that, since gold is thought to be precious, it has some magical, medicinal or other special properties. But, in truth, gold is nowhere near as useful or as valuable health-wise as the iron, magnesium, potassium and other metals which occur as minute traces in the body. Yet, until quite recent times, gold had a limited use as an ingredient in medicinal preparations. Even today, there are those who believe that rubbing a gold ring on skin eruptions can have a beneficial effects. See **mineral**.

Golden Age See **Zhou dynasty**.

golden bell *Forsythia suspensa* Herbal medicine. Distribution: China, Japan. Parts: fruits. Character: cool, bitter. Affinity: heart, gall-bladder. Effects: antipyretic, antiphlogistic, antidote. Symptoms: high temperature, thirst, rashes, irritability. Treatments: swelling of lymph glands, glandular fever, erysipelas, breast tumours, heat-injury conditions. Dosage: 6–10 g. This herb is often used in combination with Japanese honeysuckle, *Lonicera japonica*, which has similar medicinal properties.

Golden Lotus, See **Jing Ping Mei**.

golden mean Both Lao Zi and Confucius advocated a strict adherence to the *golden mean*, which is the principle that one should always take the middle way, and so avoid extremes of conduct. This is the principle of compromise. It reflects the yin-yang concept of complementary opposites, which creates harmony in society, with nature and within the human body. In many respects, it is the key to a sound state of health, which arises from moderate habits in diet, exercise and social conduct. See **moderation**.

golden rule This well-known rule, which is contained in the *Analects*, indicates the Confucian concept of the correct form of human relationships: 'What do you not want done to yourself, do not do to others.' Confucius recognized that stable individuals are largely a product of caring families within a stable society, and that harmony in society is conducive to mental health. It must surely be the case that frustration, anxiety and stress are caused in no small measure by disruptive, violent and dishonest elements in society.

gonorrhoea A venereal disease caused by the gonococcus bacterium.

The initial symptoms, which generally occur within ten days after infection, are painful and frequent urination and a discharge from the urethra or vagina. If untreated, the infection spreads to the testicles or womb and fallopian tubes, and will eventually lead to certain forms of arthritis, endocarditis and conjunctivitis. See **venereal disease**.

gota kola *Hydrocotyle asiatica* Also called Indian pennywort. Herbal medicine. Distribution: Near and Far East, especially India. Parts: whole plant. Character: cool, bitter. Affinity: liver, spleen. Effects: relaxant, digestive, diuretic, antipyretic. Symptoms: inflammation of the skin, irritability, sleeplessness, fever, aches in joints and limbs. Treatments: rheumatism, arthritis, sores, skin ulcers, poorly healing wounds, leprous sores, mental and nervous disorders. Dosage: 2–6 g.

gourmandizing See **moderation**.

gout See **podagra**.

governor-vessel Brain. See **meridian**.

grains-of-paradise *Amomum xanthioides* Herbal medicine. Distribution: South China, Vietnam. Parts: seeds. Character: warm, pungent. Affinity: stomach, spleen, kidneys. Effects: astringent, decongestant, digestive, stomachic, carminative, sedative to a restless foetus. Symptoms: diarrhoea, indigestion, nausea, vomiting. Treatments: restless foetus, fullness in chest and abdomen, excess damp in stomach and spleen. Dosage: 2–4 g.

grand mal See **epilepsy**.

Grave's disease See **thyrotoxicosis**.

gravid Pregnant.

graze See **cuts**.

great burdock There are three species of burdock, which are the great, or greater, burdock, *Arctium lappa*, the lesser burdock, *Arctium minus*, and the common burdock, *Arctium pubens*. They have similar anatomical characteristics and medicinal properties, but the lesser burdock is somewhat smaller than the others. The great burdock, *Arctium lappa*, which is generally referred to simply as 'burdock', is the species used in TCM. It is native to both China and Europe. See **burdock**.

great plantain *Plantago major* This herb has several common names: common plantain, greater plantain, waybread and rat's-tail plantain. Also, there are several species of plants which take the common name of *plantain*: great plantain, *Plantago major*; hoary plantain or lamb's tongue, *Plantago media*; ribwort plantain, *Plantago lanceolata*; sea plantain, *Plantago maritima*; buck's horn plantain, *Plantago coronopus*; lesser water plantain, *Baldellia*

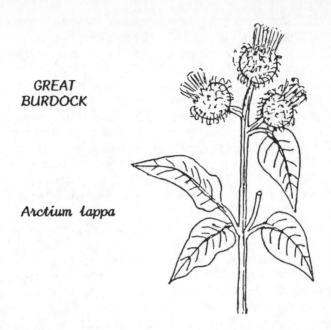

GREAT
BURDOCK

Arctium lappa

ranunculoides; water plantain, *Alisma plantago-aquatica*; floating water plantain, *Luronium natans*; lanceolate water plantain, *Alisma lanceolatum*. But these plants do not all have the same anatomical characteristics and medicinal properties, and none of them must be confused with the tree-like plantain which is allied to the banana, *Musa sapientum*, and a native of the tropics. The species used in TCM are the so-called common plantain, *Plantago asiatica*, and the water plantain, *Alisma plantago-aquatica*. See **common plantain** and **water plantain**.

Greek elements See **element**.

green consumers These are the wise and worthy people who make a practice of buying only those commodities which will do no harm to the environment, for they recognize that man cannot live healthily in an unhealthy environment. They do not purchase petrol that is not unleaded, aerosols which contain substances that could damage the ozone layer, harmful detergents, pesticides and fertilizers containing synthetic substances, garments made from animal furs, and perfumes and other toiletries made of animal products. At the same time, they are very careful about the disposal of waste, and prefer to buy goods whose packagings are made of biodegradable materials. This particularly caring attitude towards the environment is a new development in the Western world, but it is certainly not new to China, where the establishment of harmony between man and nature is central to the teachings of Taoism. The Chinese government imposes heavy penalties on those who break their stringent laws which are designed to protect endangered species, such as the panda and the tiger. See **environment**.

Green Dragon See **White Tiger**.

green ginger Fresh ginger roots, which are really rhizomes, are sold in whole pieces called races. In this form, it is commonly sliced and candied and used in confectionery.

green-stick fracture A type of fracture, usually in the soft bones of a child, in which one side of the bone is broken and the other side is bent – in the same way as a green stick would be fractured. See **fracture**.

green tea This is the uncured, or unfermented, dried leaves of the tea plant, *Camellia sinensis*, and the form in which it is usually taken by the Chinese, mainly as a mild stimulant, an aid to the digestion and a refreshing drink. They claim that tea improves the eyesight, calms the nerves, stimulates the brain, strengthens the arteries, disposes of excess fat, clears phlegm, counteracts poisons, kills harmful micro-organisms, tones the kidneys and controls diarrhoea. Therefore, there is much to be said for the tea-drinking habit. However, those substances in tea which are beneficial to the health are also damaging if in excess, as occurs when tea is over infused or too much tea is drunk. In making green tea, use 3 teaspoons tea to 1 litre boiling water, infuse for only 3 minutes, and consume without milk or sugar. See **tea**.

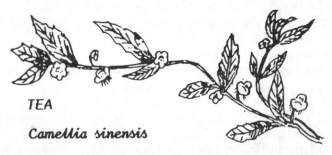

TEA

Camellia sinensis

green vegetables Those vegetables which are green, such as cabbage, spinach and runner beans, contain no fat and very little protein or carbohydrate, but they are rich in certain vitamins and iron and other minerals. They also provide dietary fibre. Some nutritionists say that they are preventive of cancer. Perhaps the truth is that, as man's natural diet is essentially vegetarian, a large intake of vegetables helps to create those natural dietary circumstances which are likely to prevent cancer and those other diseases which can be partly attributed to an unsound diet. See **carrot** and **natural diet**.

grief See **sorrow**.

gripe water A carminative to relieve flatulence in babies. One cannot afford to take risks with infants, for they are unable to speak for themselves, and so one should take proper medical advice before administering a proprietary brand of gripe water or embarking upon any other kind of treatment. In many primitive societies, a baby with 'wind' is encouraged to suck a cold ember from the ashes of a wood fire. This contains traces of potash, a crude form of potassium carbonate, which is mildly alkaline. This is not a hygienic practice, and so it is not to be recommended. The Chinese use lye water, which is a solution of potassium carbonate, as an antacid and preservative in noodles and some other foodstuffs. It is obtained by the lixiviation of vegetable ashes. See **flatulence**.

grippe See **influenza**.

gristle See **cartilage**.

growth One of the various kinds of morbid formations which sometimes occur in the body, though the term is commonly used in relation to cancer or a tumour. See **cancer** and **tumour**.

Guan Yu Historical records indicate that anaesthetics were first used in China during the time of the Han dynasty. It is very likely that Chinese surgeons were the first persons in the world to use anaesthetics. Guan Yu, a Chinese general who had been struck in the arm by a poisoned arrow, was one of the first to benefit from the use of anaesthetics. Hua To, an eminent surgeon of that period, saved the general's life by administering an anaesthetic and then cutting away the poisoned flesh. He probably used jimson, or loco, weed, *Datura metel*, as a local anaesthetic, and aconite, *Aconitum carmichaeli*, as an analgesic.

guan zhong *Dryopteris crassirhizoma* Herbal medicine. Distribution: global. Parts: rhizomes. Character: cool, bitter. Affinity: stomach, liver. Effects: antipyretic, haemostatic, antidote, anthelmintic. Symptoms: painful and distended abdomen, inflamed abscesses. Treatments: menorrhagia, inflamed thyroid glands, intestinal worms, contagious colds. Dosage: 7–15 g. This herb is slightly poisonous. For medicinal purposes, the nearest equivalent available in the West is the male fern, *Dryopteris filixmas*.

gui jing Natural affinities of herbs, which the Chinese physician takes into account, together with their energies, tastes, odours, direction, etc., when prescribing medicines. It often happens that, though two different organs, say the lungs and the liver, require the same category of medicine in matters of energy, taste, direction and yin-yang, they will probably not be treated with the same medicine, for those medicines which have an affinity for the lungs will not necessarily have an affinity for the liver. It is important to note that a medicine which has an affinity for a particular organ will also influence the meridian connected with that organ. In this way, a medication can have an indirect affinity for a part of the body which is not a vital organ. Thus, a herb which has an affinity for the liver will also affect those parts of the leg which are on the liver meridian. The affinities of herbs have been established by many centuries of experience. See **affinity of herbs**.

gulf seaweed *Sargassum fusiforme* Herbal medicine. Distribution: coasts of Japan and China. Parts: entire plant. Character: cold, bitter-salty. Affinity: stomach, liver, kidneys. Effects: diuretic, expectorant, reduces goitre. Symptoms: swollen lymph glands, excessive and lumpy phlegm, goitre, fever, sore throat. Treatments: hyperthyroidism, goitre, glandular fever. Dosage: 5–12 g. This herb contains 0.2 per cent iodine and, in China, it is an age-old remedy for illnesses due to iodine deficiency.

gumboil A small abscess on the gum. The ground kernels of the longan fruit, *Euphoria longan*, can be used as a styptic. A mouthwash is helpful. See **gingivitis**.

gums In TCM, gums are mainly used in tonic medications for the treatment of debility, fatigue, lassitude and similar conditions. They are derived from skin, bones, carapaces, horns, hooves and connective tissue generally, some exotic sources being the bones of tigers, the dried hides of asses, the carapaces of tortoises, the feet of pigs and the horns of stags. These items are scraped to remove all the flesh, thoroughly washed, simmered for two days, strained to remove sediment, simmered again until the liquid becomes viscous, strained again and then heated until all the water has evaporated and a translucent residue remains. This has the texture of rubber, and is cut into cubes or squares, and is then ready for use. For diseases of the gums, see **gingivitis** and **pyorrhoea**.

gynaecology The branch of medicine which is concerned with the anatomy, physiological functions and diseases of women. From ancient times, all physicians, Chinese or otherwise, have recognized that men and women have different physical and emotional needs, and may require different treatments even when suffering from the same disease, for women menstruate, become pregnant and undergo the menopause; but men do not. Also, men and women are not exactly alike in their hormones.

gypsum *Gypsum fibrosum* (calcium sulphate) Medicine. Distribution: global. Parts: crystals. Character: cold, sweet-pungent. Affinity: stomach, lungs. Effects: antipyretic, antiphlogistic, refrigerant, astringent. Symptoms: fever, heat rash, toothache, headache, coughs. Treatments: physical and emotional conditions caused by heat excess, particularly in the lungs and stomach, asthma and bronchitis coughs, external application to rashes, abscesses, burns and scalds. Dosage: 12–36 g. If this substance is to be taken internally, it must not be of commercial standard, which is generally impure, but of a pure standard, as are BP standard chemicals used in the West.

H

habit spasm See **tic**.

hacking See **percussion**.

haematite Brown iron oxide (Fe_2O_3). Medicine. Distribution: global. Parts: powdered mineral. Character: cold, bitter. Affinity: liver, pericardium. Effects: haemostatic, astringent, antiemetic, blood tonic, sedative to liver. Symptoms: hiccups, belching, nausea, vomiting, dizziness, headaches. Treatments: nosebleeds, tinnitus, bronchial asthma, conditions due to ascending liver-yang. Dosage: 10–15 g. This substance is an iron compound, which explains why it is used as a blood tonic, though one may wonder if the intestine would readily assimilate iron in this crude mineral form. This medicine would certainly not be used in the West.

haematoma A contusion under the skin, and which is a collection of ruptured blood vessels.

haematuria Blood in the urine, and a condition which requires immediate medical attention.

haemoglobin A pigment containing iron which occurs in the red blood cells, and which gives blood its colour. See **erythrocyte**.

haemolytic disease A severe form of anaemia due to an abnormally excessive breakdown of the red blood cells. It occasionally occurs in new-born babies, when it is known as erythroblastic foetalis. See **anaemia**.

haemophilia An inherited disease which is characterized by inadequate clotting of the blood, causing easy bruising or severe bleeding if an injury occurs. See **hereditary defects**.

haemorrhage Bleeding. See **cuts**, **haemostatic**, **san qi** and **Yunnan bai yao**.

haemorrhoids Piles. Distended, or varicose, veins just within the anus. In severe cases, they may protrude permanently from the anus, and they then have the appearance of small black grapes. Sometimes, a thrombus, or blood clot, converts a haemorrhoid into a hard and painful lump, which can be removed by surgery, using a local anaesthetic. If there are doubts about anal bleeding, medical advice should be sought. The causes of haemorrhoids are constipation over a long period, diarrhoea due to excessive use of laxatives, lack of dietary fibre, constant exposure to hot, cold or wet conditions and lack of exercise. In TCM, haemorrhoids are attributed to heat, damp and blood stagnation in the anus. The upright stance of humans is considered to be a contributory factor, for it is the case that mammals, which walk on all fours, do not have haemorrhoids. This condition can be prevented or alleviated by using soft tissues or a wet cloth instead of hard toilet paper, having a more natural diet with ample amounts of dietary fibre, including more liquid in the diet to prevent constipation, avoiding straining when passing motions, and taking exercise and maintaining a good posture as per the *qi gong*, which is explained in the *Chinese Exercise Manual*. The treatments used in TCM include a wet compress of marigold, *Calendula officinalis*, flowers, and an infusion, taken internally, of 0.3 g rhubarb, *rheum officinale*, rhizomes or 10–30 g dandelion, *Taraxacum officinale*, leaves, flowers or roots. Ear acupuncture is also helpful. A traditional Chinese remedy used by country people is to simmer 125 g rice and 30 g each of sesame seeds, walnuts, almonds, peach kernels and pine nuts in 2 litres water for an hour, and to drink the resulting liquid as a soup twice daily. This is also a good remedy for constipation.

haemostatic A medicine to arrest haemorrhage. Haemostatics in common use in TCM include the following, prepared as an infusion or decoction, and taken internally, using the parts and dosages indicated: mugwort, *Artemisia vulgaris*, leaves, 4–8 g; comfrey, *Symphytum asperum*, leaves or roots, 3–12 g; salad burnet, *Sanguisorba minor*, roots, 4–10 g. See **astringent** and **san qi**.

Hahnemann see **homoeopathy**.

hair This is the fastest-growing cellular component of the body, but there is a limit to the length to which it can grow, and so a few loose hairs should give no cause for alarm. Hair is lubricated, and so kept supple and shiny, by sebum, which is a natural oil exuded by the sebaceous glands, which are in the skin. Sebum also has antiseptic properties, and so it helps to destroy bacteria on the scalp. Generally, the hair on the head is in good condition if one's general health is good and one washes the hair regularly as a part of one's personal hygiene. However, the sebum is destroyed, and so its benefits are lost, if the hair is washed too frequently and conditioners, shampoos, grooming equipment and the other tools of the hairdresser's trade are over-used.

Occasionally, there are problems such as alopecia, dandruff, ringworm and other diseases of the scalp. Head lice can be a problem, too. These conditions not only damage the hair but also undermine one's health and general well-being. See **hair care** and **head lice**.

hair care A great deal of time and money is devoted to modern hair care. Really, the only care that the hair needs is a once-weekly wash, a varied and adequate diet to ensure a good supply of nutrients, and regular exercise to make sure that these nutrients are circulated to the head via the blood. This is the general practice in China, where a person who is bald is rarely encountered. But it must be said that the Chinese have a natural advantage here in so far as black, lank and strong hair is one of the inherited characteristics of the Mongoloid races. An infusion of 6 g sage, *Salvia officinalis*, leaves, 6 g thyme, *Thymus vulgare*, leaves, 6 g stinging nettle, *Urtica dioica*, leaves or 20 g dandelion, *Taraxacum officinale*, leaves, roots or flowers combined with water and a little soap makes a shampoo that will clean and tone the scalp, and also improve the circulation in the scalp. These same infusions can be taken internally to cleanse the blood and provide mineral nutrients which are good for hair growth. See **hair loss** and **oily hair**.

hair follicle A tubular sac in the skin containing the base, or root, of a hair.

hairiness This is a normal condition, but one which displeases some people. There is hair on all parts of the body with the exception of the soles of the feet, palms of the hands, ends of the toes and fingers, umbilicus and some parts of the genitals. It serves a useful purpose in that it provides insulation which helps to keep the body warm. The amount and nature of the hair on a person's body is largely an inherited characteristic. It is also a racial characteristic. A member of the Caucasian races has a fair amount of hair on his body, and that on his head is wavy or straight, and comes in a variety of colours – black, blond, brunette, flaxen, auburn, ginger and grey, and where the hairdressers have been at work, even green, blue, silver and gold! If we are to believe all that we read in the history books, the Vikings, who were Scandinavians, were very hairy people indeed. A person who is of the Negroid races has a fair amount of black, frizzy or woolly hair on both his head and his chest. A person who is of the Mongoloid races has jet-black, straight, coarse hair on his head, but very little on his body. Anthropologists assure us that racial differences are indicated more by the texture of the hair than the colour of the skin. Many people go to great lengths to alter the appearance of their hair. However, the Taoist view is that we should accept ourselves, and our state of hairiness, as nature has made us. That must be the best arrangement, for nature surely knows best, though there must be many people, particularly those who are congenitally ill or have some inherited defect, who might feel that nature has let them down. See **hair care** and **hereditary defects**.

hair loss Hair is constantly growing, being lost and being replaced. But when the hair does not grow fast enough to replace that being lost, which condition is largely due to imbalances in the hormone levels, baldness occurs, though this is more noticeable with the hair on the head than that on the rest of the body. The baldness may be patchy or an overall thinning of the hair. Permanent baldness, which affects men more than women, is usually hereditary, but other factors may be involved – stress, poor circulation and inadequate diet. Temporary baldness may be caused by anaemia, deficiencies in the thyroid hormones, contraceptive pills, antibiotics, steroids and scalp infections, such as alopecia, ringworm and dandruff. It may also be caused by an excessive use of shampoos and similar cosmetic preparations, but herbal shampoos containing thyme or rosemary extracts do no harm. Here, the obvious procedure is to eradicate the cause of the baldness, but this may involve a difficult decision or an element of compromise. For example, does one abandon the contraceptive pill or accept baldness? On the other hand, scalp infections can be treated, and then the baldness should depart. Some of the hair restorers being sold are of doubtful value, but others are fairly effective and are offered in good faith. For even the best of the hair restorers, there is only a 40 per cent success rate. Where there are no hair roots, it is impossible to make the hair grow again, for it has completely ceased to exist. And where there are hair roots, but the conditions which inhibit the growth of hair cannot be counteracted by hair restorers, the hair may grow for a short time, but it is likely to be weak and straggly, and then baldness returns. The Chinese have shown that temporary loss of hair on the head may be prevented by regularly massaging the scalp with almond oil, which improves circulation in the scalp. In the West, rosemary oil is used for this purpose. Chinese physicians recommend tonic medicines, such as ginseng, wolf-berries, sesame seeds and royal jelly, which will provide the scalp with nutrients. In TCM, the most effective medicine for the promotion of hair growth is *han lian cao*, *Eclipta prostrata*.

The juice of the fresh herb is rubbed into the scalp. An infusion of 8–15 g of this herb, taken internally, prevents premature greying and will completely darken the hair, beard and eyebrows. One of the traditional Chinese folklorish remedies for hair loss and greying hair is an apple, a carrot and a quarter of a lemon, all finely chopped, infused together in 1 litre water, and consumed once daily. Mulberry wine is also considered to be good for hair loss. See **hair care**.

hair restorers See **hair loss**.

hairweed See **facai**.

halitosis An unpleasant odour of the breath. Its causes are infections and upsets of the teeth, mouth, nose, sinuses, throat, lungs and stomach, including gingivitis, pyorrhoea and septic tonsils. Medical advice should be sought if the condition persists, for there could be an underlying cause which urgently needs attention. Otherwise, an infusion of any of the following, using the parts and dosage indicated, can be used as a mouthwash and breath sweetener. Sage, *Salvia officinalis*, leaves, 2–4 g; sweet marjoram, *Oregano marjorana*, leaves, 2–4 g; cardamom, *Elettaria cardamomum*, crushed seeds, 2–6 g; agrimony, *Agrimonia eupatoria*, flowers, 10–15 g. A saline solution – 2 g salt dissolved in 1 litre water – makes an effective mouthwash. Caraway seeds can be chewed as a breath sweetener.

hallucination Illusion. The apparent perception by sight, smell or sound of something which does not exist. Hallucinations are a feature of delirium. See **drug**.

hallucinogen See **drug**.

hallux valgus A deformity of the big toe in which the toe is turned inwards. It is usually caused by wearing shoes that are too tight. See **pigtail**.

hammer toe A deformity in which a toe points upwards and backwards. It is often caused by wearing shoes that are too tight.

Han dynasty During the period of the Han dynasty (206 BC–AD 200), China's economy and trade flourished, and roads and canals were constructed, which not only helped the merchants but also encouraged the communication of ideas, so giving a stimulus to the development of Chinese medicine. The literature of this period contains many references to longevity and the people who had mastered the secret of long life, some of whom lived to be over 150 years of age. New medicines became available as a consequence of the Han emperors' conquest of the fertile southern regions of China. New medicines also became available through China's trade with India and Persia. Scholars of the early Han period compiled *Huang Di Nei Jing*, or 'The Internal Book of the Yellow Emperor', which describes the exploits and medical discoveries of the Yellow Emperor, and *Shen Nong Ben Cao Jing*, or 'The Pharmacopoeia of Shen Nong', which recorded all herbal knowledge from the time of Shen Nong, one of the legendary rulers of early China. Zhang Zhongjing wrote *Shang Han Lun*, or 'Discussions on Fevers'. Anaesthetics came into use, and they were probably the first in the world. Veterinary medicine also came into being at this time, for one of the Han relics discovered in the Gansu province contains a prescription for treating a horse. See **Yellow Emperor**, **Guan Yu**, **Zhang Zhongjing** and **Gansu books**.

hangnail Also called an agnail. A piece of torn skin at the base or side of a finger-nail, and a condition which is prevalent among people who, in the course of their occupations, are constantly handling rough materials. The dead skin should be cut off and the fingertips immersed in a mixture of warm water and olive oil to keep them soft, and then covered with a sterile pad until healed.

hangover This is very much a self-inflicted injury, and a good example of one of those many conditions where prevention is certainly easier than a cure. In view of the immense damage done to the health of many of the people of the West, together with the man-hours lost to industrial production, by alcohol-addiction, the hangover is deserving of special mention in a book concerned with health. The Chinese have few problems in this respect because, being of moderate habits, they partake of alcoholic drinks, but only rarely to excess. In this connection, it is interesting to note that one of the characteristics of the Chinese race is that a Chinese person's face becomes very flushed after he has imbibed only a small amount of alcohol; and so, perhaps, it is the fear of being embarrassed by this tell-tale sign of inebriation which helps to maintain the Chinese in their frugal habits in regard to alcohol. A hangover will be more intense if the alcohol has been consumed with large quantities of cigarettes and rich food. The effects are likely to be felt more keenly by someone who drinks only occasionally than by a habitual drinker. But what is a hangover? Alcohol in the body triggers off a mechanism in the brain which creates a desire to drink. This is why an individual who can boast about drinking eight pints of beer in an evening could not be induced to drink the same quantity of water in the same time. But alcohol is a diuretic, and so a large amount in the body produces excessive and frequent urination. This, in turn, produces dehydration, which is usually accompanied by acidity, and occasionally by toxaemia, which is manifested first by confusion and sleepiness, and later by nausea, a headache, blurred vision, a dry mouth, shaking and depression. Some of these effects are due more to the additives in the drink than to the alcohol itself. See **congener**. A hangover can be prevented, and without interfering with the essential pleasure, by drinking moderately, and never on an empty stomach. Food absorbs the acidic and toxic substances in the alcoholic drinks, so assisting their evacuation from the bowel on the following day. More water with drinks will help to reduce dehydration. Tonic water and drinks containing saccharin and other artificial sweeteners should be avoided. The quinine in the former is a depressant, and the latter increases the absorption rate of alcohol. Before the drinking session commences, a suitable food or beverage, such as plain-cooked rice or noodles, porridge or milk, should be consumed in order to make an absorbent and non-irritant layer that will protect the delicate membranes of the digestive tract. Four tablespoons of olive oil, if one has the courage to take them, could be helpful. Immediately after waking on the morning after a hectic night, one should drink copious quantities of water to replace that lost by dehydration during the night. It will be less insipid if flavoured with grapefruit or lemon juice – or even orange peel – which will help to settle the stomach. A 'hair of the dog', that is, taking another alcoholic drink, gives some measure of relief, but it is deceptive, and only serves to postpone the outcome; and, when the final hangover does occur, it will be more intense than it might otherwise be. Aspirin and coffee should be avoided. The former is an irritant to the stomach, and the latter is a stimulant and diuretic, and so, though it will clear the head for a short time, it will also increase dehydration, so doing more harm than good. Many drugs, including opium derivatives, cannot be safely taken with alcohol, so they must NOT be taken as a cure for a hangover. On the other hand, fruit juice can be helpful, for it contains fructose, which will assist in reducing the alcohol by the normal metabolic process of oxidation. A meat broth or fish soup will help to replace the sodium and potassium salts lost by perspiration. A hangover is likely to be accompanied by diarrhoea if the drinks consumed contained impurities, which is often the case with cheap wine and beers. This should be allowed to take its course to some extent, for it is nature's way of ridding the bowel of toxic or irritating substances. But if the condition becomes too distressing or persists, white rice porridge will provide gentle relief. A headache accompanying a hangover is only a symptom, and it should disappear along with the hangover if the cause of the condition, which is dehydration, is effectively treated. However, a small cup of sage tea sipped gently should provide instant relief for a splitting headache. To make this, infuse 10 g dried leaves of common sage, *Salvia officinalis*, in ½ litre boiling water for 5 minutes. It takes about 3 days for alcohol to be completely eliminated from the body. During this period, the diet should consist of foods which are absorbent, non-irritant, easily digested and easily assimilated. Some suitable items are boiled rice, plain-cooked noodles, porridge oats, dry toast, yoghurt, milk, lightly poached eggs, steamed fish, barley water, white rice porridge and taro starch jelly. Fresh orange juice will replace the ascorbic acid (vitamin C) which has been lost during carousing, and honey will do the same for blood sugar, so creating a more energetic and wide-awake attitude to the world at large. Agrimony, *Agrimonia eupatoria*, has an affinity for the heart, lungs and liver, and an infusion of 10 g of its dried flowers can be taken internally as a treatment for hangovers. It can also be used as a gargle and mouthwash for the treatment of halitosis (bad breath). This species of agrimony must not be confused with *Agrimonia pilosa*, which is commonly used in TCM, but whose properties and applications are somewhat different. An infusion of 6 g haws, the fruit of the hawthorn, *Crataegus monogyna* or *Crataegus laevigata*, is also helpful. The Chinese use a decoction of two herbs as a block-busting treatment for hangovers. Unfortunately, these herbs do not grow in the West, and can only be obtained from a Chinese herbalist. To make this decoction, boil 15 g dried leaves of *Hovenia dulcis* and 7 g each of roots and flowers of *Pueraria lobata* in ½ litre water until the volume of the liquid is about 160 ml. Strain and take as two separate doses – ½ cup each – on an empty stomach. In the Western world, the remedies for a hangover include peppermint cordial, oil of evening primrose, soda water, weak tea, vinegar, lime flowers, rosemary leaves, lemon juice and nux vomica (which contains strychnine, and cannot be obtained off prescription). *Radix puerariae*, a Chinese medicine, reduces the craving for alcohol, but that is hardly a treatment for a hangover. See **white rice porridge.**

han lian cao *Eclipta prostrata* Herbal medicine. Distribution: China, Japan, Taiwan. Parts: entire plant. Character: cold, sweet-sour. Affinity: liver, kidneys. Effects: haemostatic, astringent, blood refrigerant, tonic to kidneys. Symptoms: dizziness, blurred vision, headaches, premature hair loss and greying. Treatments: spermatorrhoea, menorrhagia, blood in urine and sputum, deficiency of liver-yin and kidney-yin. Dosage: 8–15 g. See **hair loss**.

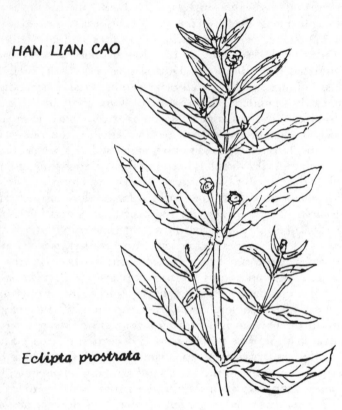

HAN LIAN CAO

Eclipta prostrata

happiness See **joy**.
harelip See **hereditary defect**.
hare's ear *Bupleurum falcatum* Herbal medicine. Distribution: North China, Northern Europe. Parts: roots. Character: neutral, bitter. Affinity: pericardium, liver, gall-bladder, triple-warmer. Effects: antipyretic, sedative to liver. Symptoms: sporadic chills and fevers. Treatments: malaria, blackwater fever, prolapse of rectum, womb and other internal organs. Dosage: 2–5 g.
harmony If one had to choose a single word which would completely and effectively describe the Chinese way of life, the word would be *harmony*. The concept of harmonious relationships permeates all the thinking of the Chinese, and is manifested in all their activities. Health, they believe, is the outcome of

harmony with nature, within the body and in society. This is an extension of the yin-yang principle of complementary opposites, which is the basis of the Tai Chi, or Supreme Absolute. See **Tai Chi**.

harmony fuel This is an apt term used in Chinese literature to describe foods, and health foods in particular, which supply energy and help to maintain the body in a state of harmony. The physicians of ancient China knew nothing of the chemical nature of vitamins, but they were certainly aware that food has constituents, which they would have regarded as vital energies, that are necessary for the health of the body. See **vitamin**.

haw tablets See **hawthorn**.

hawthorn *Crataegus pinnatifida* Herbal medicine. Distribution: China, Japan. Parts: fruits (haws). Character: warm, sweet, sour. Affinity: stomach, liver, spleen. Effects: stomachic, digestive, prevents diarrhoea, eliminates stagnant and excess food. Symptoms: diarrhoea, postnatal abdominal pain and distension, scrotal pain. Treatments: accumulations of meats, fats and undigested food, hypertension. Dosage: 7–15 g. This herb functions as a vasodilator, so reducing blood pressure. It also reduces cholesterol deposits. There are several species of hawthorn. No doubt, the species which are native to Europe, such as *Crataegus monogyna* and *Crataegus laevigata*, could be used similarly to the Chinese species. In China, dried and powdered haws are mixed with starch and sugar and then compressed to make disc-shaped tablets which are consumed as a medicated confection. An infusion of hawthorn fruits is considered to be a good treatment for a hangover.

hay fever This condition, which is not a fever, is a form of rhinitis, or inflammation of the mucous membrane in the nose and throat, and is caused by allergens, resulting in a running and itchy nose, a sore and itchy throat, watering of the eyes and blocked sinuses. The main cause of hay fever is allergy to pollen, which explains why it is particularly prevalent during the spring and summer months, but it may also be caused by dust, fur, feathers, mites, moulds, chemicals and plant and animal parts. These allergens induce the body to release chemical substances called histamines, which cause some of the symptoms mentioned above. In the West, physicians usually prescribe antihistamine tablets, which cause drowsiness, so they must be used with caution by people who handle machinery or need to make responsible decisions. Cortisone injections, inhalers and nasal sprays are used to reduce inflammation and swelling of the membranes. But the treatment of hay fever can be a complicated business. Chinese physicians recommend a two-part treatment for hay fever: blood cleansers to remove allergens and toxic waste from the bloodstream, and emollients to soothe the sensitive membranes in the mouth, throat and nasal cavities. Additionally, they might recommend acupuncture as a treatment for stress. For blood cleansing, one should drink copious quantities of water and garlic tea, made as an infusion of 2 cloves, crushed and finely chopped, in ½ litre water, or nettle (*Urtica dioica*) tea, made as an infusion of the dried herb, using any parts. For an emollient, use an infusion of 3–4 g dried flowers of one of the following, taken orally and sipped slowly, and also as a mouthwash and gargle. Marigold, *Calendula officinalis*; chrysanthemum, *Chrysanthemum leucanthemum*; corn marigold, *Chrysanthemum segetum*; tansy, *Chrysanthemum vulgare*; feverfew, *Chrysanthemum parthenium*. Chinese physicians claim that, with care and perseverance, hay fever can be cured. But, for this, they need to use herbs, some quite rare, which are indigenous to China and Japan. Therefore, hay fever sufferers who want to be completely cured might do well to consult a Chinese physician or herbalist.

headaches The main causes of headaches are tension due to stress or concentration, wrong diet, alcohol abuse, colds, influenza, menstruation, concussion, sinus problems and, rarely, eyestrain. If the condition persists, medical advice should be sought, for there may be a serious cause, such as a tumour or kidney disease. A headache which is intensified by bright light and accompanied by stiffening of the neck and fever is a symptom of meningitis. In treating a headache, the patient's dietary habits should be considered. Cheese, chocolate or alcohol can cause a headache. Two common causes of a headache are constipation and breathing the foul air in a stuffy room. A cathartic and diet high in fibre are the obvious treatments for the former condition, and a brisk walk around the block will clear the head. Tension headaches are generally due to muscular contractions, for which massage and acupuncture are the most effective treatments. Reflexology provides effective treatment for some types of headaches. An infusion of any of the following taken internally, using the parts and dosage indicated, is a suitable treatment for most headaches: wolfberry, *Lycium chinense*, fruits, 4–10 g; dandelion, *Taraxacum officinale*, all parts, 10–30 g; self-heal, *Prunella vulgaris*, flowers and seeds, 5–7 g; chrysanthemum, *Chrysanthemum morifolium*, flowers, 4–10 g; corn mint, *Mentha arvensis*, leaves, 2–4 g; stinging nettle, *Urtica dioica*, young shoots,

2–4 g; sweet flag, *Acorus calamus*, leaves, 3–7 g; feverfew, *Chrysanthemum parthenium*, flowers and leaves, 2–4 g. A suspension of gypsum in water can be similarly used. Chewing fresh leaves of basil, *Ocicum basilicum*, will sometimes relieve a headache, as will an infusion of 20 g fennel, *Foeniculum vulgare*, seeds if applied externally. A traditional Chinese remedy is to simmer four bulbs of the Chinese spring onion *Allium fistulosum*, in ½ litre water for 5 minutes, and then drink the resulting liquid. 15 g honey added to this drink will help to maintain the correct level of blood sugar, lack of which can sometimes cause a headache. If the headache is accompanied by nausea or a cold, 20 g ginger should also be added. See **hangover**, **migraine** and **reflexology**.

head lice At one time, head lice, *Pediculus humanus*, and their nits, or eggs, commonly infected the hair of children, and those whose hair was regularly washed and neatly groomed were just as susceptible as any other children. An effective treatment is to rinse the hair with an infusion of walnut leaves, rubbing the liquid into the scalp, and to continue with this process until the lice are eradicated. To make this infusion, pour 1 litre boiling water on to 2 g chopped fresh walnut leaves, and allow to stand for 10 minutes. A TCM treatment is external application of an infusion of 5–10 g roots of *bai bu*, *Stemona tuberosa*.

heal-all See **self-heal**.

healing The *tao* of healing, which is called *tui na* by the Chinese, is one of the Eight Pillars of Taoism. Its ancient wisdom teaches how one can regulate and improve vital energy by massage and manipulation of the meridians, and its techniques may be applied to repositioning internal organs which have moved out of position. The five elements – wood, fire, earth, metal and water – are involved, with acupuncture and moxibustion being two of the metal and fire methods. Shiatsu, in its various styles, is commonly used to manipulate the meridians, though the approach must initially be gentle, otherwise 'curative reactions', which may be headaches or influenza-like, may occur. It is important to remember that certain exercises are the most effective, and the organs which they stimulate are the most responsive, at certain times of the day. See **zodiac exercises** and **shiatsu**.

healing arts Many centuries ago, the Greek physician Hippocrates (*c.* 460–*c.* 370 BC) pointed out that the human body is essentially self-reliant and largely self-healing except where it is in a particularly weakened state, and that those who are skilled in the healing arts are merely assisting nature in its efforts to maintain the balance of the body and effect a cure when illness arises. In fact, it could be said that the physician does not heal sickness so much as assists nature to heal sickness. His opinion would be shared by Chinese physicians, who would contend that the human body is resilient and self-regulating and has its own immunity system, so that, when it is in a good state of health, it is well able to throw off most minor infections. Chinese physicians would also contend that disease-organisms which invade the body can do harm only where the organs are weak. Thus, if two men, one with healthy lungs, and the other with weak lungs, are exposed to identically damp and otherwise non-salubrious climatic conditions, it will be the one with weak lungs who will be the more likely to succumb to bronchial ailments. This, of course, is an example of one of the fundamental differences between TCM and Western medicine. Where there is a disease or defect of a particular organ, the Chinese physician will provide treatments to strengthen that organ, whereas the Western physician will provide treatments to eliminate the invading organisms. Chinese physicians do not exactly equate the healing arts with medicines, for many of their treatments are dietary, and so the healing arts have much in common with the culinary arts. They also use manipulative treatments, involving massage and physical and breathing exercises, and medicine is regarded as the last resort, being used only when all else has failed.

healing exercises Massage, manipulative techniques and physical and breathing exercises constitute an important and large component of TCM. Many of these exercises derive from the ancient wisdom contained in the Eight Pillars of Taoism and its supportive philosophy, as explained by the *Tao Te Ching*, which was written by Lao Zi, the founder of Taoism. Some of these exercises encourage relaxation and recreation, and so relieve tension, which is good for the mental health, some are for keep-fit purposes, and some are used therapeutically to prevent, relieve or cure specific conditions, including those which, in the West, would be regarded as incurable or very difficult to treat. It is surprising – and also comforting – to learn that the Chinese can alleviate and sometimes cure such difficult conditions as asthma, arthritis, emphysema and coronary heart disease by means of therapeutic exercises, and without recourse to medicines. Full details of these exercises are contained in the *Chinese Exercise Manual*, which is an official publication. It explains *tai chi chuan*, which is a keep-fit system for the young and the elderly, *yee chin ching*, which builds strength, *dao yin*, which are psycho-physiological exercises, *ta na*, which are breathing exercises, *qi gong*, which provides for breathing and concentration, *an mu*, which is massage, and some other systems. The various exercises are placed, somewhat arbitrarily, into seven categories: therapeutic exercises, therapeutic athletics, mechanically aided therapy, breathing exercises (*qi gong*), massage (*an mu*), recreational exercises and natural treatments – fresh air, water and sunlight. See **dancing** and **Chinese Exercise Manual**.

healing reaction 'Curative reaction'. See **healing**.

health The Chinese value health above all else. They recognize that one's own body is one's most precious possession, and that its proper state of health, and not money, property or power, is the true wealth. They regard a good state of health as being the outcome of a sound diet, adequate exercise, moderate habits, regard for one's personal hygiene, a wise philosophy of living, some knowledge of those herbal medicines which may be used in the self-treatment of minor ailments, and sufficient sense to consult a physician if one should become seriously ill or be unfortunate enough to have some congenital defect. They regard a sound state of health as being the *status quo*, and sickness should arise only where people live unnaturally. See **diet** and **exercise**.

health foods In the West, a sharp distinction is made between medicines and health foods. The former are regarded as non-nutritious substances with specific or general remedial properties, whereas the latter are regarded as foods which, in addition to being nutritious, have health-giving or medicinal properties, and they are considered to include such items as vitamin supplements, food concentrates, and organically grown vegetables. But the term *health food* as it is used in the West is something of a misnomer, for some of the so-called foods are simply not foods, though this is a matter of how one defines a food. Some people would regard anything that is consumed as being a food, whilst others would require a more rigorous definition, and would regard a food as being a substance which provides nutriment. But there are some anomalies. For example, dietary fibre, which is mainly cellulose, has no nutritional value; but, in stimulating the bowel muscles and preventing constipation, it is a valuable item of diet, and so it is not unreasonable to regard it as a food. Also, some so-called health foods are not particularly healthy. Although vitamins are vital to the health, which is why they are so named, and food concentrates provide a nutritional boost, a meal consisting solely of vitamins and food concentrates could be damaging to the health, for one can have too much of a good thing. And the main benefit – perhaps the only real benefit – derived from organically grown vegetables is that they are free of pesticides, artificial fertilizers and other unnatural, and possibly toxic, substances. Some foods which have a good reputation health-wise are of no great nutritional benefit. Spinach, for example, has a high content of iron, but the iron is poorly absorbed, and so spinach is of no better value than any other green vegetable as a source of iron. Some people would be inclined to define a health food as one which improves the health or does no harm to the health. For example, both beef and fish are rich in protein, but the latter is to be preferred as an item of diet, and so could be regarded as a health food, because its oils are polyunsaturated and do not lead to the formation of cholesterol with all its attendant risks, which include thrombosis and arteriosclerosis (hardening of the arteries). In China, there is no sharp distinction between medicines and health foods, for Chinese medicines often have the characteristics of foods and vice versa. But, then, Chinese medicines are herbal, and many of their herbs and spices are used for both culinary and medicinal purposes. Furthermore, in China, medicines are usually administered as special ingredients in soups, stews, and other dishes, and it is the general practice for both physicians and cooks to classify foodstuffs according to their medicinal properties. In TCM, no thought is given to vitamins, minerals and trace elements as such, but the Chinese believe that foods contain energies and essences which are vital to the health, and they know from long experience what the specific medicinal effects of certain foods are likely to be. See **diet**, **mineral** and **vitamin**.

health foods recipes The Chinese have thousands of recipes which yield dishes that are highly nutritious, very appetizing and possessed of medicinal properties. This is an effective way of combining business with pleasure, for the Chinese live to eat as well as eat to live. For detailed information about these recipes, one has only to consult a Chinese cookbook of high quality, which should present no difficulties, for there is no dearth of Chinese cookbooks in the West, such is the popularity of Chinese cuisine throughout the world.

health hazards A list of health hazards would be of enormous length, for we live in a dangerous world. In fact, we have always lived in a dangerous world, but the emphasis has changed somewhat. Whereas, in earlier ages, the hazards to human health were mainly of a natural origin – disease, wild animals, climatic conditions, tribal warfare, etc. – these days, they are generally unnatural and man-made, and often the by-products of science and technology – pollution of the environment by the toxic chemicals in waste products, accidental injuries involving machinery and electrical equipment, noise, radiation, contaminated foodstuffs, etc. The Chinese view is that, as many of the health hazards to which modern man is exposed are due to his own activities, he must change his habits considerably if he is to escape their unfortunate consequences. In this respect, the people of the West would do well to follow the Chinese example by living more naturally and more moderately in regard to diet and exercise, and to avoid accidents and social ills by living more carefully and in accordance with unassailable moral values of the kind espoused by Confucius. Here, there must be an element of compromise because, though man is imaginative and inventive, he also has a positive genius for doing injury to both himself and his environment, and so he sometimes has to make a difficult choice in dealing with a discovery or device which is immensely beneficial in one direction but also immensely damaging in another. A good example of this is the internal combustion engine, which has rendered transportation quick and easy, but whose exhaust belches out noxious fumes, so polluting the atmosphere. The Chinese approach in this particular situation is to make use of manually operated bicycles, which do no damage to the environment and, additionally, provide a means of taking healthy exercise. The Chinese are great survivors and, for thousands of years, they have been eliminating health hazards, together with their associated social ills, as per the teachings of Taoism and Confucianism. This is a part of their traditional culture. The situation is somewhat different in the West, where standards of environmental health are maintained by a formal system of regulation and inspection. See **chemicals**, **environment** and **green consumers**.

hearing This is one of the techniques employed by the Chinese physicians in making a diagnosis, and it involves the use of the ears and a stethoscope in listening to a patient's speech, breathing and coughing and any sounds emanating from the heart, stomach, lungs and other visceral organs. It will also involve the use of the nose to assess the intensity of the bodily secretions, such as perspiration and defaecation, for Chinese physicians do not distinguish between hearing and smell for diagnostic purposes. Full, or yang, ailments are characterized by confusing speech, rapid or noisy breathing, a raucous cough and a racing pulse, whereas empty, or yin, ailments are characterized by weak speech, shallow breathing, a low cough and a slow or feeble pulse. See **consultation** and **diagnosis**.

heart The heart, which is yin, is one of the *wu zang*, or five solid organs of the body. Its element is fire, and the hollow organ with which it is paired is the small intestine, which is yang. Obviously, the heart operates very much in conjunction with the small intestine, which absorbs nutrients and water from digested food, separating the pure products from the impure products in the process. The nutrients reach the tissues via the blood, whose circulation is maintained by the heart. The traditional associations of the heart in astrology – climate, emotions, etc. – are listed under **element**. In China, as in the West, the heart is regarded as the chief organ, and it is described as the 'emperor of the body'. It controls the other organs and the circulation of the blood. Without effective circulation, the body would soon become cold, and so it is understandable that the Chinese describe the heart as the 'fire organ'. In ancient times, it was thought to house the spirit, which is explained by the fact that the heart has some considerable influence, via the circulation of the blood, on a person's moods, thoughts and general well-being, and it must be the case that a healthy and robust person will have a healthy heart. It is associated with the liver, whose element is wood, by the mother-and-son rule: fire is son to wood, for wood generates fire. The symptoms of the activity of the heart are indicated by the face and tongue. Redness indicates excessive heart activity, or heart *qi*, and paleness or greyness indicates deficient heart activity. When the heart is defective, there will be circulation problems and other conditions, including schizophrenia, epilepsy and mouth ulcers. The heart is connected with the tongue, whose colouration indicates heart conditions. The heart is closely associated with the emotion of joy and, to a lesser extent, with grief and fright. It is also associated with the sound of laughter, which is called 'fire sound' because it resembles the crackling sound made by a wood fire. The heart may be briefly described as a four-chambered muscular pump with valves to ensure that blood flows in the right directions. An interesting feature of the heart is the two rhythm regulators, or pacemaker, which are two nodes of specialized nerve tissue that regulate the heartbeat. See **solid organs**, **joy** and **pacemaker**.

heart attack This is the layman's term for coronary thrombosis.

heartbeat See **pulse**.

heartburn A painful sensation in the region of the heart, though it does not indicate a heart condition. It may produce a burning sensation at the back of the throat. It could be a symptom of hiatus hernia or hyperacidity. Otherwise, it should be treated as for dyspepsia. See **indigestion**.

heart-constrictor See **pericardium**.

heart disorders Heart diseases and defects are of various kinds, which include angina pectoris, aneurysm, coronary thrombosis and heart valve disease. Susceptibility to a heart attack increases with age, and can be brought about by obesity, unhealthy diet, smoking, diabetes mellitus, hypertension, heavy consumption of alcohol, anaemia, stress and arteriosclerosis. The symptoms of a heart attack are a severe pain across the chest, radiating down the left arm or up into the jaw, and lasting for at least 30 minutes, together with breathlessness, laboured breathing, restlessness, anxiety, excessive perspiration, a cold and clammy skin, collapse and sometimes unconsciousness. Death can result from damaged heart muscle or arrhythmia (disturbed heart rhythm). Chinese physicians say that some heart conditions are due to yang-*qi* deficiency, and others to yin-*qi* deficiency. The herbal remedies they use include cinnamon twigs (*Cinnamomum cassia*), red sage (*Salvia officinalis purpurea*), aconite (*Aconitum carmichaeli*), angelica (*Angelica sinensis*), hawthorn (*Crataegus pinnatifida*), jujube (*Ziziphus jujuba*), and lotus seeds (*Nelumbo nucifera*). The exercises of *qi gong* and *ch'iang chuang kung* are preventive of some of the conditions which give rise to heart diseases. But the treatment of heart disorders should not be undertaken by unqualified persons. The risks are too great. Also, powerful purgatives, medicinal wines and violently acting medicines of any kind should not be administered to people with a heart condition. See **heart's blood** and **palpitation**.

heart failure A condition in which the heart fails to pump sufficient blood to the lungs and the rest of the body. It can occur on the left side of the heart, when its causes are anaemia, hypertension, heart valve defects, arrhythmia (irregular heartbeat), congenital heart defects and diseases of the heart muscles. On the right side of the heart, its causes are chronic bronchitis and emphysema. The symptoms are general fatigue, breathlessness and swollen limbs. Do-it-yourself medicine should not be applied here. See **heart disorders**.

heart's blood A somewhat old-fashioned term commonly used by British novelists in Victorian times. Perhaps it indicates that our forebears were aware that the heart, as well as the other organs, requires a blood supply. The heart was believed to be the seat of the emotions, and so it was associated with sexual prowess. It is a belief that is not without justification, for it is certainly the case that violent sexual activity cannot be safely undertaken by someone with coronary heart disease. On the other hand, the sperm count is much higher in those who are physically fit, a condition which must include a healthy heart. The health benefits of this combinative relationship of the heart, blood and semen have been known to Chinese physicians since the time of the Yellow Emperor. See **angina**.

heart-valve disease The heart contains four valves, and if these become diseased, sometimes as a consequence of rheumatic fever or even syphilis, the blood supply to the body is adversely affected. See **heart disorders**.

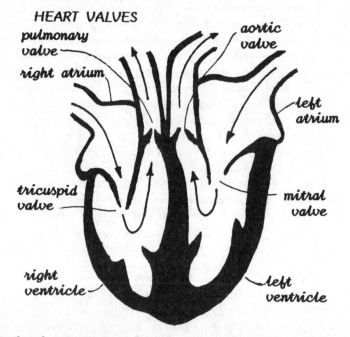

HEART VALVES

pulmonary valve

aortic valve

right atrium

left atrium

tricuspid valve

mitral valve

right ventricle

left ventricle

heart-clearing treatment In this method of treatment, antipyretics and refrigerants, which are cooling yin medicines, are used to reduce fever and temperature, stimulate the salivary glands and detoxify the body fluids. There is a very wide range of these medicines, and they include the gardenia, *Gardenia jasminoides*, reed grass, *Phragmites communis*, lotus, *Nelumbo nucifera*, and dandelion, *Taraxacum officinale*. See **antipyretic**.

heat excess See **fire**.

heat exhaustion A condition of dehydration and salt depletion that occurs in hot weather, particularly where a person is exposed to intense sunlight, and which is characterized by thirst, headaches, loss of appetite, dizziness, pallor, nausea and even vomiting. If the condition is ignored, there could be an occurence of heatstroke, which can be fatal. The treatment is to keep out of the sun, rehydrate by slowly sipping warm water, take glucose drinks, and sprinkle the head and neck with cold water. It is highly desirable that the sufferer should be persuaded to move to an air-conditioned area. See **heat-stroke**.

heating foods See **classification of foods**.

heat rash Prickly heat. This is an irritating, but harmless, pimply rash which commonly affects infants and obese people in hot weather. It generally occurs in the skin creases and where the clothing is tight-fitting. The treatment is to wear loose clothing, avoid sunlight and bath frequently. Powdered talc (magnesium silicate) or gypsum (calcium sulphate) can be applied externally to the affected parts. But this condition will disappear of its own accord when the weather becomes cooler.

heat-stroke An extremely dangerous condition, which could prove to be fatal, especially in a humid atmosphere, and which is likely to occur if heat exhaustion is allowed to go untreated. It is characterized by a very high temperature, cessation of perspiration and complete collapse. Professional medical attention is immediately required. See **heat exhaustion**.

heaven Chinese philosophy is without bigotry and blind faith, and the term *heaven* is used generically and somewhat vaguely to indicate those cosmic forces which control the universe but are not entirely understood, though we, in the West, in the light of our present knowledge, might regard them as manifestations of those universal and inexorable laws of physics and chemistry which may not totally govern the univese but do go a long way towards explaining the structure of matter and the nature of energy. 'All is chemistry,' said some biochemist. Taoism, which is probably the oldest religion in the world, and certainly the most profound, does not conceive of a universe controlled by manlike deities, which are products of the primitive mind, but one which is an integrated and harmonious whole governed by its own self-perpetuating mechanisms. Man is a tiny part of this vast universe, and his state of health and general well-being is largely determined by the extent to which he conforms with the divine pattern, albeit an inanimate one. In this respect, Taoism has much more in common with the modern science of the West than Western religions, which says much for the wisdom of the philosophers and physicians of ancient China, who perceived that man's satisfactory existence in health and all else depends upon his achieving the correct balance in his relationship, both direct and indirect, with the forces of nature – *qi*, climatic conditions, seasonal changes, the earth's magnetism, etc. Over 5000 years ago, Chinese physicians understood what the physicians of the West were not aware of until recent times, which is that diseases have natural causes and are not due to demons. The French chemist Louis Pasteur (1822–95) had great difficulty in convincing the French Medical Academy of this fact. It is the Taoist belief that man is a miniature version of the universe, and that, in his anatomy and behaviour, he reflects its nature. See **universe** and **immortality**.

hemp *Cannabis sativa* Herbal medicine. Distribution: China, India, North Africa. Parts: seeds. Character: neutral, sweet. Affinity: stomach, spleen, large intestine. Effects: laxative, demulcent, emollient, antitussive, antiseptic, antitoxic. Symptoms: constipation, coughs, sore throat. Treatments: constipation and other conditions due to fluid deficiency, especially in old age and during the postnatal period. Dosage: 8–10 g. The other parts of this plant have their medicinal uses: the stems as a diuretic, the male flowers for menstrual disorders, and the female flowers as a stimulant in the treatment of nervous disorders. The female flowers are slightly poisonous, and will cause hallucinations if taken in excess. It is important to note that the resin from the flowers yields a narcotic drug, but there are restrictions on its use in most countries. See **drug**.

hepatic Relating to the liver.

hepatitis Inflammation of the liver. Hepatitis A, or 'infectious hepatitis', is caused by a virus which is transmitted in food and drink. It is characterized by fever, sickness and jaundice. This condition lasts for three weeks, and is frequently followed by post-viral depression. It is rarely serious, but medical attention should be sought. This condition does not respond well to drugs, but it is helpful to rest, take little food and avoid fatty items of diet. Hepatitis B, or 'serum hepatitis', which is also caused by a virus, is a far more serious condition, and is transmitted by sexual intercourse, infected blood and blood products and the syringes and needles used by drug addicts. Its symptoms are headaches, chills, fever, debility and jaundice. After an incubation period of one to six months, recovery is slow even with treatment, and about one in ten cases are fatal. Measures to prevent the spread of hepatitis include avoiding both the use of contaminated needles and sexual intercourse without the use of a condom. There is no fully effective treatment for hepatitis B, for it appears to be a relatively new condition. Its causative virus has probably always existed; but, in recent years, with all the encouragement provided by the permissive society, its free development has reached near-epidemic proportions. However, Chinese physicians have done some promising research in this field. Traditionally, Chinese physicians use the fruits of the gardenia, *Gardenia jasminoides*, as a treatment for jaundice, or what they describe as liver stagnation. As a tonic for the liver, they prescribe American ginseng, *Panax quinquefolium*, liquorice, *Glycyrrhiza uralensis*, *huang qi*, *Astralagus membranaceus*, or Chinese angelica, *Angelica sinensis*. Healing exercises, such as those of *qi gong* and *tai chi chuan*, are helpful in treating insomnia, depression and other conditions associated with chronic hepatitis, but they must not be overdone, for hepatitis patients tire very quickly. See **AIDS** and **drug addiction**.

herb Botanically, a herb is defined as a plant with a non-woody stem and which dies down to ground level after flowering, and does not go on growing year after year. Thus, a tree or a shrub would not be regarded as a herbaceous plant. Medically or commercially, a herb is defined as a plant which is used for culinary, medicinal or other specific purposes, as with perfumes and dyestuffs. In this sense, certain trees, shrubs and fungi are regarded as herbs.

herbal In the West, a herbal is a book which lists medicinal herbs, together with their descriptions and healing properties, usually under their botanical names and in alphabetical order. This differs from a pharmacopoeia in so far as the latter also lists medicines which are of mineral or animal origin. In China, a herbal also lists medicines of mineral and animal origin, classifies all the items according to their healing properties rather than their botanical descriptions, and contains details about their affinities, yin and yang effects, dietary properties, and so forth. See **herbal medicines**.

herbal constituents The chemical constituents of plants are mind-boggling in their multiplicity and complexity. A biochemist can inform us that buckwheat contains rutin and other flavonoid glycosides, or that American ginseng contains triterpenoid saponins, but these chemical names are meaningless to most people, for chemistry is not an uncomplicated science. It is much easier, and probably more useful, to classify medicines by their medicinal uses than by their chemical constituents, as Chinese physicians have done since ancient times. But, then, their approach to medicine has always been more practical and empirical than purely theoretical, and one can be sure that a patient who is suffering badly will be more concerned about effective results than the whys and wherefores of pharmacy. In TCM, a medicine which is good for the liver is said to possess liver-*qi*, one that is good for the kidneys is said to possess kidney-*qi*, and so on. However, where *qi* is deficient, the organ is starved of vitality, and so may become damaged, temporarily or permanently. Damage may also occur where *qi* is in excess, for the organ is then overwhelmed. The differences between the various forms of *qi* associated with the organs are more of situation than of kind. See **qi**.

herbalism A system of medical treatment based upon the administering of herbs, together with the assumption that most diseases can be so cured, and generally without any unpleasant side-effects.

herbalist A person who deals, or trades, in herbs, for which no special qualifications are required, or a person who has been trained in the skills associated with the preparation and administering of herbal remedies, and for which, in many countries, registrable professional qualifications are required if he is to enter into practice. In China, herbalism is the main branch of medicine, though most practitioners have been trained in other skills, such as acupuncture and massage. See **herbal medicines**.

herbal medicines Chinese physicians have at their disposal a vast repertoire of herbal medicines. Li Shizhen, (1517–1593), the great physician of the period of the Ming dynasty (1368–1644), listed and described 2000 items in his herbal, *Ben Cao Gang Mu*, or 'Outlines and Branches of Herbal Medicine'. Of these, only about 300 are in common use today. Herbal medicines are natural, generally non-addictive and have no unpleasant side-effects. Chinese physicians use the whole herbs or their parts – roots, leaves, flowers, stems, etc. – and not herbal extracts, as we do in the West. The advantage of this is that the active ingredient is rendered less potent by the other ingredients, which inhibits side-effects. See **active ingredient** and **buffer**. Many herbal medicines have the same or similar properties, and so, if a patient develops an allergy to a particular medicine, his physician can usually provide him with a more suitable alternative.

However, herbal medicines are slow in action, and must be taken over a long period if they are to be truly effective. On the other hand, cures brought about by herbal medicines tend to be permanent. A few medical scientists in the West make the criticism that Chinese herbal medicines are unreliable because they have not been laboratory tested. But this is hardly a valid criticism, for some of the laboratory-tested Western-style synthetic medicines have proved to be unreliable, addictive or dangerous. One should note that some manufactured medicines contain natural ingredients. For example, digitalis, used as a heart stimulant, is extracted from the foxglove. Herbal medicine is really an offshoot of the culinary arts. It began when Shen Nong and others noticed that certain food plants have specific medicinal effects. Shen Nong put all medicines into three main categories: those which support life, those which fortify vitality, and poisons which are used to treat the most virulent diseases. Perhaps, to these, we should add those medicines which inhibit the ageing process. In TCM, the tendency is not to use medicines to combat the climatic conditions, or six excesses, and the invaders of the body, such as viruses and bacteria, but to strengthen the vital organs so that they are better able to cope with adverse conditions. See **healing arts** and **six excesses**. Herbal medicines are broadly classified as yin or yang, the former being used to cool, suppress or sedate yang illnesses, which are hot, full, external and ascending; and the latter to warm, elevate, stimulate or tone yin illnesses, which are cold, empty, internal and descending. A medicine is always of an opposite nature to the illness being treated. Problems can arise when several medicines are being used at the same time to treat more than one condition, for a yang medicine will offset the curative or alleviate effects of a yin medicine, and then the illnesses are inadequately treated. From this, it will be understood that the Chinese physician needs to be extremely skilful in achieving the correct balance when prescribing medicines. See **herbal**, **Shen Nong** and **treatment principles**.

herbal prescriptions In preparing a prescription, the Chinese physician must give much consideration to a wide variety of factors, not only in regard to the nature of the illness but also in regard to the nature of the medicine. Herbal medicines are categorized according to their four energies, five tastes and direction. Yang medicines are warm, ascending, elevating, scattering and hot, sweet or plain in taste, whereas yin medicines are cold, descending, inward-moving and sour, bitter or salty.

Yang medicines stimulate or tone, and yin medicines sedate or suppress. The affinity of the medicine must also be considered. Thus, a kidney condition where there is a deficiency of *qi* might require a warming medicine, but the medicine will not be effective if it has no affinity for the kidneys. And so, medicines are also classified according to their affinities. Each of the solid organs – heart, liver, spleen, lungs and kidneys – is associated with a colour and paired with a hollow organ, and so a simple colour code may be used to indicate the affinities of medicines. See **colour**. One should note that the solid organs are yin, and the hollow organs are yang. One should also note that a medicine which has an affinity for a certain organ will also have an affinity for the meridian associated with that organ. The colour code for the solid organs also applies to the hollow organs, as the table indicates, and so a medicine that is good for one of the solid organs is sometimes good for its corresponding hollow organ. It is clear that, with so much complexity in the diagnosis of illnesses and the classification of medicines, the Chinese physician must be possessed of that high degree of skill which can only stem from intensive training and long experience. In China, the usual practice is for the physician to write out a prescription for the medicine he deems to be necessary, which is then prepared by a herbalist. Pills, pastes and other special forms of medicine are prepared by the herbalist, but broths, teas and suchlike are prepared by the patient himself from a mixture made up by the herbalist. Some herbs need to be specially prepared by being boiled, steamed or ground into a fine powder if they are to be fully effective. The degree of concentration of a medicine is determined by the patient's physical condition. For example, weak or elderly patients will be prescribed less potent medicines, which are more slowly absorbed. See **treatment principles**.

YIN ILLNESSES cold, cool, empty internal, damp

YANG MEDICINES hot, warm, elevating, ascending, scattering, toning, stimulating, hot in taste, sweet, of plain taste, fragrant, rank, of neutral odour

YANG ILLNESSES hot, warm, full, external, dry

YIN MEDICINES cold, cool, inward-moving, descending, suppressive, sedative, sour, bitter, salty, acid, scorched, putrid

RED	heart	small intestine	fire	bitter
GREEN	liver	gall-bladder	wood	sour

YELLOW	spleen	stomach	earth	sweet
WHITE	lungs	large intestine	metal	hot
BLACK	kidneys	bladder	water	salty

herbal teas In popular use in China, both as gentle medicines and refreshing drinks, herbal teas are infusions, which are made by pouring boiling water on to a single herbal ingredient, such as sage leaves and chrysanthemum and jasmine flowers, or a mixture of herbal ingredients, and allowing to stand for 5 minutes. A wide range of these herbal teas are now readily available at Chinese pharmacies and grocery stores in the West. See **infusion**.

herbal trade The Chinese practice of herbal medicine has such a good reputation that it is hardly surprising that Chinese herbal medicines are now obtainable in all parts of the world, catering not only for the needs of the Chinese communities in the large cities in both the East and the West but also for the needs of the non-Chinese people in the West, who, during recent years, have acquired a liking for Chinese herbal medicines. Herbs of the best quality command very high prices, and so, understandably, the Chinese export trade in herbs is certainly booming. China's main commercial outlet for herbs is Hong Kong, where wholesalers supply the local shops and pharmacies, which are flourishing concerns, as well as the international market. Some of the more exotic herbs are extremely expensive because they are derived from species of plants and animals which are becoming quite rare, but it is generally possible to purchase herbs which are equally as efficacious but are common and inexpensive.

herbal treatments In TCM, there are eight categories of herbal treatments: cathartic, deflecting, diaphoretic, emetic, heat-clearing, neutralizing, stimulating and tonic. This classification is somewhat arbitrary but it holds good for most practical purposes. See **treatment principles**.

herbs of Shen Nong See **Shen Nong** and **Tao Hongjing**.

hereditary Of a disease or other condition which has been inherited. See **hereditary defects**.

hereditary defects All our characteristics, whether they be regarded as defects or fine qualities, are either acquired from our environment or inherited from our ancestors. It is important to distinguish between inherited diseases and defects and those which are congenital. A congenital defect is one which exists at the time of birth but is not necessarily inherited. Thus, a baby may be born with a harelip, or without an arm or a leg, which is an acquired characteristic resulting from its mother having taken the thalidomide drug. Both conditions are congenital, but only the former is inherited. Acquired characteristics, such as hair styles, tattoo marks, scars and warts, which are due to environmental influences, cannot be passed on from one generation to the next. It is true that a pregnant woman who has a disease may pass on that disease to her baby while it is still in her womb, and it may be affected by unhealthy influences, such as smoking, alcohol and drug-taking, which affect the woman, but these are not hereditary characteristics. Hereditary characteristics are passed on through genes, which are individual molecules of protein that are attached to the germ plasm of the reproductive cells, by which they are transmitted from generation to generation, so determining our genetic destiny. It is awesome to realize that we ourselves have very little say in what kind of persons we are. Our basic characteristics are decided for us by our parents at our conception, and generally unwittingly, for they are merely passing on to us those traits which they have inherited from their ancestors through countless generations, a process which began long before the beginning of recorded time. But, if this is the case, how is it that a couple, both with brown eyes, can produce a child with blue eyes? The simple explanation is that hereditary characteristics do not show themselves in every generation, for one, such as blue eyes, which is said to be recessive, may be masked by another, such as brown eyes, which is said to be dominant. This also explains why children sometimes bear a closer resemblance to their grandparents than to their parents. Some dominant hereditary characteristics are brown eyes, woolly hair, normal skin pigment, defective tooth enamel, lack of incisor teeth, extra teeth and night-blindness. Some recessive hereditary characteristics are blue eyes, albinism, straight hair, normal tooth enamel, normal number of teeth, epilepsy, haemophilia, deaf-mutism, adherent ear lobes, extra fingers, baldness, cleft palate, harelip and colour-blindness. Some of these conditions are treatable. For example, a harelip can be removed by cosmetic surgery, and haemophilia can be controlled with coagulant drugs. But these treatments do not eradicate the hereditary traits, and the persons so treated will pass on these characteristics to their offspring. No one knew the exact principles which govern inheritance until Gregor Mendel, (1822–1844), an Austrian monk, performed his classic experiments with garden peas, and thereby established the laws of heredity, or Mendel's laws as they are more commonly known. Nevertheless, the philosophers and physicians of ancient China saw the need for some kind of selective mating, which gave rise to the system of arranged marriages. Where marriage occurs with a man and a woman who have the same hereditary defects, which is often the case if they are closely related, as with cousins, there is likely to be a greater chance of their children inheriting those same defects. Of course, there is also likely to be a greater chance of their children inheriting their good qualities. But good qualities in this sense are hard to define and not easy to perceive, and so, in this situation, eradicating defects is more important than establishing good qualities. Experience indicates that a defect generally totally outweighs the benefits which might be derived from a good quality. The ancient Chinese also perceived that there is a tendency for healthy and worthy people to produce healthy and worthy descendants, and that, if a person is blessed with good qualities, he has good reason to be grateful to his ancestors, who have not been reckless in the mating process. This clearly indicates that the so-called ancestor worship practised by the Chinese is an expression of gratitude and a wholesome endeavour. The Chinese regard themselves as a stage in a continuous genetic process, which explains why both children and elderly people are well cared for in China. See **genetics**, **eugenics**, **inbreeding**, **fingerprints** and **ancestor worship**.

hermaphrodite See **bisexual**.

hernia Rupture. A condition in which an organ protrudes through its associated muscles or membranes. The stomach and intestines are the organs which are usually the most affected. Surgery may be required; but, where the condition is not serious, the patient should rest to allow the displaced organs to readjust themselves as far as is possible. In China, this condition is commonly treated, and most effectively, by manipulation. See **hiatus hernia**.

herpes This condition, caused by the virus *Herpes simplex*, is characterized by small blisters, called cold sores, which generally occur on or near the lips and nose, producing yellow crusts when broken. See **cold sores**. Genital, or venereal, herpes, caused by the virus *Herpes simplex* Type II, occurs on the genital area and buttocks and in the vagina and anus. It is transmitted only by direct contact, as with sexual intercourse. It may be passed from the mouth to the genitals and vice versa. It is characterized by feverishness and painful blisters, which appear after an incubation period of 2–12 days, and which burst to leave ulcers. After an attack, the virus remains dormant in nerve roots, but it may be reactivated during times of stress or illness. Chinese physicians ascribe this condition to damp-heat in the gall-bladder duct. The treatments they recommend are a diet containing plenty of chicken, fish, beans, bean sprouts and other vegetables, a saline bath or douche to reduce irritation, and infusions, taken internally, of the following, using the parts and dosages indicated. Chinese gentian, *Gentiana macrophylla*, roots, 5–10 g; rhubarb, *Rheum officinale*, rhizomes, 1–2 g; water plantain, *Alisma plantago-aquatica*, seeds, 2–4 g; common plantain, *Plantago asiatica*, leaves, 3–5 g. The herpes virus may also cause aphthous ulcers inside the cheeks and on the tongue. They are small, round, shallow and painful, and are accompanied by a sore throat. In children, they may also occur on the hands and feet. The treatment is a healthy, gluten-free diet and a mouthwash of an infusion of camomile, sage or fennel. If the symptoms persist, medical advice should be sought. *Herpes simplex* should not be confused with *Herpes zoster*, which causes chickenpox and shingles. See **gluten** and **shingles**.

heterosexual Attraction to the opposite sex, or a person who is so attracted. See **homosexual**.

hexagram See **I Ching**.

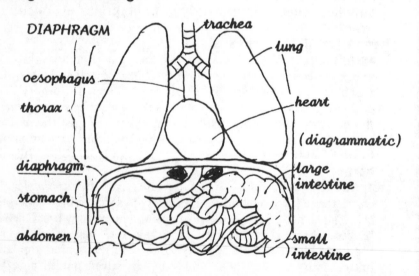

hiatus hernia A hernia in which a part of the stomach protrudes through the diaphragm, so allowing a little of its content, which is acid, to enter the oesophagus, thereby causing pain and occasional regurgitation. It is one of the causes of heartburn. Professional medical treatment is required.

hiccoughs See **hiccups**.

hiccups Hiccoughs. This condition is a contraction of the diaphragm caused by irritation of the phrenic nerve. It can be caused by stress, eating food too quickly or swallowing too much air. Chinese physicians ascribe hiccups to heat, cold or food stagnation. This condition is similar to a reflex action, and so the treatment would seem to be a matter of giving a small shock to the phrenic nerve. One can do this by holding one's breath as long as possible, and then swallowing when a hiccup seems to be on its way. Or one can put the index fingers into the ears and hold one's breath. Chinese physicians recommend an infusion, taken internally, of one of the following, using the parts and dosage indicated: fennel, *Foeniculum vulgare*, seeds 3 g, leaves 1 g; corn mint, *Mentha arvensis*, leaves 2–4 g; black mustard, *Brassica nigra*, seeds, 3 g; ginger, *Zingiber officinale*, rhizomes, 3–7 g; rhubarb, *Rheum officiale*, rhizomes, 0.3 g. Acupuncture is sometimes a helpful treatment when this condition frequently recurs. In TCM, haematite, or brown iron oxide, is regarded as an effective remedy for hiccups, but it is not one which would meet with the approval of the physicians of the West. See **flatulence** and **persimmon**.

hip See **rose**.

hip-disease A diseased condition of the hip-bone characterized by inflammation, fungus growth and caries.

hip-joint see **acetabulum** and **arthritis**.

Hippocrates A Greek physician who made substantial contributions to the practice of medicine in the West, where he is known as the Father of Medicine. He founded a medical school on the island of Cos, and put Western medicine on a scientific basis, distinguishing it from philosophy and religion. The Hippocratic Oath, which he devised, and which is taken by medical graduates, represents his ethical ideals in the practice of medicine. His system of medicine was essentially allopathic, and he perceived that co-operation between the physician and nature attains the best results. He also perceived that diet and climatic conditions have a great effect on health, and that diseases have natural causes, and are not brought about by magic or malevolent spirits. In these respects and others, his ideas were similar to those of the physicians of ancient China, who were probably the first to divorce the study of medicine from religion and superstition. Hippocrates' well-known saying, in its Latin version of the Greek original, *Ars longa, vita brevis*, 'Art is long, but life is short', expresses his regret that his life was so short that he was severely limited in what he could learn of the healing arts. He was not to know that, during his lifetime, Chinese medicine was already well established at an advanced level, whereas that of the West was still in its infancy. See **healing arts** and **heaven**.

Hippocratic Oath See **Hippocrates**.

hirsutism An excessive growth of hair on those parts of the body which are generally devoid of masses of hair, such as the palms of the hands or the face of a woman. This condition is to do with the hormones; and, no doubt, an excess of hair on a woman's face, legs or chest can be ascribed to the levels of those hormones which decide a person's degree of femininity or masculinity, or what are sometimes described as the primary sex characteristics. There are also racial factors. A person of Scandinavian or German origin, whether male or female, is likely to have a hairy body, whereas a Chinese person, whether male or female, is likely to be almost hairless. Hair is protective of the body, especially for those people who live in cold climates, and so it is an unfortunate accident of history that we have come to associate hairiness with savagery, and so regard it as being ugly and undesirable. But there are some exceptions. Among men, hairiness of the scalp or chest is regarded as a positive boon, and ranks as one of the hallmarks of manhood. But, then, human nature is very perverse. The view of Chinese physicians is simple and clear. We should accept ourselves as nature has made us, for what is natural is surely normal, and to interfere with nature too much is likely to invite her retaliation. We should also accept that, in the long term, beauty in the heart is more real and lasting than that which, supposedly, is indicated by a surfeit or deficiency of hair in certain places. See **hairiness**.

histamine A substance within the body which causes allergic reactions. It occurs in many plants and animals, and is often released when tissues are damaged. It can cause minor ailments, such as hives – or nettle-rash – or more serious conditions, such as hay fever, asthma and hypotension (low blood pressure), which may lead to complete collapse. In the West, the treatment is to administer an antihistamine, which is a medicine that counteracts the effects of a histamine in the body. Chinese physicians trained only in TCM would not know of histamine, but would readily accept that the body contains things made by itself, or taken from plants and animals, which can have beneficial or deleterious effects. These things would be described as protective-*qi*, evil-*qi*, rebellious-*qi*, and so on. Their method of treatment would be to strengthen the affected organs. One Chinese physician has made a comment in this regard: 'I am very suspicious of these theories about histamines and allergies. One could easily conclude that the Western physician invents item *x* as the cause of ailness *y*, and treats it with medicine *z*, when, in reality, he does not know the real cause of *y* nor the real effects of *z*.' See **allergy**.

history See **Chinese history** and **past history**.

HIV Human immunodeficiency virus. See **AIDS**.

hives This condition, which is also called urticaria, or nettle-rash, though it is not caused by nettles, is an allergic reaction characterized by itchy red weals on the skin, varying in size from tiny spots to raised patches several inches across, lasting for minutes, hours, days or even weeks, and sometimes changing their positions on the body. Hives results from histamines and other substances being released when the body tissues react allergically to certain foods, such as fish and strawberries, food additives, dust, pollen, coldness and sunlight. Generally, the condition is not serious. In the West, the orthodox treatment is a suitable antihistamine prescribed by a physician. In TCM, the treatment mainly consists of avoiding those food items which are suspected of being causative of the condition, though many of such food items do not feature in the Chinese diet in any case. Some relief is obtained by bathing the affected parts with an infusion of one of the following, using the parts and dosage indicated: camomile, *Matricaria chamomilla*, flowers, 3–10 g; chickweed, *Stellaria media*, whole plant, 4–10 g; Chinese gentian, *Gentiana scabra*, roots, 3–7 g.

hoarseness Generally associated with a sore throat or a common cold, hoarseness can be effectively treated by gargling with a saline solution, say 3 teaspoons table salt per litre hot water or an infusion of 3–10 g flowers of coltsfoot, *Tussilago farfara*. But, if the condition persists, there could be a serious cause, and medical advice should be sought. See **sore throat**.

'hold-back medicine' A literal translation of the Chinese name, which is most apt, for an astringent medicine. See **astringent**.

holistic medicine This approach to healing views health as a positive state, and not the mere absence of disease. It is not enough that a person should be free of disease as might be decided by a cursory medical examination. He must be 'glowing with health' – or 'fighting fit', as we might say – if he is to make the most of life and not pursue an unrewarding existence that is physically, mentally and spiritually inhibited, and if society is to regard him as a valued member and not a mere appendage. The individual should, to a large extent, take responsibility for his own health-care, so that his attention to both his physical and mental needs, coupled with the appropriate therapeutic techniques, with a special emphasis on herbal remedies, will develop within him a capacity for self-healing. Holistic medicine is a relatively modern concept in the West, but Chinese physicians are aware that many ailments have a psychosomatic quality, and they have always considered a healthy person as being one who is health-conscious and thoroughly integrated in both body and mind, and also as one who is a useful component in the natural and social scheme of things, to which he is fully related, both culturally and communally. The holistic approach is essentially one of combined caring and self-caring in matters of diet, exercise, therapy, social habits, and so on, so that, by and large, in matters of health and medicine, the individual will be attuned to nature and capable of self-help, and not a feeble dependent on a system which he barely understands. Holistic medicine treats the whole man, and not just isolated aspects of his make-up. It could be said that TCM is essentially allopathic in the treatment of individual ailments, but holistic in its wider aims.

hollow organs See **liu fu**.

homoeopathy Homoeopathy is a system of medicine in which natural remedies are used to support the body's own powers of resistance and recovery. The treatment of a disease is performed by administering drugs which, in a healthy person, would produce symptoms similar to those of the disease. Since these drugs are of natural origin and administered in highly diluted forms, they do no harm, but they do prompt the body's immunity system to go into action. Many of these drugs are of mineral origin, and experience has shown that the more diluted the forms in which they are administered, the greater are the benefits. The principle of homoeopathy, *similia similibus curentur*, 'let like be treated by like', was known to the Greek physician Hippocrates and the Swiss alchemist Paracelsus, but Samuel Hahnemann (1755–1843), a German physician and chemist, established homoeopathy in the form in which it is used today. TCM is not homoeopathic. See **allopathy**.

homosexual Attraction to the same sex, or a person who is so attracted. The Chinese authorities, who place much importance on traditional family values, regard homosexuality as being highly undesirable. See **heterosexual** and **genitalia**.

honey Obtained from the honey bee, *Apis mellifera*, which is distributed world-wide, honey is used extensively in TCM. Character: warm, sweet. Affinity: lungs, spleen, large intestine. Effects: demulcent, nutrient, laxative, emollient. Symptoms: dry mouth and throat. Treatments: bronchitis, hay fever, anaemia, kidney and circulatory complaints. Honey should be avoided by those people who have a chronically loose bowel. Honey was known to the ancient Chinese, Egyptians, Greeks and Romans as a high-energy food, and the Greeks and Romans called it ambrosia, or 'food of the gods', for they believed that it conferred immortality on those who consumed it. In the Middle Ages, it was used for making mead, an alcoholic drink, and as a salve for wounds, burns and skin eruptions. Seemingly, it does have mildly antiseptic properties. Bees make honey from nectar, a sugary fluid, which they obtain from the nectaries in the bases of the petals of flowers. Nectar has a high content of fructose and glucose, which explains why honey has been used as a food, preservative and sweetener since ancient times. It is sweeter than cane sugar because of the presence of fructose. As an item of diet, it is preferable to refined sugar, which sometimes causes allergies, and it is also preferable to artificial sweeteners, such as aspartame, saccharin and acesulfame K, which have no food value and are suspected of being causative of cancer. It contains small amounts of minerals and traces of pollen grains. The latter, being products of the male sexual organs of flowering plants, have led some people, including the Chinese, to believe that honey has some value as an aphrodisiac. It is certainly a source of high energy, which might be helpful to those who wish to improve their libido. The Chinese use a great deal of honey in their cooking. For health reasons they prefer it to refined sugar. In TCM, honey is the base for most herbal pills. See **sweetener** and **royal jelly**.

honey pills To make these pills, the herbal ingredients are finely ground and then mixed with honey, which has been previously boiled and skimmed to remove impurities, and then rolled as a dense mixture, to make long cylindrical lengths, which are divided into small, equal-sized portions that are rolled between the thumb and fingers to make pills. Honey is a medication in itself but it is absorbed slowly by the small intestine, and so honey-based pills are effective for chronic ailments where gradual and long-term treatment is required.

honeysuckle See **Japanese honeysuckle**.

hookworm *Ancylostoma*. A parasitic nematode worm which infests man and animals. The male has hooklike spines by which it attaches itself to the wall of the intestines. It occurs in contaminated water and penetrates the soles of the feet in order to enter the body. Prevention should be simple enough. Neither walk in nor drink contaminated water. But it was very difficult to convince the fellahin that there is a great disadvantage in walking barefoot in the water from the Nile. In fact, this was the case with all the peasants in the tropical and subtropical regions of the world. The Chinese were the exception: as early as about 500 BC, physicians in the south of China were warning people against the hookworm. At one time, the people living in the south of the United States were commonly infested with the hookworm.

hop *Humulus lupulus* Herbal medicine. Distribution: Asia, Europe. Parts: strobiles (conelike female flowers). Character: warm, bitter. Affinity: stomach, spleen, small intestine, large intestine. Effects: sedative, antispasmodic, digestive, antiseptic. Symptoms: restlessness, sleeplessness, irritability, dyspepsia, constipation. Treatments: colitis, insomnia, stress. Dosage: 2–3 g. Hops should not be administered where depression is associated with stress. In the West, hops are commonly used as an inhalant to induce sleep. A bag made of muslin or some other suitable material is stuffed with hops and placed under the pillow.

hordoleum See **stye**.

hormone A chemical substance secreted by one of the endocrine, or ductless, glands, and which assists in regulating the bodily functions. Hormones are sometimes called 'chemical messengers' because they are carried in the bloodstream to the places in the body where they are required. The bodily functions and emotions, particularly those of an involuntary nature, are controlled more by the hormones than the brain and nervous system. Some so-called mental disorders are really glandular disorders, for they are due to hormonal imbalances. For example, hyperthyroidism, together with the feeling of panic which it sometimes induces, is due to excessive secretion of the thyroid hormone, which regulates the rate of metabolism and so influences growth and oxidation. The hormone secretion of the pituitary gland influences the hormone secretions of the testes and ovaries, and sexual activity is certainly associated with the emotions. See **endocrine glands** and **qi**.

horny goat weed *Epimedium sagittatum* Herbal medicine. Distribution: China, Japan. Parts: leaves. Character: warm, pungent. Affinity: liver, kidneys. Effects: tonic to kidneys, reduces wind-damp conditions, vasodilator, aphrodisiac. Symptoms: impotence, premature ejaculation, coldness of hands and feet, numbness, rheumatic aches and pains, spasms. Treatments: spermatorrhoea, lumbago, deficiency of kidney-yin, wind-damp excess, hypertension, forgetfulness. Dosage: 8–15 g. This herb is a common ingredient in spring wine and other tonic wines. It induces a flow of blood to the brain, and so improves mental activity. But one might think that this could be a dangerous procedure if the prescribed dosage were greatly exceeded. The discovery of the properties of this herb has an interesting history. See **goats**.

horoscope A chart showing the configuration of the planets as they are when the night sky is observed at a certain moment, especially at the time of a person's birth, or a prediction based upon this. See **astrology** and **prediction**.

hospitalization Chinese physicians take the view that, except where special equipment is required or because of some other special circumstance, hospitalization is generally undesirable. They would argue that a hospital is a source of infection, which surely must be the case, and so it is hardly the best place for a person who is already in a weakened state. They would also argue that there are no people better qualified to take care of a sick person than the members of his own family, for they would by motivated by strong bonds of affection and loyalty, which are the outcome of Confucian teaching. Of course, overall supervision by the physician would be required.

hot One of the four energies and five tastes of TCM. See **energy** and **taste**.

hot-dryness See **climate** and **excess combinations**.

hot food For dietetic purposes, a hot food is not defined as one that is at a high temperature, but as one which has a high energy value, and so ice-cream could be classified as a hot food in the Chinese sense of the term. Among the hot foods, the Chinese list bread, potatoes, spring onions, shellfish, black tea, spirits, sesame oil and peanut oil. It is not difficult to understand why bread and potatoes, which are mainly carbohydrate, and sesame oil and peanut oil, which are fats, are so listed, for they have a high energy value; but shellfish, though a good source of protein, and black tea have little or no energy value, and so it would seem that the Chinese also define a hot food as one which is hot to the taste. Spirits raise the skin temperature, but they also lower the internal body temperature. In fact, spirits are deceptive as a source of heat. See **cold food** and **classification of foods**.

hot illness A hot illness is generally external, full and ascending, as its symptoms will indicate. See **ba gang**.

hot symptoms See **ba gang**.

house A name given to each of the endocrine glands, or energy centres, by the Taoist physicians of ancient China. See **endocrine glands**.

housemaid's knee See **bursitis**.

Hsia dynasty See **Xia dynasty**.

Hsing-I See **Xing Yi**.

Huang Di See **Yellow Emperor**.

Huang Di Nei Jing 'The Internal Book of Huang Di'. This book contains a record of the ideas, theories and experiences of the Yellow Emperor, and was compiled by scholars during the time of the early Han dynasty (206 BC–AD 220). Here is some of his advice, which still holds good. 'To administer medicines for illnesses which have already developed is akin to the conduct of a man who begins to dig a well after he has become thirsty, or begins to make his weapons after he has engaged in battle. Do not leave it too late. It is easier to prevent than to cure. Sedate fullness, and tone emptiness. Where illness is in the skin (external) sweat it out. If the illness is hot, cool it; if it is cold, warm it.'

Huang Di Nei Jing Su Wen 'The Yellow Emperor's Classic of Internal Medicine'.

huang qi *Astralagus membranaceus* Herbal medicine. Distribution: north China, Manchuria, Mongolia. Parts: roots. Character: warm, sweet. Affinity: lungs, spleen. Effects: diuretic, tones energy, cardiotonic, inhibits perspiration, improves circulation. Symptoms: fatigue, swollen face, heavy sweating. Treatments: abscesses, diabetes, external empty ailments, prolapse of rectum or womb. Dosage: 7–14 g. Incompatible with *Magnolia liliflora*.

Hua Tuo Also spelt as *Hua To*. Taoist physician and surgeon, Hua Tuo (AD 141–208), who lived at the time of the late Han dynasty, is thought to be the first person to practise anaesthesia. He was also a devotee of the martial arts, and he devised a system of therapeutic kungfu exercises, which he called *wu qin xi*, or 'five animal play'. See **wu qin xi** and **anaesthesia**.

human immunodeficiency virus HIV. See **AIDS**.

humidity Plants and animals flourish best where there is a sufficiency of nutrients, warmth and moisture. It follows that the micro-organisms which cause diseases multiply more rapidly where there is humidity than where it is dry, as also do those fungi and other plants that are sources of food and medicines, which was noticed by Chinese physicians many centuries ago. See **climate** and **hygiene**.

humour This could be defined as a bodily fluid, or essence. In TCM, the body is regarded as having four humours: *qi*, or 'essential life-force'; *xue*, or 'blood'; *jing*, or 'vital essence'; *jin ye*, or 'fluid'. Superficially, they are not unlike the four humours – blood, phlegm, melancholy and choler – which, until fairly recent times, were an accepted principle of Western medicine. These humours are toned by massage and breathing and physical exercises, and nourished by food and medicines. They are closely related, and a deficiency or poor condition of one has an adverse effect on the others. Although the TCM approach to the body fluids is different from that which obtains in the West, the principles are similar. A deficiency in the blood will affect the lymph, a deficiency in the digestive juices will affect the blood, and so on. *Qi* is the most vital of these humours. It regulates the others, and it is the only one which can be derived from the atmosphere. The others can be derived from food and medicine. The Taoist physicians of ancient China were aware of the endocrine glands, and allocated a function to each, so associating them with the humours, though they would know little or nothing of the nature of hormones. See **endocrine glands** and **qi**.

huo qi Fire-energy, which may amass in midsummer or as a consequence of consuming too much hot food. The symptoms are as one might expect: dry lips and mouth, a parched throat, a rise in temperature and constipation. This condition can easily be remedied with cooling foods: cucumber, water melon, turnips and citrus fruits. See **classification of foods**.

hydrochloric acid Hydrogen chloride (HCl). The stomach contains a little of this acid, which is necessary for digestion, for it provides the proper medium for pepsin, which is one of the stomach enzymes, and dissolves minerals that are insoluble in water. It also destroys some of the harmful bacteria in the food entering the stomach. But an excess of this acid causes stomach upsets. However, it can be counteracted by an antacid, which is the usual procedure in Western medicine. In TCM, there would be a preference for an eliminative substance, such as white rice porridge, which absorbs the excess acid and then expels it via the bowel. The physicians of ancient China would not have been aware of hydrochloric acid as such, but they would have been aware that the stomach contents are of an acid nature, and usually beneficially so. See **sweet-and-sour dishes**.

hydrophobia See **rabies**

hydropsy See **oedema**.

hydrotherapy The use of water in medical treatments, either externally, as with some physical exercises, such as swimming and sea-water bathing, or internally, as with drinking water from mineral springs. Hydrotherapy is one of the natural treatments among the seven categories of healing exercises employed in TCM. See **healing exercises** and **nature's treatment**.

hygiene The principles of maintaining health by cleanliness, which is as important to the Chinese as it is to the people of the West, except that the methods used by the Chinese in this respect are not riddled with fetishism. It is useful to remember that all micro-organisms, including those which cause diseases, multiply rapidly where there is moisture, warmth and a supply of nutrients, which means that, in the interests of food hygiene, a kitchen should be kept cool and dry as far as is possible. It should also be regularly cleansed in order to remove grease and dirt, etc., which contain nutrients for micro-organisms. The same common-sense thinking should be applied to personal hygiene. A toilet seat recently vacated is usually warm, moist and fouled, if only slightly, with excreted substances, which makes it an ideal place for the breeding and transmission of micro-organisms. See **humidity, personal hygiene** and **food hygiene**.

hymen A membrane which covers the opening in the vagina, and which is usually ruptured when sexual intercourse occurs for the first time.

hyperactivity Excessive restlessness, together with sleeplessness, excited speech and lack of balance. It could be a symptom of a full illness, which needs to be sedated or suppressed. See **full illness**.

hyercholesterolaemia This is an Anglicized version of a Chinese term which describes a condition where there is great excess of cholesterol in the circulatory organs. Chinese physicians regard tienchi, *Panax pseudo-ginseng*, as an excellent treatment. See **tienchi**.

hyperglycaemia An abnormally excessive amount of glucose in the blood, and a symptom of diabetes mellitus. See **endocrine glands**.

hyperhidrosis Excessive perspiration. It may be associated with one of a number of conditions, such as fever, heat exhaustion and hyperthyroidism. A TCM treatment for this condition is an infusion, taken internally, of 7–14 g roots of *huang qi, Astralagus membranaceus*. See **diaphoresis**.

hypermenorrhoea See **menorrhagia**.

hypermetropia Long-sightedness. See **optical defects**.

hypersensitivity Intolerance. An abnormally high sensitivity of the body in its reactions to foreign matter and external influences, though it does not necessarily constitute an allergy. See **allergy**.

hypersomnia A condition in which a person tends to sleep too much, and which, in an opposite direction, can be as bothersome as insomnia. The cause may be depression or lack of energy, as would be the case after an illness or severe shock. Generally, there is no cause for alarm, for almost all people have stages in their lives when they are excessively tired, and so become irritable and lose all interest in their work, leisure, friends and family. Age may play a part in this. It is often the case that young people, especially teenagers, need more sleep than elderly people because they take more out of themselves in physical and sexual activity. Where hypersomnia is due to debility or the after-effects of an illness, Chinese physicians would recommend a wholesome and energy-giving diet to help the body to get back to normal. This could be supplemented with a tonic medicine from the wide range available in TCM: Asiatic ginseng, *Panax ginseng*; eucommia, *Eucommia ulmoides*; longan, *Euphoria longan*; wolfberry, *Lycium chinense*; tienchi, *Panax pseudo-ginseng*; huang qi, *Astralagus membranaceus*; royal jelly. But, if the condition persists, medical advice should be sought because there may be a serious underlying cause. See **tiredness**.

hypertension High blood pressure, which must NOT be confused with hypotension, or low blood pressure. It has a mild form, which is said to be benign. Its severe form, which is said to be malignant, causes complications which affect the heart and circulatory system, and may lead to kidney complaints, strokes, angina and heart attacks. Generally, there are no symptoms, but headaches, dizziness and tinnitus occur in a few cases. Its causes include a constant excess of salt in the diet, too much alcohol, obesity, lack of exercise, smoking, the contraceptive pill, pregnancy and arteriosclerosis. It is helpful to have a diet containing fruit, vegetables, brown rice and other wholegrain cereals, pulses, chicken, fish, garlic, onions and honey, and omitting red meat, animal fats, tea, coffee and alcohol. One should not smoke or use the contraceptive pill, and one should lose weight and take part in non-competitive exercise, such as walking, swimming and cycling. One should also try to reduce stress. Acupuncture is sometimes successful in this respect.

Infusions or decoctions of the following, taken internally, using the parts and dosages indicated will help to lower blood pressure: *huang qi*, *Astralagus membranaceus*, roots, 7–14 g; peach, *Prunus persica*, kernels, 4–10 g; morning star, *Incaria rhychophylla*, stems, 6–10 g; antelope, *Saiga tatarica*, horn, 1–3 g; self-heal, *Prunella vulgaris*, flowers, 4–6 g; wolfberry, *Lycium chinense*, skin of roots, 10–15 g; common plantain, *Plantago asiatica*, seeds, 5–9 g; chrysanthemum, *Chrysanthemum morifolium*, flowers, 4–10 g; wheat, *Triticum aestivum*, grains, 15–30 g; hawthorn, *Crataegus pinnatifida*, haws (fruits), 6–14 g; lotus, *Nelumbo nucifera*, leaves, 10–15 g. *Ch'iang chuang kung*, or 'invigorated breathing', and *qi gong* exercises are helpful, but must be conducted under medical supervision. See **hypotension** and **arteriosclerosis**.

hyperthyroidism Overactivity of the thyroid gland, which must NOT be confused with hypothyroidism. It is characterized by an increase in blood pressure, heart action, body temperature and perspiration. The patient becomes nervous and irritable and, in some cases, will have bulging and staring eyes. In the West, the treatment is by thyroid hormone extracted from the dried thyroid glands of sheep. A similar technique was used by Sun Simiao, one of the great physicians of the period of the Tang dynasty (618–907), who prescribed extracts from the thyroid glands of lambs and calves for this condition. In TCM, the usual treatment is an infusion, taken internally, of 5–15 g gulf seaweed, *Sargassum fusiforme*. See **goitre**.

hyperventilation Overbreathing, that is, breathing too hard and rapidly as a consequence of great anxiety. Too much carbon dioxide is exhaled, leading to a loss of carbon dioxide in the blood, which becomes alkaline, so producing a state of panic. This condition commonly occurs at a time of social tension, as when making a speech in public or being interviewed for a job, which can be quite an ordeal for some people. This condition is basically harmless, but it can be accompanied by fainting, dizziness, tingling or numbness in the fingers or toes, sweaty palms, excessive sighing and yawning, and tightness or even pain in the chest. Occasionally, the victims becomes so panicky that they hyperventilate until they collapse. These symptoms are sometimes mistakenly thought to be indicative of angina or a heart attack. The treatment is to try to relax and breathe slowly, say, one breath every six seconds. It is helpful to breathe into a paper bag – NOT a plastic bag – so that the exhaled carbon dioxide is returned via the lungs to the blood. In TCM, acupuncture is generally used to treat this condition, particularly where the sufferer is highly nervous by temperament. See **stress**.

hypnosis A trance-like state of sleep that is artificially produced. It should not be confused with catalepsy, which is not artificially induced. See **catalepsy**.

hypnotherapy This is a technique by which a therapist takes temporary control over a person's mind when he is in a trance-like state of consciousness between sleep and wakefulness, and which is not unlike the state of mind of a person who is sleep-walking or day-dreaming. The therapist will use various devices, such as a swinging object, a bright source of light or soothing and quietly spoken words to lull the patient into closing his eyes. The patient may even fall into a deep sleep, which does no harm, and could give him a rest which may be much needed. Then, with great skill, the therapist will make suggestions that will reduce anxiety, build confidence, relieve pain or elicit diagnostic-type information. Hypnotherapy has been used quite successfully to treat stress-related disorders, such as eczema, migraine, peptic ulcers, hysteria, asthma and insomnia. It has also been used with some degree of success as a treatment for tobacco, alcohol and drug addiction. During the early part of the nineteenth century, a few European surgeons were using hypnosis as a form of anaesthesia. But hypnotherapy, or mesmerism, as it was once called, fell out of favour when its founder, Franz Anton Mesmer (1734–1815), an Austrian physician, was declared to be a charlatan. However, hypnotherapy is regaining its popularity, and mainly because it is now understood that many illnesses are psychosomatic, and the emotional states which were once thought to be solely products of the mind, are largely determined by secretions from the endocrine glands. If a person can be persuaded to relax, whether by drugs or suggestion, his breathing and pulse will become normalized, which will improve the circulation of the blood, so beneficially affecting all the organs of the body, including the brain, nervous system and endocrine glands. Hypnosis in various forms is practised on a limited scale in the rural areas of China, but its practitioners are generally charlatans who are taking mean advantage of credulous peasants. But hypnotherapy, which is hypnosis used to heal, has no great role in TCM, though Chinese physicians would readily claim that the benefits of hypnotherapy can be achieved on a far wider scale by acupuncture and physical and breathing exercises. On the other hand, self-hypnosis, or auto-suggestion, is a vital component of those meditative exercises which feature prominently in Taoist healing systems, and which discipline the emotions by a sheer effort of will, or provide an escape from the harsh realities of life, so establishing a greater serenity of mind and a much healthier body. See **meditation** and **self-hypnosis**.

hypnotic See **soporific**.

hypnotism A technique for inducing hypnosis – a trance-like or semi-conscious state in which the subject responds only to external suggestions. See **hypnotherapy** and **self-hypnosis**.

hypochondria Abnormally excessive anxiety, and even morbid depression, about one's state of health and trifling or imaginary ailments. Hypochondriacs tend to be superstitious and credulous, and often make a practice of buying patent medicines which serve no purpose, other than providing self-confidence, to treat ailments which do not exist. The hypochondriac is the kind of person who, lying quietly in bed, listens fearfully to his own heartbeat, and wonders if a heart attack is imminent. He is also the kind of person who takes up some kind of bizarre religion in the hope of finding a miracle cure, and there are always those who are ready to pander to his whims – at a price! But anxiety can be very damaging to the health, and so hypochondria is, in itself, an illness requiring treatment. Chinese physicians would recommend acupuncture, which can often effect a cure, in preference to sedation, which merely alleviates the condition, and only temporarily. One might think that, since the Chinese are so health conscious, there would be a high incidence of hypo-chondria in China, but that is not the case, probably because Confucianism, Taoism and some of the other traditional beliefs of the Chinese do not breed fear and superstition, for chronic anxiety is often a bad habit which derives from unhealthy social habits and an unsound philosophy of living.

hypoglycaemia An abnormally low amount of glucose in the blood, which means that the brain is starved of glucose. This condition is characterized by profuse perspiration, a rapid pulse, confusion, hunger and irritability. Without treatment, there will be unconsciousness and even brain damage. The condition is associated with diabetes which is untreated. Sleep, food and an intake of sugar quickly remedy this condition. Diabetics will generally carry a supply of glucose tablets for use in this situation. See **diabetes mellitus** and **insulin**.

hypomenorrhoea A decrease in the duration or quantity of the flow of blood during menstruation. This may indicate conception, the onset of the menopause or a low state of health. It may be no more than a temporary irregularity; but, if there are doubts, medical advice should be sought.

hypotension Low blood pressure, which must NOT be confused with hypertension, which is high blood pressure. It is generally not a serious condition, and its effects, such as faintness and giddiness, are usually only temporary, and often follow a severe shock, but do not require special treatment. People with hypotension generally live longer than those with hypertension, and there is less likelihood of a stroke. Chinese physicians would recommend a wholesome diet and a yang tonic for this condition, which they regard as a yin ailment, empty and descending, but certainly not disastrous. Asiatic ginseng, *Panax ginseng*, Chinese jujube, *Ziziphus jujuba*, and royal jelly could be helpful.

hypothermia A body temperature of less than 35°C, which is brought about by exposure to severe cold, and which mainly affects babies and elderly people. It inhibits the bodily functions, and metabolism slows down. If a person is accustomed to cold conditions, the fall in body temperature may go unnoticed. Shivering ceases at about 33°C, and then the victim becomes confused and unsteady. At about 30°C, he will sink into unconsciousness, and death will follow if he is alone, for there will be no one to take action on his behalf. The treatment is to move the victim to a warm environment, wrap him in blankets and give him warm drinks to begin with. He can be given hot drinks when his body temperature rises. He must NOT be given alcoholic drinks, for they only create an illusion of warmth, and will reduce the temperature of his internal organs. In Britain, there have been many deaths from hypothermia during recent years. This is because many British people pin their hopes on the possibility of a mild winter, and so do not take adequate precautions against cold weather. It is also the case that many of the pensioners on low incomes try to economize by spending too little on fuel. There is a low incidence of hypothermia in China, and for two main reasons. In the south of China, the weather is mild during the winter months; and, in the north, the weather is always bitterly cold during the winter, and so the inhabitants make proper provision. Windows and doors are sealed, many layers of clothing are worn, and fires of wood, coal, charcoal, peat or dung are kept burning night and day. And it goes without saying that the Chinese are not neglectful of elderly people in this or any other respect.

hypothyroidism Underactivity of the thyroid gland, which must NOT be confused with hyperthyroidism. A baby born with this condition has constipation, sleeps and eats badly, and will suffer from slow physical and mental development, growing short and fat with a protruding tongue and scanty hair. Such a baby is called a cretin. With an adult, the condition develops slowly, and the patient sleeps more, puts on weight and becomes listless. Also, the skin becomes dry, the hair becomes brittle and may fall out, and the voice deepens. There is some doubt about the cause of hypothyroidism, though inflammation of the glands is the cause in some cases, and the pituitary gland, at the base of the brain, which secretes a hormone that stimulates the thyroid gland, may also play a part. In the West, hypothyroidism is detected by a blood test; and, if caught in time, it is treated with thyroxine tablets. In TCM, it is treated by acupuncture, the meridians relating to the gall-bladder and the large intestine being used for this purpose, or by putting iodine-rich foods, such as seaweed, into the diet, as is done with all thyroid disorders. For the latter treatment, gulf seaweed, *Sargassum fusiforme*, is very suitable. See **hyperthyroidism**.

hyssop *Agastache rugosa* Herbal medicine. Distribution: China, Japan, Laos, Vietnam. Parts: leaves, stems. Character: warm, sweet-pungent. Affinity: stomach, spleen, lungs. Effects: astringent, expectorant, stomachic, carminative, diaphoretic. Symptoms: nausea, vomiting, diarrhoea, slight fever, tightness of chest. Treatments: damp-excess in stomach and spleen, damp summer-heat conditions, external wind-cold injuries, summer colds, heat exhaustion, heat stroke, influenza, respiratory infections. Dosage: 4–7 g. Perhaps this herb would be better named as Chinese hyssop, for there is a European species of hyssop – *Hyssopus officinalis* – which has similar properties.

hysteria This term is used rather loosely and in an everyday sense to describe the state of a person who laughs, screams or weeps loudly and uncontrollably as the consequence of a sudden fright. It is a panic reaction. But, used in its strict medical sense, hysteria is a psychoneurosis which may produce convulsions, temporary loss of sight or memory, and even apparent paralysis of a limb, together with disturbance of the moral and intellectual faculties. It arises from a state of anxiety or frustration built up during the formative years, and which can only be expressed by bodily symptoms. Too much rigid discipline in childhood is largely responsible for this deep-seated disorder, which is far more serious than is generally realized. People with this illness become hysterical to avoid a difficult situation, to divert attention away from their inadequacies, or to satisfy their craving for love or recognition. Children need discipline, it is true, for they need to be trained, but discipline without any discernible purpose is frustrating to a child. Hysteria certainly needs proper treatment, which must NOT include slapping the face of a hysterical person, for the shock only produces more psychological unrest. In dealing with an immediate attack of hysteria, one should attempt to remove what appears to be the immediate cause. In the West, the long-term treatment could involve psychotherapy or hypnotherapy. Chinese physicians would recommend acupuncture and meditative exercises to induce self-confidence. They would also recommend an attempt to remove the underlying cause of the condition, which would appear to be the obvious course of action. It is probably the case that hysteria is less common in China than elsewhere, for the Chinese approach to life is more pragmatic, natural and leisurely, and Chinese society does not suffer from over-regulation or lack of natural moral values. It says much for the perspicacity of the physicians of ancient China that they associated excitable laughter, which they called 'fire-sound', with heart defects and hysteria, and not with blissful happiness. There is no doubt that, over a long period, the stress due to hysteria could produce a heart condition. See '**fire-sound**'.

I

iatrogenesis Illnesses and abnormalities which develop as a consequence of medical treatment. They may arise from the human errors in the diagnoses and treatments made by physicians and surgeons. Errors in diagnosis occur because some illnesses have the same or similar symptoms, or the physician does not always distinguish between what is a real illness and what is only a symptom. For example, taking aspirin for a headache will not necessarily cure the condition for which a headache may be merely a symptom. Sometimes, the wrong drugs are prescribed, or drugs may be taken as an overdose. Since drugs and surgery often interfere with the normal functioning of the body, it sometimes happens that both the physician and the patient have to consider the risks involved, and decide whether the advantages of a treatment outweigh the risks. Iatrogenic illnesses may be unavoidable, as with those severe illnesses, such as cancer, which may require drastic treatment producing undesirable side-effects. It is estimated that as many as one in six persons are admitted into hospital as a consequence of iatrogenic illnesses. During recent years, there have been some unfortunate side-effects resulting from the use of manufactured drugs, some of which are addictive. TCM has much to offer in this regard, for its herbal remedies are natural and generally non-addictive and without side-effects, Chinese physicians are extremely skilful in diagnosis, and a medical examination by a Chinese physician is always thorough, and never cursory.

IBS See **irritable bowel syndrome**.

I Ching Also spelt as *Yijing*, which is the Pinyin Anglicized version of this title. Those Chinese who feel that they have need of a 'salve for sickness of the soul' or would like to have some knowledge of what the future holds for them, consult the *I Ching*, or 'Book of Changes', which is briefly but accurately described in the following quotation: 'Semi-sacred, a legacy from ancient China, a classical work of great antiquity, fount of profound wisdom, the most reliable of all divinatory oracles, supportive of

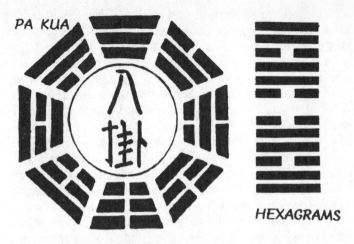

PA KUA

HEXAGRAMS

the all-important art of living, founded by the Taoists, studied by Confucius and improved by his followers, and, in its inspiration, the oldest and one of the most valuable books in the world, the *I Ching* is amazingly GOOD NEWS!' The *I Ching* is a source of wisdom for the talented and ambitious, consolation for the afflicted and desperate, and encouragement for all who value health, longevity and peace of mind; and the Chinese have as much respect, even reverence, for it as the people of the West have for the Bible. The *I Ching* consists essentially of 64 six-line figures, or hexagrams, which have been made by pairing the eight trigrams of the Pa Kua, a mystic device, of which a copy is shown here. A complete line is positive, or yang, and represents one in the binary system of numbers, and a broken line is negative, or yin, and represents zero. Sixty-four is a multiple of two, which is the base number in the binary system. This, of course, is the principle of the electronic computer, and it is one of the many instances where, by over 5000 years, the sages of ancient China anticipated some of the recent scientific and technological developments in the West; from which it may be gathered that those people of the West who consider themselves to be intellectually superior to the Chinese certainly have much to learn. A prediction, together with some explanations is attached to each of the hexagrams. It is this arrangement which has led people to use the *I Ching* for telling fortunes. It has been described, in ignorance, as a book of magic spells. But the truth is that these so-called predictions are snippets of informaion which advise a person how to cope with a particular type of situation, and how to anticipate the problems and/or benefits which might arise from it, and so the *I Ching* could be described as an 'encyclopaedia of the emotions'. It owes its accuracy to the fact that the sages of ancient China had discovered that every human thought could be expressed as a question to which the answer must be either 'yes' or 'no', though there are degrees of positivity and negativity, with not much difference between a weak 'yes' and a weak 'no'. The soundness of their thinking has been confirmed by modern scientific research in the West, which has shown that the brain functions in a similar way to a computer, with impulses that are electrochemical. C.G. Jung (1875–1961), the Swiss psychiatrist and psychologist, used the *I Ching* in treating his patients, and Baron von Leibnitz (1646–1716), the German mathematician and philosopher, was inspired by the *I Ching* when he invented a mechanical calculator and a form of the calculus, which is a branch of mathematics that is indispensable to the needs of modern engineering. This is a valuable testimony to the validity of the *I Ching* as a divinatory oracle and book of wisdom, which is of undoubted usefulness in the field of mental health. See **Pa Kua** and **prediction**.

icterus See **jaundice**.

id See **ego**.

idiocy In its idiomatic usage, *idiocy* means 'foolishness' or 'craziness'; but, as a medical term, it indicates mental deficiency in its severest form. See **mental illness**.

ileum Small intestine. This term must not be confused with *ilium*. See **ilium**.

ilium Haunch-bone. The upper part of each half of the pelvis. See **skeleton** and **ileum**.

illness A dictionary would define an illness as an unhealthy state of the body, and so, in its widest sense, an illness could be any disease or defect, physical or mental, congenital or acquired, minor or serious, commonplace or rare, chronic or acute, whatever its cause. The term *ailment* is generally reserved for illnesses that are of a minor or chronic nature, such as toothache, acne, indigestion and asthma. The term *disease* is generally reserved for those illnesses which have a specific organic cause. Some diseases are due to dietary deficiencies, especially of vitamins and minerals, and abnormal growths and functions, as with tumours and diabetes, but most are due to pathogens, which are micro-organisms – viruses, bacteria, protozoa and fungi – that produce toxins or do damage in other ways. Such conditions as a nervous breakdown and a fractured bone would be regarded as illnesses or defects, but not as diseases. Chinese physicians categorize illnesses quite differently, and put them into four main classes: those due to climatic and environmental conditions, which would include infectious diseases; those due to emotional factors, which would include mental and nervous disorders and psychosomatic conditions; those due to weaknesses of the organs, whose causes, among others, are poor diet, lack of exercise and immoderate habits; and miscellaneous items, such as fractured bones, food poisoning and insect bites. Of course, these are not clear-cut categories. For example, a mental illness can have a climatic or dietary cause as well as an emotional cause, and rabies is an infectious disease which leads to a mental condition, though its initial cause is being bitten by an infected dog, which could rank as a miscellaneous item. In TCM, it is assumed that the healing effects of medication reach the organs and tissues where they are required as much by the meridians as through the blood. Illnesses are partly explained in terms of qi, or 'vital energy', that is, its amount, nature and location. That in air is called air-qi, that in the body is called human-qi, or person-qi, that in the kidneys is called kidney-qi, that which causes illness is called evil-qi or rebellious-qi, and so on. The concept of qi is difficult for people of the West to understand, but it can be explained in terms of Western medicine, and then it might be readily understood. See **qi** and **symptom**.

illusion A deception of the sight, hearing, touch, taste, smell or mind. It is a medical condition where there is a dysfunction of the brain or a sense organ or some other organ concerned, directly or indirectly, with acuity. See **delusion**.

imbecility A condition of weak intellect, especially that of an adult with a mental age of about five years. See **mental illness**.

immortality Although man's intelligence has given him many advantages, it has also given him one great disadvantage, for he is the only animal which has foreknowledge, well in advance, of his own demise. But he has never relished the prospect of death, and so, rather than face up to its harsh reality, he has sought for some kind of immortality, which has generally manifested itself as a religious belief in an afterlife where all will be good and beautiful. The rulers of ancient Egypt were so convinced of the reality of a future life that they arranged for their personal possessions to be left in their tombs so that they might have some measure of comfort in the next world. And *The English Prayer Book* makes mention of the hope of eternal life. But, since the time of Confucius, the Chinese have had a much more mature and realistic attitude in matters of this kind, as is indicated by this quotation, often attributed to Confucius and contained in the *I Ching*: 'Our main purpose in life should not be to hanker after a heaven in the sky, which probably does not exist, but to create a heaven on earth for each other by effecting complete harmony of the yin and yang forces around us and within us.' However, ancient China was not without its superstitions, and its emperors regarded themselves as demigods, and were wont to set their physicians and other learned men the difficult task of searching for herbs and other devices which they might use to achieve immortality. The physicians and alchemists concocted a wide range of strange elixirs, containing such ingredients as sulphur, mercury and scorpions; but, when administered, the consequences were often disastrous, and sometimes fatal. But it could be said that, in an odd sort of way, some of these emperors did realize their ambition, for they did not grow old! This quest for immortality was abandoned when it became evident that its objective could never be attained. But it had not been an entirely unfruitful exercise, for its researches had yielded a wide range of health foods and herbal medicines which improve the general health, increase virility and inhibit the ageing process, so extending the life span and producing more than a little peace of mind. And so, although the Chinese did not find the means of attaining a youthful immortality, nor was that likely, they did contrive the means to attain the next best thing, which is a long and healthy life of vigorous youthfulness. That there might be some special food or medicine, a sort of super-tonic, that would confer youthfulness and virility on its users is not a new concept, nor is it one that is confined to China. The gods and goddesses of Greek mythology were sustained by a special food, called *ambrosia*, and a special drink, called *nectar*. In medieval times, the alchemists sought an elixir which would confer eternal youth. The Aztecs, who lived in what we now call Mexico, considered cocoa to be good for the libido. And the ancient Romans were energetic worshippers of Ceres, their goddess of corn and harvests, showing that they saw a connection between food and fecundity. However, it is only the Chinese who have managed to transform some of this wishful thinking into near-reality. It is consoling to know that there is a kind of immortality which is due to the genetic process by which characteristics are passed on from one generation to the next. In that sense, though humanity is not immortal, it has existed for a very long time when compared with the life span of an individual person. See **ageing**, **youth** and **hereditary defects**.

immune system The system of the body which acts to prevent disease or malfunction. Actually, the body has more than one immune system, and it is their combined functions which provide what is loosely described as the immune system. Thus the natural oil on the skin both destroys micro-organisms and prevents their entry into the body. Leucocytes, or the white cells in the blood, and lymph, which originate in the bone marrow and have an amoeba-like appearance, provide protection against infection by destroying bacteria which enter the body. Some do this directly by engulfing the invaders, and some do it indirectly by forming antibodies, which are substances that neutralize foreign substances or make them inactive. The hydrochloric acid in the stomach destroys micro-organisms in the food that is consumed. Chinese physicians describe the immune system as the 'defence system', and it has been shown that some Chinese herbal medicines function effectively as boosters for the immune system. They include ginseng, *Panax ginseng*, wolfberry, *Lycium chinense*, astralagus, *Astralagus membranaceus*, and tienchi, *Panax pseudo-ginseng*. Chinese physicians would have the opinion that some of the measures taken by the environmental health inspectorates in the West impede rather than assist the immune system. Their view is that a little of what is bad for us may also be good for us providing there is not too much of it, which is the essential principle of immunization. Attempts to attain a state of complete cleanliness only serve to undermine the immune system and make the body too dependent on artificial aid. See **immunization** and **interferon**.

LEUCOCYTES

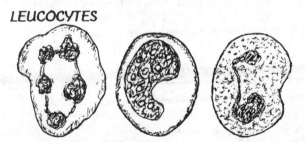

immunity The protection conferred on the body by its ability to resist infection. Where there is an infectious disease, the body produces antibodies, which help to counteract the disease. Some of these antibodies remain to provide protection against a further infection. This protection may last for many years. Thus, if a child contracts measles, the chances are that he will not have measles as an adult. His attack of measles as a child has given him immunity against further attacks, which is just as well, for measles in an adult is much more serious than it is in a child. See **immune system** and **immunization**.

immunization A medical technique used to make the body immune to a particular infection. With active immunization, the disease-causing organisms are administered by injection in a weakened or altered form so that they will not cause disease but will stimulate the development of anti-bodies, so producing an immunity which will last from several months to many years. With passive immunization, an antitoxin prepared from the disease-causing micro-organisms, but which may contain no living material, is administered. This offers immediate protection, but it lasts for only a short time. There is a third type of immunization, called acquired immunity, which the body creates for itself as the consequence of an infection, which is often picked up in childhood. See **immunity**, **immune system** and **immunology**.

immunology The scientific study of resistance to infection in man and animals. Edward Jenner (1749–1823), an English country doctor, is regarded as being the first person in the West to practise immunization. His technique is used as a treatment for smallpox, a potentially fatal disease affecting humans. For this, he used a vaccine prepared from vaccinia, or cowpox, a virus affecting cows, which is similar to smallpox but much milder in its effects, for he had noticed that milkmaids who had contracted cowpox were immune to smallpox. The vaccine is not introduced into the body by an injection, but by rubbing it into a scratch made on the arm or leg. This technique is called vaccination. The Chinese were using immunization methods similar to vaccination at the time of the Song dynasty (960–1279), long before Jenner, but these were later abandoned for a variety of reasons. By tradition, the Chinese have great respect for the human body, and so are not greatly in favour of techniques which might involve its mutilation, no matter how slight, and prefer to use those herbal remedies which boost the immune system. What is more, they contend that if a person is in a good state of health, which can be achieved by diet, exercise and tonics to strengthen the vital organs, he should be able to throw off most infections, but if he does happen to fall victim to an infection, the acquired immunity is likely to be more effective than that obtained by unnatural means. This is an attitude with which Western physicians would not entirely agree, but the stark reality remains that the Chinese are very healthy and live to a great age. Perhaps the simple truth is that the Chinese have less need of immunization techniques than the people of the West because they are healthier. See **immune system**, **immunity**, **immunization** and **Jesuits**.

impaired digestion Providing there is no serious underlying cause, white rice porridge and taro starch jelly are excellent treatments for an impaired digestion, particularly with invalids and elderly people. See **indigestion**.

impetigo A common and highly contagious skin disease in children which is caused by staphylococcus bacteria. It is characterized by red spots with yellow crusts, which mainly affect the face, hands and knees, though other parts of the skin are vulnerable. Medical advice should be sought because of the risk of spreading the infection. Underwear and bedclothes should be sterilized, separate face cloths and towels should be used, and the hands should be frequently washed and then rinsed in alcohol or an antiseptic fluid. In the West, it is usual for antibiotics in tablet or ointment form to be prescribed. Chinese physicians would recommend garlic, *Allium sativum*, which is a natural antibiotic, to be taken internally in a dosage of 3 or 4 cloves, fresh and finely chopped. They are not unappetizing if eaten in a salad. An infusion or decoction of one of the following should be applied to the affected area twice daily, using the parts and dosage indicated: thyme, *Thymus vulgare*, leaves, 4–12 g; marigold, *Calendula officinalis*, flowers, 3–12 g; camomile, *Matricaria chamomilla*, leaves and flowers, 3–6 g. A poor diet may be a contributory factor to this condition, and so a wholesome diet with plenty of fresh fruit and vegetables, but no sugar and fats, would be helpful.

impotence Erectile insufficiency. In men, this is the inability to achieve and sustain an erection. In both men and women, sexual arousal leads to an increase in the flow of blood to the genital region. In a man, the spongy erectile tissue in the penis fills with blood, and so the penis becomes erect. Sexual arousal involves the nervous system, the hormone balance and an erotically centred state of mind, but an erection cannot be achieved where there are adverse physical, chemical, neurological and psychological influences, which can be due to age, fatigue, alcohol, tobacco, inadequate diet, stress, anxiety, antihistamines, tranquillizers and other drugs, social concerns and moral and religious considerations, such as repression and feelings of guilt. There are so many factors involved that a man can be both proud and apprehensive of his prowess with his penis, and such a mixed state of mind can inhibit his ability to achieve an erection. In TCM, impotence in young men is regarded as being due to weakness of the liver and kidneys. Anxiety or stress cause liver-*qi* stagnation, which, in turn, weakens the kidneys. Chinese herbal remedies include infusions or decoctions of the following, taken internally, using the parts and dosages indicated: Asiatic ginseng, *Panax ginseng*, roots, 2–8 g; blackberry, *Rubus coreanus*, unripe berries, 6–10 g; eucommia, *Eucommia ulmoides*, bark, 9–14 g; horny goat weed, *Epimedium sagittatum*, leaves, 8–12 g; broomrape, *Cistanche salsa*, stems, 8–14 g. Sexual potency tends to decrease with age, but this can be offset by sound diet, adequate exercise and avoidance of stress, which helps to maintain a state of health and youthfulness. As one becomes older, it is important to relax, so that the nervous system will allow more blood to enter the penis. It is also important not to expect too much, for one cannot get an erection or regain it as quickly at the age of 50 or 60 as one did in one's youth. In the West, where some people adopt a curious moral stance in matters of sex, an elderly man who has erections and sexual inclinations may be referred to, somewhat offensively, as a 'dirty old man'. In China, he would be regarded as a healthy old man, and a fortunate one at that. See **libido**.

inbreeding Mating between people who are closely related. Inbreeding has been practised in the past as a form of selective breeding, but often with disastrous results. In Europe, it was once the common practice for members of the various royal families to intermarry. This was done to preserve the royal status and the purity of the royal blood, though, in fact, inherited characteristics, whether desirable or otherwise, are not passed on by the blood, but by the chromosomes in the germ plasm of the reproductive cells. The offspring which result from inbreeding often have undesirable characteristics, such as colour-blindness and deaf-mutism. The members of the European royal families are usually cousins, and so it is hardly surprising that there has been a high incidence of haemophilia and imbecility among the royalty of Europe. This situation has changed somewhat in recent years, for those of royal birth now tend to marry commoners. No doubt, the stories we read and hear about village idiots have a basis in fact because, years ago, when villages were smaller and people travelled very little, marriages between persons who were related – cousins and second cousins – occurred quite commonly. It is quite understandable that incest, which is a sexual relationship between two members of the same family – brother and sister, father and daughter, mother and son, etc. – which was practised by the Pharoahs of ancient Egypt, is regarded as a highly immoral act, and it is strictly forbidden by law in most countries. The Chinese have never had any illusions in this regard, and they have always tried to prevent inbreeding and other marital problems by a system of arranged marriages. It was generally the case in ancient China that an emperor had many concubines, but the one who was to bear him a son to be the heir to the Dragon Throne was likely to be chosen more for her sound state of health than for her desirability in other directions, and one can be sure that most of his concubines were of lowly birth. The Chinese view here is that a healthy family line without any undesirable traits not only helps to secure the smooth continuity of the Chinese race but also helps to ensure the peace of mind and sense of purpose of each of the individuals who make up the race. In matters of this kind, the Chinese display a remarkable insight. See **genetics, eugenics, hereditary defects** and **ancestor worship**.

incest See **inbreeding**.

incompatible Those drugs, including herbal medicines, which cannot be administered together or with certain foods because of the possibility of adverse reactions are said to be incompatible. For example, ginseng is incompatible with alcohol, coffee and turnips: and clematis, *Clematis chinensis*, is incompatible with tea.

incontinence A person's inability to control his bowel and bladder functions. This condition has a variety of causes, including stress, and it is advisable to consult a physician. A common cause of faecal incontinence is constipation, which strains the bowel muscles so much that they become slack, and so are unable to control the bowel movements. Urinary incontinence in children is generally due to emotional insecurity. In women, it may be due to a prolapse, or organ displacement, resulting from childbirth. In men, problems with the prostate gland may be the cause. It can also be caused by a stroke which inhibits the operation of the part of the nervous system which controls the bladder. According to TCM, the cause is kidney-yang deficiency coupled with internal coldness, and the treatments recommended are similar to those for enuresis, or bed-wetting, in children. In the West, sufferers are advised to avoid high-liquid diets and foods which have diuretic properties, such as grapes, coffee and alcohol. They are also advised to strengthen the muscles in the bowel by holding back on a bowel movement for a short time, and those in the bladder by double voiding, which means to urinate and then, after a short lapse of time, to attempt to urinate again. One might think that such practices would exacerbate these conditions rather than alleviate or cure them. The TCM treatment for urinary incontinence is an infusion, taken internally, of blackberry, *Rubus coreanus*, unripe berries, 5–10 g, or agrimony, *Agrimony pilosa*, leaves and stems, 12–28 g. For faecal incontinence, it is an infusion, taken internally, of marigold, *Calendula officinalis*, flowers, 3–12 g, or meadowsweet, *Filipendula ulmaria*, leaves and flowers, 3–8 g. A traditional and homely Chinese remedy for urinary incontinence is a pig's bladder steamed with dried hops and consumed as an ordinary item of diet. See **enuresis**.

incubation period The time between a patient being infected and the appearance of the first symptoms. Thus, the incubation period for measles is 10–14 days.

Indian bread *Poria cocos* In the United States, it is also called tuckahoe or Virginia truffle. Herbal medicine. Distribution: global. Parts: entire body. Character: neutral, sweet. Affinity: heart, lungs, stomach, spleen, kidneys. Effects: stomachic, digestive, diuretic, sedative. Symptoms: lack of appetite, excess phlegm, abdominal distension, diarrhoea, difficult or painful urination, irritability, sleeplessness. Treatments: coughs, debility, palpitations. Dosage: 4–9 g.

Indian corn See **maize**.

indication See **symptom**.

indigenous Native. A plant or animal which belongs naturally to a certain region is said to be indigenous, or native, to that region. As a consequence of the activities of man, many plants and animals have been transferred to regions where they are not indigenous; but, where the climatic and other conditions are suitable, they have thrived. For example, rabbits are not indigenous to Australia, but since they have been introduced there, they have multiplied very rapidly and become a positive menace, consuming much of the vegetation which the farmers require for grazing sheep. Cultivated non-indigenous plants sometimes 'escape' from gardens and parks, and then grow successfully in the wild. This is the case with the wolfberry, *Lycium chinense*, which is indigenous to China and Japan, but which, since its introduction into some of the countries in the West, where it now grows wild in the hedgerows, is regarded as a troublesome weed. It has been found that many of the medicinal herbs that are indigenous to Japan and the temperate regions of China can be cultivated quite successfully in the West. No doubt, with the present interest and increasing dependence on herbal medicines, the cultivation of non-indigenous herbs in suitable regions throughout the world will become big business. See **herbal trade**.

indigestion Dyspepsia. It is characterized by discomfort, and sometimes pain, in the upper abdomen and chest, and occasionally accompanied by heartburn or flatulence, and followed by nausea, a headache, a coated tongue, loss of appetite, depression and clouded urine. Indigestion has a variety of causes, which include eating too much or too quickly, smoking, drinking too much alcohol, consuming rich and fatty foods and drinks containing caffeine, such as tea and coffee, nervous tension and taking drugs which irritate or inflame the stomach, such as aspirin. The symptoms of indigestion are also associated with hernia, obesity, ulcers and gallstones. Indigestion can be caused by stomach cancer, though this is extremely rare in young people. But if indigestion becomes chronic in a person over 40 years of age, medical advice should be sought. Indigestion can generally be prevented by regular exercise and small meals containing moderate amounts of spicy and fatty ingredients and no synthetic additives, chewing food thoroughly, and avoiding stress, tobacco, alcohol, coffee, tea, aspirin and postprandial physical exercise. It is also important to get enough sleep. In the West, physicians generally prescribe an antacid to neutralize the excess acid in the stomach. See **acidity**. But indigestion is not always caused by acidity. In fact, it is sometimes due to a deficiency of stomach acid, for the stomach enzymes will not function effectively without an acid medium. This no doubt explains why the Chinese include sweet-and-sour dishes in their meals. These dishes contain vinegar, which is an organic acid. Chinese physicians recommend acupuncture, acupressure and *qi gong* exercises to prevent or relieve nervous tension, and massage of the stomach to assist the muscular movements involved in the digestive process. They also recommend that the diet should include haws, which are hawthorn fruits, and wheat and bean sprouts to absorb acids and grease and provide dietary fibre. For an impaired digestion, as sometimes occurs with invalids and elderly people, there is much to be said for white rice porridge and taro starch jelly, both of which, being foods, are gentler and more natural in their action than many of the remedies available. Chewing the pith from a mandarin orange is a traditional Chinese remedy. If the cause of the indigestion is stress, a sedative, such as camomile or nut grass, could be administered. See **sedative**. If there is flatulence, a carminative, such as parsley, cinnamon or ginger, could be administered. See **flatulence**. Other treatments include infusions of the following, taken internally, using the parts and dosages indicated: marigold, *Calendula officinalis*, flowers, 4–12 g; Indian bread, *Poria cocos*, entire plant, 4–9 g; meadowsweet, *Filipendula ulmaria*, leaves and flowers, 3–8 g; comfrey, *Symphytum officinale*, roots or leaves, 3–10 g; yarrow, *Achillea millefolium*, flowers, 3–10 g; gentian, *Gentiana scabra*, roots, 4–7 g. Gentian must be administered before a meal, NOT after. Also, it must NOT be administered to pregnant women. See **Chinese gentian** and **heartburn**.

industrial dermatitis Detergent eczema. See **eczema**.

industrial disease See **occupational disease**.

infantile paralysis See **poliomyelitis**.

infection A condition within the body due to its being penetrated by harmful micro-organisms. They can enter the body via the skin, lungs, digestive tract and genital orifices, which are those parts of the body where there are 'openings' to the exterior. Micro-organisms can enter the skin more easily where there are stings, scratches and other wounds. Food poisoning is caused by those which enter the digestive tract. Those which cause venereal diseases enter the body via the genital orifices, but other routes are possible. There are those who say, 'You can't get it by kissing.' But they are quite mistaken. The physicians of ancient China were not aware of the existence of micro-organisms as such, but they were of the opinion that food, water and the atmosphere contain energies and climatic influences, both beneficial and harmful, which can enter the body by the routes mentioned above. Considering that they had no microscopes or other means of knowing of the existence of micro-organisms, their understanding of the situation was remarkably accurate. See **infectious diseases**.

infectious diseases Diseases have a variety of causes, but those that are due to pathogens, which are micro-organisms – viruses, bacteria, fungi and protozoa – that produce toxins or do damage in other ways, are said to be infectious. Pathogens are transmitted to the body by water, food, water droplets in the atmosphere, the skin and animals, such as rats and fleas, which are called vectors. Those infectious diseases which can only be spread by direct contact, are said to be contagious. Thus, influenza and the common cold are infectious but not contagious, whereas impetigo and scarlet fever are both infectious and contagious. The spread of infectious diseases is prevented by clean water supplies, fresh food, adequate disposal of sewage, the destruction of vectors, vaccination, immunization, food hygiene and personal hygiene. See **contagious disease**, **food hygiene** and **personal hygiene**.

infectious hepatitis Hepatitis A. See **hepatitis**.

infectious mononucleosis Glandular fever. A virus infection, mainly affecting adolescents, whose symptoms are a sore throat, rashes and enlargement of the lymph glands. Jaundice may occur, but it is rare. Treatment is always slow, requiring a long period of convalescence and diet and medication to improve the general health. In TCM, the treatment is an infusion or decoction of one of the following, taken internally, using the parts and dosages indicated: Japanese honeysuckle, *Locinera japonica*, flowers, 10–16 g; golden bell, *Forsythia suspensa*, fruits, 4–10 g; gulf seaweed, *Sargassum fusiforme*, entire plant, 6–10 g.

inferiority complex An idea or belief derived from forgotten or repressed experiences from the past by which a person is convinced, but without good cause, that he is inferior socially, in health, achievement or some other respect. An inferiority complex, as with most complexes, generally develops during the formative years, when the mind is very receptive and very much open to suggestion. The obvious treatment would seem to be to eradicate the deeply rooted belief which has given rise to the condition. This is best done by a psychiatrist so that errors due to subjective thinking can be avoided. Chinese physicians might recommend acupuncture or meditative exercises, which contain elements of self-hypnosis. One suspects that, in Britain, an inferiority complex related to social affairs is sometimes one of the unfortunate by-products of a class-structured society. One may also suspect that many of those people who are said to have an inferiority complex and be lacking in self-esteem are really just timid, self-effacing, courteous, kindly and over-sentient beings who wish to steer clear of aggressiveness, acquisitiveness, bombast, insincerity and impropriety. But so many illnesses and so much unhappiness can be attributed to stress and anxiety that it is imperative that those who do quite genuinely have an inferiority complex should receive effective treatment. The Chinese probably have few problems in this regard, for Chinese society has always been essentially egalitarian. In ancient times, apart from the emperor and a few feudal lords, the ruling class of China was made up of mandarins – officials selected on their merits by a civil service examination – and not hereditary aristocrats. Confucius taught that a rich man should not boast of his wealth, and a poor man should not complain about his poverty, so the Chinese do not use wealth as the measuring rod of success. Taoism teaches that health, longevity and peace of mind are the keys to happiness and self-fulfilment. Such a philosophy effectively obviates the possibility of the development of a wide range of anxieties, frustrations and complexes.

infertility The inability of a woman to conceive or a man to father a child. This condition is quite common in the West, where it affects about one in ten couples. It has a variety of causes, which include illness, alcohol, smoking, drug-taking, stress and anxiety, particularly that which arises from trying to have a baby. In women, the condition may be due to age, dysfunction of the ovaries, inflammation of the fallopian tubes, or taking too much strenuous exercise. In men, it may be due to impotence, a low sperm count or premature ejaculation. Conception is more likely to occur if both partners take care of their general health, have a balanced and wholesome diet, take a fair amount of exercise and do not miss out on sleep, rest and relaxation. In addition, the woman should try to put on some weight because the fat in the body produces and stores the hormone which is involved in pregnancy. But it is as well to bear in mind that it is quite natural for some women to take longer than others to conceive. The human egg survives for about 36 hours, and the sperm for two to three days, and so the best time to have sexual intercourse to achieve pregnancy is about 12–24 hours before ovulation, though this cannot always be easily estimated. It is also advisable to use the man-on-top, or missionary, position, and the woman should remain in that position for 15–20 minutes after her partner has ejaculated, which allows the sperm to drain into the place where it is required. In TCM, there are a number of herbal remedies for impotence. See **impotence** and **aphrodisiac**. The Chinese set great store by Asiatic ginseng and rhinoceros horn as aphrodisiacs, but Western physicians have doubts about the efficacy of the latter. Certain foods are reputed to have aphrodisiac qualities. They include oats, almonds, cress, fennel, celery, bananas, nutmeg, chilli, ginger, cardamom, fish oils and oysters. TCM also has a number of herbal remedies for premature ejaculation. See **premature ejaculation**. A couple may become anxious in their desperation to have a baby, and they may also worry about the things that could go wrong during pregnancy, and so, perhaps, they should not rely too much on DIY treatments or listen to old wives' tales, but should consult a physician. See **miscarriage** and **uterine disorders**.

inflammation A condition in which the skin or a membrane becomes swollen, red, warm, painful and reduced in function. It is a defensive reaction to infection or injury, causing blood vessels to release leucocytes and other protective substances which will combat bacteria and other foreign bodies. Diseases whose names have the suffix '-itis', such as dermatitis, laryngitis, gastritis and nephritis, will have an inflamed condition.

influenza Grippe. Influenza, or flu, as it is termed colloquially, is a viral infection, which often occurs as an epidemic, and whose symptoms are cold sensations, sweating, headaches, aching muscles, weakness, coughs, loss of appetite and pain behind the sternum. The symptoms last for about a week and are usually followed by depression. There is more than one strain of the influenza virus, which makes it difficult to treat. Influenza is often confused with a common cold, which is a great error, for influenza is a much more serious condition, and there can be complications if it is not properly treated. According to TCM, influenza falls into three categories which are attributed to climatic conditions of excess: wind-cold, wind-heat and damp. It is important that the patient should rest, take plenty of drinks to 'flush out' the toxins and replace the water lost by sweating, and not be in too much of a hurry to get back to work, for that only spreads the infection. The Chinese consider moxibustion to be

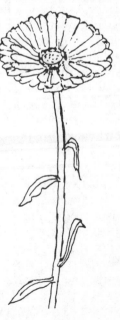

MARIGOLD

Calendula officinalis

an excellent treatment. Also helpful as alleviatives are infusions of the following, taken internally, using the parts and dosages indicated: dandelion, *Taraxacum officinale*, all parts, 10–30 g; marigold, *Calendula officinalis*, flowers, 3–12 g; garlic, Allium *sativum*, 3 cloves; onion, *Allium cepa*, bulb, 20–40 g; cardamom, *Elettaria cardamom*, crushed seeds, 2–6 g; corn mint, *Mentha arvensis*, leaves, 2–4 g; cinnamon, *Cinnamomum cassia*, bark, 2–5 g; yarrow, *Achillea millefolium*, leaves, 2–4 g; sorrel, *Rumex acetosa*, leaves, 3–5 g; chrysanthemum, *Chrysanthemum morifolium*, flowers, 4–9 g; Japanese honeysuckle, *Lonicera japonica*, flowers, 10–15 g. A pinch of cayenne pepper (*Capsicum frutescens*) added to the infusion of corn mint is considered to be very helpful. Japanese honeysuckle will not be readily available in the West, but a European species, *Lonicera periclymenum*, also called the woodbine in Britain, has similar medicinal properties. During recent years, in the West, the marigold has become quite popular as a treatment for influenza.

infusion This is the simplest of the preparations used in TCM, requiring only that boiling water be poured on to the prescribed dosage of the dried herb, and allowing it to stand for 15–20 minutes. While steeping, it should be covered to prevent the loss of volatile oils by evaporation. The resulting liquid is strained to remove the debris. The amount of water used is decided by convenience, but it must not be so small that it fails to extract all the active ingredients from the herb, or so large that there is more liquid than can be consumed in one day. In TCM, a dosage of a medicine to be taken internally is generally expressed as the weight of the dried herb to be taken in one day, either as an infusion or a decoction. But, if the fresh herb is used, the weight must be doubled. Thus, 10 g fresh dandelion leaves in ½ litre water is equivalent to 5 g dried dandelion leaves in ½ litre water; and the whole ½ litre must be consumed in one day. A supply of an infusion can be prepared in advance, but it must be sealed and stored in a refrigerator so that it will keep fresh. In this instance, a supply for five days would require 25 g dried dandelion leaves and 2½ litres water. Dried herbs are used in medicine because, unlike fresh herbs, they can be stored for long periods and, as their fibres are brittle and easily broken when crushed, their ingredients dissolve more readily in water. The medicinal properties of some herbs are destroyed by hot water, and so, in these cases, the infusions are made with cold water. Herbal infusions are also called herbal teas. But a tea must not be confused with a ptisan, or tisane, which is a milder infusion prepared in the same way as a tea but drunk immediately and not stood to steep. See **dosages**.

ingestion The intake of food. With all animals except the simplest, this is done through the mouth. It must not be confused with digestion, which is the process by which food undergoes chemical decomposition. For example, the cellulose in green vegetables is ingested but it is not digested, at least not in the alimentary canal of a human.

ingrowing toe-nails A condition in which the cut end of a toe-nail grows into the surrounding flesh, and which is caused by badly-fitting shoes, accidents or cutting the nails too short and with a sharp edge. The treatment is to avoid wearing tight socks and tight or pointed shoes, apply an antiseptic to prevent infection, and wear sandals until the condition has been cured. Jagged edges of the nails should be smoothed with a file. If the condition persists, professional medical treatment will need to be obtained. There must have been a high incidence of ingrowing toe-nails in China prior to 1912, when China became a republic, for it was the established practice in imperial China for young girls to have their feet tightly bound so that their feet would be of a delicate appearance and they would be compelled to walk gingerly to create an impression of daintiness and poise. These tightly bound feet were considered to be one of the hallmarks of feminine beauty, but it was a painful procedure which produced deformities.

inhalation See **breathing**.

inherited defect See **hereditary defects**.

inherited disease See **hereditary defects**.

inner-cold See **cold**.

inner-dampness Internal dampness. See **dampness**.

inner-dryness Internal dryness. See **dryness**.

inner-fire See **fire**.

inner-wind See **wind**.

inoculation The injection, with a hypodermic needle, of infective substances into the body as a means of immunization. See **immunization**.

insect bite See **bites**.

insecticide See **chemicals**.

insect sting See **stings**.

insecurity See **nervous disorders**.

insight A term used in psychiatry to indicate the extent to which a mentally ill person is aware of his own condition. One of the main differences between psychosis, which is mental illness, and neurosis, which is nervous illness, is that the psychopath often has no insight about his condition, whereas the neuropath is acutely aware of his. The man who thinks that he is Emperor Napoleon, or the woman who claims that she has a personal relationship with God, is not likely to be convinced that matters could be otherwise, though a psychopath sometimes has periods of lucidity, when, faced by the reality of the situation, he is greatly distressed. But the person undergoing a nervous breakdown will have both physical and mental symptoms, of which he will be totally aware, causing depression and distress, and his frustrating attempts at self-analysis may exacerbate his condition, so making it even more difficult to treat. See **mental illness** and **nervous disorders**.

insipid See **taste**.

insomnia Chronic sleeplessness. Everyone suffers from mild bouts of sleeplessness at some time or other, and for one or more of a wide variety of reasons, which include lack of exercise, noise, pain, drugs and coffee and other drinks containing stimulants, anxiety, shock, depression, overtiredness, coldness, unfamiliar surroundings, smoking, alcohol, jet lag, changing shifts at work, a heavy or sugary meal before retiring, and other interferences with the circadian rhythm and the biorhythms, or 'body clocks', which regulate the internal functions of the body. Biorhythms are not a concept which is confined to Western medical science, for the Taoist physicians of ancient China were aware of their existence, and they had divided the day into twelve two-hour periods, for they had discovered that some healing exercises were most effective when performed at certain times of the day. See **circadian rhythm** and **zodiac exercises**. Age plays a part in a person's sleeping habits. Young people generally need more sleep than elderly people, for they are more active, and so take more out of themselves. One can often relieve sleeplessness by trying to relax and taking plenty of exercise in the fresh air during the day, and by taking a warm, but not hot, bath, consuming a light meal and a warm drink and allowing oneself time to unwind before retiring. It also helps if the bedroom is quiet, dark and well ventilated and the bed is warm and comfortable. One should try to get into the habit of retiring at a regular time. However, there is no point in tossing and turning in bed if one cannot sleep. One should read or perform some other activity until one is naturally tired. But, once in bed, one should concentrate one's mind on pleasant things, and fantasize a little as a way of escape from troublesome thoughts if anxiety is the cause of the sleeplessness. Sexual activity will also promote sleep, but more so in men than in women, for women often remain in an excited state for several hours after intercourse. Sleeping tablets, which are usually benzodiazepines or barbiturates, are not to be recommended, for they cause drowsiness and lack of concentration on the following day, and one feels just as wide awake on the following evening. They are also habit forming. When sleeplessness becomes a chronic condition, it is called insomnia. Its causes include persistent stress and anxiety, defective diet, menstrual or menopausal difficulties and diseases of the internal organs. There may be underlying causes which are difficult to detect, and so the sufferer should seek professional medical advice. In TCM, there is a wide range of tonics, sedatives and soporifics which may be used to treat insomnia. They include infusions or decoctions of the following, taken internally, using the parts and dosages indicated. A medication which suits one person may not suit another, and so each should be tried out, in turn, to find out which is the most suitable for one's needs. Garlic, *Allium sativum*, 3 cloves; ramsons (wild garlic), *Allium ursinium*, fresh leaves, 8 g; valerian, *Valerian officinalis*, root, 5–6 g; cowslip, *Primula officinalis*, flowers, 1–5 g; meadowsweet, *Filipendula ulmaria*, flowers, 3–4 g; camomile, *Matricaria chamomilla*, roots, 3–5 g; hawthorn, *Crataegus monogyna*, fresh leaves and flowers, 6–8 g; deadnettle, *Lamium album*, all parts, 3–4 g; wheat, *Tricitum aestivus*, crushed grains, 15–30 g; sweet flag, *Acorus calamus*, leaves, 3–7 g; hop, *Humulus lupulus*, strobiles (cone-like flowers), 1.5–3 g; basil, *Ocimum basilicum*, leaves, 2–4 g; onion, *Allium cepa*, bulb, 20–40 g; Asiatic ginseng, *Panax ginseng*, roots, 2–8 g; *dang shen*, *Codonopsis tangshen*, roots, 8–14 g; angelica, *Angelica sinensis*, roots, 8–14 g; *dan shen*, *Salvia miltiorrhiza*, roots, 5–6 g; *tienchi*, *Panax pseudo-ginseng*, roots, 2–4 g. A suspension of 6–10 g powdered shells of the oyster, *Ostrea rivulalis*, is effective as a sedative. A traditional and homely Chinese remedy is an infusion of equal quantities, say 5 g, of the fresh roots of liquorice, *Glycyrrhiza uralensis*, and pre-cooked seeds of the lotus, *Nelumbo nucifera*. Another such remedy is the water in which a lettuce has been boiled, sweetened with honey. It is also the practice in China to alleviate insomnia by sleeping with one's head on a pillow stuffed with hops, gypsum (calcium sulphate), black tea leaves and angelica leaves. For insomnia due to depression and emotional disturbances, Chinese physicians would recommend acupuncture or a suitable healing exercise. The latter is simple enough. Before retiring, take a leisurely walk or perform one set of the *tai chi chuan* exercises, self-massage the body all over, and then massage the acupoint *yung chuan*, which is in the middle of the sole of the foot. They might also recommend meditation, which has a component of self-hypnosis. See **sleep disorders** and **medication**.

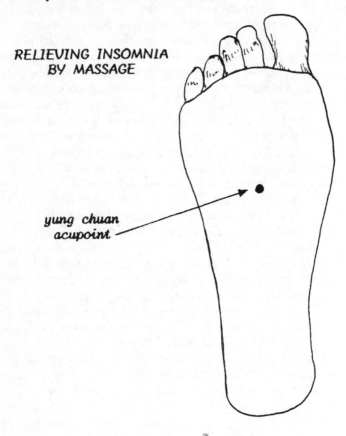

RELIEVING INSOMNIA
BY MASSAGE

*yung chuan
acupoint*

inspiration See **breathing**.

insulin A hormone produced by the pancreas, and without which the body cannot store or oxidize sugar effectively, and so the tissues are deprived of energy, and sugar accumulates in the blood. See **diabetes mellitus**.

interferon Also called interleukin. A dictionary defines this as a protein produced within the body and which inhibits the development of disease-causing micro-organisms in the blood and body tissues. Its recent discovery by the medical scientists of the West confirms the view, long held by Chinese physicians, that the body is largely self-regulating and self-healing and provides its own immunity to disease. See **immune system**. For its main defence against infection, the body relies upon lymphocytes and antibodies. The former are types of leucocytes, or white blood cells, and the latter are substances which attach themselves to invading micro-organisms or their toxins and neutralize them. Lymphocytes occur in great concentration in the thymus gland and pancreas. The dead micro-organisms and their toxins are then engulfed by macrophages, which are similar to leucocytes but larger. This process is considerably assisted by T-lymphocytes, some of which, called cytoxic T-lymphocytes, destroy micro-organisms directly, while the others produce interferon, which stimulates the B-lymphocytes to make and release more antibodies. The body fluid and remains of dead micro-organisms and leucocytes which accumulate at areas of infection is called pus. Lymphocytes occur not only in the blood but also in lymph and connective tissue. There is some correspondence between the four humours of TCM and the behaviour and various sources of lymphocytes and interferon. *Xue*, or blood, contains lymphocytes; *jing ye*, or fluid, is the

DESTROYING THE INVADERS OF THE BODY

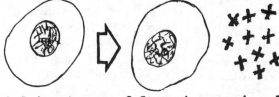

1 A B–lymphocyte detects invading bacteria.

2 It produces and releases antibodies.

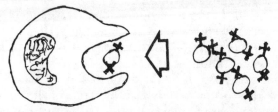

4 A macrophage engulfs the marked bacteria.

3 The antibodies lock on to and mark the invading bacteria.

lymph, or sticky fluid which occurs in connective tissue; *jing*, or vital essence, which contains interferon, is the sum total of the effects of the hormones which prevent disease and retard the ageing process; and *qi* regulates and nourishes the other humours. Modern research has shown that men with dense semen and a high sperm-count, which are encouraged by a high level of sex hormone, are immune to many diseases and highly resistant to others. This is a fact which has been known to Chinese physicians for thousands of years. The physicians of ancient China had no knowledge of interferon as such, but they did know that the immune system is dependent upon blood, fluid, vital essence and connective tissue, which are the sources of interferon. They also realized that these humours need to be fortified by food and preventive therapy. This explains why chicken's feet, pig's feet and eels feature prominently in the Chinese diet. They are rich in connective tissue and *jing ye*. The scales of the pangolin, or scaly ant-eater, which are used as a medicine to improve circulation, promote the development of those lymphocytes which produce interferon. See **leucocyte**.

interleukin See **interferon**.

intermittent claudication Severe pain in the calves when walking, and due to narrow arteries in the leg restricting the supply of blood to the muscles. The pain is only a symptom of a more serious underlying condition, and a physician should be consulted. As with most circulatory ailments, this condition is more easily prevented than cured. Prevention requires a Chinese-style diet, that is, one which is balanced and varied and high in vegetables, fruit, cereals and fish, and low in red meat, animal fats and sugar. It also requires regular exercise of a strenuous kind, such as walking, cycling and one of the martial arts. But, of course, once this condition has become established, one should not take strenuous exercise unless advised to do so by one's physician. In TCM, a recommended treatment is an infusion, taken internally and regularly over a long period, of 6–14 g fruits of the hawthorn, *Crataegus pinnatifida*. It is helpful to be a non-smoker. See **smoking**.

internal A term use in TCM diagnosis to indicate the location, extent and direction of a disease. It is one of the eight principles of *ba gang*, or differential diagnosis. If a disease moves towards the inside of the body and the bones and vital organs, the symptoms become internal, which indicates that the condition is worsening. Internal symptoms and ailments are regarded as being yin, but they must be considered together with yin tonics, which nourish the kidneys, liver, lungs and stomach, and yang tonics, which nourish the heart, spleen and blood. The other principles of diagnosis must also be considered. See **ba gang**.

Internal Book of Huang Di See **Huang Di Nei Jing**.

internal exercises The Taoists of ancient China devised a system of internal exercises which would benefit the vital organs, and which, as a self-healing system, would encourage the body to adhere closely to its natural arrangement, and thereby produce a sound state of health. These exercises promote freedom from pain, disease and stress, and so create a state of general well-being coupled with a positive attitude towards ageing. By strengthening the vital organs with these exercises, the body develops a condition of harmony, and so is able to cope with adverse external influences, and the mind is more able to control the emotions by means of its vitality and alertness. These exercises, which fall into many categories, must be performed daily and regularly if they are to take full effect. Many of them are contained in the *Chinese Exercise Manual*. These exercises balance the complementary and antagonistic forces within the body, which are a miniature reflection of those contained throughout the universe. These relationships are explained by the theory of the five elements. See **five elements, element, movement** and **revitalization**.

internal-external symptoms See **diagnostic combinations**.

internal illness See **internal**.

internal symptoms and treatments The internal symptoms of illness are not quite so obvious as the external symptoms, and they fall into four categories: internal-full, internal-empty, internal-hot and internal-cold. Each of these categories has its set of symptoms. Generally, the treatments involve administering tonic medicines to strengthen the vital organs, bones and connective tissue. See **internal, ba gang** and **diagnostic combinations**.

internal therapy This is not so straightforward as external therapy, for the physician is often dealing with a condition which is worsening and whose symptoms are less manifest. The medications used will include emetics, carthartics and heat-clearers to remove toxins, reduce heat excess and eliminate waste from the vital organs. Tonics, both yin and yang, are also used. See **internal** and **external therapy**.

intervertebral discs Thick pads of fibrous cartilage between the vertebrae, which are the 33 small bones of the vertebral column, which is known commonly as the backbone or the spine. The spinal cord, which consists of nerve tissue, runs down the middle of these vertebrae, and is thereby enclosed and protected by them. The discs, which absorb shocks, are attached to each other by ligaments, and so the vertebral column is strong and flexible, holding the body erect but also allowing movement. A prolapsed, or 'slipped' disc, is one that has been partly damaged or moved out of position by a strain on the vertebral column. This condition is most common among elderly people. If the disc presses against the nerves in the spinal cord, there is pain and disablement. In the West, the orthodox treatment is to bed-rest to take pressure off the disc and so allow natural healing to occur, which generally takes about six weeks. Manipulative treatment by osteopaths or chiropractors is sometimes effective. Chinese physicians would recommend acupuncture, in which the meridians of the kidneys, spleen, gall-bladder and small and large intestines are 'needled' to reduce pain. They would probably also point out that, as a 'slipped disc' is a rare occurrence among young persons,

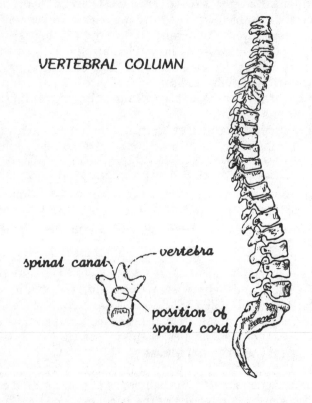

VERTEBRAL COLUMN

spinal canal — vertebra

position of spinal cord

elderly people should keep themselves physically youthful by regular exercise in order to prevent this condition. See **skeleton**.

intestinal worms See **parasite** and **anthelmintic**.

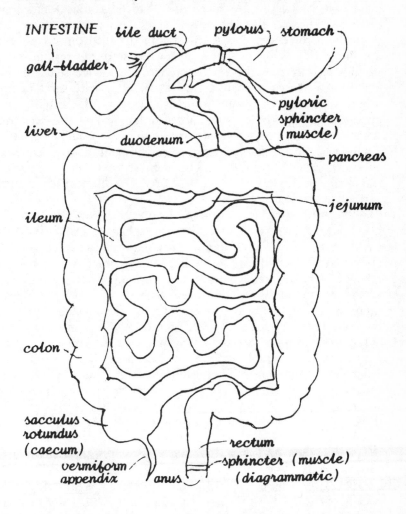

INTESTINE   bile duct   pylorus   stomach
gall-bladder
liver
duodenum
pyloric sphincter (muscle)
pancreas
jejunum
ileum
colon
sacculus rotundus (caecum)
vermiform appendix   anus
rectum
sphincter (muscle) (diagrammatic)

intestine The part of the alimentary canal, or digestive tract, between the lower, or pyloric, region of the stomach and the anus. It has two main parts, which are the small intestine, consisting of the duodenum, jejunum and ileum, and the large intestine, consisting of the colon, vermiform appendix and rectum. The duodenum, which is the first part of the small intestine, completes the process of digestion which began in the mouth and stomach. The ileum assimilates the products of digestion. The small intestine has a total length of about 8 metres. In the colon, moisture is absorbed from faecal material prior to its evacuation by the rectum, which has muscles for that purpose. The sacculus rotundus, which is the point where the ileum joins the colon, has a protuberance, called the vermiform appendix, that is vestigial and serves no useful purpose in man, though it is one of the many pieces of evidence that, in the evolutionary process, man shares his ancestry with some of the other mammals. In some animals, such as the rabbit, the appendix would be a much larger organ, called the caecum, where cellulose undergoes decomposition, and so can be partially assimilated. An inflamed or diseased appendix produces the condition called appendicitis. The ileum and the colon are two of the *liu fu*, or 'hollow organs', of TCM. See **alimentary canal** and **appendicitis**.

intolerance An adverse reaction by the body, and which may have psychological effects, to a food or some other substance. It is not a true allergy, in which histamines are released, nor is it the same condition as sensitivity, in which the degree of the body's reaction is determined by the amount of food or other substance, though these conditions are often closely allied. In the West, there is much confusion in the use of these terms because the differences between these conditions, as indicated by symptoms, are not always strikingly apparent. Thus, the body may react unfavourably to substance A under all conditions and whatever the amount. This is intolerance. But it may react unfavourably to substance B only under certain conditions or when it is present in a large amount. That is, the reaction is directly proportional to the amount of substance. This is sensitivity. Chinese physicians do not have any problems in this regard, for their understanding and approach in these matters is fundamentally different. See **allergy** and **hypersensitivity**.

introvert A term used in psychology to describe a person who is socially restrained, timid and retiring, and who tends to turn inwards in his thinking and interests. The Chinese would say that he has a yin personality. See **yin** and **nervous disorders**.

invalid diet In China, as in other parts of the world, cooks and physicians arrange an invalid's diet in a way which best suits his needs – cooling foods for hot illnesses, warming foods for cold illnesses, non-irritating foods for stomach upsets, the avoidance of items of diet which may cause allergies, and so on. But, in any case, the normal Chinese diet is so varied that the eater generally cannot have too much of what is bad for him, nor too little of what is good for him, and the Chinese are certainly aware that a sound diet does away with much of the need for medicines. See **diet**, **health foods**, **classification of foods**, **white rice porridge** and **taro starch jelly**.

invigorated breathing See **ch'iang chuang kung**.

involuntary movement Involuntary reaction or reflex. This is a movement or reaction which occurs spontaneously without deliberate direction by the mind. For example, if a person's hand accidentally comes into contact with a hot surface, sensory nerves will carry a message from the sense organs in the skin to a nerve centre in the spinal cord, and then, instantaneously, motor nerves carry a message from the spinal cord to the muscles in the arm, which quickly move the person's hand away from the hot surface. At the same time, sensory nerves carry a message from the nerve centre to the brain, and so the activities of the motor nerves are monitored and the person is made aware of the movement even though he has not initiated it. These nerves should not be confused with those in the autonomic, or sympathetic, nervous system, which regulate those activities, such as the heartbeat, digestion and breathing, that are not controlled by the mind and of which the mind is usually unaware. A physician uses the knee-jerk test to find out if a person's reflexes are functioning. He uses a soft-headed hammer to tap a patient's bent and relaxed leg just below the kneecap. If the leg kicks upwards, the reflexes are in order. In a voluntary movement or reaction, the movement is deliberately initiated by the mind. A message is carried by motor nerves from the brain via the spinal cord to the muscles concerned. An involuntary movement or emotional reaction may be produced by experience

NERVE CONTROL OF MOVEMENT

or association of ideas. This is known as a conditioned reflex. Many of the movements of the hands and feet of a motorist in driving a vehicle are conditioned reflexes. The success of acupuncture and acupressure depends to a large extent, though not entirely, on the acupuncturist's skill in 'needling' the groups of sensory nerve endings on the meridians in such a way that they stimulate the brain or the motor nerves leading to organs in other parts of the body. In fact, the acupuncturist sometimes alters the natural functioning of the nerves, and so what would normally be regarded as an involuntary response becomes an externally controlled response, but controlled by the acupuncturist not the patient. It is very revealing that the point just below the kneecap which is used by the physicians of the West in their well-established knee-jerk test is also used by acupuncturists in the treatment of a wide range of disorders, including insomnia and indigestion, and so it is clear that Chinese physicians are quite knowledgeable about the reflexes. In fact, they were being studied in China long before they were known to the physicians of the West. Some chemical substances have effects on the sensory nerves that are similar to those of acupuncture, and spinal injections are now commonly used as a form of anaesthesia. What is more, Chinese physicians have successfully demonstrated that, in certain circumstances, acupuncture can be used to induce anaesthesia. In this connection, it is important to understand that the brain and nervous system do not control all the bodily functions, for the hormones, which produce chemical reactions, also play a part, as do the enzymes, which function as catalysts in chemical reactions. See **autonomic nervous system**, **nervous system**, **meridian** and **reflexology**.

involuntary reaction See **involuntary movement**.

involution The contraction of the uterus in returning to its normal size after childbirth.

inward-moving A term used in TCM to describe yin medicines which descend and suppress, for they tend to move vital-energy downwards and inwards, so producing an effect of concentration.

iodine A trace element which, in the human body, is contained mainly in the thyroid gland, where it is necessary for the production of the thyroid hormones. Good sources of iodine in the diet are kelp and fish, but the former is not consumed in large quantities. Other sources are meat, milk and dairy products. For medicinal purposes, the Chinese use gulf seaweed, *Sargassum fusiforme*, as a source of iodine. See **mineral** and **kelp**.

iodine deficiency See **goitre** and **mineral**.

iris The flat, coloured membrane behind the cornea of the eye, with a circular aperture, called the pupil, at its centre and in front of the lens.

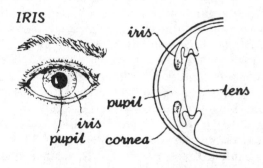

IRIS

iris diagnosis There are alternative therapists, called iridologists, who claim that the iris of the eye may be used to provide accurate diagnosis of a wide range of illnesses, but their claims seem to have very little scientific foundation. However, the eye as a whole, by its condition of yellowness, dullness or unusual brilliance, can be indicative of ill health. No doubt, it is for this reason that a certain Chinese physician described the eyes as the 'windows of the body'.

iron A trace element which is an important constituent of haemoglobin and essential to the health of women who are pregnant or in lactation. Good sources of iron in the diet are liver, kidneys, meat, molluscs, game animals, wholemeal bread, cereal products, and green vegetables. See **mineral**.

iron deficiency See **anaemia**, **mineral** and **molasses**.

iron oxide See **haematite** and **magnetite**.

irritability Sensitivity. Touchiness. This is a symptom of depression or debility, and it commonly follows an illness, such as influenza or a severe cold, which has a debilitating effect. When the general health improves, the irritability should depart. A helpful remedy is an infusion of 2–4 g leaves of basil, *Ocicum basilicum*, taken internally. But if the condition persists, there could be a serious underlying cause, and so a physician should be consulted. But it is important to allow that some people are touchy and impatient by temperament, and so a bout of moodiness or a sudden burst of ill temper could hardly be regarded in itself as a sure sign of illness. See **debility**.

irritable bowel syndrome IBS is the abbreviation for this term. More common among young and middle-aged persons than among older persons, and more so with women than with men, IBS, whose alternative names are spastic colon and mucous colitis, generally occurs sporadically, though it may become chronic. It restricts the normal movements of the muscles in the wall of the intestine, which produces pain, constipation and diarrhoea containing mucus, and may be accompanied by weakness, fatigue, back pain, abdominal cramps and bloatedness. The movements of the bowel muscles are involuntary, which suggests that this condition is either brought on or exacerbated by anxiety, stress or some other nervous disorder, though the cause could be an infection which has left the bowel in a weakened state. If there is any bleeding from the rectum, medical advice must be sought immediately. This condition is sometimes confused with diverticulosis, or diverticular disease; but, in any case, there is considerable uncertainty about its cause. If it is suspected that the condition is due to food or drinks or lactose intolerance, the following items can be omitted, in turn, from the diet for a fortnight, and the effects noted: milk, dairy products, spicy foods, sauces, bland foods, salad oils, coffee, tea, beer, red wine, fried foods, fatty meat, confectionery and flatulent foods – pulses, onions, sprouts, cabbage, broccoli and cauliflower. The dietary fibre in meals should be increased by adding bran, fruits, vegetables and wholegrain cereals. At least 2 litres of fluid should be taken daily in order to maintain hydration. IBS is as common in China as it is in the West, and just as difficult to treat. In TCM, the cause is attributed to an imbalance of the stomach, spleen and intestine, which sometimes affects the kidneys and liver, and which arises from a combination of weakness of the spleen and kidneys, excessive dampness in the intestine and liver-*qi* stagnation. The usual herbal remedies are infusions or decoctions of the following, taken internally, using the parts and dosages for the purposes indicated. Tone spleen, clear toxins and strengthen the immune system: dandelion, *Taraxacum officinale*, all parts, 10–30 g. Bloatedness: magnolia, *Magnolia officinalis*, bark, 5–10 g. Constipation: rhubarb, *Rheum officinale*, rhizomes, 1–2 g. Diarrhoea: Indian bread, *Poria cocos*, whole plant, 4–10 g. Flatulence: fennel, *Foeniculum vulgare*, fruits, 0.5–2 g. Sleeplessness: hop, *Humulus lupulus*, strobiles (cone-like flowers), 1.5–3 g. Stress: camomile, *Matricaria chamomilla*, flowers, 3–12 g. See **diverticulosis**.

irritant A substance, usually from an external source, which produces an adverse reaction within the body, and which may be biological, chemical, mechanical or radioactive in its effects.

Without a doubt, the wide range of irritants, many of which are man-made, with which the body comes into contact are responsible for many illnesses. See **chemicals** and **cancer**.

irritating foods See **classification of foods**.

Island of the Eastern Sea According to an old Chinese legend, which arose from the beliefs of the Taoists, and which probably has a basis in fact, there existed a region called the Island of the Eastern Sea, where grew a herb which would confer immortality on those who consumed it. One may wonder if this island is the group of islands we now know as Japan, for there are records which indicate that, at the time of the Han dynasty (206 BC–AD 220), an emperor sent an expedition, which included 6000 children, to Japan in order to locate this herb of immortality. The children did not return, and they are sometimes numbered among those people of different races who were the ancestors of the Japanese.

isolation The temporary segregation of a person with an infectious disease so that it is not transmitted to others. Isolation should not be confused with quarantine, which is the segregation of people who, having travelled from one country to another, might have an infectious disease or are merely suspected of having an infectious disease. Quarantine is usually enforced by government regulations. Chinese physicians have always recognized the need for isolation or semi-isolation of sick people who have illnesses which can be easily spread, and they have difficulty in understanding why the physicians of the West are so keen on making use of hospitals, which, by their very nature, are sources of infection.

itchiness See **pruritis**.

'itis' See **inflammation**.

J

jade Nephrite. A silicate of calcium and magnesium, and much valued by the Chinese for making ornaments and inexpensive items of jewellery. As with gold and pearls, jade has a cultural significance, and it was used as a medicine in ancient China. For this, it was ground into a powder and dissolved in black rice vinegar. It was credited with magical powers, which included restoration of the sight and immunity to poison and wounding by knives and other sharp instruments. No doubt, its benefits were mainly psychological but calcium and magnesium are among the minerals the body needs, and so, perhaps it does have some real benefit. See **nephrite** and **Nei Pien**.

Jamestown-weed See **jimson weed**.

Japanese catnip *Schizonepeta tenuifolia* Herbal medicine. Distribution: China. Parts: stems, leaves, floral buds. Character: warm, bitter-pungent. Affinity: liver, lungs. Effects: antipyretic, haemostatic, diaphoretic. Symptoms: fever, chills, pains, headaches, sore throat. Treatments: wind-cold conditions, postnatal and menstrual haemorrhage. Dosage: 4–10 g. This herb must NOT be confused with catnip, *Nepeta cataria*, also called catnep or cat mint, which is an entirely different species with different properties.

Japanese honeysuckle *Lonicera japonica* Herbal medicine. Distribution: Japan, China, Korea. Parts: flowers. Character: cold, sweet. Affinity: heart, lungs, stomach, spleen. Effects: antipyretic, refrigerant, antidote. Symptoms: inflamed and swollen throat. Treatments: blood in stools or sputum, ulcers, skin sores and infections, eczema, heat injuries, external heat becoming inner-heat. Dosage: 10–15 g. There is a European species of honeysuckle, *Lonicera periclymenum*, also called woodbine, which has similar properties but is less potent. In the West, honeysuckle is used as a treatment for catarrh.

Japanese medicine The traditional medicine of Japan is somewhat similar to that of China, and many of the medicinal herbs that are indigenous to China are also indigenous to Japan. But

Japan has become more Westernized than China – which could be its undoing – and its traditional medicines have been largely superseded by Western-style medicines or have been adapted to meet the requirements of Western medicine. But the Buddhist influence has been as strong in Japan as it has been in China, and so the Japanese, as well as the Chinese, have developed and still practise the martial arts in their various systems, many of which originated in the Buddhist temples. But there are differences. The Japanese martial arts, or karate, are more aggressive and warlike and less motivated by health and meditation than the Chinese martial arts, or kungfu. The Japanese diet is excellent in that it is preventive of defects of the heart and circulation, but it is less appetizing, though more colourful, than that of the Chinese.

Japanese medlar See **loquat**.

jaundice Icterus. A yellow discolouration of the skin and eyes due to the presence in the bloodstream of bilirubin, which is a yellow pigment produced by the spleen when red blood cells are destroyed. Obviously, if red blood cells are being destroyed in large quantities, something must be amiss within the body. Jaundice is not an illness in itself but a symptom of illness, generally of the liver, such as hepatitis A, or infectious jaundice, cirrhosis, cancer, gallstones blocking the bile duct or hepatitis B, which is less common than hepatitis A but more dangerous. Rarely, it is a symptom of glandular fever. Jaundice is often symptomatic of a serious condition, and so professional medical advice should always be sought. In TCM, jaundice is attributed to dampness of the liver and the gall-bladder. Providing there is no serious underlying cause, jaundice can be treated with an infusion or decoction, taken internally, of one of the following, using the parts and dosage indicated: dandelion, *Taraxacum officinale*, roots, 10–30 g; self-heal, *Prunella vulgaris*, flowers, 5–7 g; maize, *Zea mays*, silk of ears, 15–30 g; chervil, *Anthriscus cerifolium*, leaves, 2–4 g; gardenia, *Gardenia jasminoides*, mature fruits, 4–10 g.

jejunum See **intestine**.

'jelly fungus' See **silver wood ears**.

Jenner The English physician Edward Jenner (1749–1823) is credited with having made the first vaccination against smallpox, but he was not the first person to practise immunology. See **immunology** and **Jesuits**.

Jesuits Members of the Society of Jesus, a Roman Catholic religious order, founded in 1554. The first Christian missionaries to China arrived during the fourteenth century. The first Jesuit missionaries arrived about two centuries later. Generally, they were made welcome, for the Chinese are courteous and hospitable by temperament; and, no doubt, some Chinese found their doctrines of brotherly love and salvation to be quite attractive. However, they came to be regarded with suspicion when it became apparent that certain aspects of their behaviour were riddled with hypocrisy and acquisitiveness. Matters came to a head in 1704, when the Pope issued an encyclical forbidding participation in ancestor worship. The Chinese were greatly incensed by this, which they regarded as a direct attack on one of their most valued institutions. When the Confucians complained to the emperor that the Jesuits were a corruptive influence they were expelled from China forthwith, despite the fact that some of them had been employed as advisers at the imperial court, mainly for their scientific and medical knowledge. However, the Jesuits had performed a useful service in that they had effected a two-way transmission of knowledge between Europe and China, and Europeans received their first insight into TCM during the fifteenth century. Chinese-style medicines were in fashion in Europe during the sixteenth century, acupuncture arrived in the seventeenth century, and the Chinese method of inoculation against smallpox was introduced during the eighteenth century. Perhaps the Jesuits' sojourn in China brought greater blessings to the Europeans than it did to the Chinese. See **Jenner** and **immunology**.

jet fatigue See **jet lag**.

jet lag The fatigue, lethargy, irritability, sleeplessness, inability to concentrate and, sometimes, loss of appetite and diarrhoea which follow an east–west or west–east flight crossing any of the earth's 24 time zones, and which arises from disturbances of the body's natural daily cycle, or circadian rhythm. The body becomes accustomed to going to sleep and awaking at certain times, and it has difficulty in adjusting to the hours of sleep which are different from those at home. But other factors are involved, which include low pressurization of the aircraft cabin, exposure to radiation by flying at great heights of more than 3,000 metres, eating unusual food, breathing foul or dry air, and sitting in a cramped position without exercise for hours on end. The condition departs when the body has adjusted to the new times or, after returning home, has readjusted to the normal times. The condition is minimized if, during the flight, one avoids heavy meals, alcohol and short naps, and drinks plenty of fluids, removes one's shoes, wears loose and comfortable clothing and occasionally leaves one's seat for a few minutes to maintain a good circulation. In this connection, it is interesting to note that, though TCM originated long before air travel came into being, the physicians of ancient China were aware of the circadian rhythm and biorhythms. In fact, in Chinese astrology, the day is divided into 12 two-hour periods, which can be related to the circadian rhythm and an individual's personality and bodily functions. This is one of the many instances among Chinese beliefs and institutions where what, at first sight, appears to the Western observer to be superstition turns out to be profound thinking, and often with a scientific basis. See **zodiac exercises**, **insomnia** and **travel sickness**.

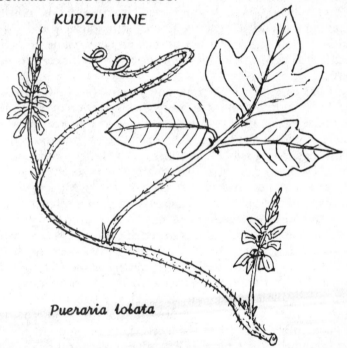

KUDZU VINE

Pueraria lobata

jimson weed *Datura metel* Also called Jamestown-weed, thorn apple or loco weed, the latter name being an Americanism. Herbal medicine. Distribution: South China, south of Asia, North America, Central America. Parts: flowers. Character: warm, bitter. Affinity: lungs, Effects: sedative, analgesic, antitussive. Symptoms: stomach ache, difficult or irregular breathing, shortness of breath. Treatments: asthma, bronchitis, coughs. Dosage: 0.1–0.2 g. This medicine is poisonous, so the dosage must NOT be exceeded, nor must it be taken without professional medical supervision. In fact, in Britain, by the terms of the Medicines Act 1968, the use of this medicine is restricted to medical practitioners, and the maximum permitted dosage is 0.05 g dried herb, or its equivalent, three times daily. It is NOT suitable for children. In China, the dried flowers are smoked in a pipe to relieve asthma. All parts of the herb – flowers, leaves and seeds – were once widely used in local anaesthetics. See **anaesthetics** and **Guan Yu**.

jin See **jin ye**.

jin bu huan This Chinese phrase, which, loosely translated, means 'money is no deal', is the name that was given to the herb *san qi*, *Panax notoginseng*, by the soldiers of ancient China in recognition of its efficacy as a healing medicine. *San qi* is powerfully haemostatic and it heals wounds, both internal and external, without clots or scars. It was of such immense value to soldiers in battle that they would not sell it, even for gold. See **Yunnan bai yao**.

jing Vital essence, or energy, and one of the four humours of TCM. It is produced by the transforming action of *qi* on the food in the stomach and small intestine, and is the creative force, or energy, within the body. This makes sense, for food, together with the oxygen which reaches it via the lungs and blood, is the body's source of energy, a fact with which the physicians of the West would not disagree. According to TCM, *jing* is of two forms – life-essence and semen-essence. Life-essence regulates growth and other developments, such as decay, or deterioration with age, and death, and it is stored in the kidneys from which it is released when required. In terms of Western medicine, it could be said that life-essence regulates metabolism, and can be equated with the hormones secreted by the suprarenal glands, also called the adrenal glands, which are situated at the upper ends of the kidneys. See **adrenal glands**. Modern medical science informs us that the cortex of the suprarenal glands secretes hormones which are essential to life, for they control the structure of connective tissue, the production of some types of white corpuscle, protein metabolism, certain phases of carbohydrate and fat, and the salt and water balance. Adrenalin, one of the hormones secreted by these glands, comes to our aid in an emergency, providing energy and courage on a temporary basis, and constricting the blood vessels so that less blood is lost in the event of a surface injury. In the West, until recent years, courage was associated with the heart, and so a brave man was a 'stout-hearted fellow', but the Chinese have always associated it with the kidneys, so coming to the correct conclusion without the aid of all the sophisticated equipment which is now available to the medical scientists of the West. Semen-essence is the spermatozoa, or male sex cells, and the ova, or female sex cells. The union of male semen-essence with female semen-essence yields eggs that develop into embryos, which draw their life-essence from that which was taken from the semen and stored in the eggs. After a child is born, it makes its own life-essence from the food it has digested. The differences between Chinese ideas and Western ideas in medicine are sometimes more apparent than real, and more to do with words than facts. Substituting English words for Chinese words shows that Chinese and English physicians may sometimes arrive at the same conclusion by taking different routes. According to TCM, girls mature somewhat earlier than boys, and women lose their sexual potency earlier than men, but there is no doubt that, during the period of sexual activity, much life-essence is required. In the West, it has been established that men with dense semen and a high sperm-count are very active and resistant to disease. See **humour**, **essence** and **maturity cycle**.

jing luo See **qing lo**.

Jin Ping Mei 'Golden Lotus'. This is the title of a novel written at the time of the Ming period, and in which there are herbal prescriptions written in verse. This is an indication of the importance which the Chinese attach to health and medicine, and also the high respect they have for physicians. Their attitude in this regard derives from Taoism, which is not only the oldest religion in the world but also the only religion which teaches that a sound state of health is our only hope of salvation. The poetic writings of the scholars of the Ming period could be regarded as hymns to nature.

jin ye Bodily fluid, and one of the four humours of TCM. According to TCM, bodily fluid is extracted from food and drink, and it differs from water and other liquids in that, after being acted upon by *qi*, it is alive. This also makes good sense by Western standards, for the bodily fluids are components of tissues, and they contain living cells, hormones and enzymes and other vital fluids. Apart from that, some of the substances in *jin ye* are of such chemical complexity that they are not likely to exist freely outside the body of an animal or plant. The amount of fluid in the body does need to be regulated. This is achieved by the intestine, which, in the process of assimilation, separates the pure liquid from the waste, and the kidneys, bladder and skin expel the waste and excess fluid. TCM also holds to the view that some organs convert *jin ye* into forms which have specific function. The liver converts fluid into tears, the spleen converts fluid into saliva, the kidneys convert fluid into urine, and the heart, via the skin, converts fluid into sweat. But there is a certain vagueness about this. It is difficult to understand just what connection there is between the spleen and saliva or the liver and tears; but, on the other hand, there is *some* connection, for a diseased liver is sometimes indicated by a jaundiced condition of the eye, and the sight or smell of food, as well as the taste of it, will stimulate secretion of saliva by the salivary glands, and so it could well be that the connection is partly emotional, as there is with overactivity of the lacrimal glands, when there is a flood of tears, which serves a useful purpose in so far as tears have mildly antiseptic properties, and help to protect the eyeballs. TCM also regards *jin ye* as being of two types: *jin*, which is clear fluid, and *ye*, which is dense fluid. *Jin*, together with protective-*qi*, circulates throughout the body, moistening the flesh and cleansing the skin, and appearing on its surface as perspiration. *Ye*, or 'dense-fluid', together with nourishing-*qi*, travels throughout the body, lubricating tendons, ligaments, muscles and joints, filling the cavities in the brain, adding to the bone marrow, and appearing on the surface of the skin as sebum, the oily secretion of the sebaceous glands. See **humour** and **interferon**.

jinzhen, or *jinzhencai*, which are dried lily flowers, is a Chinese folk remedy for nosebleeds, depression and the after-effects of hepatitis. They are also popular as an item of diet – braised, stir-fried or in soups. There is more than one species of lily in the genus *Lilium*, and the name *lily* has been given to a number of plants which are not true lilies. In Britain, the lily of the valley, *Convallaria majalis*, should NOT be used as an item of diet, and it should be noted that, as a medicine, its use is confined to medical practitioners operating under the terms of the Medicines Act 1968.

jitsu Overactive energy, as with diseases with external symptoms. See **shiatsu**.

Job's tears *Coix lacryma-jobi* Herbal medicine. Distribution: China, India, Africa, America. Parts: seeds. Character: cool, plain-sweet. Affinity: stomach, lungs, spleen. Effects: digestive, decongestant, refrigerant, diuretic, antidysenteric. Symptoms: dark-coloured and scanty urine, swollen and painful bones, joints and tendons, diarrhoea, indigestion. Treatments: illnesses due to damp exceses, damp injury to spleen, dysentery, ulcers in stomach or lungs. Dosage: 10–30 g. This herb is commonly used as a food in China and Japan, for it is very rich in protein. A liquor made by fermenting its seeds is efficacious as a treatment for rheumatism. See **medicinal wine**.

joint There are four types of movable joints: ball-and-socket, hinge, pivot and gliding. A ball-and-socket joint, such as the hip, allows movement in all directions. A hinge joint, such as the elbow, allows only forward and backward movement. A pivot joint, such as occurs between the bones in the neck, allows turning. A gliding joint, such as those in the ankle and backbone allow only slight movement. When joints become inflamed or worn, they become stiff, swollen and painful. Joints are sometimes damaged by injury, and then it is the ligaments rather than the actual bones which are most affected. But most joint problems are due to arthritis in its various forms. Osteoarthritis mainly affects the hips, backbone or knees of elderly persons, rheumatoid arthritis mainly affects the knees, hands and feet of middle-aged persons, and gout mainly affects the joints of the fingers, legs or big toes. An infusion of 10–30 g leaves, roots and flowers of dandelion, *Taraxacum officinale*, taken internally, will afford some measure of relief for inflamed joints. See **arthritis** and **podagra**.

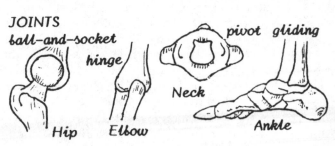

JOINTS
ball-and-socket
hinge
pivot gliding
Neck
Hip
Elbow
Ankle

joint fir *Ephedra sinica* Herbal medicine. Distribution: North China, Mongolia, Europe. Parts: stems. Character: warm, slightly bitter. Affinity: lungs, bladder. Effects: diaphoretic, respiratory stimulant, bronchi-dilator, diuretic. Symptoms: chills, fever. Treatments: wind-cold conditions, hay fever, bronchial asthma. Dosage: 1–1.8 g. As a treatment for wind-cold conditions, this herb should be used with cinnamon or corn mint. As a treatment for asthma, it could be used with almond. The roots of this herb are not diaphoretic; in fact, they are antidiaphoretic. Extracts of ephedrine, an alkaloid contained in this herb, is now widely used in the West as a treatment for asthma. It is important to note that, in Britain, by the terms of the Medicines Act 1968, this herb is available only to be used by registered medical practitioners, and the maximum permitted dosage is 0.6 g dried stems, or the equivalent, three times daily. There are two other species of this herb, which have similar medicinal properties: *Ephedra equisetina* and *Ephedra gerardiana*. See **asthma**.

joss-sticks Originally designed to be used as incense in temples, joss-sticks are now used in any place where a soothing fragrance or an air-freshener is required. The Chinese use them for the same purpose that we, in the West, would use an air-freshener aerosol. But joss-sticks do have the important advantage that they do no damage to the ozone layer. A joss-stick is a long, thin splinter of wood thinly coated with a mixture of clay, fragrant gum and a suitable oxidizing agent, such as saltpetre, or nitre (potassium nitrate), and which, when ignited, burns very slowly, emitting sweet-smelling fumes. The oxidizing agent provides oxygen in which the gum burns, and the clay acts as a dilutent, which inhibits a too rapid combustion of the gum. The word *joss* means 'idol' or 'god'. Thus, a joss-house is a temple. Seemingly, *joss* is a corruption of the Portuguese word *deos*, which means 'god', and which derives from the Latin *deus*. It does seem rather odd that a Chinese idol should come to possess a Latin name. Portugal was among the first of the European nations to make contact with China.

joule A unit of work and energy. It is too small for practical purposes, and so the energy values of foods are measured in kilojoules (kJ) or kilocalories (kcal). 1 kilocalorie = 4.18 kilojoules. See **calories** and **calorific value of food**.

joy This is one of the seven emotions of TCM, but it is used in the sense of elation or great happiness rather than mere contentment. It is associated with the heart and the element fire, and so it is understandable that laughter, which is symptomatic of a joyful heart, is called 'fire-sound' by the Chinese. According to the teachings of the early Taoists, the heart houses the spirit, and when a person is extremely joyful, his spirit cannot be contained, and so it is scattered. But, here, the Chinese use the word *spirit* to mean 'exuberance' or 'boisterousness', and not to mean 'soul' or 'ghost', as we do in the West. However, an excessive or prolonged period of joy can do damage to the heart, and uncontrolled paroxysms of laughter, as with hysteria, not only affects the heart unfavourably but is evidence of a psychopathic condition. A person who is permanently exuberant is likely to have an over-active heart, which could easily become an overworked heart. See **emotion**, '**fire-sound**' and **hysteria**.

ju ching See **fang sung kung**.

jujube *Ziziphus jujuba* Also called Chinese jujube or red date. Herbal medicine. Distribution: China, Japan, India, Pakistan, Afghanistan, Malaysia. There is a cultivated variety of this herb, of which different parts are used in medicine, and so it must be described separately. Wild herb parts: seeds. Character: neutral, sweet-sour. Affinity: heart, liver, gall-bladder, spleen. Effects: cardiotonic, yin tonic, nutrient, sedative, antidiaphoretic. Symptoms: sleeplessness, palpitations, cold sweats. Treatments: insomnia, neurasthenia, poor complexion. Dosage: 5–12 g. Cultivated herb parts: fruits. Character: neutral, sweet. Affinity: spleen. Effects: nutrient, sedative, tonic for spleen and stomach.

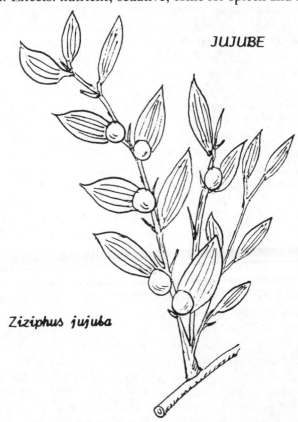

JUJUBE

Ziziphus jujuba

Symptoms: fatigue, loss of appetite. Treatments: empty conditions of spleen and stomach, hysteria. Dosage: 2–5 fruits. This herb is often included, to function as a buffer, in prescriptions for potent tonics. See **buffer** and '**cinnamon sap soup**'.

Jung The eminent Swiss psychologist and psychiatrist Carl Gustav Jung (1875–1961) made use of Taoist philosophy in treating his patients. No doubt, he was acquainted with *Ben Cao Gang Mu*, the herbal compiled by Li Shizhen. See **I Ching**.

junk food The Chinese take a great pride in their culinary skills and regard a sound diet as a main source of good health, and so they would not readily approve of the convenience foods, disparagingly described as junk foods, which have become so popular in the West during recent years, mainly because they are time-saving, attractively packaged and in fashion, and which have led to a mushroom-like proliferation of fast-food outlets and grocery chains and conglomerates. Some of these processed and pre-packed foods are prepared under the most hygienic conditions and with due regard to the best dietetic principles – of that there can be no doubt – and all is well, but only until something goes wrong in the mass-production process, and then a batch of many thousands of jars, bottles, cans or packets of contaminated food finds its way on to the shelves of grocery stores throughout the land. But some convenience foods are not of the highest standards, and their manufacture involves the use of inferior ingredients, meat substitutes and additives to boost weight, bulk and appearance. By their very nature, processed foods require the use of preservatives, acidity-regulators, emulsifiers, and so forth; and these are generally synthetic. Attractiveness in appearance, flavour and texture is often maintained to the detriment of nutriment, for manufacturers are aware that many people judge only by appearances. But, here, the real disadvantage, and even danger, lies with the consumers who are failing to treat convenience food as what it is intended to be – something quick and easy when time is at a premium – and allowing it to become a way of life. And it is important to remember that food which is quickly served and purchased is likely to be hastily ingested, and then it will not be properly digested, for the digestive process begins in the mouth. The Chinese attitude here is straightforward and uncompromising. All meals should be appetizing, nutritious, individually prepared from fresh ingredients, and consumed without undue haste. In view of the damage done by unsound diet, it surely behoves us to emulate the Chinese example. See **diet** and **health foods**.

Juvenal This Roman poet perceived, as did the physicians of ancient China, that fitness of the body is coupled with fitness of the mind and vice versa. See **mental health**.

K

kala-azar See **Leishmaniasis**.
kaoliangjiu See **wine**.
karate See **martial arts** and **Japanese medicine**.
kcal The abbreviation for *kilocalorie*. See **calorie**.
keeping fit In the Chinese view, keeping fit is more than being merely healthy. It means that one should glow with health and youthfulness and enjoy life to the full. Keep-fit activities have become quite a fetish among some of the people of the West, but the procedures they adopt are sometimes extreme or even ridiculous. Strict dieting which leads to anorexia nervosa is hardly the way to keep fit and over-strenuous physical exercise, as with weight-lifting and body-building, may lead to unnatural muscular development. Being a contortionist is not the key to good health, and one notices that athletes who have given up strenuous exercise often become flabby. Boxing, rugby football, hockey and similar pursuits create many minor injuries which generally go unnoticed when they are sustained but which may show up with tragic ill-effects in later life. Then there are the high-minded and singularly determined people who completely shun alcohol and tobacco with sanctimonious zeal, even though, providing it is taken in moderation, alcohol can be preventive of heart and circulatory conditions, and it is certainly preferable to sedatives and soporifics if one needs a good night's sleep, and tobacco with an admixture of jimson weed and coltsfoot is recommended by some Chinese physicians as an anticongestant in the treatment of some forms of asthma. The Chinese also have a desire to keep fit, and they do so extremely well without making themselves unhappy in the process. Their diet is nutritious and preventive of obesity and circulatory diseases, but it is also very appetizing. Their physical exercise is based upon the gentler forms of the martial arts, such as *tai chi chuan*. They enjoy a glass of wine, but rarely do they become intoxicated to the point of stupidity. They have no guilt-ridden complexes about sex, nor are they exponents of promiscuity. They would

argue that, with moderation, as with most things, sex is beneficial to the health. It might do some good for elderly people with rheumatism. See **sexual therapy**. The Chinese view, if expressed briefly, is that few of our practices are bad for us provided we avoid the extremes of conduct. To take but one example, lack of exercise makes the blood sluggish, which hastens the normal process of deterioration of the vital organs and connective tissue; but by contrast, excessive exercise or manual labour produces fatigue and weakness, which will also accelerate the deterioration of the vital organs. A middle-of-the-way approach is surely the correct approach in keeping fit. See **moderation**.

kelp A brown-coloured seaweed which, as a dietary item, could be a rich source of iodine and minerals for the people of the West, but they do not consume it on a large scale. See **iodine**.

keratin A hard protein which is a constituent of hair, nails, horny tissue and the thin outer layer of the skin.

keratosis A hard and horny growth, such as a wart or a corn. See **corn** and **wart**.

kidney infections See **renal disorders**.

kidneys The kidneys, which are yin, belong to the *qu zang*, or solid organs of the body. Their element is water, and the hollow organ with which they are paired is the bladder, which is what one would expect, for the two main functions of the kidneys are to maintain the fluid balance of the body – which affects blood pressure – and to filter waste from the blood, whose liquid component, or urine, is stored in the bladder, from which it will pass to the outside. The traditional associations of the kidneys in astrology, climate, emotions, etc., are listed under **element**. According to TCM, the kidneys store life-essence, which is a component of *jing*, or 'vital-essence', and which, being something received genetically from one's parents, is involved in inheritance, and should be cherished and not downgraded or damaged by excessive indulgence in sex or alcohol. The kidneys are also associated with the lungs and breathing, and some forms of asthma are treated by toning the kidneys. They influence mental activity and the growth and development of bones and marrow, and nourish the hair and teeth. Strong teeth and thick hair are indications of healthy kidneys. Weak kidneys may be a cause of infertility. Insomnia, amnesia, tinnitus, bed-wetting, oedema and back pains occur where there is a deficiency of kidney-*qi* or a kidney dysfunction. The kidneys are closely associated with the adrenal glands, which secrete a wide variety of hormones, including one of the sex hormones. The kidneys are thought to house the will-power, which makes some sense, for the adrenal glands provide determination when an emergency situation arises. The kidneys are also associated with the emotion of fear, as is caused by the loss of will-power when the kidneys are weak. But, in this sense, *fear* means 'conscious and prolonged fear', as distinct from panic or a sudden fright. The incidence of involuntary urination when there is intense fear clearly shows that there is indeed some association between fear and the functionings of the kidneys and bladder. In fact, excessive fear and inner-wind conditions may injure the kidneys. See **adrenal glands** and **jing**.

kidney stones See **calculus** and **renal disorders**.

kidney tonics As the kidneys are yin organs, weak kidneys will generally be treated with yang tonics in the hope that they will have a strengthening effect, but the particular tonic to be used will be decided by the cause and nature of the weakness; and, if there is a specific disease or defect, the treatment will require medicines other than yang tonics. Chinese physicians might prescribe an infusion, to be taken internally, of 8–14 g leaves of horny goat weed, *Epimedium sagittatum*, where the symptoms are high blood pressure or amnesia. They might also prescribe mistletoe, *Viscum album*; but, in Britain, under the terms of the Medicines Act 1968, the medicinal use of mistletoe berries is confined to registered medical practitioners. For tinnitus and urinary incontinence, they might prescribe an infusion, to be taken internally, of 8–14 g mature fruits of calthrop, *Tribulus terrestris*. An infusion, taken internally, of 8–12 g bark of eucommia, *Eucommia ulmoides*, is a good tonic for a more generalized weakness of the kidneys, and it is also a nutrient to the bones and marrow. But the kidneys are delicate organs, and it would be foolish to embark on any kind of self-treatment without an accurate diagnosis, which can only be provided by a physician.

kilocalorie See **calorie**.

kilojoule See **joule**.

kinesiology See **pressure-point therapy**.

kJ The abbreviation for **kilojoule**.

kneading See **compression**.

knee-jerk test See **involuntary movement**.

knee pain This condition is extremely common, and is due to the excessive demands made on the knee joint by the stressful activities of modern life: over-strenuous games and sports, climbing stairs, scrubbing floors and other jobs, such as carpentry and bricklaying, which entail kneeling or sitting or standing in unnatural positions. Obesity also puts additional stress on the knee joint, and the upright stance of humans is probably a contributory factor. In the West, the usual treatments are knee wraps, which are not very effective, and sometimes affect the circulation adversely, and analgesics, which reduce pain but do not cure the condition. The obvious treatment is to eliminate the cause, and so prevent the condition from worsening. For example, if the condition is due to scrubbing floors, one should give up scrubbing floors. Chinese physicians would recommend acupuncture or acupressure, which should be performed by a professional, and healing exercises of the kind contained in the *Chinese Exercise Manual*, all of which are effective. But it would be sensible to prevent this condition from arising in the first place, and it is certain that those people who participate regularly in a gentle form of the martial arts, such as *tai chi chuan*, will be far less prone to this condition.

'knifeless surgery' This is an apt term to describe those non-surgical methods of treatment used by Chinese physicians to achieve results which are just as beneficial as, and sometimes more beneficial, and certainly less harrowing for the patient, than those achieved by some of the surgical techniques used by practitioners in the West – and, in the view of Chinese physicians, used all too readily. Some examples are herbal medicines, such as comfrey, for healing broken bones, poultices and suction cups for removing pus, and manipulation to reorientate prolapsed organs. However, 'knifeless surgery' has its limitations, and surgery in the West has improved by leaps and bounds in recent years. A finger or limb detached by an accident can now be put back into place, the severed nerves, blood vessels, muscles, etc., being skilfully rejoined. A diseased hip can be replaced with an artificial hip made of plastic or metal. It is often possible to replace a damaged organ with an organ taken from a deceased person. Open-heart surgery is regarded as one of the miracles of modern medical science, though it is rather sad that the condition which it cures can sometimes be easily prevented by diet, exercise and moderate habits. See **surgery**.

knitback See **comfrey**.

knitbone See **comfrey**.

'knocking on the door of life' See **za fu pei**.

knotty yam *Dioscorea opposita* Herbal medicine. Distribution: China, Japan. Parts: tubers. Character: neutral, sweet. Affinity:

spleen, lungs. Effects: stomachic, digestive, tones the spleen and lungs. Symptoms: fatigue, lack of appetite, diarrhoea, frequent and insufficient urination, nocturnal emissions. Treatments: leucorrhoea, spermatorrhoea, empty condition of spleen and stomach, chronic coughs, diabetes mellitus. Dosage: 12–30 g. This herb lowers the level of blood sugar, which makes it effective as a treatment for diabetes. This herb is also administered to children as a treatment for sleeplessness, poor appetite and irregular bowel movements.

'Know Everything Book' See **Chinese Almanac**.

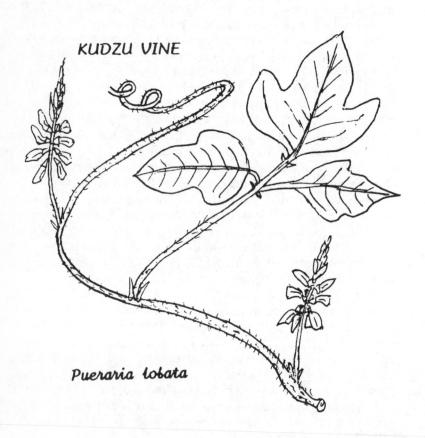

KUDZU VINE

Pueraria lobata

Ko Hung See **Nei Pien**.

kola *Cola vera* Also called cola or guru nut. This herb is indigenous to West Africa, but it is also cultivated in hot regions elsewhere, and it is used throughout the world as a gentle stimulant, tonic and diuretic in treating depression, diarrhoea, debility and weakness. Dosage: 2–9 g powdered seeds to be taken internally. Its use in China is only occasional, and it is not regarded as a prominent feature of TCM.

Kong Fuzi See **Kung Fuzi**.

Koplik's spots See **mouth diagnosis**.

kudzu vine *Pueraria lobata* Herbal medicine. Distribution: China, Japan. Parts: root. Character: neutral, bitter-sweet. Affinity: stomach, spleen. Effects: antipyretic, refrigerant, demulcent. Symptoms: coldness, dry throat and stomach, aches in shoulders, neck and back. Treatments: chills, fever, relaxes taut and painful muscles in back, neck and shoulders which are a consequence of wind-heat injury. Dosage: 4–10 g.

kungfu See **martial arts**.

Kung Fuzi Also spelt as *Kong Fuzi*, *Kung Fu-tse* or *Kung Fu-tzu*, this is the Chinese name of China's greatest philosopher. See **Confucius**.

kyo Depleted energy, as with diseases with internal symptoms. See **shiatsu**.

L

laboratory tests Some people would argue, and not unreasonably, that a Chinese medicine cannot be accepted as being efficacious and safe to use unless it has been subjected to stringent laboratory tests, for one cannot afford to take risks with medicines. It is the case that all the Chinese medicines available in the West have not undergone rigorous tests, but most of those which have been so tested are as effective as the claims which have been made for them. This was to be expected because Chinese medicines are the outcome of thousands of years of practical experience, which is likely to be a better guide than a few laboratory experiments of questionable accuracy. Some of the tranquillizers and soporifics which have appeared on the market in the West during recent years have given the authorities cause for grave concern because they have decidedly unpleasant side-effects or have proved to be unreliable and even dangerous. Thalidomide is a well-known example. Ironically, thalidomide is still being used in Brazil as a treatment for leprosy. Perhaps the sufferers think it is worth the risk – on the principle that a little relief, albeit short-lived, is better than no relief at all, and that desperate situations call for desperate measures. See **herbal medicines** and **Medicines Act 1968**.

labour The contractions of the uterus, by which means a baby is born. See **childbirth** and **uterus**.

laboured breathing Stertorous breathing. This can be symptomatic of a stroke or a heart condition. See **ba gang**.

laceration A cut that is ragged and uneven. If it is small, it can be treated in the same way as any other small wound. If it is large and there is severe bleeding, immediate first aid to arrest the bleeding and treat shock will be required prior to calling for professional medical aid. In these procedures, the Chinese approach is much the same as that in the West. See **cuts**, **ligature** and **shock**.

lack of appetite see **appetite**.

lacrimal gland A gland in the eye which normally secretes just sufficient tear fluid to keep the cornea moist. The excess fluid drains into the nose. When there is a foreign body in the eye, the lacrimal gland works overtime to produce a copious flow of tears, which washes away the foreign body and protects the cornea by its slightly antiseptic properties. See **jin ye**.

lactase See **lactose**.

lactation Suckling. The formation and secretion of milk by the breasts. Where the milk yield is low, a galactogogue may be used, though a nourishing diet, rich in iron and other minerals, is helpful. A mother breast-feeding her baby will need to eat 'enough for two'. Effective galactogogues are infusions, taken internally, of 3–18 g dried seeds of fenugreek, *Trigonella foenum-graecum*, and 2–4 g seeds of caraway, *Carum carvi*. Chewing the seeds of fennel, *Foeniculum vulgare*, in a dosage not exceeding 3 g, is considered to be helpful. For excessive lactation, a suitable treatment is an infusion, taken internally, of 10–20 g grains of barley, *Hordeum vulgare*. See **iron** and **galactogogue**.

lactose Milk sugar. This is a simple disaccharide sugar which occurs in milk and is less sweet than sucrose. In the digestive tract, it is broken down by the enzyme lactase into its two constituent monosaccharides, glucose and galactose, which can be absorbed by the intestine into the blood, where they are sources of energy. See **sugar**.

lactose intolerance The inability to absorb lactose, or milk sugar, which is a condition common among babies, but generally only temporarily following an attack of gastro-enteritis. The symptom is watery diarrhoea. The treatment is to exclude from the diet milk and foods containing lactose, such as cheese, cream and certain processed foods. Adults with lactose intolerance should avoid certain forms of confectionery, bakery products and pharmaceuticals. The people of the south of China have few problems in this respect, for milk and milk products are not a part of their diet. See **irritable bowel syndrome**.

Lao Zi Also spelt as *Lao-tse* or *Lao-tzu*. Lao Zi, who lived during the sixth century BC, at about the same time as Confucius, was one of China's great sages and, together with the Yellow Emperor, is regarded as the founder of Taoism. He is the subject of many legends, some of which have a basis in fact. Like Confucius, he believed in universal order, and that man could achieve harmony within himself by accepting the natural laws, and so being in full harmony with nature. His name, which means 'Old One' or 'Old Boy', derives from an ancient legend which tells that he was born in strange circumstances. One night, in 666 BC, a woman cried out in delight when she perceived a falling star. The shock made her become pregnant. Sixty-two years later, she gave birth to a silver-haired son who was fully capable of speech. This was Lao Zi. The theme of this story, which involves a portentous star and a human conception without a male involvement, is similar to that of legends from other parts of the world. At the age of 160, just before his demise, he wrote a book of 5000 characters, from which is derived the *Tao Te Ching*, known in English as the 'Classic of the Way and Power of Virtue and Nature'. This is regarded a the primary Taoist book, though there are many others, which are known collectively as the Taoist Patrology. Lao Zi is usually depicted holding the Peach of Immortality in his hand. But one may wonder to what extent Lao Zi himself had any serious beliefs in regard to immortality, for the *Tao Te Ching* indicates that he was a person of sound wisdom who sought for an understanding of the cosmos in terms that were more materialistic than mystical. See **Taoism**.

lard Rendered and clarified fat from the pig, and which is used in cooking. It is very high in saturated fatty acids, and so it cannot be recommended as an item of diet. However, it does have a good use in medicine. In both TCM and Western medicine, it is used as a base in preparing ointments. See **paste**.

large intestine Colon. This is one of the hollow organs, and so it is yang. Its element is metal and it is paired with the lungs. See **intestine** and **liu fu**.

laryngitis Inflammation of the larynx. In TCM, this condition is regarded as being due to heat and poison in the lungs. Western physicians would say that it is due to an infection. In TCM, the recommended treatment is an infusion, slowly sipped, of one of the following, using the parts and dosage indicated: Japanese honeysuckle, *Lonicera japonica*, flowers, 10–15 g; Chinese liquorice, *Glycyrrhiza uralensis*, roots, 2–8 g; peppermint, *Mentha piperata*, leaves and stems, 2–4 g. Additionally, one could use an infusion of one of the following as mouthwash and gargle. Sage, *Salvia officinalis*, leaves, 2–6 g; marigold, *Calendula officinalis*, flowers, 3–12 g; sorrel, *Rumex acetosa*, leaves, 2–4 g. Also, one should avoid cold drinks, smoking and cough sweets, drink plenty of liquid, which will keep the throat moist, breath through the nose and talk as little as possible for a few days.

larynx 'Voice-box'. The system of muscles and cartilage at the upper end of the trachea, which contains the vocal cords, whose movements make speech possible. Its external prominence on the front of the throat is known as the Adam's apple. See **epiglottis**.

laser treatment Technological development has entered even into the practice of acupuncture, and laser beams are now sometimes used to excite the acupoints, but it is doubtful if this technique is any more effective than the traditional technique of 'needling'.

lassitude Lethargy. Persistent tiredness. In itself, this condition indicates no more than that the weather is sultry, or a person has been 'burning the candle at both ends', and so is in need of a few good nights' rest. But, taken in conjunction with other symptoms, it can be indicative of a wide variety of diseases and defects, such as anaemia, debility and menstrual and menopausal problems, which Chinese physicians would describe as internal, empty and yin conditions. If this condition persists for a long time, a physician should be consulted. See **tiredness**.

lateral inversion See **optical illusion**.

Latin The language of ancient Rome was once the lingua franca of the educated classes – priests, lawyers and physicians – of Europe; and, even today, it still serves the needs of those professional workers who require a means of communication which is precise and commonly understood by them if not by the world at large. In medical work, it is most important that there should be no confusion, and so the names of plants, animals, illnesses, medicines, etc., have been given Latinized names which are understood by physicians and pharamacists through-out the world. This system of nomenclature is highly desirable, for the common names of plants and animals vary from region to region and country to country, and some are misleading. The cuckoo-pint, *Arum maculatum*, has over 50 common names. The guelder rose, *Viburnum opulus*, is not a rose, and the sea holly, *Eryngium maritimum*, is a herbaceous plant and not related to the holly, *Ilex aquifolium*, which is a small tree. It should be possible for a British physician who does not understand one word of Japanese to make out a prescription which could be dispensed by a Japanese pharmacist who does not understand one word of English. The advantage is obvious. Chinese physicians, including those who do not practise outside TCM, use this Latin-style system of names, for they are aware of its advantages. If one purchases a herbal mixture which has originated in China, one will find that the ingredients, as listed on its container, will be given in their Latinized names.

laudanum Tincture of opium. At the beginning of this century, laudanum was on free sale in Britain, and there were no restrictions on its use as a sedative and pain-killer. But it is addictive and dangerous when administered without proper medical supervision, as Chinese physicians have long recognized. See **law**.

laughter Like sleep and food, laughter is something we take very much for granted, though it is sometimes an excellent medicine, being good for both the mental and physical health. When people join together in laughter, there is a strengthening of the social bonds and an abandonment of mutual suspicion and hostility. It also increases the rate of breathing, stimulates the circulation, relaxes the muscles, sharpens the intellect and induces the secretion of adrenalin, the so-called 'arousal hormone'. Certainly, when one can laugh about one's problems, they seem to be far less menacing, and one's enemies or rivals seem to be far less formidable. Those morose and ill-tempered people who rarely laugh create loneliness and a mental prison for themselves, and they indirectly damage their physical health. On the other hand, as Chinese physicians would point out, forced laughter is unhelpful, for it is unnatural and promotes suspicion and produces no health benefits; and uncontrolled laughter, as with hysterics, can be indicative of an undesirable mental condition and damaging to the heart. And so with laughter, as with sleep and food and drink, one can have too much of a good thing. See **'fire-sound'**, **heart** and **joy**.

lavage A medical term used to describe the washing or irrigation of a body cavity, such as the stomach or bladder. See **enema**.

law In most countries, there are laws which are designed to protect the health and safety of the community and the interests of those who are engaged in the practice of medicine. In Britain, these laws deal with such matters as the sale and distribution of poisons and narcotics and other dangerous drugs, the pollution levels in drinking water, the notification of certain diseases, the protection of rare and near-extinct plants and animals, safety in the workplace, food hygiene, the qualifications and registration of persons involved in medical practice – physicians, surgeons, pharmacists, midwives, dental surgeons, etc. – restrictions on the uses and dosages of toxic drugs, the registration of births and deaths, and the vending of tobacco and alcoholic drinks. Of course, some of the laws which apply in Britain would not necessarily apply in China, and vice versa. See **drug** and **Medicines Act 1968**.

laxative A medium-strength cathartic to induce evacuation of the bowel. Some laxatives in TCM are infusions or decoctions of the following, taken internally, using the parts and dosages indicated: apricot, *Prunus armeniaca*, kernels, 4–9 g; peach, *Prunus persica*, kernels, 5–9 g; dandelion, *Taraxacum officinale*, all parts, 10–30 g. The fruits of the fig, *Ficus carica*, eaten raw, are effective as a laxative. See **constipation** and **cathartic**.

lead This is a poisonous metal which can damage the brain and nervous system, and is suspected of causing hyperactivity in children. It can be a danger to pregnant women and their unborn babies. In the West, most of the lead which poisons the atmosphere is emitted by motor-car exhausts. Lead poisoning is a problem in any part of the world, including China, where water is supplied through lead pipes, for the lead dissolves in the water – quite readily if it is soft water – and then slowly accumulates in the body until it reaches a dangerous level.

League of Nations In 1931, at Geneva, a conference of the League of Nations set up a committee to review and undertake research into traditional Chinese medicine, and so bring some of its benefits into Western medicine. Time has shown that the two systems can be made to complement each other, and in a way which is beneficial to the peoples of both the West and the East.

lecithin This substance occurs in foods, but it can also be made in the body, where it is contained mainly in the bloodstream and the sheaths of nerves. It was once thought that it reduces cholesterol levels, but recent research has shown that this may not be the case. As a nutrient, it rebuilds damaged cells and tissues, assists the brain in retaining information, and partly inhibits the ageing process by keeping the skin soft and supple. Commercially, it is derived from soya beans, and soya bean products feature prominently in the Chinese diet, for they are known to be highly nutritious.

leech *Hirudo medicinalis* Until quite recent times in the West, this blood-sucking parasitic worm, which is closely related to the earthworm, was used extensively as a device for blood-letting, the theory being that it would remove the poisoned blood which is causative of disease. But the practice was abandoned when it was discovered that leeches can be a source of infection, and that the loss of a large amount of blood is very weakening. Also, from the mouths of leeches comes an anticoagulant, called hirudin, which prevents the blood from clotting, and so it is difficult to stop the bleeding once it has started. The Chinese employ a system of blood-letting which is more hygienic and safer than 'leeching'. See **blood-letting**.

leek *Allium porrum* A close relative of the onion and garlic, and with similar medicinal properties. It can be used as a treatment for age spots. See **complexion**.

legendary emperors Very little is known about the first emperors of China, for they lived at a time when there were few written records, and such records that existed were destroyed on the orders of Qin Shi Huang Di, the first emperor of the Qin dynasty (221–206 BC), and so they are legendary figures and occasional heroes in the remote fabric of China's early history. By tradition, the Xia dynasty (*c.* 2100–1600 BC) is regarded as the first imperial dynasty of China, and Yu the Great, who is credited with harnessing the power of water, is mentioned as its first emperor. But there were other men of great stature on whom the title of emperor was bestowed. One of these was Huang Di, or 'the Yellow Emperor', also called 'the Sovereign Emperor', who made a study of herbal medicines, and whose wife, Lei Zu, is said to have discovered how to cultivate silkworms. Yellow has always been one of the symbols of the emperors of China, and until recent times, no one outside the imperial family was allowed to decorate his property with yellow paint, nor was anyone allowed to erect buildings higher than the imperial palace in Beijing (Peking), for such an action would have been an affront to the Dragon Throne. Another of these legendary emperors was Shen Nong, who introduced agriculture and made a study of medicinal herbs, and tested and recorded their properties. But some sources give the date of Shen Nong's discoveries as being about 3490 BC, and so it could be that he lived in an earlier period, which would indicate that Chinese medicine has been in existence for at least 5000 years. At a much later date, the discoveries, theories and exploits of Huang Di and Shen Nong were described and compiled in book form by some of the eminent scholars of the Han dynasty (206 BC–AD 220). It is interesting to note that discoveries made in recent excavations by archaeologists have indicated that the so-called legendary emperors were real people. See **Yellow Emperor** and **Shen Nong**.

legends The Chinese have many old legends, which is to be expected, for China has a very ancient civilization and its people love and respect traditions. These legends include many references to the dragon, peacock and tortoise, divination, health and medicines, so indicating the importance which the Chinese attach to these matters. Many of these legends and references to them are contained in the 'Book of Records', the historical annals of China. Ko Hung, a Taoist scholar, refers to these legends in the *Nei Pien*, a collection of writings which he compiled. There is mention of medicines made of gold, pearls, jade, verdigris, brown mica, cinnabar, bear's gall, bat's faeces, tiger's bones, silkworms, centipedes, scorpions, beetles and other unusual things. But, since some of these medicines are still in use, one may conclude that these old legends often have a factual basis. See **tea legends** and **Nei Pien**.

leg meridians There are six meridians on each leg, that is, four on the front and two on the back. In order to influence an organ so as to stimulate its activity or block pain, the appropriate points on the meridian to which it relates are influenced by needles, as with acupuncture, or the fingertips, as with acupressure. The organs controlled by the leg meridians are arranged in complementary pairs, so that a solid and yin organ is coupled with a hollow and yang organ: liver with gall-bladder, kidneys with urinary bladder and spleen with stomach. See **meridian**.

LEG MERIDIANS

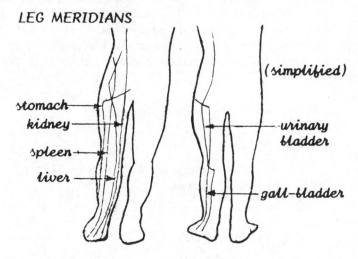

legumes These are such plants as peas, peanuts, lentils, chickpeas, soya beans, mung beans, haricot beans, broad beans and adzuki beans. The seeds are called pulses. They are good sources of protein, calcium, dietary fibre and the vitamins thiamin, riboflavin and niacin. They are an important item of diet in China, where they are regarded as one of the more nutritious and healthier foods. Mung beans and soya beans can be eaten as sprouts, and they are then rich in vitamin C. Some people say that legumes have aphrodisiac properties. Perhaps the simple truth is that weight for weight, they contain more protein than most other vegetables. As a regular item of diet, they help to maintain a good complexion. See **peanut**.

Leibnitz German philosopher and mathematician who drew some of his inspiration in regard to mental activity and binary numbers from Chinese sources. See **I Ching**.

Leishmaniasis A group of infectious diseases of the oriental tropics caused by the protozoan parasite *Leishmania*, which is transmitted by infected sandflies. The symptoms include weakness, fever, anaemia, bleeding, enlargement of the liver and spleen and skin ulcers, which have various common names, such as oriental sore, tropical sore, Baghdad sore, Delhi boil and kala-azar, that are generally determined by the region in which they occur. The treatment is as for debility, anaemia and ulcers. See **ulcer**.

Lei Zu See **legendary emperors**.

lemon The juice of this citrus fruit is used throughout the world as a source of ascorbic acid, or vitamin C. Lemon juice has mildly antiseptic properties, and the Chinese apply it to infected areas on the skin. Lemon juice undergoes unusual chemical changes within the body, as a consequence of which it can sometimes be included in special diets from which citrus fruits are specifically excluded.

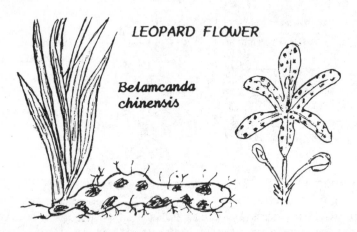

LEOPARD FLOWER

Belamcanda chinensis

leopard flower *Belamcanda chinensis* Also called blackberry lily. Herbal medicine. Distribution: South China, Japan, Korea, Laos, Vietnam. Character: cold, bitter. Affinity: liver, lungs. Effects: antipyretic, antiphlogistic, expectorant, antidote. Symptoms: cough, excess phlegm. Treatments: asthma, bronchitis and inflammation of the respiratory organs. Dosage: 3–5 g. This herb is slightly poisonous, and so, in its usage, one should take into account the terms of the Medicines Act 1968.

leprosy A chronic infectious bacterial disease of the tropics and subtropics which mainly affects the skin and nerves, and which is characterized by red nodules on the skin in the initial stages, thickness and loss of colour of the skin, thickness of the nerves, burning or tingling sensations, loss of the sense of touch, partial paralysis and deformity of the hands and limbs. This condition requires expert medical attention. See **laboratory tests** and **ulcer**.

lesbian A homosexual woman. A lesbian is sometimes defined as a female homosexual, which is hardly a valid definition if a person's sexuality is determined by the sex hormones rather than the genitalia. See **homosexual**.

lesion Local damage due to injury or disease.

lethargy See **lassitude**.

lettuce *Lactuca sativa*. A salad plant used in a Chinese folk remedy to relieve sleeplessness. See **insomnia** and **wild lettuce**.

leucocyte A white blood cell of which there are three main types: granulocytes, lymphocytes and monocytes. They have various functions. The granulocytes, which are distinguished by conspicuous granules in their cytoplasm, can move from the bloodstream into tissues in order to destroy bacterial invaders, and the lymphocytes produce antibodies. See **interferon**.

leucorrhoea An excessive discharge of white mucus from the vagina. A TCM treatment is an infusion, taken internally, of one of the following, using the parts and dosage indicated: knotty yam, *Dioscorea opposita*, tubers, 10–30 g; dodder, *Cirsium japonicum*, seeds, 10–14 g; foxnut, *Euryale ferox*, seeds, 10–28 g; water plantain, *Alisma plantago-aquatica*, tubers, 4–12 g.

leukaemia This is an uncommon type of cancer which causes the leucocytes to increase rapidly but in an immature form. The condition may be acute or chronic. The most common childhood form is acute lymphoblastic leukaemia, whose symptoms, which develop rapidly, are fever, headaches, anaemia and excessive nosebleeds. With adults, there is a loss of energy, appetite and weight, and women may menstruate excessively. This condition requires urgent medical attention. If untreated, it is likely to be fatal. In TCM, the condition is attributed to internal blood and *qi* stagnation, and the treatment is with herbs such as safflower, *Carthamus tinctorius*, and notoginseng, *Panax notoginseng*, which get the blood moving. Acupuncture and massage are also used. But this is hardly the kind of illness which could be expected to respond to do-it-yourself treatments, nor should such treatments be attempted.

libido This term is commonly used to mean 'sexual desire'; but, as used in psychology, the term refers to psychic energy, particularly that associated with sexual motivation. Obviously, the libido is influenced by the general health and mental outlook, together with the accepted standards of social behaviour. Impotence could be regarded as a weakness in the libido, but which might be eradicated by an improvement in health or the use of an aphrodisiac, though Chinese physicians would point out that aphrodisiacs no more cure a weakness of the libido than crutches cure lameness, but a bit of help is sometimes encouraging. See **impotence** and **aphrodisiac**.

lice See **head lice**.

Li Ching Yun This Chinese gentleman, who died in 1133, lived to be 256, which has been confirmed by the Chinese government after a thorough investigation by Chengdu University, although one may wonder how such a claim could be substantiated. The secret of his success has been ascribed to ginseng, *Panax ginseng*, and so, perhaps, the claims made for this popular Chinese medicine are not exaggerated, and there is hope for those who aspire to a long life. See **life-span**.

life This is a term which defies a simple explanation, and the dictionary definition that life is the state of functional activity of an animal or plant does not tell us very much, and yet we need to know much about life if we are to maintain it in a sound condition, which is the purpose of the study of medicine. Certainly, the growth and development of a large and magnificent tree from a tiny seed, or a splendidly beautiful peacock from a seemingly inanimate egg, is really quite remarkable even by the standards of those who are indifferent to the processes of nature, and it cannot be explained in simple terms. The explanations, if we wished to look for them, probably reside somewhere in the study of the substance of viruses, which sometimes exhibit properties which suggest that they are a stage between the living and the non-living – the biologically simple and the chemically complex. The ancient Chinese saw life in all things, as is evidenced by this comment made by one of the contemporaries of the legendary emperor Shen Nong: 'Life is an everlasting flux, and the universe is the outcome of the mutual influence of yin and yang, the recessive and the dominant, the negative and the positive, the female and the male.' The ancient Chinese saw life as a product of the union of male and female, and they saw similar forces at work in other parts of the natural order. The ancient Chinese also valued life, and the thought of death did not please them, and so they made attempts to achieve immortality. Needless to say, they were not successful; but, as they matured as a race, they came to accept a revision in Taoist thinking, which enjoins us to live as healthily as we can, for as long as we can, and as contentedly as we can. Confucius added weight to Taoist thinking by pointing out that rather than hanker after a heaven in the sky, we should concentrate on establishing a heaven on earth for each other, which must surely be the soundest bit of social philosophy. The Chinese physician certainly values life. The sanctity of life is the basis of his code of practice. On the other hand, he also accepts the inevitability of death, for age must make way for youth, but the postponement of death is often possible if sound preventive measures are used, and that is the basis of TCM. See **death** and **immortality**.

life-essence One of the two forms of vital essence. See **jing**.

life-force Vital energy. See **qi**.

life-span Some medical experts are of the opinion that the human life-span could be extended to between 110 and 120 years, and that, at present, longevity is inhibited by the poor quality of our life-style. The kidneys store life-essence and semen-essence, and so, for long life, there needs to be a correct functioning of the kidneys, and many of the Chinese herbal medicines which are inhibitive of the ageing process have an affinity for the kidneys. Premature ageing is due to 'emptiness of the kidney-glands', as a Chinese physician would say. See **ageing**, **youth**, **jing** and **Le Ching Yun**.

ligament A short band of tough and flexible fibrous tissue binding bones together or keeping an organ in place. It is sometimes confused with a tendon. See **tendon**.

ligature A thread of silk, wire, catgut or some other suitable material used in surgery to tie or constrict a blood vessel or some other part of the body. Catgut is made of the intestine of a sheep, horse or ass, and not that of a cat, as is popularly believed. A type of ligature, called a tourniquet, is used all over the world to arrest bleeding in an injured limb. A bandage or something similar is passed around the limb at a point which is nearer to the heart than the point where bleeding is occurring. The bandage is then twisted until the bleeding is staunched by compression. However, the ligature must be loosened every 15–20 minutes. Otherwise, the blood supply will be cut off completely, and the tissues in the limb will be damaged. These days, there is a tendency for first-aiders to be discouraged from using a tourniquet because of the danger that, mistakenly, it might not be loosened periodically. See **cuts** and **laceration**.

light See **survival**.

lily turf *Liriope spicata*. Herbal medicine. Distribution: China, Japan. Parts: tubers. Character: cool, bitter-sweet. Affinity: lungs, heart, stomach. Effects: cardiac refrigerant, stomachic, demulcent, antitussive, galactagogue. Symptoms: irritability, dry coughs, excessive thirst, blood in sputum. Treatments: lung-yin deficiency, dehydration, low lactation. Dosage: 5–9 g. This herb is also called creeping lily turf.

lime *Tilia europea*. This tree is not regarded as one of the usual herbs in TCM, but it does grow in temperate regions throughout the world, and an infusion of its flowers taken internally in a dosage of 3–12 g is effective as a gentle relaxant in the treatment of tension, anxiety, nervous irritability, hypertension and atherosclerosis. It is also considered to be an effective treatment for a hangover.

linctus A syrupy and mucilaginous liquid, and type of demulcent, which relieves coughs by providing a soothing and protective layer in the throat and trachea.

liniment Embrocation. A liquid or paste, usually in an oil base, which is rubbed into the skin as a rubifacient, local anaesthetic or for its soothing effects, and used in the treatment of sprains and aching muscles and joints. The oils of garlic, marigold, almond and chillies are effective as liniments. See **paste**.

Linnaean A term which describes the Latinized binomial nomenclature used in the classification of plants and animals, and which derives from the name of the innovator of this system of classification, the Swedish naturalist Carl von Linné (1707–78), or Carolus Linnaeus, as his name is given in a Latinized form. See **Latin**.

Li of the Iron Crutch One of the Eight Immortals, who were fairylike spirits in Chinese mythology. He is often regarded as the patron and symbol of Chinese pharmacists.

Li Taibo (*c*. 700–62). Also written as Li Tai Po. One of the great Chinese poets of the period of the Tang dynasty (618–907). His works reflect the Chinese respect for nature and wisdom.

liquorice *Glycyrrhiza uralensis* Herbal medicine. Distribution: North China, Mongolia, Siberia. Parts: roots. Character: neutral, sweet. Affinity: all organs and meridians. Effects: antipyretic, analgesic, expectorant, demulcent, antidote, tonic. Symptoms: lack of energy, sore and swollen throat, coughs, abdominal pains. Treatments: abscesses, asthma, blood deficiency, empty condition of spleen and stomach, fungus poisoning, peptic

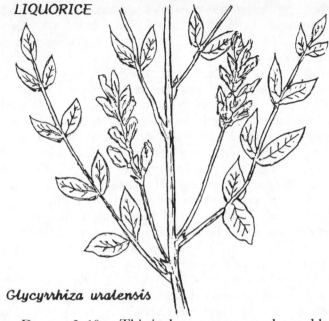

LIQUORICE

Glycyrrhiza uralensis

ulcers. Dosage: 2–10 g. This is the most commonly used herb in TCM, and it enters into many prescriptions, benefiting all organs, imparting a pleasant taste, and functioning as a buffer in potent tonic medicines. But it should not be used in cases where there is hypertension. There is a European species of liquorice, *Glycyrrhiza glabra*, which has similar properties, and it is the one that will be used in the West. It has been described as a 'magic root' which is eminently suitable for the treatment of hepatitis, jaundice, nausea, depression, constipation and muscular tension. It must NOT be confused with wood liquorice, *Polypodium vulgare*, which is a fern and an entirely different species, though its bitter-tasting rhizome does have the smell of liquorice. It is used as a strong purgative.

Li Shizhen One of the great Chinese physicians of the period of the Ming dynasty. See **Ben Cao Gang Mu**.

li shou A system of hand-swinging exercises which builds up physical strength and resistance to disease. It may also be used therapeutically to treat certain chronic diseases, such as hypertension, bronchitis, depression and anxiety, and it is suitable for the elderly and those who are physically weak. The exercises are intended to be gentle, and so their object is defeated if too much force or too many swings are used. In fact, overdoing these exercises can cause dizziness, nausea, chest pains or extreme fatigue. In doing these exercises, there must also be some movement of the legs and at the waist. The body must not be kept rigid. The *li shou* exercises are fully explained in the *Chinese Exercise Manual*.

listening One of the basic techniques employed by a Chinese physician in making a diagnosis. See **hearing**.

listeria A bacterium occurring in soil, water and the alimentary canal of animals, and which enters the human body via unwashed vegetables, certain soft cheeses and stale food. It causes the condition called listeriosis, which generally affects only those with a lowered immunity, such as babies, pregnant women, the elderly and the sick, particularly those with cancer or AIDS. It can lead to meningitis or a miscarriage. The symptoms are flu-like, with dizziness and a high temperature. There is likely to be a higher incidence of listeria where processed and pre-packaged foods are improperly prepared. But there need be no problems if the rules of food hygiene are strictly observed and one is in a sound state of health. There is much to be said for the Chinese attitude towards the preparation of meals, which is that the ingredients should be fresh and adequately cooked.

litter Empty food cans and cartons, discarded wrappings and other forms of litter provide excellent breeding grounds for micro-organisms and insects and encourage rodents, and so will lead to the spread of diseases unless they are properly disposed of. China does not have a 'waste economy', and the Chinese are not very enthusiastic about preserved foodstuffs, and so litter is less of a problem in China than it is in the West. See **food hygiene**.

Liu Ching A seventh-century Chinese physician who made an important pronouncement about the regulation of sexual activity. See **essence**.

liu fu This is a Chinese term meaning 'hollow organs', or 'bladder organs', which TCM designates as the gall-bladder, stomach, small intestine, large intestine, bladder and triple-warmer. The triple-warmer, or triple-heater, for which the Chinese name is *san jiao*, meaning 'three-points', is made up of the openings into the stomach, small intestine and bladder, and is not an organ in the Western sense of the term, though it is certainly vital to the bodily functions, for it deals with the passage of food and fluid. Obviously, the name *triple-warmer*, derives from the fact that the contents of the stomach, small intestine and bladder are warm. The triple-warmer has more significance in acupuncture treat-ments than it has in herbal therapy. The hollow organs are yang, and each is paired with one of the solid organs, which are yin: the gall-bladder and liver, small intestine and heart, stomach and spleen, large intestine and lungs, and bladder and kidneys. Illnesses which affect a solid organ will generally affect its corresponding hollow organ. Likewise, those herbal medicines which have an affinity for a solid organ will generally have an affinity for its corresponding hollow organ. Each solid organ and its corresponding hollow organ are associated with the same element. See **herbal prescriptions** and **vital organs**.

liver The liver, which is yin, is one of the *wu zang*, or solid organs of the body. Its element is wood, and the hollow organ with which it is paired is the gall-bladder, which is yang. Obviously, the liver operates in conjunction with the gall-bladder, which stores the bile made by the liver. The liver also breaks down and re-synthesizes proteins, neutralizes toxins and stores glycogen, iron, copper and vitamins. The traditional associations of the liver in climate, astrology, emotions, etc., are listed under **element**. If the heart is the 'emperor' of the body, the liver is its 'commander-in-chief', for it both stores and maintains the flow of blood and *qi*, and blood diseases and defects need to be treated via the liver. It is the centre of the metabolism, playing a great part in health and longevity, a view with which most Western physicians would probably agree. According to Chinese tradition, the liver houses the soul, and so there is a connection between the liver and the heart, for the latter houses the spirit. However, in Chinese philosophy, *soul* and *spirit* are symbolic terms, and they do not have the same significance as they have in the religions of the West. The liver is related to the heart by the mother-and-son rule: fire, the heart element, is son to wood, the liver element, for wood generates fire. Disharmony in the liver, which is called stagnant liver-*qi*, causes depression, anxiety, anger, sleeplessness, headaches, dizziness and even suicidal tendencies. In the West, a person who is irritable and not his usual self is said to be liverish. Liver-*qi* may assist the functions of the stomach and spleen; on the other hand, it may move in the wrong direction, thereby damaging the spleen and stomach, which can cause abdominal pain, nausea, eructation and diarrhoea. This view roughly corresponds with medical opinion in the West. Bile, made in the liver and reaching the stomach via the gall-bladder, is necessary to the digestive process in that it emulsifies fats, but an excess causes sickness, which is sometimes indicated by jaundice. The liver is sensitive to psychosomatic injury, and it may be damaged by prolonged bouts of anger or depression, or the excitability –

or lack of it – which Chinese physicians describe as an inner-wind condition. The health of the liver is reflected in the eyes, muscles and nails. Stiff or aching joints and muscles, fragile and brittle finger-nails and toe-nails, itching and dry or sore eyes are attributed to liver weakness. The functions of the liver are many, and it does seem rather surprising that according to TCM, the liver, among its many functions, converts *jin ye*, or vital fluid, into the tears which fall from the eye. But, perhaps, here there is a mistaken association of ideas based on the principle that people are sad when they have a liver disorder, and sadness is sometimes manifested by a copious flow of tears. The ailments and other problems associated with a defective liver include premenstrual tension, obesity, gastric ulcers, stiff joints, cramp, eye weaknesses, depression and herpes. Herbal medicines commonly used in the treatment of liver conditions are Chinese gentian, *Gentiana scabra*, Chinese angelica, *Angelica sinensis*, and white peony, *Paeonia lactiflora*. In acupuncture, the function of the liver is regulated, via the meridians, by the areas on the side of the head, the breasts and genitals. See **'liver-fire'** and **solid organs**.

'liver-fire' A Chinese term meaning 'anger'. See **anger** and **liver-qi**.

liver-qi According to TCM, an excess of blood causes anger, or 'liver-fire', which, in turn, weakens the blood and liver, so causing an increase in liver-*qi*, which further weakens the blood and liver. Unless self-control is exercised, the liver-*qi* and anger increase so much that the liver is severely damaged. See **anger**.

liver sedation In TCM, many serious nervous disorders are thought to be due to liver dysfunction, which is manifested as ascending liver-yang, or liver-wind, of which the symptoms are blurred vision, feverishness, excitability, convulsions, dizziness, ill temper and delirium. There are sedative medicines which act specifically on the liver, so reducing the liver-wind, or nervous energy. Where there is a blood deficiency, warm liver sedatives should be used. They could include centipede, *Scolopendra subspinipes*, and *tian ma*, *Gastrodia elata*. Where there is a weak spleen and chronic spasms, cold and cool liver sedatives should be avoided. They include abalone, *Haliotis gigantea*, antelope horn, *Saiga tatarica*, and scorpion, *Buthus martensi*. But most of these medicines are poisonous, and so they should not be used without proper medical supervision. Furthermore, some of them would not meet with the approval of the medical authorities of the West. See **liver** and **sedative**.

liver-stagnation A term used in TCM to describe sluggishness of the blood and *qi* in the liver, and which is the cause of hepatitis, feverishness, irritability, depression, anxiety, sleeplessness, headaches, dizziness and reckless behaviour, which the Chinese describe as *gan ho*, meaning 'ill-considered actions'. See **liver** and **liver sedation**.

liver-wind A term used in TCM to describe the nervous excitation associated with liver dysfunction. See **liver sedation**.

local anaesthetic See **anaesthesia, Guan Yu** and **acupuncture treatments**.

lockjaw See **tetanus**.

loco weed See **jimson weed**.

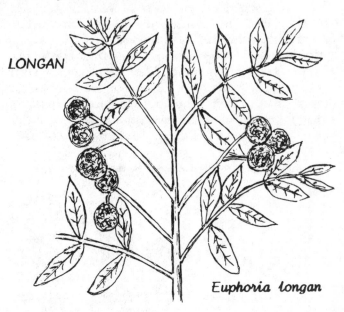

LONGAN

Euphoria longan

longan *Euphoria longan* Herbal medicine. Distribution: South China, Japan. Parts: flesh of fruits. Character: warm, sweet. Affinity: heart, spleen. Effects: cardiotonic, blood tonic, digestive, sedative. Symptoms: insomnia, anaemia, weakness, fatigue. Treatments: anaemia, weakness of heart and spleen, premature greying, amnesia. Dosage: 10–14 g. Dried longans are valued as both a food and a medicine, and they are consumed to nourish the nerves, as a tonic for the blood, to reinforce the body in a run-down condition, and to combat sleeplessness and premature ageing. They are of value to a mother during the postnatal period. Longan and rice porridge is a remedy for elderly people and invalids who are weak and do not sleep well. A powder made by grinding the kernels can be applied as a styptic to sores, abscesses and small wounds.

longevity In ancient times, the Chinese emperors sought immortality. In this, they were not successful, but their physicians and other advisers did discover that a long life of youthful vigour could be achieved by a sound diet, physical and breathing exercises, moderate habits, including regulated sexual activity, attention to personal hygiene, and health foods and medicines which inhibit the ageing process. Coriander, *Coriandrum sativum*, ginseng, *Panax ginseng*, wolfberry, *Lycium chinense*, garlic, *Allium sativum*, and red tea fungus are considered to be helpful in this respect. Longan, *Euphoria longan*, and *han lian cao*, *Eclipta prostrata*, combat premature greying. See **immortality**, **life-span**, **ageing-inhibitor** and **essence**.

long-sightedness Hypermetropia. See **optical defects**.

long yam *Dioscorea hypoglauca* Herbal medicine. Distribution: Central China. Parts: tubers. Character: neutral, bitter. Affinity: stomach, liver. Effects: diuretic, eliminative. Symptoms: stiff and painful joints, muscles, knees and back, leucorrhoea, cloudy urine. Treatments: wind-damp conditions, urethritis. Dosage: 9–14 g.

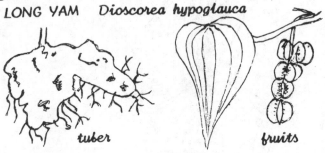

LONG YAM *Dioscorea hypoglauca*

tuber   fruits

loquat *Eriobotrya japonica* Also called the Japanese medlar. Herbal medicine. Distribution: South China, Japan, Europe. Parts: leaves. Character: neutral, bitter. Affinity: stomach, lungs. Effects: expectorant, antitussive, antiemetic. Symptoms: nausea, vomiting, thirst, eructation, coughs. Treatments: difficult breathing, heat excess in lungs. Dosage: 8–14 g.

loss of appetite Anorexia. A decoction of 3–5 fruits of Chinese jujube, *Ziziphus jujuba*, is effective as a nutrient where loss of appetite is due to debility or fatigue. See **appetite**, **digestive** and **anorexia nervosa**.

loss of memory Amnesia. A decoction of 8–14 g dried fruits of longan, *Euphoria longan*, or 8–14 g leaves of horny goat weed,

Epimedium sagittatum, is helpful where this condition is no more than the absent-mindedness associated with age or fatigue. Severe amnesia may be associated with dementia, and will require professional medical treatment. See **amnesia**.

lotus *Nelembo nucifera* Herbal medicine. Distribution: Asia, Australia. Parts: leaves. Character: neutral, bitter. Affinity: liver, stomach, spleen. Effects: antipyretic, refrigerant. Symptoms: headache, thirst, heaviness in chest, scanty and cloudy urine. Treatments: summer-heat ailments. Dosage: 10–15 g. Parts: seeds. Character: neutral, bitter. Affinity: stomach, spleen. Effects: sedative, astringent. Symptoms: sleeplessness, diarrhoea. Treatments: spermatorrhoea. Dosage: 1–5 g. The stamens are used as a treatment for premature ejaculation.

lotus seed sprouts An infusion of lotus seed sprouts has a cooling and sedative effect, and is of particular value as a mild cardiotonic.

love See **lust**.

lu chong A stag's genital organs, that is, its penis and testicles. For medicinal purposes, the fat and meat are removed, and the residue is wind dried. This medicine is highly valued for its efficacy as a treatment for male impotency and female infertility. About 50 g of the dried organs are steamed with chicken and ginger and other herbs, and then consumed as a food. But the Chinese always take this medicine under proper medical supervision, and it is avoided by those people who have high blood pressure, impaired digestion, a cold or a fever. But one would doubt if, despite its unquestionable benefits, many people in the West would welcome the macerated penis and testicles of a deer as an item of diet.

lumbago A form of fibrosis which affects the muscles and tendons in the lumbar, or lower, region of the back, producing painful swellings in the tendon sheaths. In the West, bed-rest, heat treatment and massage have been found to be generally effective as a means of alleviating this condition. But, if it persists, medical advice should be sought. In TCM, the treatments are acupuncture, manipulation and a tincture of herbs to relieve the pain. Two traditional Chinese remedies are wolfberry wine, which is strongly alcoholic, and 4–10 g fruits of the hawthorn, *Crataegus pinnatifida*, administered in a soup. The Chinese will use a species of hawthorn that is indigenous to China and Japan, and therefore readily available to them. But *Crataegus monogyna*, a species that is native to Europe, is equally as effective. See **wolfberry wine**.

'lump in the throat' See **globus hystericus**.

lumps Swellings and lumps sometimes occur in the body, and for a wide variety of reasons. Generally, there is no cause for alarm, for a swelling is often nature's way of dealing with a localized infection or a small injury in the body. On the other hand, the sudden appearance of a lump can have a serious underlying cause. A lump in the breast, for example, could be indicative of a malignant growth. Therefore, where there is any doubt, medical advice should be sought. But, even with these more serious conditions, there need be no cause for alarm if treatment is obtained without delay. Many of the lumps which occur in the body, and whatever their immediate causes, are due to the way in which we misuse our bodies. Heavy punches to the body, as occur in boxing and wrestling, kicks to the legs, as occur in football and hockey, and the fondling of breasts, which is sometimes regarded as one of the joys of sex, are effective ways of producing lumps which, after many years of latent development, could do irreparable damage in later life. A traditional Chinese remedy for non-malignant lumps, especially those associated with breast tension, is to steep 250 g fruits of the hawthorn, *Crataegus pinnatifida* or *Crataegus monogyna*, in 1 litre red wine for a week, and then to drink a little, say 30 ml, each day.

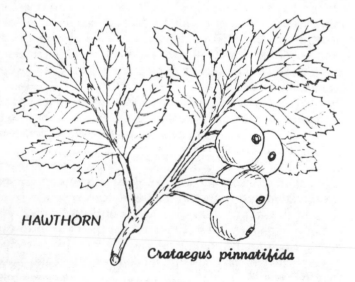

HAWTHORN

Crataegus pinnatifida

lung-qi See **qi**.

lungs The lungs, which are yin, are one of the *wu zang*, or solid organs of the body. Their element is metal, and the hollow organ with which they are linked is the large intestine. The relationship between these two organs is that they are both responsible for the removal of waste. Diseases of the lungs, such as bronchitis, pneumonia and influenza, are accompanied by constipation, which is a condition of the large intestine. The traditional associations of the lungs in climate, astrology, emotions, etc., are listed under **element**. The lungs control breathing, that is, the intake of air, moisture and *qi*, which they distribute throughout the body, and so affect the skin and hair and strengthen the joints and muscles, and transmit waste to the kidneys to form urine, which is discharged from the body via the bladder. According to tradition, the lungs house the animal-soul, which enters the embryo at the very moment when conception occurs. If lung-*qi* takes the wrong direction, the consequences are coughing, sneezing, swollen eyes, influenza and tonsillitis. If the lungs are strong, the skin is also strong, and so its pores are able to expel waste and excess coldness from the body. During very cold weather, the Chinese take ginger or spring onion tea, which encourages the pores to open, and then the lungs are more able to expel coldness from the body. The lungs are associated with the emotion of anxiety, which can injure the lungs if it is in excess. Some common symptoms of anxiety are shallow and irregular breathing and holding the breath. The large intestine, which is the lungs' 'paired organ', is also affected by anxiety, of which diarrhoea is a symptom. The conditions associated with malfunctions of the lungs include sneezing, colds, influenza, hay fever, asthma, bronchitis, nephritis and oedema. If the lungs cannot deal with excess water, the physician will prescribe a diuretic. TCM herbal remedies commonly used in the treatment of lung conditions are skullcap, *Scutellaria baicalensis*, mulberry, *Morus alba*, and fennel, *Foeniculum vulgare*. See **solid organs** and **intestine**.

Lunyu Analects. A collection of the sayings of Confucius, and which should be studied by those who realize that a sound state of health derives in no small measure from moderate habits and social harmony.

lust The Chinese are keenly aware of the distinction between love and lust. Their attitude here draws its inspiration and authority from the teachings of Confucianism and Taoism. Confucius pointed out that sex is a healthy activity providing that it is pursued within the framework of a caring and loyal relationship, and without the treachery, selfishness and immodceracy which are so destructive of social harmony. Lao Zi taught that sex should be pursued as nature intended, and not allied to conduct which can lead to the transmission of disease, abuse of the genital organs, unwanted children and sickness of both mind and body. Thus, despite the Western influences, there is still a tendency for the young Chinese to pursue their courtship in a romantic and unspeedy manner with coitus being the least consideration, and on the principle that with sex, as with most pleasures, more is gained from the anticipation than from the realization. In China, arranged marriages are still fashionable, but the marital arrangements are not made in a cold-blooded way. The parents concerned, who have the benefits of the wisdom that comes with age, ensure that the young man and girl concerned are compatible socially and by temperament, and some regard is paid to hereditary defects and diseases and other matters of health. The outcome of this approach is successful and happy families, together with individuals who are in a sound state of health and have complete serenity of mind. To destroy this satisfactory *status quo* by acts of lust would be foolish in the extreme. Lust may bring some immediate carnal pleasure; but, in the long term, it can only bring ill health, a short life and an insecure state of mind. And so, for the Chinese, who value health above all else, the difference between love and lust is the difference between health and ill health. See **sex**.

Lu Yu See **Cha Ching**.

lye water See **gripe water**.

lymph A colourless alkaline fluid which occurs in all the tissues and organs of the body. It is similar to blood in its composition but it contains no erythrocytes, or red corpuscles. It is what Chinese physicians describe as *jin ye*, or 'fluid', though their notions about its origins, structure and functions are somewhat different from those of the physicians of the West. See **jin ye** and **lymphatic system**.

lymphatic system This is a network of thin vessels which carry lymph to all parts of the body, and which drain into large veins in the neck. At the points where they meet, there are lymph glands, or nodes, consisting of fibrous tissue, which act as filters to remove bacteria and other foreign bodies, and so assist in preventing the spread of infection throughout the body. These glands also produce lymphocytes and antibodies. A virus infection of the lymph glands causes glandular fever, or infectious mononucleosis. See **lymph** and **infectious mononucleosis**.

lymph glands A traditional Chinese health food to strengthen the lymph glands is to steam together, for 15–20 minutes, 250 g shredded or sliced lean chicken, 60 g chopped dried mushrooms, 30 g chopped dates, 2 chopped spring onions and 2 g ground ginger, together with a little salt, white sugar, soy sauce, rice wine and sesame oil. It can be eaten along with a dish of boiled rice. See **lymphatic system** and **infectious mononucleosis**.

lymph node See **lymphatic system**.

lymphocyte See **leucocyte** and **immune system**.

M

maceration See **essential oil**.

macrobiotics A dietary system of treatment, initiated by Sagen Ishizuka, a Japanese physician, towards the end of the nineteenth century, and later developed by George Ohsawa, a Japanese writer, by which common health problems can be cured or prevented by a food intake of wholegrain cereals, fruit and vegetables, and without white rice, sugar and meat products. It is a strictly vegetarian diet, but it is also one that is balanced on the Chinese yin-yang principle of complementary opposites, and so a person's food intake is arranged in a way that best suits his condition. Thus, a yin person, who is calm, relaxed, peaceful, thoughtful, shy and introverted, and may also be subject to lethargy and depression, will need a diet in which yang foods are predominant. Some moderate yang foods are brown rice, wholegrain bread and flour, root vegetables, pulses, fish, shellfish and cream cheese. A yang person, who is active, energetic, exuberant, headstrong, outgoing and extroverted, and may also be subject to tension and ill temper, will need a diet in which yin foods are predominant. Some moderate yin foods are fruit, leafy green vegetables, nuts and seeds. Foods which are extremely yang, such as meat, chicken, cheese and eggs, and foods which are extremely yin, such as sugar, cakes, confectionery, spices, tea, coffee and alcohol, are avoided altogether. If this diet is to be fully effective, it must be supported by physical exercises, and allowances need to be made for climatic conditions. Thus, yang foods, which are warming, are more suitable for cold weather; and yin foods, which are cooling, are more suitable for hot weather. Those Japanese who practise macrobiotics generally include seaweed in their diet, for it improves the flavour and nutritional value of other foods. The macrobiotic diet is similar to the normal Chinese diet, which is essentially vegetarian and with emphasis on the balance between *fan* and *cai*, but it would not meet with the full approval of Chinese physicians, for they recognize the need for the inclusion of a small amount of fish,

meat and eggs in the diet. See **classification of foods**.
macrophage See **interferon**.
'mad-cow disease' See **bovine spongiform encephalopathy**.
magnesium See **mineral**.
magnetite Magnetic iron oxide. (Fe_3O_4). Also called lodestone because of its magnetic properties. Medicine. Distribution: global. Parts: crushed ore. Character: cold, pungent. Affinity: kidneys, liver. Effects: sedative, tonic. Symptoms: palpitation, insomnia, hysteria, dizziness, tinnitis, deafness. Treatments: hypertension, trauma, anaemia, weak kidneys, prolapse of the rectum.

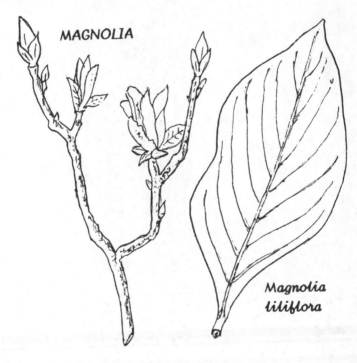

MAGNOLIA

Magnolia liliflora

magnolia *Magnolia liliflora* Herbal medicine. Distribution: China, Japan, North America. Parts: floral buds. Character: warm, acrid. Affinity: stomach, lungs. Effects: analgesic, decongestant. Symptoms: sneezing, itchy or blocked nose. Treatments: all nose conditions, sinusitis, catarrh. Dosage: 4–8 g. Magnolia is not compatible with liquorice, *Glycyrrhiza uralensis* or *Glycyrrhiza glabra*, or astralagus, *Astralagus membranaceus*. Another species of magnolia, *Magnolia officinalis*, with different medicinal properties is also commonly used in TCM.

ma huang Joint fir, *Ephedra sinica*. See **ephedrine** and **joint fir**.

maize *Zea mays* Also called Indian corn or sweet corn. Herbal medicine. Distribution: China, North America. Parts: pistils and stamens of the young flowers, silk from the mature ears. Character: neutral, sweet. Affinity: kidneys, bladder. Effects: diuretic, antidote. Symptoms: difficult or painful urination, swellings, jaundice. Treatments: hepatitis, hypertension, gallstones. Dosage: 15–30 g.

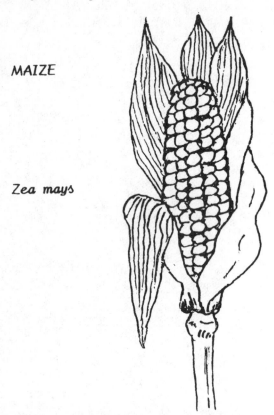

MAIZE

Zea mays

malaria A disease caused by the malarial parasite, *Plasmodium vivax*, an amoeba-like protozoon. It has a complicated life cycle, spending part of its life in the female of a species of mosquito, *Anopheles gambiae*, and part in the blood and liver of a human. It feeds on red blood corpuscles, and the toxins so produced cause a fever. The male mosquito plays no part in the transmission of malaria. It feeds on plant juices. In those regions where malaria is endemic, people adopt various measures to avoid being bitten by mosquitoes. They include wearing long-sleeved shirts and long trousers and using insect repellents. To some extent, mosquitoes are controlled by spraying their breeding grounds with insecticides, and by spraying oil on the surface of the water containing their larvae. In the West, the remedies are quinine, a natural medicine obtained from cinchona bark, and mepacrine and paludrine, which are synthetic medicines. In TCM, the treatment is an infusion or decoction taken internally of 5–10 g leaves and stems of sweet wormwood, *Artemisia annua*, or 4–9 g nuts of betel palm, *Areca catechu*. Blackwater fever is a severe but rare complication of malaria. It damages the kidneys and discolours the urine.

male fern See **guan zhong**.

male semen-essence See **jing**.

malfeisan A herbal anaesthetic which was once used by Hua Tuo (141–208), an eminent physician and surgeon, in performing abdominal operations and removing tumours. See **Hua Tuo**.

malfunction Abnormal and impaired functioning of an organ. See **dysfunction**.

malignant This term describes a severe illness which is progressive or recurring. It is used particularly in relation to growths. See **tumour**.

malignant growth An abnormal growth of cells in a tissue, and which will be disseminated throughout the body. See **cancer**, **tumour** and **lumps**.

malnutrition A condition in which the body either lacks food or is not being provided with nutrients in the proportions necessary for health. Providing there is no disease or defect to inhibit the normal processes of digestion, assimilation and metabolism, there are some health foods which will hasten the recuperative process: honey, maltose, soya bean products, brown rice, bitter gourd, longans, figs, knotty yam, silver wood ears, sesame seeds and oil, winter mushrooms, white rice porridge, pig's feet, citrus fruits, leafy green vegetables, sunflower seeds, chicken and oily fish. See **facai**.

maltase See **maltose**.

maltose As used in TCM, maltose is the malt extract, sticky and brown, a type of sugar but less sweet than cane sugar, obtained from sprouted wheat or barley, maize or sweet potatoes. It is formed by the action of diastase, an enzyme contained in seedlings, which converts starch into sugar. It is easy to digest and does not aggravate the stomach. This explains why the Chinese prefer bean sprouts to ordinary beans as an item of diet.

A small amount of maltose occurs naturally in honey. Maltose is used as a binder in making pills. The enzyme ptyalin, in the mouth, and the enzyme amylase, in the small intestine, convert starch into maltose. In turn, the enzyme maltase, in the small intestine, converts maltose into glucose, which is easily assimilated by the small intestine. See **sugar**.

malt vinegar See **vinegar**.

mammary glands The correct medical term for the breasts, which are the milk-secreting organs in mammals. See **mastitis**, **lactation** and **lumps**.

Manchu See **Qing dynasty**.

Mandarin In the old imperial China, prior to the establishment of the Chinese republic, a mandarin was one of nine grades of important government officials. Their title became the name of the kind of Chinese language they spoke, which was the lingua franca of the officials and educated classes. These days, Mandarin, together with English as the second language, is taught in all the schools in China. Obviously, a standard form of language is of considerable benefit in a country in which there are over a hundred languages and dialects. The Chinese words absorbed into the English language, some of which are medical terms, have been derived from more than one of the languages of China. For example, *char*, meaning 'tea', derives from the Mandarin word *cha*, and *tay*, or *tey*, a seventeenth-century English word, meaning 'tea', derives from the Fujianese word *t'e*.

mandarin orange *Citrus reticulata* Herbal medicine. Distribution: South China, Taiwan, Vietnam. Parts: peel. Character: warm, pungent-bitter. Affinity: lungs, spleen, stomach. Effects: digestive, stomachic, antitussive, expectorant, antiemetic, astringent. Symptoms: nausea, eructation, vomiting, cough, mucus discharge. Treatments: abdominal pain and distension, dyspepsia, flatulence. Dosage: 3–7 g. Chinese physicians attribute the above conditions to stagnant-*qi* in the stomach and lungs. The peel contains vitamins A and C and most of those in the B-complex. Chewing the pith is considered to be a most effective treatment for indigestion. The seeds are used as an analgesic.

manic-depression Alternating periods of elation and depression. See **mental illness**.

manipulative techniques Chinese physicians employ a wide range of manipulative techniques. They may be used in conjunction with poultices, compresses, ointments, liniments and the medications which are taken orally. With some illnesses, treatments by these manipulative techniques are often just as effective, and sometimes more effective than those achieved by herbal medicines, and they are one of the main features of TCM. One of the curious aspects of medical practice in the West is the conviction held by some patients that they are not being properly treated unless the doctor provides a prescription for a bottle of medicine or a packet of pills, when, in fact, they might benefit more from a manipulative treatment or a few words of timely advice. See **medicine**, **placebo** and **external therapy**.

Marco Polo Cultural exchange, including medical knowledge, between China and the West began when the Venetian explorer Marco Polo (1254–1324) returned from China, in 1295, after a journey which had taken him three-and-a-half years. He had been in China for about 20 years, first as an honoured guest and court attendant, and then as an official of the Kublai Khan, the Mogul emperor of China. He learned some of the languages of China, and was appointed as a governor of a city. When in Genoa, he related his experiences to a writer he had met, Rusticano of Pisa, who wrote about them under the title *The Adventures of Marco Polo*. This is fascinating reading, the first really great story of exploration, and one of the first recorded accounts of a cultural exchange between nations, and with mutual benefits of a positive kind, as was to be proved. Pasta products, such as spaghetti, macaroni and lasagne, and rice dishes, such as risotto, originated in Italy as a consequence of information brought back from China by Marco Polo. It is not difficult to perceive that the transition from the *miensien*, or threadlike wheat noodles, of China to the noodles and spaghetti of Italy was not a mere coincidence. Inspired by the example set by Marco Polo, other Venetian adventurers visited China, taking Western knowledge of science, technology and medicine to the court of the Ming emperors. At the same time, the pharmacopoeia of Chinese medicine was made available to the people of the West, and such herbs as gentian, rhubarb, liquorice, ginger and monkshood entered into European pharmacology. Medical books in European languages were translated into Chinese, and vice versa.

marigold *Calendula officinalis* Herbal medicine. Distribution: Mediterranean lands, but naturalized in temperate regions throughout the world. Parts: flowers. Character: warm, bitter. Affinity: stomach, spleen. Effects: astringent, antipyretic, antispasmodic, heals damaged tissue. Symptoms: bruises, cuts, scratches, burns, sore throat. Treatments: as a wet compress or as an ointment to treat ulcerated tissues or similar conditions, burns, varicose veins, and fissures, haemorrhoids, chilblains and insect stings. As an infusion, used as a mouthwash and gargle, to treat gum disease, mouth ulcers and throat infections, or, used as an eyewash, to treat tired or sore eyes. Dosage: 3–12 g. A hot infusion sipped slowly is soothing and relaxing and will sweat out a cold or influenza. It is also a treatment for glandular fever, measles and age spots.

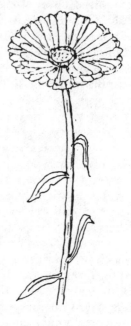

MARIGOLD

Calendula officinalis

marriage The Chinese attitude towards marriage is essentially practical. They do not regard it as a sacred institution but as a convenient partnership, sometimes regulated by law, and sometimes not, which is designed to prevent the transmission of diseases and hereditary defects, provide affection and security for children, guard against the possibility of unwanted children, ensure a fair and sensible division of labour and sharing of responsibility in the home, and provide for the sexual needs of the partners, and so protect the health and well-being of both society and the individual. The Chinese regard sex as being not only normal and healthy but also very necessary for a sound state of health. However, they also reecognize that sexual activity can have disastrous effects if it is conducted in an irresponsible manner. The Chinese eagerness to avoid disruptive influences in the family that could create disharmony in society explains their preference for arranged marriages. There is a far lower divorce rate in China than in the West, which suggests that arranged marriages are conducive to loyalty and trust. The Chinese characteristics of patience, willingness to compromise and respect for traditional values also play a part. It must be the case that the stress and anxiety associated with marital problems is not good for the mental health. See **hereditary defects**, **lust** and **sex**.

marrow The soft, waxlike red or yellow substance in the cavities of bones. The red marrow is responsible for the formation of red blood corpuscles. See **bones** and **jin ye**.

marsh woundwort See **woundwort**.

martial arts One may wonder why people so peace loving and sober minded as the Chinese should indulge in the martial arts, which, by definition, are warlike pursuits. The simple truth is that, though they may occasionally employ these skills in self-defence, they generally do not use them for purposes of aggressive combat, but only as physical and meditative exercises, which provide pleasure and are also an aid to health, and a healthy diet in particular. Many of the exercises described in the *Chinese Exercise Manual* are components of the martial arts. One finds that most Chinese, even the very young and the very elderly, participate in the martial arts. These activities are an essential component of the keep-fit regimen which the Chinese follow in order to achieve a long life of youthful vigour. Despite the blood-curdling yells and the rapidity of the movements involved, the martial arts are essentially gentle sports in which all the movements are governed and patterned by certain rules and laid-down procedures. Of course, this has not always been the case, for the martial arts were evolved in an age when warfare was commonplace, and it was the exponent's purpose to put his enemy out of action without too much effort on his own part, and even with little or no injury to his enemy, for a badly injured prisoner of war was not likely to be of much use as a slave. There are hundreds of different systems of the martial arts, or kungfu, as they are popularly known in the West, each with its own style and traditions, but all have certain features in common. *Kungfu* is a Chinese term which means 'skill produced by training', and it is as much applicable to carpentry, needlework or any other skilled activity as it is to the martial arts; but it is used more specifically to denote the skills of the martial arts, though *wushu* is the more precise term. To the Westerner, the various systems of kungfu appear to be strange combinations of wrestling and boxing, together with the occasional use of weapons. The people in the north of China often live in mountainous regions, and so they are taller in stature and often have longer legs than the people of the south, which explains why the exponents of the so-called northern styles of kungfu use their feet as much as their hands when engaged in combat. They 'box with their feet', as we might say. The meditative aspect of any of the kungfu systems is good for the mental health in that it relieves tension and anxiety and encourages people to think carefully in dealing with problems and making decisions. The various systems of kungfu are classified as styles: northern or southern, hard or soft, and external or internal. Exponents of the hard styles use their own strength directly, and as this is clearly seen in their techniques, their styles are said to be external, that is, not hidden. By contrast, the exponents of the soft styles, using will-power and skill, yield to their opponents' strength but turn it to their own advantage, which is not clearly seen, so their styles are said to be internal, or hidden. Three popular hard styles are *wing-chun*, *tang-lang* and *Shaolin*. Three popular soft styles are *hsing-1*, *pa kua* and *tai chi chuan*. The traditions and meditative aspects of the hard styles are firmly rooted in the tenets of Buddhism. The soft styles are based on the teachings of Taoism. The system of kungfu that is most suitable for elderly people, and which is commonly used for remedial purposes, is *tai chi chuan*. The Japanese forms of the martial arts are called *karate*. They are more violently aggressive than the Chinese forms, from which they have been developed. See **exercise** and **Chinese Exercise Manual**.

massage There are many systems of massage, which include aromatherapy, reflexology and shiatsu; but, in recent years, there has been a tendency for them to borrow from each other. The orthodox system of massage as used in the West relaxes, stimulates and invigorates the mind and body, relieving tension and depression, improving circulation and treating heart disorders, hypertension, hyperactivity, migraine, insomnia and sinusitis. It achieves these objects mainly by toning the blood, nerves and muscles, and aiding the body to assimilate food and eliminate waste products. It is of particular benefit to athletes and others involved in strenuous physical activity, for it helps to 'draw off' those toxic wastes which cause stiffness of the muscles. However, massage must not be applied to those persons suffering from thrombosis, varicose veins, phlebitis or a fever. In fact, where a person has any kind of severe illness, it is always as

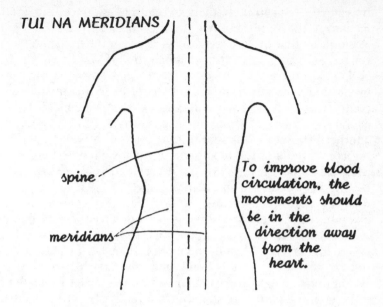

TUI NA MERIDIANS

spine

meridians

To improve blood circulation, the movements should be in the direction away from the heart.

well to obtain professional medical advice before applying massage. The four basic techniques of movement involved in orthodox massage are effleurage, friction, petrisage and percussion. Effleurage is a stroking movement, which is either light or deep. See **effleurage**. Friction, or pressure, and petrisage, or kneading, are generally used in combination, and are then known as compression. See **compression**. Percussion is a drumming motion. See **percussion**. *Tui na*, or Chinese massage, produces benefits similar to those of the systems of the West, but the techniques are simpler and more direct. They clear the meridians of waste and blockages, stimulate circulation of the blood and *qi*, loosen stiff joints and muscles, and increase energy and resistance to disease. It is mainly used, often in combination with acupuncture or acupressure, to treat sprained joints, pulled tendons, rheumatism, arthritis, sciatica, paralysis and prolapse of the internal organs, but it is sometimes used quite successfully to treat a wide variety of other conditions, which include asthma, catarrh, cramp, insomnia, migraine, nervous disorders, palpitations, premenstrual tension, shock, fatigue and bursitis. With the usual technique, the ball of the thumb and the heel of the hand are used to push and rub along the meridians, especially those on either side of the spine, which extend from the base of the neck to the heels, though there is one technique in which the movements are confined solely to the head and face, and another in which they are confined to the soles of the feet, on the assumption that the nerves and meridians in the head and feet are related to the organs in all parts of the body. Massage of the head and neck is often very effective in treating insomnia. Massage is often used in conjunction with other forms of treatment, such as compresses and herbal poultices, on the principle that what cannot be achieved by one form of treatment can be achieved by another. Massage is thought to tone the four humours, and in so far as it stimulates the blood and *qi*, this is likely to be the case. Massage could be regarded as 'exercise in reverse' because, in that it improves the circulation of the blood and tones the muscles and other organs, it provides the same benefits as exercise, but the energy is being expended by the environment, which is the masseur, and not against the environment, as is the case with exercise. Most of the work is done by the masseur, and not by the subject. It is sometimes the lazy person's way of taking exercise. It is of particular benefit to martial artists, whose muscles and tendons are sometimes severely strained, and also to elderly people who, for one reason or another, cannot indulge in vigorous exercise. A system of self-massage, called *dao yin*, which is a type of gymnastic exercise, was evolved in ancient China. *An mu*, a system of massage described in the *Chinese Exercise Manual*, involves emphasis on violent movements: patting the legs, beating the waist and hitting the shoulders with the fist or palm. The aim is to stimulate the acupoints. See **healing, reflexology, shiatsu** and **Chinese Exercise Manual**.

masculinity Traditionally, in China, the husband is the head of the family, but this is no more than a sensible division of labour, which is in accordance with Confucian teachings, and it is very much a case of the husband being no more than the 'first among equals'. See **femininity**.

mastery See **supremacy**.

mastic *Bosnellia carterii* Herbal medicine. Distribution: Mediterranean lands. Parts: resin from under the bark. Character: warm, pungent, bitter. Affinity: heart, liver, spleen. Effects: analgesic, antitussive, improves circulation, promotes growth of muscle tissue. Symptoms: lower abdominal pains and discomforts. Treatments: dysmenorrhoea, amemorrhoea, wind-damp conditions, traumatic injuries, halitosis. Dosage: 3–5 g. The resin may be applied to abscesses, furuncles and carbuncles which are not responding to other treatments.

mastitis Inflammation of the breasts. Chinese physicians attribute this condition to stagnant blood and *qi*, and recommend that heat and poisons be removed by administering an infusion or decoction of one of the following, to be taken internally, using the parts and dosage indicated: dandelion, *Taraxacum officinale*, entire plant, 10–30 g; madder, *Rubia cordifolia*, roots, 5–8 g; Chinese gentian, *Gentiana scabra*, roots, 3–7 g. To ease pain and promote healing, a mixture of olive oil and the finely ground dried rhizome of rhubarb, *Rheum officinale*, may be applied externally.

materia medica The science or study of the substances used in medical treatments. The *materia medica* of China is based largely upon the classic work of the renowned Ming physician Li Shizhen. See **Ben Cao Gang Mu**.

maturity cycle The human life cycle can be divided into stages: birth, infancy, childhood, teenage, adulthood, middle age, old age and death. But these are somewhat arbitrary divisions. According to Chinese tradition, the maturity cycle of a girl has seven seven-year periods. She matures sexually at 14, which is twice seven, and begins to deteriorate, as is manifested by the menopause, at 49, which is seven times seven. For a boy, the cycle has eight eight-year periods. He matures sexually at 16, which is twice eight, and begins to deteriorate at 64, which is eight times eight. This may be a sound working rule, but there are certainly some exceptions, for many men in their eighties are still sexually active, and some women still have strong sexual desires long after the menopause.

ME The abbreviation for **myalgic encephalomyelitis**.

meadowsweet *Filipendula ulmaria* Also called queen of the meadow and bridewort. Herbal medicine. Distribution: Europe, Asia, North America. Parts: flowers, leaves. Character: warm, sweet. Affinity: stomach, spleen, liver. Effects: diuretic, diaphoretic, demulcent, antiseptic, antipyretic, astringent. Symptoms: fever, aching limbs, nausea, vomiting, headache, diarrhoea. Treatments: rheumatism, arthritis, hyperactivity, intestinal upsets, skin eruptions. Dosage: 5–12 g.

measles See **morbilla**.

meat The Chinese view is that some meat should be included in the diet, for it is rich in certain substances which are essential to the health – iron, zinc and a variety of vitamins – and which are not so readily available in non-meat foods. It is also a good source of protein. However, it should not be consumed to excess, for its fat contains a high proportion of saturated fatty acids. A normal meal should not contain more than 10 per cent meat by weight.

The lean meat from poultry has a low fat content, and so it is preferable to other forms of meat. The fat in meat can be removed by boiling, but this destroys some of the vitamins. Where meat is included in the diet, it should be fresh, and then adequately cooked to break down its muscle fibres so that they are more digestible, and to ensure that any parasites it might contain are completely destroyed. Processed meat products, such as luncheon meat, beefburgers, hamburgers, mince, patés and sausage, should be regarded with suspicion, for they may contain preservatives, colourings and other additives which, in the Chinese view, could be harmful.

meat parasites Animals are the hosts for a wide variety of parasitic worms, and so meat should never be consumed raw, and should always be thoroughly cooked to ensure that, if it does contain worms, they will be destroyed.

mechanically aided therapy A term which describes those Chinese-style healing gymnastics in which the limbs and joints are exercised or assisted by mechanical contrivances, such as bicycles to strengthen the leg muscles, and weighted wheels to strengthen the shoulders. Bicycles are one of the main means of transport in China, and so the Chinese are well served in mechanically aided therapy.

medical books Some of the medical books of China are as follows. Each title is followed by the name of the author/compiler, where known, and the name of the dynastic period in which he lived. 'The Pharmacopoeia of Shen Nong', Han; 'The Internal Book of Huang Di', Han; 'Precious Prescriptions', Sun Simiao, Tang; 'Principles of Longevity', Liu Ching, Tang; 'Discussion of Febrile Diseases', Zhang Zhongjing, Han; 'Outlines and Branches of Herbal Medicine', Li Shizhen, Ming; 'The Herbs Studied by Shen Nong', Tao Hongjing, Sui; 'The Sayings of Celebrated Physicians', Tao Hongjing, Sui; 'The Book of Changes' (*I Ching*), Xia onwards; 'Chinese Almanac', Emperor Yu, Xia; 'The Book of Tea', Lu Yu, Tang; 'Pulse Studies of Binhu', Li Shizhen, Ming; 'Synopsis of Prescriptions of the Golden Chamber', Zhang Zhongjing, Han.

medical education The thorough training of Chinese physicians is a paramount aspect of Chinese medicine. Many are trained in the medical schools attached to the universities, where they study medicine in both the Western style and the traditional style of China. In the country areas, many are trained in the traditional way, which is by serving as an assistant or apprentice to an established practitioner, as apothecaries were once trained in Britain, and still are in Spain. The apprenticeship system has much to commend it, for it involves on-the-job training which is practical and lengthy, unsuitable entrants to the profession are soon weeded out, there is a close relationship between the teacher and the taught, often with a 1:1 pupil-teacher ratio, and the teacher is a highly skilled practitioner of long and wide experience. Anyone who has been on holiday in Spain and required medical attention will know that apothecaries trained in this way are competent and versatile, giving advice, dispensing medicines, extracting teeth, performing minor operations, and so on. See **'barefoot doctors'**.

medical examination In China, a medical examination is conducted very thoroughly, and the diagnosis by observation, listening and touch is preceded by an interview at which the patient provides the physician with information about his personal habits, past history, etc. See **consultation** and **diagnosis**.

medicament See **medicine**.

medication See **medicine**.

medicinal oils These are essential oils which are extracted from plant materials and used for medicinal purposes or as flavourings and fragrances for cosmetics and confectionery. Some examples of medicinal oils in common use are almond, rosemary, garlic, sage, lemon, juniper, peppermint and bergamot. Their medicinal properties are similar to those of the infusions and decoctions made from the same plants; but, because of their aromatic properties, they may be used to add flavour to other medicines, particularly those applied externally, such as liniments and ointments. They are also used in aromatherapy and other forms of massage, but aromatherapy is not employed on a large scale in China. See **essential oil** and **aromatherapy**.

medicinal properties of herbs Whether Chinese or in the Western style, a herbal will provide information about the anatomical structures, natural distribution and habitats of herbs. This is done mainly for the purpose of identification and collection. But there will also be a strong emphasis on the medicinal properties of herbs, and that is the means by which they are classified. Prior consideration is given to the character, or nature, of a herb, that is, its energy, taste and fragrance. A herb which does not fall into one of the categories of the four energies – hot, warm, cold and cool – is said to be neutral. Those herbs which are of a sour, bitter or salty taste are yin; and those of a sweet, hot or plain taste are yang. Another property of a herb is its affinity for certain organs, and it may be classified according to the colour or element associated with the organs for which it has an affinity. For example, a herb which is of sour taste and has an affinity for the gall-bladder is associated with the colour blue/green and the element wood. In this connection, it is interesting to note that some of the drugs manufacturers in the West use a form of colour coding with tablets and capsules. See **herbal prescriptions**. Generally, medicines of hot or warm energy are of sweet, hot or plain taste, and those of cold or cool energy are of sour, bitter or salty taste. Those of neutral energy can be of any taste. One of the properties of a herb is its medicinal effects. This table shows the relationships between the organs and the tastes and effects of herbs. Fragrances are not a precise way of classifying herbs, for they are varied and sometimes vague, but they are sometimes closely associated with taste, as with lemons and fennel, and, if very distinct, they are a useful guide when a herb is of plain taste. See **energy**, **taste** and **classification of medicines**.

Organ	Taste	+/−	Effects
spleen	sweet	yang	sedative, tonic
lungs	hot	yang	stimulative, carminative
kidneys	plain	yang	diuretic
heart	bitter	yin	antipyretic, drying
liver	sour	yin	astringent
kidneys	salty	yin	purgative

medicinal teas In Western medicine, the word *tea* is widely defined, and infusions of beef extracts and suchlike might be regarded as teas. But, in China, a tea is an infusion of a herb or a mixture of herbs, and is generally employed medicinally. See **herbal teas**.

medicinal wine Home-made medicinal wine features quite prominently among the folk remedies which the Chinese use in treating a great variety of ailments. To imbibe a flavoursome wine with medicinal properties is an effective way of combining medical business with worldly pleasure. There are hundreds of kinds of traditional medicinal wine, which are in the nature of tinctures, for they are made by steeping herbs in wine or spirit. The usual base is *shaojiu*, or rice wine, but brandy and gin, imported from the West, have been found to be excellent for this purpose. Gin, which is made by distilling beer, is one of the purest of the spirit drinks. The advantages of medicinal wine are that the alcohol effectively extracts the active ingredients in dried herbs, functions as a dilutent for those herbs which are too potent to be taken in the raw state, acts as a stimulant and facilitates the absorption of the active ingredients into the bloodstream. However, medicinal wines must not be confused with *chang*, which are the wines directly fermented from herbs in the same way as wines are made in the West. Some of the popular medicinal wines are made from wolfberries, figs, chrysanthemum flowers, persimmons, mulberries and red dates (jujubes). Medicinal wines are used to alleviate many conditions, which include neuralgia, nervous debility, indigestion, flatulence, rheumatism, arthritis, disorders of the kidneys and liver and antenatal weakness. Some have a tonic effect, stimulating the brain, increasing male virility and inhibiting the ageing process. However, medicinal wines are very potent, and so they must be taken with great care. Generally, the daily dosage must NOT exceed 90 g (90ml/3 fluid ounces), and they must NOT be taken for a period of more than three months, which must be followed by a rest period of at least one month before the treatment is resumed. They must NOT be taken by people with a weak constitution, a poor digestion or a heart condition, nor by people being treated for cancer or suffering from a common cold, influenza, a fever or a similar illness. Nor must pregnant women partake of these wines. Proprietary brands of medicinal wines are available in the West, but they are not made in the same way as the traditional medicinal wines of China, and they are generally no more than a cheap wine, such as port, to which phosphates and iron and other medicinal substances of doubtful value have been added. See **wine**.

medicine Remedy. Medication. Medicament. For practical purposes, these terms are generally regarded as being interchangeable, though, in fact, there are some differences of meaning. A medicament and a remedy, whether taken internally or externally, are regarded as being curative but not alleviative or preventive, and a remedy may not even be a medicine. It can be a form of exercise or meditation, for example. A medication, whether taken internally or externally, can be curative, alleviative or preventive. A medicine is generally thought of as being a substance to be taken internally but not externally. It is important that one should not be misled by these names, for errors in using medicines can lead to disaster. See **dangers with medicines**. The Chinese attitude towards medicines is that they are a last resort, and should be used only when there is a complete failure with other forms of treatment: diet and health foods, breathing and physical exercises, meditation, acupuncture, massage, etc. There are many excellent curative and alleviative medicines in TCM, but these should be used only when preventive medicines have failed. The situation is very different in the West, where many people take medicines unnecessarily or excessively on the deceptive principle that one cannot have too much of a good thing. Taken to excess, a medicine may do more harm than good, for dosages are often critical, and there may be other remedial techniques which are far more effective. What is more, medicines are not always a good thing. Often, it is a case of compromise, and choosing the lesser of the two evils, as when a narcotic drug is administered to a patient who is terminally ill. A person who keeps himself in a sound state of health by taking proper care of his body will generally have little need of medicine. So often do people say, 'Take your medicine. It will make you better.' But, in fact, it may offer no more than a temporary respite. It is probably true to say that, in the West, there are far more alleviative medicines than curative or preventive medicines. All too often, it is a case of matching a chronic illness with continual alleviation. One of the advantages of Chinese herbal medicines is that, once a cure has been effected, it is likely to be permanent. The Chinese have remedies for some illnesses which, in the West, are regarded as being virtually incurable. Chinese physicians have been treating asthma and diabetes successfully for over 2000 years, and they have a successful prescription for haemorrhoids which is at least 400 years old. But, then, Chinese physicians have a vast repertoire of medicines on which to draw, and they are in such a wide variety that they may be broadly classified according to their main sources: fish, insects, turtles and shellfish (animals with exoskeletons), birds, dragons and snakes (reptiles), minerals and stones, and animals (mammals). See **hypochondria** and **herbal medicines**.

medicine-dew This is a TCM liquid medicine similar to a broth or a decoction but much more concentrated. The herbal ingredients are put into an earthenware or porcelain dish, and a little water is added. The dish is then covered and steamed. A culinary-type steamer is suitable for this purpose. This technique is ideal for extracting the active ingredients from roots and rhizomes, and the medicine-dew so produced is quite potent.

medicine-juice This is a Chinese-style liquid medicine similar to a broth but more concentrated. It is more suitable for fresh herbs than dried herbs. The herbs are mixed and crushed with a little water, and then the juice is squeezed out. Fresh herbs are more potent than dried herbs. A Western-style juice-extractor could be used for whole fruits and roots.

Medicines Act 1968 Most countries have laws which govern the distribution, sale, preparation, testing and prescribing of medic-ines, whether herbal or otherwise, and, in this respect Britain is no exception. For example, the distribution of narcotics is severely restricted, the gathering of near-extinct herbs is controlled, and medicines which have toxic effects can only be prescribed by registered medical practitioners. These laws are intended for our protection, and so, in general, they should be welcomed. Unfortunately, they are sometimes marred by the damaging hand of an unimaginative and stultifying bureaucracy. Some Chinese herbal medicines which have been shown to be both efficacious and safe by many centuries of experience cannot be prescribed for British people, to whom they would be of considerable benefit, because they have not yet been subjected to certain laboratory tests. The irony is that some of the drugs which have passed these tests are now causing some alarm because they are addictive or have injurious side-effects. But, in using medicines of any kind, including those obtainable over the counter, and regarded as being safe, one should take no risks. It is also important to ensure that one is not behaving illegally. In particular, one should note that, under the terms of the Medicines Act 1968, certain medicines, including medicinal herbs, cannot be prescribed by anyone other than a registered medical practitioner; and, where they are prescribed, the permitted dosage must not be exceeded. See **medicine** and **dangers with medicines**.

meditation This is one way of dealing with problems, tension and anxiety, and their associated conditions, such as fatigue, insomnia, blood pressure, headaches and migraine, and achieving a tranquil state of mind without the use of sedatives, soporifics and antidepressants. Eliminating tension can help to eliminate the aches and pains which it causes or worsens. To meditate, one should sit comfortably in a quiet room with the eyes open and the hands resting in one's lap for a period of about 10–20 minutes each day. Some people try to meditate when lying in bed, but, more often than not, they fall asleep before anything is achieved. Meditation achieves results in three main ways. In a quiet room without distractions, the meditator may think deeply about his problems, and then decide, coolly and rationally, how he may best dispose of them. Or, he may shut out unpleasant thoughts and concentrate his mind on comforting and pleasure-giving items, as people do when they are day-dreaming or fantasizing. Or, he may try self-hypnosis and, by a colossal effort of will, convince himself that his affairs and life-style are in a better state, or could be in a better state, than they really are, and so he may become what he wants to be psychologically, and even physically, if he is suffering from a psychosomatic disorder. A philosopher once said that 'We are what we eat'. It is also true that we are what we think. This is really a form of auto-suggestion, a simple type of hypnotherapy developed in Europe by Emile Coué (1857–1926), a French apothecary. The Chinese have always recognized that many ailments are psychosomatic, and so they combine meditation with physical and breathing exercises, and the patient benefits thereby in a variety of ways. It is certainly the case that meditation influences the pulse and breathing rates. See **hypnotherapy**, **psychotherapy**, **self-hypnosis** and **meridian meditation**.

medulla oblongata See **brain**.

melancholy One of the four humours of traditional Western medicine. It is associated with bile and the liver. See **humour**.

melancholia Severe depression. See **depression**.

membrane 'Internal skin'. Thin and sheetlike connective tissue in an animal or plant.

memory The brain functions in much the same way as a computer, and its memory system is good if it is efficient in its input, storage and retrieval. In physiological terms, there is some doubt about the way in which the memory functions, but it seems that there are two kinds of memory: short-term and long-term. Only about seven items can be stored in the short-term memory, which lasts for about 30 seconds. With the long-term memory, the items most easily recalled are those which made a deep impression during input or are related to other items retained within the memory. Associations of ideas may cause an inaccurate or faulty recall, and this, no doubt, explains why stories from the past become embroidered in the telling, albeit unwittingly. Temporary loss of memory can be caused by fatigue, distress, alcohol, tobacco and certain drugs. Acute or chronic loss of memory can be caused by head injury, blood pressure and hysteria. See **amnesia, loss of memory** and **I Ching**.

menarche The onset of the first menstruation. See **maturity cycle**.

Mencius The Latinized name of Meng Zi (*c*. 371–*c*. 288 BC), a Chinese scholar who urged people to accept and follow the teachings of Confucius.

Mendel See **hereditary defects**.

meningitis Cerebro-spinal fever. Inflammation of the meninges, which is a layer of tissue that covers the brain and spinal cord. Its symptoms are fever, a severe headache, stiffness of the head and back, and the inability to bend the head forward. It is generally due to infection by the meningococcus bacterium, when it may be accompanied by a rash which is commonly called 'spotted fever'. Immediate medical attention is required, for the condition is often fatal. In TCM, the treatment is a mixture, taken internally, of decoctions of *zhu ye*, which are various species of bamboo (of the genus *Phyllostachyi*) and gypsum (*gypsum fibrosum*, or calcium sulphate). But this is a treatment which would not meet with the approval of the physicians of the West.

menopause Climacteric. 'Change of life'. The time when menstruation and the hormonal cycles cease. The process is sometimes sudden but usually takes two to three years. Initially, the woman ceases to ovulate, that is, produce eggs, and later there is a cessation of the output of oestrogen, which is the hormone that regulates the female reproductive organs. Generally, with a healthy woman, there should be few problems, but it is not surprising that the end of ovulation sometimes leads to emotional and other disturbances, which include depression, nervous irritability, weight gain, water retention, 'pins and needles' and hot flushes. But the psychological effects outweigh the physical discomforts, and there is sadness and fear that fertility and sexual attractiveness are at an end. But this fear is often misplaced because, apart from vaginal dryness and shrinkage, there need be few difficulties, and most women can have a full and active life, both sexually and otherwise, without the bother of menstruation and contraceptives, or the fear of pregnancy, and so, in some respects, the 'change of life' could be a change for the better. According to TCM theory, menopausal problems are due to imbalance between the kidneys and liver, kidney weakness and blood deficiency. Chinese physicians may recommend acupuncture as a treatment for the nervous conditions associated with the menopause, but they generally have a preference for an infusion or decoction, to be taken internally, of one of the following, using the parts and dosage indicated, either as a blood tonic or a relaxant: sage, *Salvia officinalis*, leaves, 2–6 g; Chinese angelica, *Angelica sinensis*, roots, 8–14 g; white peony, *Paeonia lactiflora*, roots, 4–8 g; camomile, *Matricaria chamomilla*, flowers, 3–19 g; parsley, *Petroselinum crispum*, root, leaves, 3–10 g; vervain, *Verbena officinalis*, leaves, stems, 3–10 g. It is important to note that bleeding outside the normal menstrual period during or before the menopause needs professional medical attention. See **maturity cycle**.

menorrhagia Hypermenorrhoea. Heavy bleeding during menstruation. This condition is weakening and inconvenient and may cause some discomfort, but there is generally no cause for great alarm. However, if the condition persists, medical advice should be sought in order to ensure that its cause is correctly diagnosed. The possible causes include hormonal imbalance, infection and inflammation of the uterus and uterine tubes, the use of an IUD (intra-uterine contraceptive device), circulatory congestion in the pelvic region, fibroids in the uterus, and capillary fragility due to anaemia. Fibroids are non-cancerous growths. Circulatory congestion is alleviated by exercise, and is likely to cease after the first pregnancy. In TCM, the herbal treatments are infusions or decoctions of the following, taken internally, using the parts and dosages indicated: shepherd's purse, *Capsella bursa-pastoris*, entire plant, 3–9 g; yarrow, or milfoil, *Achillea millefolium*, flowers, 3–12 g; parsley, *Petroselinum crispum*, 3–12 g roots or leaves, 3–6 g seeds; white deadnettle, *Lamium album*, entire plant, 3–12 g; mugwort, *Artemisia vulgaris*, leaves, 2–6 g; burnet, *Sanguisorba officinalis*, roots, 3–10 g; sage, *Salvia officinalis*, leaves, 2–6 g; agrimony, *Agrimonia pilosa*, leaves, 8–28 g. A suspension of 5–10 g powdered shells of the oyster, *Ostrea rivularis*, taken internally is also helpful. But it is as well to remember that these herbal remedies were adopted into TCM in an age when there were no intra-uterine contraceptive devices as we know them today. In addition to herbal medicines, Chinese physicians might recommend acupuncture, moxibustion and meditation. They would also advise against consuming heating foods, for they ascribe menorrhagia to heat in the blood. See **menstruation**.

menorrhoea Normal menstruation. See **amenorrhoea**.

menses Menstruation. Monthly periods. These are lunar-monthly, and so they occur every 28 days. This means that they occur two or three days earlier in every calendar month, which contains 30 or 31 days, so creating an impression of menstrual irregularity. See **menstruation**.

menstrual cramps See **meridian massage dysmenorrhoea**.

menstruation Menses. Monthly periods. This is the periodic bleeding, lasting for about four days, and which occurs about every 28 days, from the vagina of a sexually mature woman who is not pregnant. It is the discharge of unfertilized ova and the broken-up lining of the uterus. Menstruation does not occur during pregnancy because, at that time, an ovum has been fertilized to form an egg, and the lining of the uterus is enlarging to protect and feed the embryo which is developing from the egg. Although menstruation is a perfectly natural process, it creates problems for those people who live unnaturally. In TCM, menstrual problems are ascribed to imbalances in the liver, kidneys and spleen. Menorrhagia, or hypermenorrhoea, which is excessive bleeding from the vagina, is said to be due to heat in the blood, and dysmenorrhoea, or difficult menstruation, is said to be due to coldness in the blood. For these conditions, Chinese physicians would recommend acupuncture, moxibustion and meditation. They would also recommend the avoidance of hot foods when the blood is heated, and cold foods when the blood is cool. An infusion, taken internally, of 6–20 g leaves of raspberry, *Rubus idaeus*, is considered to be an effective tonic where there are conditions associated with the female reproductive organs – menstruation, premenstrual tension, menopause and pregnancy. See **amenorrhoea**, **dysmenorrhoea** and **menorrhagia**.

mental health In his *Satires*, the Roman poet Juvenal (c. AD 60–130) wrote, *Orandum est ut sit mens sana in corpore sano*, which means 'Your prayer must be for a healthy mind in a healthy body.' Chinese physicians would certainly go along with this quotation, for they regard mental health and physical health as being interdependent. For countless centuries, they have always taken the view that many ailments are psychosomatic, that is, possessed of physical features but originating in the mind and the emotions. This should seem to be all too obvious, for a person may shake and become red faced when he is angry, or become ashen faced and perspire freely when he is afraid, or have a 'lump in his throat' when he is grieving. This has always been obvious to Chinese physicians, so that in TCM, the seven emotions are associated with the five solid organs: joy – heart, anger – liver, anxiety – lungs, fear – kidneys, concentration – spleen. Sorrow and panic can be associated, according to the circumstances, with

THE SOLID ORGANS

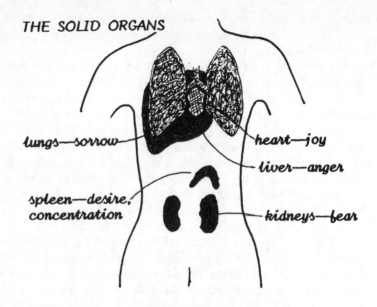

any of the solid organs. Panic differs from fear in being of a sudden and unexpected character, and concentration may take the form of desire or yearning. This is an over-simplification of the true state of affairs, but it does indicate that the physicians of ancient China had perceived that the emotions are governed as much by the body as by the brain. This differs from the traditional Western religious belief that the body and soul are separate entities. In both Christianity and Buddhism, it is held that the soul continues to exist after death. Of course, this cannot be the case, for the soul – or personality, or psyche, as it was called by the ancient Greeks – is the manifestation of the sum total of all the functionings of the body. The brain may be the organ of reasoning and stored thoughts, but it requires a nervous system and sense organs if it is to be supplied with data, and a blood supply, provided by the heart, if it is to function at all. It is also influenced by those chemical secretions, called hormones, from the endocrine glands. Strong feelings of joy, sadness and anger are registered by the brain, but they are prompted by the chemistry of the body. One might think that there would be less ignorance and superstition in this regard if the brain were regarded as what it is – just another organ – for all the organs of the body make some contribution, directly or indirectly, to the mind, or personality. No doubt, it is the indications of hormonal activity, but not the hormones themselves, of which the physicians of ancient China had little or no knowledge, which prompted the TCM theory that the emotions derive from the five solid organs and the absence or presence of *qi* in its various forms. See **hormone, endocrine glands** and **qi**. Mental unhealthiness should not be confused with mental illness. There is a distinction between mental illness on the one hand and unhealthy or antisocial attitudes – towards sex, diet or social affairs – on the other, although the dividing line may not always be clear. But, if an unhealthy attitude is not mental illness, it can sometimes lead to mental illness and nervous disorders. For example, an over-interest in food can result in anorexia nervosa. 'Big things, whether good or bad, have small beginnings.' Chinese physicians advise people to avoid the onset of mental illness and nervous disorders by taking care of both their mental health and their bodily health, which involves moderate habits and a more regulated way of life, and to be aware that food, exercise, sleep and laughter are good medicines. One can be sure that Taoism, which places emphasis on harmony with nature, and Confucianism, which places emphasis on harmony in society, have done much to keep the Chinese free of mental and nervous disorders and out of the clutches of the psychiatrists. A most useful tool in this regard is the *I Ching*. This remarkable classic work provides sound advice which could be applicable to almost any person at any time in any place, and is often of a divinatory nature, so enabling its users to cope with almost every emotive or emotional situation which might arise. See **mental illness, nervous disorders, I Ching** and **philosophy of health**.

mental illness This is a term which cannot be simply defined, for it is sometimes difficult to distinguish between a disorder of the mind and a disorder of the body. For example, nervous debility is essentially a disorder of the body, but its effects are registered in the brain. And the brain is so strongly influenced by the chemical activities of the body that it is sometimes difficult to decide whether and to what extent the mind should be regarded as a function of the brain or the body. Many of the so-called nervous disorders are bodily disorders which are merely reflected as an unfavourable functioning of the nervous system. The term *mental illness* is best reserved for those conditions which are dysfunctions of the brain itself. Alzheimer's disease, amnesia, autism, schizophrenia and manic-depressive disorders fall into this category. Alzheimer's disease is due to loss of nerve cells and shrinkage in the brain; amnesia is due to head injury or the shock resulting from hysteria or drink or drug addiction; and autism, which affects children, is an inability to communicate by speech, which is accompanied by temper tantrums and a display of indifference, so creating an impression of deaf-mutism. Schizophrenia is a condition in which the sufferer has delusions and hallucinations, hears imaginary voices and feels that he is being persecuted, and is depressed and uncommunicative, so giving the impression that he has more than one personality. Manic-depressive disorders are manifested by over-confidence, talk-ativeness, extravagance and hyperactivity, followed by bouts of depression and contemplations of suicide. The symptoms of manic-depression resemble those of schizophrenia. There are also genetic factors, and some mental illnesses, such as imbecility and schizophrenia, may be inherited. The brain can be affected in a way which constitutes an illness but is not necessarily a mental illness as per the usual definitions. A tumour in the brain, for example, is not likely to be very much different from a tumour in any other part of the body. There are many other examples of this kind. Cerebral haemorrhage, or stroke, is an organic condition, and not a form of insanity. But, in any case, the animal body is complex and integrated, and definitions are only valid within certain limits. *Psychopath* is the term used to describe a person who is truly mentally ill, as distinct from a neuropath, who has a nervous disorder. But, for the physician, there is a subtle but very meaningful difference between the psychopath and the neuropath. The former is generally totally unaware of his condition, though he may have short periods of lucidity, whereas the latter is very much aware of his condition – he has insight – which is why nervous disorders are generally far more distressing than mental disorders. On the other hand, the neuropath does make an attempt to recover because, to a large extent, he is still the master of his own destiny. In fact, his recovery depends very much on the effort he makes himself. But the psychopath cannot alter his own condition, for he has lost control, and he may be perfectly content to accept his condition because he knows no better. In TCM, the treatments for mental illness involve acupuncture, acupressure, moxibustion and medic-inal herbs, but they are of the kind which cannot be safely administered as do-it-yourself medicine, and must be conducted by professional practitioners. The various types of mental illness mentioned in this section are explained in more detail as separate entries. See **nervous disorders**, **mental health**, **hereditary defects** and **insight**.

mercury Quicksilver, its older name, derives from the once-held belief that it is a liquid form of silver. Chinese alchemists included mercury in some of their preparations, which was certainly a dangerous practice where they were used as medicines. Many centuries ago, Chinese physicians were using calomel, or mercurous chloride, as a purgative and a treatment for venereal diseases. Many centuries later, it was used for the same purposes in the West, though it has now been abandoned in favour of penicillin and other antibiotics, which are much safer. Some mercury compounds, such as cinnabar, or red mercuric sulphide, are still being used in Chinese medicine. See **cinnabar**.

meridian This may be briefly described as a bodily channel which conveys *qi*, or 'vital energy'. There are 59 meridians, or *jing luo* (also written as *qing lo* or *ching lo*), as the Chinese call them, and, in TCM, they are regarded as being more important than the nerves, blood or lymph because they circulate *qi*, which is vital to life, and illness may be caused if they become filled with waste or are blocked so that *qi* cannot circulate. The meridians make up an invisible network which connects all the organs and tissues of the body; and, as Chinese physicians treat the whole person when combating an illness, it is important that there should be no obstructions to prevent complete communication in the meridian network. There are acupoints, or vital-energy points, which could be groupings of nerve endings, on the meridians, and these are stimulated by acupuncture, acupressure, moxibustion or massage to effect beneficial changes in the body. There are over 800 acupoints, and some experts say that there could be as many as 2000, but only about 150 are utilized in most acupuncture treatments. Until recent years, the physicians of the West were very sceptical about the meridians, and they generally contended that they either do not exist or are no more than fibres of the autonomic nervous system. Yet the meridians are conceptually familiar to the equator. Both the equator and the meridians exist only by definition, the former being an imaginary line forming a great circle which is equidistant from the poles, and the latter is an imaginary line joining a series of acupoints. But TCM physicians would argue that the meridians are not imaginary, and that it would be erroneous to say that they do not exist simply because they cannot be seen with the naked eye. There is evidence to support the view of the Chinese physicians. Electro-acupuncture techniques, which have been developed in recent years, clearly indicate that there are areas of reduced skin-resistance on the body, and the undoubted success of acupuncture treatments adds considerable weight to their view. It is significant that stimulation of areas where there are very few nerve endings may produce a massive involuntary response. This suggests that the meridians are something other than nerve endings. The classical theory of TCM recognizes 12 main meridians, but modern theory recognizes 14, of which there are 12 paired and two unpaired. Each pair contains a yang meridian, which connects with one of the hollow organs, and a yin meridian, which connects with one of the solid organs. The hollow organs are the stomach, gall-bladder, small intestine, large intestine and bladder. The solid organs are the heart, lungs, liver, spleen and kidneys. On models of the human body used by acupuncturists, the meridians are often shown in the colours which are traditionally associated with the organs to which the meridians relate: heart, small intestine – red; lungs, large intestine – white; liver, gall-bladder – blue/green; spleen, stomach – yellow; kidneys, bladder – black. See **yang meridians** and **yin**

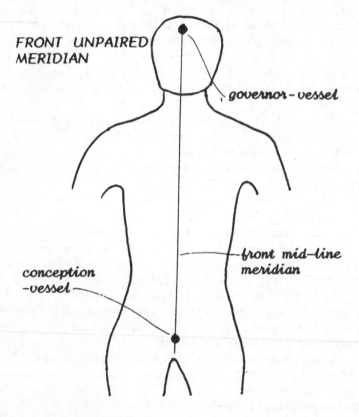

FRONT UNPAIRED MERIDIAN

governor – vessel

front mid–line meridian

conception –vessel

meridians. Of the two unpaired main meridians, one runs down the front mid-line of the body, and the other runs down the back mid-line. They are connected to the conception-vessel, which is the genitalia, and the governor-vessel, which is the brain. If there is a disorder in one of the main meridians, its connected organ will be affected, so producing bodily disharmony. Conversely, if there is a disorder in an organ, its meridian will be affected superficially or in its internal course, and some of the minor meridians may be affected also. Breathing exercises encourage or deflect the flow of *qi* along the meridians, and the healing effects of medicinal herbs travel throughout the body as much by the meridian network as by the bloodstream. See **acupuncture**, **electro-acupuncture**, **meridian research** and **meridian safety**.

meridian massage This is a form of massage which was developed by the Taoists in ancient China, and which was designed to improve the circulation of *qi*, or 'vital energy', by

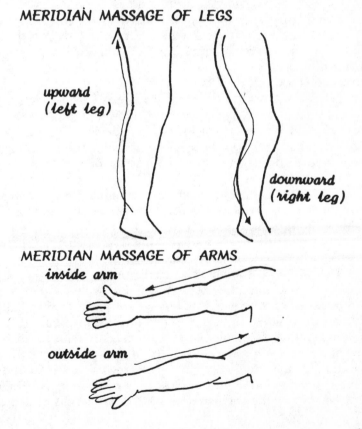

MERIDIAN MASSAGE OF LEGS

upward
(left leg)

downward
(right leg)

MERIDIAN MASSAGE OF ARMS
inside arm

outside arm

massaging the meridians. It also improves the circulation of the blood. This technique is based on the fact that the meridians which regulate the liver, spleen and kidneys meet together on the inside of the thigh, passing through the pelvic region near to the genital organs; and those which regulate the stomach, gall-bladder and bladder meet together on the outside of the thigh. In upward massage, the palms are placed on the insides of the legs at the ankles, and then slowly brought up the legs, inside the knees and up the thighs into the genitals. This is repeated 11 more times, making a total of 12 strokes. This treatment improves the circulation in the lower part of the body, so preventing varicose veins and menstrual cramps. In downward massage, the palms are placed on the outside of the thighs, and then slowly brought down the legs, outside the knees and over the calves and into the ankles. This movement is carried out 12 times. This treatment prevents blood pressure, water retention, obesity and bursitis. Similar effects on the organs can be achieved by massaging the arm meridians – on the inside of the arm and stroking away from the body for the heart, lungs and pericardium, and on the outside of the arm and towards the body for the triple-warmer, large intestine and small intestine. See **meridian**.

meridian meditation Chinese preventive medicine is based largely on the principle that, if weaknesses are neglected, they will become worse, but if they are eradicated, illnesses will not develop. In Western medicine, various devices, such as X-rays, blood and urine tests, scanners, and screening for cervical cancer, are used to detect the onset of illnesses, or weaknesses which could develop into illnesses. In TCM, weaknesses are detected by meridian meditation, which is a technique that was developed by the Taoists in ancient China. The person who wishes to use this technique must first memorize the meridians, and then, by gently feeling them, try to detect the flow of energy. Failure to detect a flow of energy indicates either a blockage in a meridian or lack of concentration. The meditation is repeated, and if a blockage is again indicated, it can be assumed that a false impression is not being created by lack of concentration, and that there is a weakness in the organ to which the meridian is related. And then that organ must be strengthened by remedial exercises or herbal medicines. Of course, this technique requires patience and skill, and it would not be easily learned by a person from the West who, from the outset, closes his mind to its possibilities. Although, by the standards of the West, meridian meditation may seem to be a bit far-fetched, it has been providing the Chinese with accurate indications for thousands of years, and the Chinese are the healthiest people in the world. See **meridian research** and **meridian safety**.

meridian research Until recent years, the medical scientists of the West had regarded the meridians of TCM as being no more than products of the imagination, but the research conducted by institutions in various parts of the world has thrown much new light on the subject. Perhaps the most spectacular research is that which was done by Dr Kim Bong Han at the University of Pyongana, in North Korea, and which has shown that the meridians do exist. They are composed of histological tissue, and are symmetrical bilateral channels with a diameter between 20 and 50 millimicrons, which is very small indeed, considering that a micron is a millionth part of a metre, or 0.001 millimetres. They occur below the surface of the skin, have membraneous walls and are filled with transparent fluid. The main meridians have subsidiary branches which unite at single points, where they are often surrounded by blood vessels, and which explains why there may be a little bleeding when an acupuncturist 'misses his target'. Other research has revealed that the meridians convey electro-chemical impulses, which could lead the sceptic to believe that the meridians are really the tiniest extensions of the tiniest nerve fibres. It has been suggested that the meridians might be indicative of the transitional stage between a complex combination of chemical substances and the simplest form of living material, but the same thing has been said about viruses, and so this is only a matter of conjecture. The question one could ask is why is it that Chinese physicians are so convinced. Perhaps it is just a matter of time and maturity. The system of medicine in China has gradually evolved over a period of more than 5000 years, whereas that of the West as we know it today is no more than about 200 years old. Prior to the beginning of the nineteenth century, much of Western medicine was a heterogeneous mixture of folklore herbal remedies, bits of medical knowledge bequeathed to us by the physicians of ancient Egypt, Greece and Rome, alchemical ideas borrowed from the Arabs and superstition posing as tradition. See **meridian** and **meridian meditation**.

meridian safety If it is the case, according to the theory of TCM, that the meridians regulate some of the activities of the vital organs and provide for the circulation of *qi*, or 'vital energy', what happens if a main meridian becomes completely blocked or damaged in some way? Is the related vital organ severely

QI FLOW IN MERIDIANS

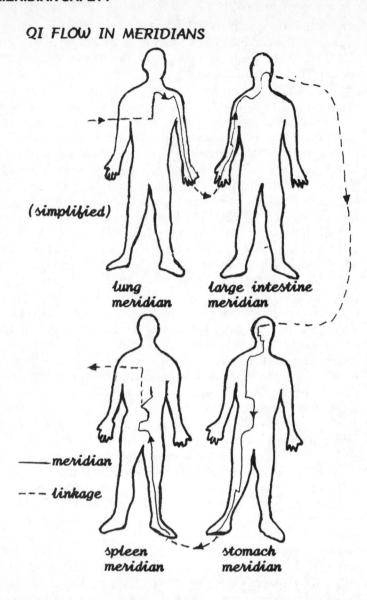

(simplified)

lung
meridian

large intestine
meridian

—— meridian

--- linkage

spleen
meridian

stomach
meridian

damaged or rendered inactive? And does a damaged or diseased organ affect its related meridians to such an extent that *qi* is unable to flow through the body? There are some damaging effects, it is true, but the damage is rarely irretrievable, for the meridian network has its own in-built safety system, which consists essentially of eight special meridians which supplement the functions of the main meridians by providing alternative pathways for *qi* should they be needed. In addition to bypassing diseased organs or blocked meridians, these special meridians provide an escape for *qi* when it occurs in excess. Furthermore, the 12 paired meridians are linked together at their ends in the hands, feet, head or elsewhere, so providing a continuous flow of *qi* throughout the body. Thus, beginning with, say, the lung meridian, *qi* flows from the lung meridian via the hand into the large intestine meridian, from the large intestine meridian via the head into the stomach meridian, from the stomach meridian via the foot into the spleen meridian, and so on. This means that if the flow of *qi* is blocked in one direction, it will be available in the opposite direction. This arrangement is similar to that of a ring-main electrical circuit, in which there is always a flow of current even when some of the lamps or other appliances fail to function. The order of flow of *qi* in the 12 paired meridians can be shown diagrammatically, as below. See **meridian**.

DIAGRAMMATIC QI FLOW

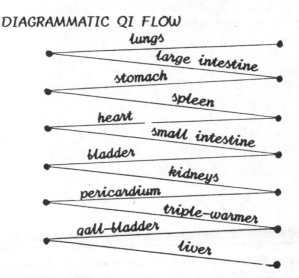

mescaline See **drug**.
mesmerism See **hypnotherapy**.
metabolic catalyst A medicinal ingredient, usually herbal, which influences metabolism, mainly by assisting biochemical changes, in much the same way as do enzymes, which are catalysts that occur naturally within the body. One of the great advances in TCM, many centuries ago, was the realization that some of the chemical substances contained in the animal body, and vital to

the health, are also contained in plants, though one can be sure that the physicians of those ancient times thought of them as energies and essences. See **enzyme**.

metabolism The sum total of all the chemical and energy changes in a plant or an animal, and which are concerned in its growth, repairs and other activities. It involves catabolism, which is the conversion of complex substances into simpler substances, as when starches are converted into glucose, and anabolism, which is the synthesis of complex substances from simpler substances, as when carbohydrates and nitrates combine to form protein. One of the several purposes of medicines is to influence metabolism beneficially by reducing, increasing, supplementing or replacing some of these chemical processes. In TCM, metabolism would be considered in terms of the four humours, particularly *jing*, or 'vital essence'. See **humour** and **jing**.

metal One of the five symbolic elements of Chinese philosophy and medicine. It is yang and is associated with the lungs and the emotion of anxiety. See **element**.

metaphysics The theoretical philosophy of human existence. This is a form of study which is not despised by Chinese scholars, who take a pragmatic view of life, and tend to reserve judgement on the big issues of human endeavour. The two motivating intellectual forces in the West are religion and natural science. Religion does provide a code of ethics, and an ill-thought-out code of ethics is better than no code of ethics at all; but, alas, religion tends to enforce its rules by superstition, wishful thinking and blind faith. Science has provided us with technological advancement, high-speed transport and improved health care, for which we should be grateful, but some of its plain facts and figures are no more than statistical misrepresentations and convenient assumptions, accompanied by a lack of faith in common sense and the nobler aspirations of mankind. Perhaps the Chinese attitude towards metaphysics may be succinctly summarized by a quotation from *Hamlet*, by William Shakespeare: 'There are more things in heaven and earth, Horatio, than are dreamt of in your philosophy.' Confucius confessed to being totally ignorant about many things. He was a wise man. But, then, it does seem that Confucius and Lao Zi between them, and by giving their attention to the knowable rather than the unknowable, have provided the Chinese with the means to master the art of living, which includes the pursuit of health, longevity and peace of mind.

methanoic acid (HCOOH). Known as formic acid in an older system of chemical nomenclature, this acid is contained in the fluid emitted by ants.

methanol See **alcohol**.

methyl alcohol See **alcohol**.

methylated spirit See **alcohol**.

metrorrhagia Heavy bleeding from the uterus, and which should not be confused with menorrhagia, which is bleeding from the vagina, though the conditions may be associated. *Dang shen*, *Codonopsis tangshen*, is usually an effective treatment, but the sensible procedure would be to seek professional medical advice, for there could be complications.

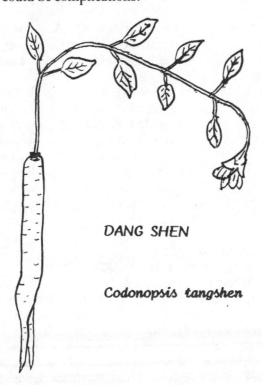

DANG SHEN

Codonopsis tangshen

microbe See **micro-organism**.

micro-organism Microbe. This is a plant or animal which is so small that it can be seen only with the aid of a microscope. Micro-organisms include bacteria, fungi, protozoa and viruses. Bacteria and fungi are plants. Bacteria are single-celled organisms, as are some of the moulds and other fungi. Protozoa are single-celled animals. Viruses are the simplest forms of life, and they are so small that they cannot be seen with an optical microscope, and can only be detected with an electron microscope. Those micro-organisms which cause diseases are called pathogens or pathogenic agents. Some of the diseases of plants, animals and humans caused by pathogens are shown in the table below. Most micro-organisms are harmless, and some are a necessary and beneficial part of the environment, as, for example, those which decompose organic material to form the humus and minerals in the soil. A few are of particular benefit to man. Examples of these are the bacteria which sour the milk used in making cheese, and yeast, which converts sugar into alcohol. See **bacterium**, **amoeba** and **virus**.

PATHOGENIC MICRO-ORGANISMS

humans	influenza	virus
humans	tuberculosis	bacterium
humans	measles	virus
humans	tonsillitis	bacterium
humans	ringworm	fungus
humans	malaria	protozoon
humans	dysentery	protozoon
rabbits	myxomatosis	virus
cattle	anthrax	bacterium
dogs	distemper	virus
cabbage	clubroot	fungus
tobacco	necrosis	virus

micturition See **urination**.

middle way See **golden mean** and **compromise**.

mid-line meridians See **meridian**.

migraine The condition which is often described as a migraine is generally no more than a headache. A migraine is a specific type of headache, and is much more than an ordinary headache, being accompanied by pain in the eyes and on one side of the head, flashing lights, nausea, vomiting and photophobia. The condition is thought to be due to alternate constriction and deflation of blood vessels in the brain, which may become inflamed. The flashes, or aura, are caused by lack of blood following a constriction. Certain dietary items may trigger off a migraine, and so migraine sufferers should try omitting cheese, eggs, chocolate, pork, peanuts, tomatoes, citrus fruits and wheat products from the diet. Chinese physicians ascribe this condition to imbalance between the liver and stomach, stagnation of liver *qi*, imbalance in the liver meridian and stomach weakness. They would recommend acupuncture, acupressure and massage. It is helpful to consume fresh leaves of feverfew, *Chrysanthemum parthenium*, in a salad. A decoction of 20 g seeds of fennel, *Foeniculum vulgare*, may be applied externally to relieve pain. See **headaches**.

milaria See **prickly heat**.

milfoil See **yarrow**.

milk and milk products Milk is a liquid formed and secreted by the mammary glands of female mammals as a source of nutrition for their young. It contains fat with a high proportion of saturated fatty acids, protein, minerals which include calcium, zinc, potassium and phosphorus, and a wide variety of vitamins, including thiamin, pyridoxine, niacin, biotin, folic acid, cobalamin, retinol, riboflavin and tocopherol. The proportions and character of the constituents of milk vary from mammal to mammal, and so it seems sensible that a baby mammal should be fed on the milk from a female mammal of its own species if it is to receive the type of nutrition that is best suited to its needs. It is certainly the case that a human baby fed on human milk rather than cow's milk is less likely to develop eczema or suffer from lactose intolerance. In various parts of the world, people consume cow's milk, ewe's milk, goat's milk and mare's milk, but cow's milk is the kind most commonly consumed in the United Kingdom. Yet cow's milk can be a source of infection, and so apart from that from accredited herds, all milk is required by law to be subjected to some form of heat treatment, such as pasteurization, sterilization and ultra-heat treatment, in order to destroy harmful micro-organisms. Milk products do not have the same constituents as whole milk, for some of the fat will have been removed, and some of the vitamins will have been destroyed by the treatments to which it has been subjected. Apart from Mongolia and the most northern parts of China, where butter and mare's milk are commonly consumed, very little milk and few milk products are consumed by the Chinese, for they are sources of animal fat, which the Chinese consider to be harmful to the health. But the Chinese do consume an excellent milk substitute, which is made from soya beans. See **eczema, breast-feeding** and **lactose intolerance**.

milk teeth See **teeth**.

mineral A metallic or non-metallic element which is essential to the body, and which is derived from the diet, but as a compound, and not in the pure elemental form. The main functions of minerals are as regulators of the body fluids, components of enzymes and constituents of the bones and teeth. The body contains about 25 essential minerals, of which those required in large amounts are calcium, magnesium, potassium, sodium, sulphur, phosphorus, iron, zinc and iodine. Those which are required in only the tiniest amounts, but which are no less essential, are called trace elements. A deficiency of a mineral may give rise to an adverse bodily condition. Thus, a deficiency of iron or copper may cause anaemia, and a deficiency of phosphorus may cause nervous disorders. The usual treatment for a deficiency disease is to correct the deficiency by adding to the diet some of those foods containing the mineral of which the body is deficient, though mineral supplements may be required in severe cases. The person who diets to lose weight or for whatever other reason should take steps to ensure that his body is not deprived of the minerals which are essential to health. TCM does not recognize minerals, and they were not known to the physicians of the West until recent times, but there is an awareness that certain foods contain energies and essences that are essential to the health, which amounts, more or less, to a similar interpretation of the same state of affairs. Thus, a physician of the West will say that an anaemic person needs iron-rich foods, such as liver, red meat, figs, green vegetables and nuts, whereas a Chinese physician will say that an anaemic person needs such foods as liver, pulses, figs and nuts to fortify the blood and prevent stagnation of liver-*qi*. The approach is different, but the end result is the same. Most of the problems and complaints which arise from dietary deficiencies can be circumvented by adopting the Chinese style of diet, which is balanced and varied so that one cannot consume too much of what is harmful, nor too little of what is beneficial. See **dieting**.

mineral acids See **acid**.

mineral medicines Although we tend to think of Chinese medicines as being herbal, as indeed most of them are, some derive from animal sources, and a few are of mineral origin. Some examples of the latter are Glauber's salt (hydrated sodium sulphate), gypsum (calcium sulphate), talc (hydrous magnesium silicate) and haematite (ferric oxide).

Ming dynasty The period of the Ming dynasty (1368–1644) was one of great cultural development and changes, political and otherwise. The Ming empire reached the height of its power under Emperor Yong Le, during which time a magnificent Chinese fleet, commanded by the eunoch Zheng He, explored the west coast of Africa. Agriculture was improved, irrigation systems were introduced, handicrafts, including weaving and spinning and the manufacture of porcelain, were developed, and maritime trade with the West was established. The first Portuguese ships arrived at Guangzhou (Canton) in 1516. They were soon followed by the French, Dutch and English. Western technology and scientific ideas were introduced into China, and medical science flourished. Li Shizhen, the greatest of the physicians of this period, compiled a superb pharmacopoeia, *Ben Cao Gang Mu*, which is still in use today, and which, after translation into various Western languages, instituted an exchange of ideas between Chinese medical science and that of the West. Many Chinese medicinal herbs were introduced into Europe, where they were cultivated on quite a large scale.

mint Various species of mint are used in Chinese medicine, two of the commonest being corn mint, *Mentha arvensis*, and peppermint, *Mentha piperita*. The latter is used extensively as a flavouring.

mirabilite See **Glauber's salt**.

mirrors In various parts of China, one will see small hexagonal mirrors on the walls of buildings and in other places. These *pa kua*, or *bhat gwa*, mirrors, as they are called, once had a certain significance for the peasantry, who believed that they would reflect evil influences back to where they came from. This is a part of the strange belief called *fung shui*. However, the mirrors had a much deeper significance for Chinese scholars. The eight sides of a *pa kua* mirror represent the eight trigrams which are paired to make the 64 hexagrams of the *I Ching*, which are associated with binary numbers and the optical principle of lateral inversion. Is this not a case of the peasants drawing a conclusion which is different from that held by their intellectual betters? There is a parallel here with the different interpretations of the Christian Bible: while some regard it as the literal truth, others consider much of it to be allegorical. Beliefs sometimes have powerful psychological effects; and, in China, there have been cases of people suffering from depression or anxiety being cured by the erection of a *pa kua* mirror to reflect away the evil influences to which their illnesses were attributed. Of course, some people would say that a belief in the healing power of mirrors is indicative of feebleness of mind. But one should not condemn too readily what appears to be superstition, for many disorders are psychosomatic, and so a study of the metaphysical aspects of human behaviour can sometimes produce remedial benefits. See **fung shui** and **I Ching**.

miscarriage The popular alternative term for an abortion. But the term *abortion* should be used where the condition is artificially induced. In China and elsewhere, it is often associated with female infertility, though the condition can occur where a woman is fertile and healthy and as a consequence of a traumatic shock or some other form of external cause. Listeria is suspected of being causative of an abortion. In TCM, eucommia, *Eucommia ulmoides*, is regarded as a sound treatment for a restless foetus, which could lead to an abortion. But this is an area where do-it-yourself medicine is totally inadvisable. If there are doubts, seek professional medical advice. See **abortion** and **uterine disorders**.

mishmi bitter *Coptis sinensis* Herbal medicine. Distribution: China, India. Parts: rhizomes. Character: cold, bitter. Affinity: heart, large intestine, liver, stomach. Effects: antipyretic, refrigerant, astringent, antidote. Symptoms: fullness in chest, diarrhoea, jaundice, nosebleeds. Treatments: dysentery, abscesses, heat stroke, ailments due to full or hot excess. Dosage: 2–5 g. The juice of the fresh rhizomes, which has strongly antiseptic properties, may be used as a wash for sore and swollen eyes, and as a mouthwash and gargle for abscesses in the mouth.

mistletoe *Viscum album* Herbal medicine. In the traditional herbal medicine of both China and the West, mistletoe leaves and stems have the reputation of being effective in the treatment of tumours, but there could be dangers in their use. By the terms of the Medicines Act 1968, mistletoe berries cannot be prescribed by anyone other than a registered medical practitioner.

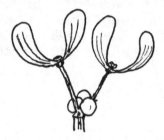

MISTLETOE

Viscum album

mixed nerve See **nervous system**.

mixing medicines In mixing medicines, which, in TCM, generally means mixing dried herbs to be administered as an infusion or decoction, it is important to understand that some dosages are critical, particularly where the medicines are poisonous or have unpleasant side-effects. One may wonder why Chinese pharmacists do not make life easier for themselves, and avoid all the complications of measuring dried herbs, by using the active ingredients in a refined and concentrated form. The simple explanation is that the crude herbs are medicinally more beneficial than tablets and capsules in the Western style. See **dosages**, **active ingredient**, **buffer** and **dangers with medicines**.

moderation The Chinese are calm by temperament, and of moderate habits, and they try to establish harmony in all their endeavours, which are a few of the reasons why they are healthy and have great peace of mind. It does follow that the person who is not reckless in his habits will be less prone to illness and accidents; and, if he has peace of mind, he will surely sleep better, eat better and generally feel better. In this respect, both Lao Zi and Confucius advocated a strict adherence to the *golden mean*, which is the principle that one should always take the middle way, and so avoid violent extremes of conduct. In the West, gourmandizing is one of the commonest forms of immoderacy. In fact, it is a positive vice, for it is certainly the case that more people die from overeating than under-eating. Unfortunately, the people of the West tend to adopt an 'all-or-nothing' approach in many of their activities, and so immoderacy abounds. With many, it is either total self-indulgence or total abstinence. The Chinese see no virtue in greed; on the other hand, they see no virtue in complete self-denial. See **compromise** and **golden mean**.

moist Damp. A term used in TCM to describe those ailments and their symptoms which are associated with an excess of moisture. See **dampness** and **six excesses**.

moisture See **water**.

molar See **teeth**.

mole See **naevus**.

molasses Treacle. The residue of uncrystallized syrup from the refining of raw cane or beet sugar. It has a high energy value – 278 kcal/100 g – and is a rich source of calcium and iron. It also provides some copper, magnesium, potassium and zinc. It has a mildly laxative effect. As a source of energy, the Chinese prefer to use the actual sugar cane, which is cut into short pieces, immersed in water and gently simmered. For anaemic people, molasses makes a good addition to the diet because it contains twice as much iron as ox liver and is more easily digested. It increases virility and counters the ageing effect. See **sugar**.

mollusc This is an animal with a soft and simple body, a muscular creeping foot and a shell. But there are exceptions. Some molluscs, such as mussels and oysters, are stationary, and octopuses and slugs do not possess shells. Some well-known molluscs are snails, slugs, whelks, limpets, oysters, cockles, winkles, mussels, octopuses, escallops and abalone. Molluscs such as the snail and the limpet, which have a ventrally positioned locomotive organ, are called gastropods. Those such as the mussel and the oyster, which have a hinged double shell, are called bivalves. See **shellfish**.

monkshood See **aconite**.

Monilia See **Candida albicans**.

Mongoloid races Two of the characteristics of the Mongoloid races, to which the Chinese belong, are stamina and longevity, but it is difficult to say to what extent these characteristics are influenced by their way of life, which includes a sound diet and an adequate amount of exercise. See **race**.

Mongols Genghis Khan conquered China in 1260, from which time the Mongols ruled the empire, with Beijing (Peking) as its capital, for 108 years. During this period, Chinese medicine and other forms of learning went into a decline because, though the Mongols were great warriors, they had little culture and were poor administrators. However, China was restored to a position of intellectual activity when the Ming dynasty assumed sovereignty of the empire in 1368. See **Ming dynasty**.

monosodium glutamate Taste powder. Nowadays, this substance, which was first isolated from seaweed by a Japanese scientist in 1908, and which is manufactured under a variety of proprietary names, is used throughout the world as an additive to enhance the flavour of food. A wide variety of processed and precooked foods contain the permitted amount of this substance. The Chinese themselves are averse to the use of food additives, particularly those of the synthetic kind, but it is often added to the food served in Chinese restaurants in the West, and on the principle, one may suppose, that 'when in Rome, do as the Romans do'. But its use is not to be recommended, for it sometimes produces an allergic reaction, accompanied by a headache, palpitations and severe thirst, which is called 'Chinese restaurant syndrome', and if it is added to food before it is cooked, it is liable to be rendered toxic by the high temperature of cooking – and it is very potent.

mons pubis See **mons Veneris**.

mons Veneris Mons pubis. The mount of Venus. The rounded mass of fatty tissue on a woman's abdomen above the vulva.

moon The ghostly presence of the moon in the night sky has always been a source of inspiration for poets and dreamers, which is especially the case in China, where the moon is of great significance in astrology and mythology, and is yin, or feminine, to which the sun is yang, or masculine. There are 13 lunar months, each of 28 days, in a year, which is the basis of the Chinese lunar calendar. Today, officially, the Chinese calendar is the same as that of the West, with its 12 months of varying lengths, which is called the Gregorian calendar after Pope Gregory XIII (1502–1585), who ordered a revision in 1582. But in the rural areas and for unofficial purposes in China, the ancient lunar calendar is still in common use. Seemingly, the lunar calendar is better related to seasonal changes than the Gregorian calendar, which has some significance in a country whose economy is basically agricultural, and whose system of medicine is dependent upon herbs, which come into maturity at certain times of the year. It is interesting to note that in China, as in the West, mental illness is associated with the moon. See **Chinese Almanac**.

morality Chinese physicians and scholars take the not unreasonable view that many mental illnesses and nervous disorders, particularly those whose symptoms are anxiety and depression, are due to the way in which we live, and could be ascribed as much to a lack of morality as to any overtly medical cause. Confucius advised people to avoid immoderacy and live by the five cardinal virtues of wisdom, justice, charity, honesty and propriety. Without a doubt, much illness, both physical and mental, is caused by immoderacy with diet, sex and alcohol. The person who behaves without wisdom will not be successful in his affairs, which could lead to frustration and anxiety, though there is an element of truth in the old saying, which derives from the poetic works of Thomas Gray: 'Where ignorance is bliss, 'tis folly to be wise.' The person who behaves without justice or charity will generally invite reciprocal acts of injustice or lack of charity, which could also lead to frustration and anxiety. Dishonesty may bring success in the short term, but only disaster in the long term, for a reputation for dishonesty and hypocrisy once gained is rarely lost, and it is usually the case that vice, as well as virtue, brings its own rewards. Impropriety leads to disloyalty, confusion, an unenviable reputation and the transmission of venereal diseases, none of which are good for the health of society or the individuals within it. Those who feel that they need some good advice in these respects should consult the *I Ching*. See **moderation** and **I Ching**.

morbid depression A state of mind in which the sufferer has morbid fears and thoughts of death, and may even be tempted to commit suicide. The obvious treatment is to eradicate the problem which is causing this state of mind. But this is not always possible, and then the sufferer must 'learn to live with it', as we are told by the popular and not very helpful saying. Unfortunately, anxiety can become a habit, and it may persist long after its cause has ceased to be. Furthermore, depression may be due to hormonal and other chemical changes within the body. For this condition, Chinese physicians would recommend a wide variety of treatments, which include acupuncture, acupressure, moxibustion, meditation, massage and herbal tonics. But some sound advice from a worldly wise and understanding person could also be very helpful. See **mental illness** and **nervous disorders**.

morbilli Rubeola. Measles. This is a disease of childhood which is characterized by a fever, a running nose, watery eyes, a dry cough and a rash of large pink spots. Caused by a virus, it has an incubation period of 10–14 days; and, after the rash has cleared, the other symptoms continue for four days. The condition lasts for about 10 days, and there are generally no complications, but it is highly infectious and is one of the main causes of death in less developed countries. Measles contracted in childhood confers an immunity which lasts into adulthood, but when it is contracted by an adult who has not had it as a child, it lasts for four weeks and is much more severe, being accompanied by complications, such as ear infections, acute photophobia, pneumonia and even encephalitis (inflammation of the brain). It is a notifiable disease, and so a suspected case must be reported to a medical practitioner. Strictly speaking, *rubeola* is the correct medical term for measles, *morbilli* being the term for the large pink spots, but the two terms are used as if they were interchangeable. According to TCM, measles is caused by heat in the blood and stomach. The spots are brought out and the fever reduced by including duck meat in the diet, and internally administering infusions or decoctions of the following, using the parts and dosages indicated: Japanese honeysuckle, *Lonicerum japonica*, flowers, 8–15 g; safflower, *Carthamus tinctorius*, flowers, 2–4 g; peppermint, *Mentha piperita*, leaves, 3–12 g; yarrow, *Achillea millefolium*, flowers, 3–12 g; marigold, *Calendula officinalis*, flowers, 3–12 g. Itching can be relieved by the external application of a cool infusion of 1.5–6 g flowers of lavender, *Lavandula officinalis*.

morning glory *Pharbitis nil* Herbal medicine. Distribution: China,

India. Parts: seeds. Character: cold, bitter. Affinity: lungs, large intestine, kidneys. Effects: diuretic, cathartic, expectorant, anthelmintic, reduces swellings. Symptoms: constipation. Treatments: intestinal parasites, oedema. Dosage: 1–2 g. This herb is slightly poisonous, and so the dosage must NOT be exceeded, and it must NOT be taken regularly, but only occasionally. See **Medicines Act 1968**.

morning sickness A condition which is due to an increase in hormone production, and which is characterized by nausea and sickness with occasional vomiting. It generally occurs during the first three months of pregnancy, but it sometimes persists into late pregnancy. Hyperemesis gravidarum, or excessive vomiting, causes severe dehydration, which could be dangerous, and so professional medical attention should be sought. One should avoid fatty food and consume plenty of fluids other than milk, such as broth and fruit juices, to counter dehydration. One should also consume dry biscuits to prevent hunger pangs without inducing vomiting, and drinks containing glucose, which will replace the energy lost by vomiting and dehydration. One cannot avoid food altogether, for the foetus needs to be fed. In TCM, suitable alleviative treatments are infusions, sipped slowly, of the following, using the parts and dosages indicated: ginger, *Zingiber officinale*, fresh rhizome, 3–8 g; fennel, *Foeniculum vulgare*, fruits, 2–4 g; camomile, *Matricaria chamomilla*, flowers, 3–10 g; raspberry, *Rubus idaeus*, leaves, 2–8 g; peppermint, *Mentha piperita*, leaves, 3–10 g. According to TCM, severe morning sickness is due to too much heat and weakness in the stomach and liver. Chinese physicians would recommend massage or acupuncture, but this must be done with great care by a professional masseur or acupuncturist, otherwise a miscarriage might be induced. They would also advise the consumption of warm foods and the avoidance of cold foods. One of the Chinese folklore remedies for morning sickness is ginger tea, which is made by adding 60 g sliced fresh ginger to 1 litre water, bringing to the boil, and then simmering for 10 minutes. This remedy is quite effective.

morning star *Uncaria rhynchophylla*. Distribution: China. Parts: stems. Character: cool, sweet. Affinity: liver, pericardium. Effects: antipyretic, sedative, antispasmodic. Symptoms: dizziness, blurred vision, headaches, body heat, children's spasms, convulsions in last months of pregnancy. Treatments: conditions due to ascending liver-yang, hypertension. Dosage: 4–9 g. This herb is also of value as a vasodilator.

morphia A popular name for morphine. See **morphine**.

morphine Alkaloid narcotic substance derived from opium. It is available only to registered medical practitioners. See **opium**.

mortar and pestle This extremely useful device, which is made of earthenware, and which may be purchased from a pharmacy, is ideal for grinding seeds, roots, bark and the other hard parts of herbs. It is an indispensable tool for those people who prepare their own herbal medicines.

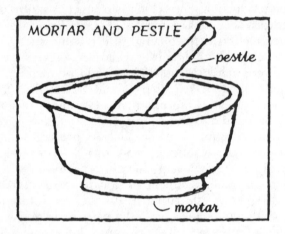

MORTAR AND PESTLE — pestle — mortar

mosquito There is more than one species of mosquito. Those which occur in cold and temperate regions, and which are usually called gnats, belong to the genus *Culex*. Their bites can cause a little pain and skin irritation, but otherwise they are generally harmless. A gnat bite very occasionally leads to septicaemia, which will require medical attention, but it is usually sufficient to treat the skin irritation by applying an antiseptic ointment. The mosquitoes of the wet, tropical and subtropical regions, which belong to the genus *Anopheles*, transmit various diseases. The female of *Anopheles gambiae* feeds on blood and transmits malaria in the process. The male feeds on plant juices. The Chinese use sweet wormwood, *Artemisia annua*, in the treatment of malaria. The yellow fever virus is transmitted by a mosquito of the genus *Aëdes*. See **bites** and **malaria**.

mother-and-son rule See **element**.

mother-of-pearl See **nacre**.

motion sickness See **travel sickness**.

motor nerve See **nerve**.

motor neurone disease Any disease of a motor nerve which produces a loss of power in the associated muscles.

moulds Tiny fungi which grow on organic substances, such as food, wood, paper and leather, and which thrive in situations that are warm, dark and moist. Their spores, by which they reproduce, escape into the atmosphere, where they are carried by air currents. In contact with humans, they produce allergic reactions which are sometimes causative of hay fever and asthma, or so it is believed by the physicians of the West, though Chinese physicians have very different ideas about the causes of hay fever and asthma. But moulds have their uses. *Penicillium* moulds are used in the ripening of cheese, and penicillin, the antibiotic, is a secretion from some of the *Penicillium* species. See **antibiotic**.

moulting Ecdysis. The process by which an animal sheds its feathers, hair, shell or some other outer covering. Zoologists describe the material so shed as exuviae. Moulting has some significance in TCM, for the exuviae of the cicada, a type of insect, is used in the treatment of cataracts. See **cicada**.

'mountain varnish' See **Yunnan bai yao**.

mount of Venus See **mons Veneris**.

mouse A small rodent and a disease-carrier. See **vector**.

mouth diagnosis A physician's examination of a person's mouth will yield some information about the person's state of health. For example, gingivitis, or inflammation of the gums, could indicate that the body is overheated; pyorrhoea, which is a discharge of pus from the gums, indicates an infection of the mouth and, possibly the presence of toxins in the bloodstream; white spots on the inside of the cheeks, called Koplik's spots, indicate the onset of morbilli, or measles. However, most of the information that is obtained by mouth diagnosis is from the tongue, and this is just as true for the physicians of the West as it is for Chinese physicians. See **tongue diagnosis**.

mouth infections The various infections of the mouth and its associated organs are dealt with as separate entries, but a good all-round mouthwash and gargle for minor infections and other problems in the mouth, such as bleeding gums and excessive salivation, is an infusion of 2–6 g leaves of sage, *Salvia officinalis*. A saline solution also makes an effective mouthwash.

mouth ulcers Aphthous ulcers. Small, shallow, round or oval ulcers, usually with a grey bottom and a yellow edge, which occur inside the cheeks or lips, or on the tongue or other parts of the mouth. They can be very painful, and they may be caused by poor diet, stress, badly fitting dentures, abrasions due to excessive brushing of the teeth, or herpes. They are likely to be symptomatic of a run-down condition. In TCM, a sound diet is regarded as the best form of treatment, and so the diet should be arranged to include fresh vegetables and fruit, brewer's yeast and foods containing vitamin C and zinc. Chewing a piece of liquorice root has an effect which is both soothing and healing. It is also helpful to use a mouthwash of an infusion of a mixture of 5 g leaves of thyme, *Thymus vulgare*, and 5 g flowers of marigold, *Calendula officinalis*. A Chinese folk remedy for mouth abscesses is to apply a mixture of charcoal and the gizzard of a chicken, *Gallus gallus domesticus*, which has been dry-fried and powdered. See **ulcer**.

mouthwash See **mouth infections**.

movement According to Taoist philosophy, man engages in two basic activities in order to be healthy and prolong his life. They are the processes of consuming food and drink and bodily movement, or motion. Of course, this is just another way of saying that if one wishes to be healthy and live long, one must have a sound diet and an adequate amount of exercise. But what is true for humans is also true for other animals. In this respect, the other animals have no problems, for they hunt for their food, and so combine food intake with movement. They also go about it in the right way. Herbivorous animals, such as cattle and goats, do not eat meat, and carnivores, such as tigers and wolves, do not eat vegetation. Also, they run when they are in danger, but otherwise they prefer to walk. It is only the human animal who is neglectful of diet and exercise. Although he is essentially a vegetarian, he consumes large quantities of meat, together with other items which cannot be good for him, such as alcohol, fizzy drinks, synthetic food additives and canned foods. As far as movement is concerned, many people either take no exercise at all, or expose themselves to the risk of injury by participating in over-strenuous activity or potentially dangerous contact sports. The Taoists of ancient China gave much thought to food-intake and movement, as did the Buddhists at a later stage in Chinese history. This explains why the Chinese diet is essentially vegetarian, as is that of all the primates except man. The Taoists separated movement into three components – thought, bodily movement and sex. Clearly, they had recognized that exercising the mind is as important as exercising the body, and so it is not surprising that the Chinese have a fondness for such games as chess. The Taoists evolved a number of sets of activities in which meditation is combined with breathing exercises and bodily movements. Westerners are generally surprised when they learn that the Chinese achieve a sound state of health and a long life by diet and exercise, and not, as is often supposed, by pills and potions of magical quality. There are 39 sets of activities, or internal exercises, as the Chinese describe them, whose purpose is to protect and strengthen the internal organs, such as the heart, liver and kidneys, and to assist the body in its relation to time, space and direction and its meridians, nervous system and houses, or endocrine glands. These exercises are components of what the Chinese describe as *yang sheng shu*, or '*tao* of revitalization', which was built around four basic common sense assumptions. Without food, life will cease within about 10 days. Without proper food, life will shorten. Without movement, the body will go to waste. Without proper movement, the body will become weak. In this connection, it is interesting to note that these principles are now recognized by Western medicine. Whereas, some years ago, an illness was usually followed by a long period of convalescence in which the patient was confined to a bed, the convalescent person is now encouraged to be up and about, taking exercise and living as normally as is possible. The internal exercises differ from external exercises in that the former benefit the internal organs naturally, quietly, smoothly, precisely and slowly, so producing sound health, immunity to disease and vigorous youthfulness, whereas the latter, which include the martial arts, dancing, body-building and sports of the kind practised in the West, such as football and hockey, may waste energy and weaken the internal organs by fatigue, pain and stress, and so impair their ability to throw off diseases, which can cause premature ageing. The internal exercises are the basis of the therapeutic exercises – *qi-gong* and *nei-gong* – in the *Chinese Exercise Manual*. The Taoists regard sex as a separate form of movement because it is more concerned with the survival of the race than that of the individual. See **diet** and **exercise**.

moxa weed *Artemisia capillaris* Herbal medicine. Distribution: North China, Taiwan, Japan. Parts: young leaves and stems. Character: neutral, bitter. Affinity: liver, gall-bladder, stomach, spleen. Effects: diuretic, antipyretic. Symptoms: jaundice. Treatments: insufficient bile, water-retention ailments. Dosage: 8–12 g. This herb must NOT be confused with mugwort, or Chinese wormwood, *Artemisia vulgaris*, the latter being the *moxa* that is used in moxibustion.

moxibustion *Chen chiu*. This is a form of therapy which is similar to acupuncture and acupressure in its effects, but a glowing wick, instead of needles, is the source of stimulation for the vital-energy points on the meridians. The wick consists of mugwort, or Chinese wormwood, *Artemisia vulgaris*, and other herbs, which are called *moxa*, a term devised by the Japanese. The glowing wick is slowly rotated above a vital-energy point about 2 cm away from the skin. Alternatively, acupuncture needles are first inserted into the skin, and then small pieces of herb are placed on the heads of the needles and ignited. If the needles are pushed through cardboard discs before insertion, the ash from the burning weed will not fall on the patient's skin. Moxibustion is an effective treatment for menstrual problems. See **acupuncture** and **meridian**.

MSG The abbreviation for **monosodium glutamate**.

mucilage A viscous substance obtained by maceration of seeds and other plant materials. It may have a soothing effect when applied to the skin or a mucous membrane, and it is one of the active ingredients in most demulcents. Good sources of mucilage are chickweed, *Stellaria media*, slippery, or red, elm, *Ulmus fulva*, comfrey, *Symphytum officinale*, coltsfoot, *Tussilago farfara*, meadowsweet, *Filipendua ulmaria*, marshmallow, *Althaea officinalis*, Iceland moss, *Cetraria islandica*, and linseed, *Linum usitatissimum*.

mucous colitis See **irritable bowel syndrome**.

mucous membrane A delicate mucus-secreting membrane which lines the body cavities, such as the nose, bronchi and digestive tract. See **mucus**.

mucus A viscid fluid secreted by mucous membranes. It keeps the membranes and body cavities moist, but becomes dense where there is inflammation or an allergic reaction. It is a component of *jin ye*, which is one of the four humours of TCM. See **jin ye**.

mugwort *Artemisia vulgaris* Also called Chinese wormwood. Herbal medicine. Distribution: Asia, Europe. Parts: leaves. Character: warm, hot-bitter. Affinity: liver, spleen, kidneys. Effects: astringent, haemostatic, analgesic, warms meridians and reduces internal coldness. Symptoms: blood in sputum, vomit or stools, nosebleeds, menorrhagia. Treatments: dysmenorrhoea, metrorrhagia. Dosage: 4–10 g. Mugwort is the source of the *moxa* used in moxibustion. It must NOT be confused with moxa weed, *Artemisia capillaris*, or sweet wormwood, *Artemisia annua*, or other species of wormwood, such as absinthe, or green ginger, *Artemisia absinthium*. Mugwort is a good treatment for tired and swollen or blistered feet. To apply this treatment, bathe the feet in an infusion of the leaves, then dry the feet well and dust with dried, powdered mugwort leaves. Mugwort must NOT be administered to a woman who is pregnant or suspected of being pregnant.

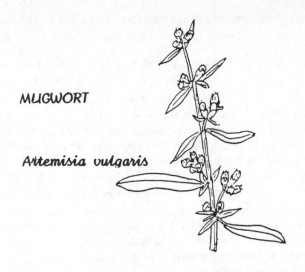

MUGWORT

Artemisia vulgaris

mukyi 'Wood ears'. An ear-shaped fungus which grows on old tree trunks. The Chinese value them as a health food, for they cool the liver, clear bloodshot eyes and clean the digestive tract and lungs. They are stir-fried or added to soups. Wood ears must not be confused with silver wood ears.

mulberry *Morus alba* Herbal medicine. Distribution: China, Japan, Vietnam. Parts: leaves. Character: cold, bitter-sweet. Affinity: liver, lungs. Effects: antipyretic, refrigerant, liver sedative, improves sight. Symptoms: headache, colds, cough, swollen and painful eyes. Treatments: asthma, bronchitis, wind-heat injury. Dosage: 4–9 g. The root may be used as an expectorant and antitussive.

mulberry wine This wine, which is made from mulberry fruits in the same way as any other medicinal wine, is considered to be helpful for hair loss. See **medicinal wine**.

multiple sclerosis A disease in which the protective sheaths of the nerves deteriorate so that the nerves develop sclerosis in various parts of the body. The condition is slowly progressive, and the symptoms, which may include dizziness, numbness, vision problems and weak or stiff limbs, vary according to which nerves have been affected. There are periods of remission and relapse. In TCM, the treatments are acupuncture, massage and remedial exercises, which are sometimes alleviative but not curative. See **sclerosis**.

mumps See **parotitis**.

mung beans See **bean sprouts**.

murmur An abnormal heart sound heard by a physician when using a stethoscope, and possibly indicating a heart defect. See **pulse**.

muscle An organ which, by its contraction, produces movement in a part of the body. There are three types of muscle: striated, which is involved in voluntary movement, and is under conscious control; smooth, which is involved in involuntary movement, and occurs unconsciously, as with the muscles which control the movements of the oesophagus; and cardiac muscle, which has the special quality of controlling the rhythm of the heartbeat. TCM recognizes the strong relationship between the lungs and the muscles. The latter require a plentiful supply of oxygen and *qi*, or 'vital energy', which the lungs provide. Muscles can be toned by some of the exercises contained in the *Chinese Exercise Manual*. See **lungs**.

muscular aches and pains These are due to over-using muscles, which require at least 48 hours to recover after doing strenuous exercise or work. The capacity of a muscle is not increased by use, but only by being built up by protein, as is done by body-builders, which can be a risky proceeding. It is generally the healthier practice for would-be body-builders to accept their limitations. Some relief from aches and pains in muscles can be obtained by hot baths, hot towels, hot compresses, massage and analgesics externally applied, and which will penetrate the skin. In TCM, the treatment would be massage, preferably by a professional, and an infusion of one of the following, taken internally, using the parts and dosages indicated: gentian, *Gentiana macrophylla*, roots, 3–7 g; clematis, *Clematis chinensis*, roots, 4–8 g; cassia, or Chinese cinnamon, *Cinnamomum cassia*, bark, 1–4 g; fennel, *Foeniculum vulgare*, fruits, 2–4 g.

muscular dystrophy A hereditary disease involving weakness and wasting of muscles. In TCM, the treatments are massage and remedial exercises, which are only alleviative.

mushroom See **fungi**.

mushroom poisoning Mushrooms of many different species feature prominently in the Chinese diet, and so there is always the risk of mushroom poisoning, for which the usual TCM treatment is an infusion, taken internally, of 2–8 g roots of liquorice, *Glycyrrhiza uralensis*. See **mustard**.

musk-deer *Moschus moschiferus* Medicine. Distribution: Tibet, North India, Siberia. Parts: dried secretion of preputial follicles. Character: warm, pungent. Affinity: heart, spleen. Effects: stimulant, resuscitive, cardiotonic, promotive of circulation.

Symptoms: fainting, delirium, shock. Treatments: amenorrhoea, retained placenta or foetus, traumatic injury. Dosage: 0.2–0.4 g. This medicine must NOT be administered to women who are pregnant. For obvious reasons, this medicine would not meet with the approval of the animal lovers of the West.

mussel See **mollusc**.

mustard The seeds of this herb, which is of Asiatic origin, are now used throughout the world for both culinary and medicinal purposes. There are three main species: white or yellow, *Brassica alba*; black, *Brassica nigra*; brown, *Brassica juncea*. A poultice of black mustard seeds relieves chest congestion, bronchitis, pneumonia and neuralgia. Chewing black mustard seeds relieves toothache, and a decoction is a treatment for mushroom poisoning. An infusion of white mustard seeds, taken internally, is a treatment for digestive disorders and bronchitis, and may also be used as a gargle to treat a sore throat.

mutation See **genetics**.

myalgia Pain in the muscles. See **muscular aches and pains**.

myalgic encephalomyelitis This is a state of complete exhaustion, for which the cause is neither simple nor immediately apparent. It is characterized by a wide variety of symptoms, which include a skin rash, itchiness, muscle pains, chest pains, excessive perspiration, a strong body odour, twitching of muscles and limbs, fever, headaches, tinnitus, visual disturbances, nausea, insomnia, enuresis, swollen glands, loss of memory and depression. It is sometimes attributed to slowness of recovery after an infection, the chicken-pox virus, the after-effects of glandular fever or a breakdown in the immune system. But some of the physicians of the West have been inclined to regard ME as no more than malingering or a mental state. Chinese physicians, however, recognize this condition, and consider its causes to be a weakness of *qi*, a blood deficiency and damp-heat. They recommend rest, a modicum of exercise, the avoidance of stressful situations and a course of acupuncture. Additionally, they recommend herbal medicines to treat the conditions as indicated by the symptoms: an antipyretic for a fever, an analgesic for a headache, a tonic for weakness, and so on.

myocarditis Inflammation of the heart muscle. This is a serious condition requiring expert medical attention. But, in any case, it could not be diagnosed by anyone other than a medical expert.

myopia Short-sightedness. See **optical defects**.

myositis Inflammation of the muscle tissue. See **muscular aches and pains**.

N

nacre Mother-of-pearl. The hard iridescent lining of the inside of the shells of certain molluscs, such as oysters and abalone. Crushed and dissolved in black vinegar, as with pearls, it was once used in TCM as a source of calcium for the body.

naevus Mole. Birthmark. An abnormal pigmented prominence or a mass of tiny blood vessels on the skin. An unsightly naevus can be removed surgically, but the Chinese view is that naevi are best left alone. A naevus must NOT be confused with a wart. See **wart**.

narcosis Sleepiness or stupor induced by drugs. See **drug**.

narcotic See **drug**.

'narcotic soup' See **anaesthesia**.

nasal spray This device is commonly used in the West to introduce a medicinal substance into the sinuses, nasal cavities or lungs. But much of the substance is wasted, for it does not always reach its target. Chinese physicians use an entirely different technique if the medicinal substance is volatile and not poisonous. It is consumed, and then it reaches the lungs via the small intestine and bloodstream. A good example of this is in the use of ephedrine in the treatment of asthma. In the West, the ephedrine is introduced into the lungs by means of a nasal spray. In TCM, the stems of joint fir, *Ephedra sinica*, which contain ephedrine, the active ingredient, are consumed. See **asthma**, **active ingredient** and **buffer**.

natural affinity of herbs See **gui jing**.

natural diet One might think that the most natural and healthiest diet for man would be one which is similar to that of his simian relatives, which is essentially vegetarian. But he has lived unnaturally for so long in matters of diet and other respects that he would now find it difficult to change his habits completely. Nevertheless, he should ensure that his diet is as natural as possible. He would do well to adopt the Chinese style of diet, which is high in fruit, vegetables and cereals, and low in meat, synthetic additives, preserved foods and sugar. See **diet, health**

foods, foods to avoid and **foods to include**.
natural distribution of herbs See **distribution**.
natural food colours See **food colours**.
natural foods These could be briefly described as foods and their sources which have not been subjected to too much of man's interference, and briefly listed as those which are grown naturally, without artificial fertilizers and pesticides, and are not preserved, processed or over-cooked. See **organic farming**.
natural immunity This is the immunity to disease which the body achieves by natural means, and not by the immunization techniques developed by medical science. See **immunity**.
natural treatments In the widest sense, this term refers to those remedial treatments which involve the use of diet, exercise, herbal medicines, and so forth, and which do not involve the use of synthetic medicines and other unnatural devices. More specifically, it refers to the direct use of the remedial effects of air, water and sunshine, as with breathing exercises, aerobics, sauna baths and sunbathing. The Chinese have a preference for natural treatments. See **weather** and **nature's treatment**.
nature The attainment of full harmony with nature is one of the cardinal principles of TCM, and it is an appreciation of nature and an understanding of man's place in nature which are the solid foundations of Taoism, from which TCM derives most of its inspiration and much of its knowledge. See **Taoism** and **Eight Pillars of Taoism**.
nature's treatment This is one of the seven categories of healing exercises which have been evolved by the Chinese over a period of about 5000 years. It comprises air treatments, water showers or baths, and sunbathing, which are fully explained in the *Chinese Exercise Manual*. See **healing exercises**.
naturopathy A system of medicine, now becoming very popular in the West, in which the body is encouraged to heal itself by diet and physical methods without resorting to drugs. It has many specialized branches, including exercise, breathing techniques, hydrotherapy and massage. Naturopathy attempts to find the underlying cause of an illness, and treat it, rather than merely attempting to suppress or alleviate the symptoms. Sweating out a fever, refraining from food to rest an empty stomach, and immersing a sprained ankle in cold water are three simple everyday examples of naturopathic treatment. Many common ailments can be effectively relieved or even cured by naturopathic treatments. But naturopathy cannot perform miracles. There are strong elements of naturopathy in TCM, with its

emphasis on acupuncture, meditation and other non-medicinal treatments.

nausea This is a feeling of sickness which may lead to actual vomiting. Its causes include disturbing movements, claustrophobia (fear of enclosed places) and other phobias, unpleasant smells, discordant sounds, resentment and an empty or acid stomach. When the cause is digestive, there is much to be said for giving the stomach a rest by fasting for 24 hours. The queasiness due to an empty stomach can be offset by eating a small amount of dry cereal food, such as toast or biscuits. The TCM herbal treatment for nausea is an infusion of one of the following, taken internally, using the parts and dosage indicated: ginger, *Zingiber officinale*, rhizomes, 3–7 g; camomile *Matricaria chamomilla*, flowers, 3–10 g; cassia, or Chinese cinnamon, *Cinnamomum cassia*, bark, 1.5–4 g; loquat, *Eriobotrya japonica*, leaves, 8–14 g; cardamom, *Elletaria cardamomum*, crushed seeds, 2–6 g. For this, one could also use a water-suspension of 10 g haematite (brown iron oxide), but this is not a remedy which would be acceptable to Western physicians. Chewing the pith or peel of a mandarin orange (*Citrus reticulata*) is helpful, as also is white rice porridge.

ACUPRESSURE FOR NAUSEA

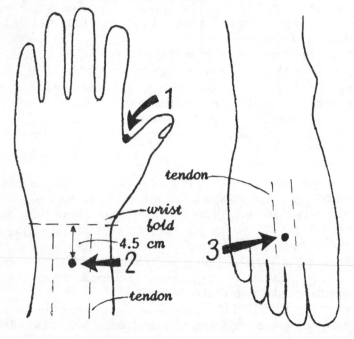

Chinese physicians would say that the treatment of nausea requires the lowering of stomach-*qi*, and would recommend acupuncture for this. Do-it-yourself acupressure can be carried out very easily on three acupoints as follows:

1. Press the point between the thumb and the forefinger on either hand, using a deep and firm pressure with a massaging movement.
2. With the palm upwards, use the same pressure and movement on the point which lies 4.5 centimetres from the wrist fold and between the two tendons.
3. Use the thumb to apply the same pressure and movement to the region between the tendons of the second and third toes on either foot.

naval Umbilicus. See **reproductive systems**.

neck acupressure The Chinese have evolved an effective acupressure technique for alleviating headaches and pain and stiffness in the neck. It is suitable for do-it-yourself treatment providing that the neck pain is due to muscular inflammation or injury, and there is no serious underlying cause, such as spinal injury. The procedure is as follows:

1. Hold the head in the hands so that the thumbs are pressing against the occipital bone behind the ears. Rotate the thumbs firmly at this point for about two minutes.
2. Hold the forehead with one hand, and the back of the head with the other so that the thumb is pressing into the hollow at the base of the skull. Rotate the thumb firmly for about two minutes.
3. Press firmly on the acupoint at the top of the arm on the edge of the shoulder.
4. Press very hard on the point on the inside of the arm at the elbow. A sensation should be felt in the hand. Do this for about 30 seconds.
5. Press firmly for about 30 seconds on the point on the forearm which is about 6 cm down from the point on the inside of the arm near the elbow.
6. Press the point on the back of the hand which is halfway between the knuckle of the forefinger and the wrist line. Do this for about one minute.

See **neck massage**.

neck massage The Chinese have evolved an effective massage technique for alleviating headaches and pain and stiffness in the neck. It is suitable for do-it-yourself treatment providing that the

NECK ACUPRESSURE

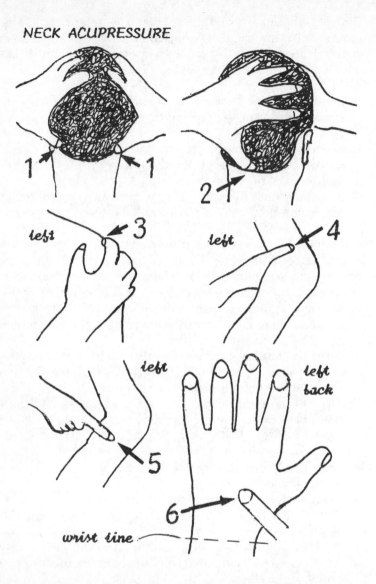

neck pain is due to muscular inflammation or injury, and there is no serious underlying cause, such as spinal injury. The procedure is as follows:

(a) Grip the left shoulder, and with the forefinger, massage the muscle firmly about 10 times, using downward strokes only.

(b) Use a dry towel to massage the neck for about two minutes.

The motion of the towel should be as if the neck is being dried after a bath.

(c) With the fist loosely clenched drum hard down the back of the neck and down the side of the arm.

(d) Move the head left to right and forwards and backwards about 20 times.

(e) Stand with legs apart and arms down at the sides, and then relax. Shake the hands, allowing free movement of the shoulders, for about five minutes.

(f) Pummel the back of the neck with both fists for about two minutes.

This neck massage can be combined with neck acupressure to make one smooth sequence, and then the correct order will be 1, 2, (a), (b), 3, 4, (c), 5, 6 (d), (e), (f). See **neck acupressure**.

neck pain This is usually due to one's occupation or some activity which requires that the head be kept in a certain position for lengthy periods. If the condition persists, medical advice should be sought, for it could be symptomatic of a spinal injury or disease. Otherwise, the treatment is to apply ice or cold water to the neck to reduce inflammation, and then take a hot bath or apply a hot towel. It is helpful to sleep in a foetal position on a flat bed without a pillow. It is highly desirable that the neck should be exercised by tossing and turning the head. But Chinese physicians would recommend acupressure and massage, which is best done by a professional, but as a temporary measure, one can massage the neck with a towel for about two minutes, and then pummel the back of the neck with both fists for about two minutes. See **neck acupressure** and **neck massage**.

necrosis The death of an organ or tissue, especially a bone.

negative cycle See **element**.

Nei Ching See **Nei Jing**.

nei gong See **nei kung**.

Nei Jing Also spelt as *Nei Ching*. This remarkable book, 'The Classic of Internal Medicine', which must not be confused with *Huang Di Nei Jing*, or 'The Internal Book of the Yellow Emperor', appeared during the middle of the period of the Han dynasty (206 BC–AD 220). It explains the theory of the circulation of the blood, which suggests that, over 2000 years ago, Chinese medicine was already in an advanced state. Together with *Tsien Ching Fang*, or 'The Thousand Prescriptions', *Nei Jing* chronicles the history of the healing exercises – *nei gong*, or 'internal exercises', and *qi gong*, or 'breathing exercises'. It could be that much of the information it contains was gleaned from a treatise on acupuncture and health in general which came into existence about 400 BC. The *Nei Jing* emphasises the importance of the meridians, as this quotation indicates: 'It is the device by which man is created, the device by which diseases occur, the device by which people are healed, and the device by which diseases are cured: the 12 meridians are the basis for all medical principles and treatments. The meridians decide all matters of life and death. It is through the meridians that the hundred diseases are treated.' See **Tsien Chin Fang** and **meridian**.

nei kung Also written as *nei gong*. The internal exercises of Taoist medical philosophy. See **Nei Jing**.

Nei Pien This book, which was compiled by Ko Hung, a Taoist scholar, and published about AD 320, contains secret teachings, hitherto unrecorded, about the protection which can be provided by occult forces. It describes how gold, silver, jade and pearls and other precious stones may be used medicinally to protect the health and confer immortality. This book makes wildly exaggerated claims for the efficacy of cinnamon and onion juice as medicines. It also lists about 300 items of diet which can improve the health, increase virility and prolong life. But, apart from these exotic prescriptions and fanciful claims, this book contains much common-sense advice, especially in regard to moderate habits and a wise philosophy of living. See **jade**, **wound** and **philosophy of health**.

nei yang kung 'Internally nourishing breathing exercise'. It constitutes one of the exercises in the *qi kung*, or 'breathing exercises', and the *nei kung*, or 'internal exercises', which are components of Taoist medical philosophy. It is appropriate for treating gastric and duodenal ulcers, hepatitis and chronic constipation. It is fully explained in the *Chinese Exercise Manual*.

nematode worm A member of a class of roundworms whose bodies are long, slender, smooth and unsegmented. Many species are parasites in both plants and animals, and it has been estimated that more than one third of the human race is infected with parasitic roundworms of one kind or another. See **hookworm** and **pin-worm**.

neoplasm See **tumour**.

nephrite Jade. This name derives from the Chinese belief in the efficacy of jade as a treatment for renal disorders. This belief was not without foundation, for jade is a mixture of silicates of calcium and magnesium, and silicon, calcium and magnesium are among the mineral needs of the body. What is more, compounds of calcium and silicon are used quite extensively in homoeopathic medicine for the treatment of a wide variety of ailments. See **jade** and **Nei Pien**.

nephritis Bright's disease. Inflammation of the kidneys, which is characterized by fever, hypertension, headaches, backache, oedema and blood and protein in the urine. It is generally caused by a disorder of the immune system or an allergic reaction to a streptococcal infection. If the condition becomes chronic, it can be insidious, and may lead to nephrosis and complete kidney failure, and then a transplant or regular treatment on a dialysis machine would be necessary. According to TCM, nephritis is associated not only with the kidneys but also with the lungs and spleen, and so all three organs will require treatment. Both the kidneys and the lungs are excretory organs, and they are interdependent in their functions to some extent. Acute nephritis will often follow influenza or tonsillitis, the kidneys being affected by the heat from those conditions. Weakness of the spleen and tiredness may also be contributory factors in the establishment of oedema. The kidneys are delicate organs, and so medical advice should be sought where nephritis or any other kidney disorder is suspected. There is some similarity between the symptoms of kidney disorders, and it is important, therefore, that nephritis should be correctly diagnosed. Many people with backache take proprietary brands of diuretic medicines, but they are taking risks, for backache also has causes other than nephritis. See **nephrosis** and **renal disorders**.

nephrosis Nephrotic syndrome. A group of conditions of the kidneys arising from several different but associated dysfunctions, including nephritis, cystitis and kidney stones. The symptoms are oedema and albuminuria, which is a large amount of protein in the urine. This is a serious condition requiring expert medical attention. See **nephritis** and **renal disorders**.

nephrotic syndrome See **nephrosis**.

nerve A bundle of fibres which has the appearance of a white thread, and which carries messages in the form of electrochemical impulses either to or from the brain or the spinal cord. A motor nerve generally carries only those impulses which activate the muscles, and a sensory nerve carries only those impulses which indicate sensation. But it still seems that some nerves are equipped to carry both sensory and motor impulses. Some nerves, such as the optic nerve from the eye and the olfactory nerve from the nose, lead directly from the sense organs to the brain, whilst others, such as those from the skin and muscles, enter the spinal cord. The nerves form a network of communication throughout the body. According to TCM, the meridians form another network of communication, but one which is mainly concerned with the transfer of *qi*. See **involuntary movement**, **nervous system** and **meridian**.

'nerves' An everyday term which is used loosely, and often misleadingly, to describe those conditions of the mind or body which are due to fatigue or debility or are stress-related, and which include those so-called mental and nervous disorders which are variously named as nervous breakdowns, nervous debility, anxiety states, neuroses, psychoses, complexes, phobias and so forth. Perhaps this term is commonly used because there is still some stigma attached to mental illnesses and nervous disorders. But the term 'nerves' is misleading because the conditions which it describes are generally not disorders of the nerves or brain, but are due to hormonal imbalances, fatigue or other disturbances. The nerves are likely to be in a sound working order because, if they were not so, they would not be able to report to the brain that something is amiss within the body. Chinese physicians have always regarded many illnesses as being psychosomatic, and they do not make a sharp distinction between sickness of the mind and sickness of the body, as we tend to do in the West, and probably because they recognize that there are no sharp distinctions. For thousands of years, they have known that emotional conditions are largely determined by the houses of the body, which we know as the endocrine glands, and are strongly influenced by the vital organs. In strict medical terms, diseases of the actual nerves, as opposed to conditions of the body which are described as 'nerves', should be described as 'neurological'. Three commonly used TCM sedatives for irritability, excitability, sleeplessness, anxiety and the other manifestations of 'nerves' are infusions, taken internally, of the following, using the parts and dosages indicated: hop, *Humulus lupulus*, strobiles, 1.5–3 g; basil, *Ocimum basilicum*, leaves, 2–4 g; camomile, *Matricaria chamomilla*, flowers, 3–10 g; sage, *Salvia officinalis*, leaves, 15–8 g. Sage must NOT be administered to a woman who is pregnant. The fruits of the wolfberry, *Lycium chinense*, added to soups and stews, in a dosage of 4–10 g, makes an effective general tonic. See **mental health**, **nervous disorders**, **neuropathy** and **neurology**.

nervine A medicine to alleviate a nervous disorder. Generally, nervines are either relaxants or stimulants. See **sedative** and **stimulant**.

nervous bowel See **colitis**.

nervous breakdown See **nervous disorders**.

nervous debility A feebleness and generally poor condition of the body, which may be accompanied by a disturbed state of mind and a lack of interest in normal affairs. Irritability, timidity, sleeplessness, depression, tiredness and feelings of helplessness, which may be collectively described as 'nerves' or nervousness, are among its symptoms, but they are more indicative of hormonal changes at puberty, unsound diet, lack of exercise, fatigue or immoderate habits than any fundamental defects in the nervous system, and so *debility*, and not *nervous debility*, is the preferable term. One of the traditional Chinese treatments for this condition is a medicinal wine, of which many are available. Whatever their medicinal effects may be, they do give a little pleasure and have a soporific effect, and so, providing they are not taken to excess, they could provide some form of relief for a person who is not bursting with enthusiasm for life in general. Some medicinal wines, such as fig and wolfberry, are strengthening to the body. Tonic wines are also a common feature of popular medicine in the West. See **debility**, **neurasthenia**, **nervous disorders** and **medicinal wine**.

nervous disorders Those nervous disorders which are called neuroses, anxiety states, nervous breakdowns, nervous debility, depression and so forth, and which are generally manifested by irrational anger or acute anxiety, and which evoke the desire to fight or take flight, are more likely to be due to malfunctions and other conditions of the body – tiredness, hormonal imbalance, glandular disturbances, obesity, dietary deficiencies, over-pre-occupation with sex, etc. – than any serious malfunction of the brain or nervous system, though the brain will react unfavourably to an abnormal condition of the body, so creating the erroneous impression of mental illness or even insanity. A nervous breakdown is one of the most distressing forms of nervous disorders. The sufferer feels anxious and insecure, or even distraught with unaccountable fears, his sleep may be disturbed by nightmares, he becomes mistrustful even of his closest relatives and friends, he becomes over-introverted and he is acutely aware of his condition, which adds to his distress. And yet, when he has recovered, as sufferers from nervous breakdowns almost invariably do, he will wonder why he was so concerned. Some nervous disorders, particularly those which induce depression or debility, may be due to dietary deficiencies, which, if uncorrected, may lead to a very serious illness, or even prove to be fatal, as with beriberi and pellagra. Deficiencies of phosphorus and niacin may be corrected by including plenty of fish in the diet, and brewer's yeast would do the same for a deficiency of thiamin. Nervous disorders are psychosomatic – the mind influencing the body, and the body influencing the mind. An example of this is Da Costa's syndrome, which is a condition of anxiety whereby a person develops palpitations and other chest conditions because he fears that his heart is diseased, though it is perfectly sound. But if the imagination and this kind of negative thinking can induce an anxiety state of this magnitude, there must surely be occasions when a bit of positive thinking could reduce anxiety or even cure a nervous disorder completely. And there is no doubt that if the treatment of a nervous disorder is to be fully effective, the patient must co-operate fully with his physician. With nervous disorders, a tragedy may occasionally occur, as when a person in a depressed state of mind decides to escape from his misery by committing suicide, though the sufferers who feel suicidal rarely do commit suicide, for the instinct for self-preservation is very strong even among those who feel desperate in their afflictions. It would seem that a very necessary part of the treatment for a nervous breakdown is the companionship of a person who is patient, understanding and firm. According to TCM, some nervous disorders are due to stagnation of liver-qi, which is feasible since the liver is the largest gland in the body. In this respect, a varied and low-fat diet and an adequate amount of exercise would be helpful. Chinese physicians would contend that, as preventive treatment is preferable to curative treatment, people should live normally in order to remain normal, eschewing immoderate practices in matters of diet, exercise, alcohol and sleep. The theory is that nervous disorders can be addressed as effectively by changes in behaviour as by medicine. If there is a lower incidence of nervous and mental disorders in China than in the West, it is because the Chinese abide by the teachings of Confucius and Lao Zi. In TCM, the usual treatments for nervous disorders are massage, acupuncture, acupressure and meditation. One of the secondary benefits of manipulative techniques is the feeling of security – that someone cares – which is created by the nearness of the practitioner to the patient. The meditation involves a complete rejection of unpleasant thoughts, and some positive thinking on the lines of auto-suggestion, or self-hypnosis. The meditator could repeat over and over again the maxim for which Emile Coué became famous: 'Every day, in every way, I am getting better and better.' It is likely that the real benefit of this exercise is that it directs the patient's mind away from unpleasant thoughts and makes him feel that he is doing something positive on his own behalf, which helps to create self-confidence. TCM also has a wide range of sedatives, soporifics, stimulants and tonics which the physician can apply according to the patient's needs. A traditional remedy for the severer forms of mental and nervous disorders, such as hysteria, epilepsy, manic depression and uncontrollable anger is a mixture of 20 g liquorice, *Glycyrrhiza uralensis*, 55 g grains of wheat, *Triticum aestivum*, and 8 fruits of jujube, *Ziziphus jujuba*, added to 1 litre water in a covered vessel, and boiled until it decocts to ⅓ litre. It is strained and then sipped slowly. But it is important to understand that the symptoms of nervous disorders are also the symptoms of many organic disorders, or a nervous disorder can be the outcome of a serious underlying condition. It is imperative, therefore, that a nervous disorder should be correctly diagnosed, which can only be done by a professional medical practitioner. Depression is one of the effects of many illnesses, and it would be unnecessary to treat a patient with a tranquillizing drug when he is only recovering from a cold or influenza. One of the interesting features of nervous disorders is that it is the intelligent and sensitive who are most likely to succumb to a nervous breakdown or an anxiety state because they are most likely to react sensitively to difficult or emotive situations. See **mental health**, **insight**, **neurosis**, **neurology**, **morality**, **moderation** and **self-hypnosis**.

nervous indigestion This is a psychosomatic condition which is more likely to be effectively treated by adopting normal habits and avoiding stressful situations than by the usual herbal remedies for indigestion. See **concentration** and **sedative**.

nervous irritability This is an everyday term of vague meaning which could describe the moroseness of a person who is liverish and generally out of sorts or the itchiness which is characteristic of some skin disorders, such as eczema and hives. A TCM treatment for itchiness of the skin is an infusion, applied externally, of 2–4 g leaves of chickweed, *Stellaria media*. See **pruritis**.

nervous system The nervous system consists of the brain, spinal cord, nerves and sense organs. It obtains and stores information and, together with the hormones, or secretions of the endocrine glands, controls the activities of the body. The larger nerves are of two main kinds, which are those that connect directly to the brain, such as the olfactory nerve in the nose, and those, such as the sciatic nerve in the leg, whose impulses reach the brain via the spinal cord. The branches of the main nerves are of three kinds – motor, sensory and mixed. The mixed nerves are unusual in that they can carry impulses either to or from the brain or spinal cord. A matter for speculation is the extent to which the mixed nerves are stimulated by acupuncture or acupressure, for there are situations where a reversal of the direction of the nerve impulses could have a beneficial effect – in inhibiting pain, perhaps. The network of nerves is really two systems. One controls the voluntary movements of the body, as when one throws a ball or speaks to someone. The other, called the autonomic, or sympathetic, nervous system, controls the involuntary movements, such as the reflexes and heartbeat. The brain is fully conscious of the former system but not the latter, at least not fully. In TCM, the meridians are also regarded as a network of communication within the body. The *Chinese Exercise Manual* contains exercises for the treatment of sciatica, paraplegia and other diseases and defects of the nervous system. See **brain**, **nerve**, **involuntary movement**, **autonomic nervous system** and **meridian**.

nettle-rash See **hives**.

neuralgia The pain due to inflammation of a nerve, and which is not felt in the nerve itself but seems to stem from the organ or tissues that are served by the nerve. Thus, inflammation of the trigeminal, or fifth cranial, nerve, which enters the skull near the ear, is felt in the forehead, chin or either cheek, so producing the condition called trigeminal neuralgia, or tic douloureux, which is a particularly painful type of neuralgia. A nerve becomes inflamed as a consequence of exposure to cold or as a reaction to a condition in some other part of the body. For example, neuralgia in the shoulder is commonly due to inflammation of the gall-bladder. Some relief can be obtained by applying hot compresses or a hot-water bottle to the affected area. According to TCM, neuralgia is due to wind, fire and heat in the meridians, and the usual treatment is acupuncture to unblock the meridians, and herbs to clear the wind and heat. The acupoints stimulated are those on the meridians associated with the governor-vessel, liver, gall-bladder, bladder, stomach, kidneys and large intestine. A suitable herbal remedy is an infusion, taken internally, of 1–3 g leaves of feverfew, *Chrysanthemum parthenium*. Crushed seeds of black mustard, *Brassica nigra*, and crushed capsules of corn poppy, *Papaver rhoeas*, can be applied in a compress or poultice. See **neuritis**.

neurasthenia A vague term which describes lassitude and a general weakness of the body. It is sometimes defined as debility of the nerves. It is best regarded as a more persistent form of debility. A TCM remedy for this condition is an infusion, taken internally, of 3–5 fruits of jujube, *Ziziphus jujuba*.

neuritis Inflammation of a nerve. If the condition causes intense pain, it is described as neuralgia. TCM attributes neuritis to wind, damp and heat in the meridians. But it can be a complex condition, and so medical advice should be sought. See **neuralgia**.

neuro-endocrine theory This is one of several theories which explain the mode of operation of acupuncture. Recent research has shown that the needling of acupoints induces the nervous system to release endorphin, which is a protein that has a great potency as a pain-killer. Endorphin has some relationship with the endocrine glands, which explains the use of the term *neuro-endocrine*. See **endorphin**, **gate control theory** and **electro-acupuncture**.

neurological disorders These are diseases and defects of the nerves and other parts of the nervous system, and should not be confused with nervous disorders, which are diseases and defects of the body that are manifested by nervous reactions. Neurological disorders include neuralgia, sciatica, shingles, neuritis and multiple sclerosis. See **'nerves'** and **nervous disorders**.

neurology The scientific study of nervous systems. It is NOT a specific study of nervous disorders, though they will be involved.

neuropath A person of abnormal nervous sensibility, but whose condition is more likely to be a reaction to disturbances in other parts of his body, and without any organic changes in his nervous system. This condition can be likened to a telephone exchange in which the lines have become crossed but are not irretrievably damaged. See **neurosis**, **mental illness**, **nervous disorders** and **psychopath**.

neuropathy. An abnormal condition of the nervous system, but not necessarily one in which organic changes are involved.

neuropeptide See **endorphin**.

neurosis An abnormal mental condition whereby there is a change in behaviour and beliefs but no loss of sense of reality and no organic changes. See **neuropath**, **mental illness**, **nervous disorders**, **insight**, **psychosis** and **psychoneurosis**.

neutral A term which is used in TCM to describe those medicinal plants that do not possess any of the four energies – hot, warm, cold and cool. It is also used to describe those medicinal plants which do not possess any of the five tastes – hot, sweet, sour, bitter and salty. See **energy** and **taste**.

neutralizing treatment This is one of the eight methods of herbal treatment in TCM. It is an allopathic approach, and is firmly rooted in the yin-yang principle of complementary opposites, which is the basis of all Chinese herbal medicine. The effects of an illness or other bodily condition are neutralized by a medicine whose effects are of an opposite character. Thus, a cold illness is neutralized by a warm medicine, a hot illness by a cool medicine, dryness by dampness, emptiness by stimulation, fullness by sedation, sourness or bitterness by sweetness, and so on. This method is commonly used to encourage the elevation of internal illnesses, which are generally more serious than external illnesses. It is particuary effective in treating diseases and other conditions of the liver and kidneys, which have profound effects on the other organs.

New Medicine This is the name which the people of the Far East have given to the newly emerging combination of traditional Chinese and modern Western medical techniques. It is significant that, though New Medicine has adopted much of the Western medical technology – X-rays, microscopy, chemical analysis and scanners and other electronic devices – it has retained the traditional Chinese system in regard to the theories of health and disease and the practical methods of therapy. All the signs are that New Medicine will be a most effective combination of new knowledge and ancient wisdom. See **new medicines**.

new medicines Most Chinese medicines are of ancient origin, and are valued because they have stood the test of time and, by long experience, are known to be reliable. Nevertheless, a few new medicines have been introduced into Chinese pharmacopoeias during recent years. A good example of a new medicine is the pumpkin, *Cucurbita moschata*, which is used in the treatment of intestinal worms. It is such a recent newcomer that its natural affinities have not yet been established. Some Western-style medicines are now included in TCM pharmacopoeias. Chinese physicians are not bigoted or prejudiced in this, for their first consideration is the health and welfare of their patients and not matters of national pride. They have a preference for herbal medicines, it is true, for they regard them as being much safer and far more reliable, but they also recognize that some synthetic medicines have their merits. See **New Medicine**.

niacin Nicotinic acid. Vitamin B_3. It must NOT be confused with nicotine, which is a poisonous alkaloid in tobacco. See **pellagra** and **vitamin**.

nicotine See **niacin**.

night-blindness See **nyctalopia**.

nightmare See **dreams**.

night sweats See **sweats**.

nipple See **teat**.

nit See **head lice**.

nitrates The nitrates in the soil are a source of the nitrogen which plants utilize in the synthesis of protein. Proteins are complex organic compounds, and all contain carbon, hydrogen, oxygen and nitrogen, and some also contain phosphorus and sulphur. See **fertilizer** and **nitrogen**.

nitrogen An odourless and colourless gas which makes up about 78 per cent of the atmosphere. It is only slightly reactive, but it is present in all proteins and is essential to life. See **nitrates**.

nocturnal emission This is an involuntary emission of semen during sleep. It is often accompanied by an erotic dream, which explains why it is commonly called a 'wet dream'. This is a perfectly natural occurrence, and it is hardly one that needs medical treatment, though many of the Taoists of ancient China held the view that the sperm must be conserved in order to achieve longevity. The TCM treatment for this condition is 10–28 g tubers of knotty yam, *Dioscorea opposita*, administered in a soup or a stew. But its purpose is not to prevent emissions but to tone and strengthen a body which has become weakened by too many emissions. See **spermatorrhoea** and **Yellow Emperor**.

nocturnal sweats See **sweats**.

node Nodule. A lymph gland or a small mass of tissue. See **tumour**.

noise We do not think of noise as being a form of pollution, but it certainly is that; and it is more than just a nuisance, for at high levels and over long periods, it can be a cause of stress and a danger to the hearing. Much of the noisiness of our modern world is due to machinery, vehicles and communications devices. Above a certain safety level, noise can cause a ringing in the ears and temporary loss of hearing. Four hours of noise at over 93 decibels can cause permanent damage to the hearing. Noise causes shocks, for a person reacts instinctively to sudden loud noises, and his muscles tense and his heartbeat and breathing rate increase, which can lead to stress, fatigue, headaches, hypertension and even insomnia and ulcers. The effects of noise can be minimized by insulating buildings and avoiding those situations where noise levels are likely to be high. In this respect, the Chinese have fewer problems than the people of the West, for the rural areas of China are of great quietude and there are few motorized vehicles in the cities. China has not yet fallen victim to the perils of mechanization. But, in any case, the Chinese are peaceful and peace-loving by temperament, and so, for them, excessive noise is one of those violent extremes which are best avoided.

non-critical dosage The dosage of most Chinese medicines is non-critical, which means that no harm is done if the prescribed dosage is exceeded, and so one does not need to work to fine limits in preparing a medicine. But there are a few medicines which will only be efficacious if the dosage is within certain prescribed limits or will be injurious if the upper limit is exceeded. See **critical dosage** and **dangers with medicines**.

non-irritant soap See **soap**.

noodles According to the history books, the Chinese invented noodles over 2000 years ago, and the first emperor to sample them was Wang Mang, who reigned for only 14 years, from AD 9 to AD 23, during the period of the Han dynasty (206 BC–AD 220). Being made from wheat or rice flour, noodles are a rich source of carbohydrate. Also, they are inexpensive and economical in use, for nothing is wasted, and the dried varieties keep so well that they can be stored almost indefinitely without any deterioration. In the north of China, they are a useful stand-by for the winter months, when fresh vegetables are not readily available. They are quickly and easily cooked, and they may be fried or boiled. They have the same sort of versatility as rice, for which they are often a convenient substitute. The Italians are the only people of the West who have seen the value of noodles, from which they have developed a wide range of pasta products. See **Marco Polo**.

normal dosage The dosage of a herbal medicine may be expressed in a variety of ways – by weight or by volume of the dried or the fresh herb – but it is generally accepted by herbalists that a normal dosage is the prescribed daily intake of the dried herb measured by weight in grams, and irrespective of the amount of water used to make an infusion or decoction. See **dosages**.

north In Chinese tradition, the direction north is symbolically associated with the kidneys. See **direction**.

nosebleed The cause of a nosebleed is a ruptured blood vessel inside the nose, on the septum, and which results from a dry atmosphere, a blow to the nose, a cold, hypertension, blood complaints, violent coughing or sneezing, catarrh or other sinus problems or picking the nose. The usual treatment in the West is to plug the bleeding nostril with cotton-wool soaked in a mildly antiseptic fluid such as white vinegar, apply an ice-pack or pinch the fleshy part of the nose with the thumb and forefinger for about 10 minutes. One should breathe through the mouth until the blood vessel has completely healed. Aspirin should be avoided, for it inhibits clotting of the blood. If nosebleeds are frequent, medical aid should be sought, for the cause could be hypertension, which would require treatment. Women should be aware that oral contraceptives can cause nosebleeds. According to TCM, nosebleeds are due to excessive heat in the blood, but with women who are menstruating, it is due to blood ascending instead of descending. The treatment is herbal, and an infusion of one of the following, taken internally, using the parts and dosage indicated, is considered to be suitable: *gan di huang*, *Rehmannia glutinosa*, root, 4–6 g; peony tree, *Paeonia moutan*, skin of roots, 4–8 g; yarrow, or milfoil, *Achillea millefolium*, flowers, 3–10 g; gardenia, *Gardenia jasminoides*, fruits, 4–8 g; mugwort, *Artemisia vulgaris*, leaves, 4–8 g; wild turmeric, *Curcuma aromatica*, roots, 4–8 g. Also helpful is a suspension of 10–20 g haematite (brown iron oxide), but this is not a medicine which would meet with the approval of the physicians of the West.

notifiable diseases In most countries, it is a legal requirement that certain infectious diseases be notified to a medical practitioner or the health authorities. This enables the authorities to take preventive action against the spread of the diseases, and the statistical information so obtained will assist the government in matters of health policy and legislation. In this respect, Chinese health regulations are similar to those of the West, but they are far less bureaucratic.

notoginseng See **san qi**.

nourishing breathing See **nei yang kung**.

nourishing foods These are the foods which supply all the bodily requirements in terms of energy, growth, tissue repair and health. Milk is one of the few foods which can fully satisfy these requirements; but, for reasons of health, the Chinese are not strong advocates of the consumption of cow's milk. For full nourishment, the body requires a varied combination of foods. See **diet**, **classification of foods** and **milk and milk products**.

nourishing-qi See **qi**.

nucleus See **cell**.

numbers Traditionally, in Chinese medicine, the five solid vital organs have symbolic numerical relationships: heart, seven; liver, eight; spleen, five; kidneys, six; lungs, nine. See **symbolism**.

nursing See **hospitalization**.

nursing mothers TCM has a number of tonic medicines which serve the needs of nursing mothers, often by producing an increase in lactation. One of these, which is commonly used in the south of China, is a stew of pork, chicken, ginger, rice wine and wood ears – a type of fungus. Another is pig's feet cooked in black rice vinegar. There are also medicines to treat excessive lactation. See **lactation**, **galactagogue** and **pig's feet**.

nut grass *Cyperus rotundus* Herbal medicine. Distribution: Asia, Europe, Australia, North America. Parts: roots. Character: neutral, pungent and slightly bitter-sweet. Affinity: liver, heart-constrictor (pericardium). Effects: sedative, analgesic, emmenagogue, regulates liver-*qi*. Symptoms: stomach ache, fullness in chest, pain in ribs, indigestion. Treatments: amonorrhoea, dysmenorrhoea, stagnation of liver-*qi*. Dosage: 4–8 g.

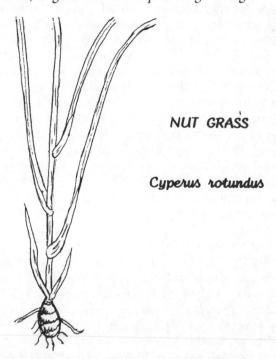

NUT GRASS

Cyperus rotundus

nutmeg *Myristica fragrans* This plant is indigenous to the islands of South-east Asia, but its kernels are used as a spice and a medicine in all parts of the world, including China. Medicinally, its kernels are used mainly as a carminative, digestive tonic and gastric stimulant in the treatment of nausea, vomiting, flatulence, colic and nervous dyspepsia. It has some reputation as an aphrodisiac, but large doses are dangerously stimulating to the nervous system.

nutrient A nutrient is a substance in food which provides energy, material for growth and repairs, and the means to regulate the bodily processes. The nutrients are carbohydrate, fat, protein, minerals and vitamins. Water and dietary fibre are not nutrients, though they are essential to the digestive and assimilative processes. In TCM, there are several herbal medicines which are valued as nutrients. Two of these are eucommia, *Eucommia ulmoides*, and jujube, *Ziziphus jujuba*. See **diet** and **food**.

nutrition The provision of food or the study of food and its purposes and health-effects. See **nutrient**, **diet** and **food**.

nux vomica *Strychnos nux-vomica*. This plant yields strychnine, a vegetable alkaloid which is highly poisonous, but which, in small amounts, is used as a stimulant and a tonic. By the terms of the Medicines Act 1968, nux vomica cannot be prescribed by someone who is not a registered medical practitioner.

nyctalopia Night-blindness. This condition is defined as both a recurrent loss of vision in twilight and darkness and the inability to see clearly at night. The condition may be inherited, or it may be due to a deficiency of retinol, or vitamin A, which is contained in yellow-orange vegetables, especially carrots. It is also contained in tomatoes, green vegetables, liver, eggs and dairy products. See **hereditary defects**.

nymphomania Abnormally excessive sexual desire in women.

nystagmus An eye disease in which there is a continual and rapid movement of the eyeballs, from side to side and up and down. It is associated with certain nervous disorders.

O

oats In the West, this cereal is regarded as a valuable item of diet because it is high in starch, fat and dietary fibre, and it also contains protein, minerals and some B-complex vitamins. It lowers cholesterol levels in the blood, which action is attributed to the presence of soluble dietary fibre and polyunsaturated fatty acids. Very little oats is consumed in China, but it is sometimes included in the diet as a means of increasing virility.

obesity This is a condition in which excess fat accumulates in the body. To some extent, it is caused by overeating. It can generally be prevented or corrected by adopting a diet which contains healthy and wholesome food. In this respect, one could not do better than to adopt the Chinese diet. It is certainly not advisable to adopt a 'crash diet' or take medicines to induce vomiting or keep the bowel in a constant state of evacuation, for these can be harmful and may lead to anorexia or bulimia. Some people have an inherited predisposition to obesity, and so, even if they are abstemious in eating, they still put on weight very easily; and, by contrast, some people consume enormous quantities of food, but do not put on weight. The people in the latter group are likely to be active – taking exercise or working manually – and so they 'burn off' their excess fat by the normal oxidation process in the tissues of the body. But the people in the former group are likely to be inactive and in a sedentary occupation. Perhaps, to some extent, we should accept ourselves as we are, and in the way that nature has made us. Psychological factors are involved here – many people's view of what is an acceptable weight is dictated by fashion, and this seems to be particularly true for women. By and large, current thinking seems to be that 'thin is beautiful'. But, if one takes a look at some of the paintings of nude women which were so tastefully executed by the artists in medieval Italy, one learns that there was a time when 'fat was beautiful', at least in Italy, if not elsewhere. However, if fatness becomes excessive, it can be damaging to the health, causing circulation problems, hypertension, heart complaints, gout, diabetes and liver and gall-bladder disorders. Excess weight may cause haemorrhoids or damage the joints of the knees and hips, causing osteoarthritis. According to TCM, the causes of obesity are complex. They include overeating, inactivity, problems with metabolism and the glands, weaknesses in the spleen and kidneys, and too much phlegm and dampness in the body. TCM treatments are a balanced and varied diet with moderate amounts of food, meridian massage, acupuncture, including ear acupuncture, and a regular intake of green tea and fennel tea to strengthen the kidneys. Fennel tea is an infusion of 2–4 g fruits of fennel, *Foeniculum vulgare*. Although much fuss is made about people being overweight, would-be slimmers should bear in mind that emaciation is not a particularly healthy state. But, in fairness, it must be said that more people die from overeating than under-eating. See **dieting**, **anorexia nervosa** and **bulimia**.

observation This is one of the four basic techniques employed by a Chinese physician in making a diagnosis. He will observe the colour and texture of the patient's tongue and skin, and examine his eyes and bodily excretions and secretions. He will observe the patient's movements in walking, sitting and lying, and how he talks and breathes. He will notice whether the patient is lively, alert and self-confident, or listless, moody and nervous. The skin, tongue, eyes, stools and urine are good guides to a person's state of health. A cold and sweaty skin, a pale complexion, bloodshot eyes, hard or watery stools, blood in the stools, murky or sugary urine, discoloured phlegm and a red or furry tongue are all indications of a poor state of health. See **tongue diagnosis**, **stools** and **urine diagnosis**.

obsessive fixations and compulsions A fixation is similar to a complex in being a fixed idea in a person's mind, and which may become an obsession, and is then persistent, intrusive and often illogical. A compulsion is an action or habit, often quite unreasonable, which a person feels compelled to perform even though the outcome could be undesirable or damaging to himself. Fixations and compulsions, which are usually allied in their origins and effects, generally develop in childhood, when the mind is receptive, and become a part of a person's daily routine. Often, they do no harm, and are sometimes beneficial, as, for example, when they are to do with rules for health and safety, or are social acts which assist the community. But they can be very harmful when they arise from superstition, irrational beliefs or unwholesome influences in the social environment. One notices that religious beliefs, no matter how irrational or ridiculous, are rarely questioned because they are generally acquired in childhood when the authority and knowledge of adults is not questioned, and so they have the character of fixations and compulsions, and they are sometimes very powerful. As far as treatment is concerned, sensible parental guidance is obviously crucial in bringing up well-adjusted and responsible children. Some minor fixations – such as compulsive cleaning – can be addressed by psychotherapy or hypnotherapy. In Chinese philosophy, developing harmony in society is one of the cardinal precepts of Confucianism, and sensible parenting to encourage rational thought and instil responsible habits is an extension of this principle. The Taoist teaching that life should be lived naturally and the Confucian teaching that superstition should be avoided are also relevant. It is often the case that, if a person is unable to satisfy his fixations by yielding to his compulsions, he becomes anxious and depressed, which can lead to mental illness and nervous disorders of a serious kind. The TCM alleviative and curative treatments for obsessive fixations and compulsions are acupuncture and meditation with a strong element of self-hypnosis. By its nature, self-hypnosis tends to produce fixations and compulsions, but if it is properly applied, they will be desirable and will counteract the undesirable fixations. The TCM preventive treatment is a wise philosophy of living, as is provided by Taoism and Confucianism, which are nothing if not practical, together with the sound advice and security provided by a caring family. See **nervous disorders**, **psychotherapy**, **meditation**, **self-hypnosis** and **morality**.

occipital bone The bone at the base and the back of the skull. It is of significance in TCM because it is one of the sites where pressure is applied in neck acupressure and massage. See **neck acupressure** and **neck massage**.

occupational disease Industrial disease. A disease which is due to unhealthy or adverse working conditions, as with exposure to poisonous chemicals in the manufacture of paints, or silicosis and nystagmus, which were once quite common among coal miners. The Chinese have few problems in this regard, for their economy is still essentially agrarian and not over-industrialized. As far as the Chinese are concerned, the chief occupational disease is idleness, which impoverishes both the individual and the community to which he belongs. What is more, a person who is slothful or in a sedentary occupation tends to be unhealthy. But this condition is uncommon among the Chinese because they are industrious people by temperament.

HUMAN SKULL

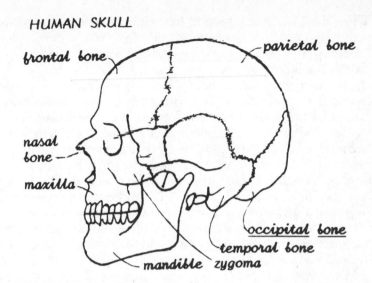

frontal bone

parietal bone

nasal bone

maxilla

occipital bone

temporal bone

mandible zygoma

occupational hazard A disease or other risk associated with one's occupation. See **occupational disease**.

occupational therapy The treatment of a sick person by some type of organized and supervised work. The work may provide some special exercise for specific muscles or joints, or, with a person who is mentally or nervously sick, it may divert his attention from his anxieties and depressing thoughts and give him confidence in his own ability to cope with problems. Chinese physicians would argue, and with much justification, that all persons, whether healthy or sick, should be fully occupied with some task or activity because everyone needs exercise for both the body and the mind. In this, the Chinese are fortunate, for few Chinese are engaged in sedentary occupations. See **philosophy of health**.

odour Traditionally, in Chinese medicine, each solid vital organ is associated with an odour: heart, burnt; liver, pungent; spleen, sweet; lungs, fetid; kidneys, putrid. But these associations are not entirely symbolic, for they also have some medicinal associations. For example, the liver, wherein lies the gall-bladder, which produces bile, an emulsifier, is associated with fats, which can become rancid; exhaled air often has a fetid odour; and the spleen is adjacent to the pancreas, which secretes insulin, the hormone that controls the amount of sugar in the blood. Furthermore, the odour associated with a solid organ is often characteristic of the herbal medicines used in its treatment.

Thus, those medicines used to treat the heart often have a burnt odour, and those to treat the spleen often have a sweet odour. Chinese physicians use odours in diagnosis and as a means to classify medicines, but only on a limited scale, for there is a lack of precision. It is sometimes difficult to distinguish between a characteristic odour and a characteristic taste; some odours cannot be identified with complete accuracy; and many herbal medicines simply have no odour at all. Thus, a herb which has a burnt odour could also be said to be pungent or bitter, which are two of the tastes of TCM. Apart from the foregoing, the English language is rich in synonyms, and so the odours of TCM can be described in a confusingly wide variety of English words, but not always in a way that expresses the exact meaning of the original Chinese words. For *odour*, one could also use *aroma*, *smell*, *fragrance* or *stink*, but *fragrance* could hardly be expressive of noxious odours, and *stink* could hardly be expressive of sweet smells. *Fetid*, *rotten*, *rank*, *raw*, *putrid* and *goatish* are the same or similar in meaning, as are *burnt* and *scorched*, *acrid* and *bitter*, *pungent* and *rancid*, and *sweet* and *fragrant*. Therefore, in general, odours should be regarded as an unreliable guide in diagnosis or selecting herbal medicines. Perhaps they are best used as no more than an occasional supplement to tastes and energies in describing the properties of herbal medicines. One should note that the characteristic odours of the solid organs are also associated with the corresponding hollow organs and the traditional elements and colours. See **taste**.

Solid organ	Hollow organ	Odour	Element	Colour
heart	small intestine	burnt	fire	red
liver	gall-bladder	pungent	wood	blue-green
spleen	stomach	fragrant	earth	yellow
lungs	large intestine	fetid	metal	white
kidneys	bladder	putrid	water	black

oedema Dropsy. Hydropsy. Water retention. Puffiness which is due to water escaping from the blood and accumulating in the tissues. It occurs mainly in the feet and ankles. Its mildest forms may be caused by varicose veins and slow or interrupted circulation, as when tight-fitting socks are worn. It is common during pregnancy and in women who suffer from premenstrual tension. Its more severe forms are caused by hypertension, toxaemia and disorders of the heart, liver or kidneys. Its symptoms include breathlessness, swellings of the legs, ankles and abdomen, very high blood pressure and jaundice. A healthy diet and regular exercise may be preventive of premenstrual water retention. If oedema is severe, medical advice should be sought so that the cause can be accurately diagnosed. In TCM, oedema is associated mainly with the kidneys, but also with the spleen and lungs. Sometimes, the kidneys are unable to remove excess water because of a deficiency of kidney-*qi*. There can also be a failure in the function of the spleen, which normally metabolizes food and blood and removes excess dampness. Oedema may also be caused by a blockage in the lungs. If the cause is problems with the kidneys, the recommended treatment is aconite, *Aconitum carmichelli*, ginger, *Zingiber officinale*, or water plantain, *Alisma plantago-aquatica*. With the spleen, it is Indian bread, *Poria cocos*, ginseng, *Panax ginseng*, or *dang shen*, *Codonopsis tangshen*. With the lungs, it is joint fir, *Ephedra sinica*, or cinnamon, *Cinnamomum cassia*. For mild forms of oedema, Chinese physicians would recommend an infusion of one of the following, taken internally as a diuretic, using the parts and dosage indicated: dandelion, *Taraxacum officinale*, all parts, 10–30 g; burdock, *Arctium lappa*, roots or seeds, 3–10 g; water plantain, *Alisma plantago-aquatica*, tubers, 4–10 g; ginger, *Zingiber officinale*, rhizomes, 3–8 g. But the use of diuretics should be regarded as a temporary measure, for damage will be done if their use is prolonged. With severe oedema, the use of diuretics will only treat the symptoms. Therefore, it is important that the real cause of this condition should be diagnosed, and then treated appropriately. See **nephritis**.

oesophagus See **alimentary canal**.

oestrogen One of the female hormones produced by the ovaries, and which determines the secondary sexual characteristics of a woman and assists in regulating the menstrual cycle. Oestrogen is a fairly recent discovery in Western medicine; but, for over 2000 years, Chinese physicians have been aware of semen-essence, which determines the femininity and pubertal and menopausal changes in a women, and which is a component of *jing*, or 'vital essence'. See **jing** and **primary sex characteristics**.

oil Many vegetable and animal oils serve as items of diet. The only physical difference between an oil and a fat is one of temperature. In fact, an oil can be defined as a fat which is liquid at room temperatures. Lower the temperature of an oil, and it will solidify; raise the temperature of a fat, and it will liquify. Edible fats must NOT be confused with mineral oil, or petroleum, which is a mixture of naturally occurring hydrocarbons – compounds of hydrogen and carbon – and which yield petrol, paraffin, diesel oil, paraffin wax, etc. Edible oils are sometimes hardened by hydrogenation, which is a process by which hydrogen is made to combine with an unsaturated oil to produce a saturated fat. Nutritionally, edible oils have the same value as edible fats, although where the former are derived from peanuts, sunflower seeds, maize and olives they are healthier items of diet, for they contain polyunsaturated fatty acids, which inhibit the formation of cholesterol. Fish-liver oil is an excellent item of diet. Unlike the fat in meat, it is high in polyunsaturated fatty acid, and is also rich in minerals and vitamins. In China, corn (maize) oil, sunflower oil and peanut oil are commonly used in cooking. See **fat**, **fish liver** and **liniment**.

oily fish Oily fish such as herrings, pilchards, sprats, sardines, skate, anchovies, mackerel, salmon, trout and tuna, are thought to be nutritionally superior to white, or non-oily fish. See **fish**.

oily hair Oily hair is regarded by some people as a nuisance. However, rather than treat it with cosmetic solutions, an effective treatment is as follows: wash the hair daily, using shampoos which have few additives to clog the hair, reduce oiliness by washing the hair in the juice of two lemons added to a litre of hot water, use oil-free or low-oil conditioners, and avoid brushing the hair too much and too often so that oil does not spread to the tips of the hairs. As far as Chinese physicians are concerned, oily hair is a symptom of stress, and so it follows that an effective treatment for stress will eliminate oily hair partly if not fully. See **oily skin** and **stress**.

oily skin Oily skin and hair have a variety of causes, which include unsuitable cosmetics, some kinds of oral contraceptives and stress, which encourages the production of androgen, the male sex hormone, which, in turn, encourages excessive secretion of sebum by the sebaceous glands at the bases of the hair follicles. Hereditary factors also play a part. The condition cannot be cured completely, but it can be alleviated by frequent washing in hot water, using special astringent soaps instead of ordinary soaps, which block up the skin pores, and using water-based, rather than oil-based, cosmetics. Chinese physicians treat stress, and thereby reduce the secretion of oil. However, an oily skin is not an illness, though it may be regarded as undesirable by the beauty conscious. See **oily hair** and **stress**.

ointment Unguent. In TCM, an ointment, or 'medicine-paste', as the Chinese describe it, is made by mixing the powdered herbal ingredients in a base of animal fat, petroleum jelly or vegetable oil. Using lard, an ointment can be made quite simply as follows: put the powdered herbs and lard in a pan, bring to the boil, simmer for a short time, remove from the heat, cover and leave to stand overnight. Then reheat the mixture, strain through muslin, put into screw-top jars and store in a refrigerator until required. A healing ointment is also called a salve, and one made with aromatic herbs is called a balm. See **paste** and **paste-medicine**.

olfactory nerve First cranial nerve. This nerve links the nose to the brain.

oliguria An abnormal decrease in urination. See **diuretic**.

olive *Olea europaea* The fruits of this tree, which are green or black, are a source of edible oil, and contain a little iron, copper and carotene. It is indigenous to the Mediterranean region and must NOT be confused with the Chinese olive, *Canarium album*, which is an entirely different species, and belongs to a different genus. See **olive oil** and **Chinese olive**.

olive oil This edible oil, obtained from the fruits of the olive, contains mono-unsaturated fatty acids, including linoleic acid, and has a high energy value of 900 kcal/100g. In the West, it is used for both medicinal and culinary purposes. It is said to be an oil which can be safely consumed by those with stomach ulcers. Olive oil, together with garlic and fresh fruit and vegetables, makes the diet of the peoples of the Mediterranean countries much healthier than that of the peoples in the other parts of Europe. There is a much lower incidence of heart and circulatory complaints in Italy than elsewhere in Europe. See **olive**.

o.m. The abbreviation for the Latin words *omni mane*, meaning 'every morning', and used in prescriptions.

Omega 3 See **fish liver**.

omnivore An animal which feeds on both plants and flesh. Humans are omnivorous, but this is not always a healthy state of affairs. See **vegetarian diet**.

o.n. The abbreviation for the Latin words *omni nocte*, meaning 'every night', and used in prescriptions.

onion *Allium cepa* Among the most useful of the vegetables and herbs are those which are close relatives of garlic: onion; shallot, *Allium ascalonicum*; leek, *Allium porrum*, chives, *Allium schoeno-prasus*. They have health-giving properties which are similar to those of garlic, but are far less potent, which makes them a valuable addition to the diet. On a limited scale, they are employed in herbal medicine. They are mildly antiseptic, aperient, stomachic and diaphoretic in their effects. They are good for the complexion, and so, if they are included as a regular part of the diet, there should be no constipation and fewer pimples. Like garlic, they impart a distinct odour to the breath, which some people find to be offensive, but that is a surely a small price to pay for health. The Chinese use onions in large quantities, but they have a preference for scallions, or shallots, *Allium ascalonicum*, for culinary purposes, and *cong bai*, or Chinese spring onions, *Allium fistulosum*, for medicinal purposes. Because of their diaphoretic and antiseptic properties, all the members of the onion family, prepared as infusions or decoctions, or added to salad and stews, are helpful in treating colds and influenza. See **garlic** and **cong bai**.

onion green See **cong bai**.

open-heart surgery This is one of the big advances in the surgical techniques of Western medicine. It has been claimed that acupuncture could be used effectively as a form of anaesthesia for this type of surgery, as it has been with thyroidectomies and tonsillectomies. See **acupuncture**.

'open spirit-gate' This is the Chinese term which describes the resuscitative medicines that are used to restore consciousness, and which are applied in cases of fainting, convulsions or epilepsy. Two of the best of these medicines are the sweet flag, *Acorus gramineus*, and musk from the musk-deer, *Moschus moschiferus*. There is a European species of sweet flag – *Acorus calamus*. However, these medicines must be used with great caution, especially in treating epilepsy. TCM has a most effective acupressure technique for reviving a person who has fainted. See **epilepsy** and **fainting**.

opiate A narcotic or soporific drug, especially one containing opium or an opium derivative. Although China has been described as 'the Land of the Opiate', opium was little used in China until the British and French insistence on free trade in Chinese ports, which led to the Opium Wars, 1839–42 and 1856–58, and resulted in the legalization of the opium trade and the importation of opium from India. As a result, large numbers of Chinese lives were undoubtedly cut short. See **opium**.

opium A reddish-brown, heavily scented and bitter drug derived from the juice of the opium poppy, *Papaver somniferum*, and smoked or eaten as a stimulant, intoxicant or narcotic. In medicine, it is used as a sedative. Morphine is its active narcotic principle, its action being sedative, hypnotic, astringent, anti-spasmodic and analgesic. It is the source of codeine, an alkaloid used as a hypnotic and analgesic. In most countries, the use of opium is strictly forbidden by law, and morphine and its other medicinal derivatives are available only to registered medical practitioners. See **opium poppy** and **drugs**.

opium poppy *Papaver somniferum* Herbal medicine. Distribution: China, India, Mediterranean countries. Parts: dried capsules from which the latex ('milk') has been extracted. Character: sour-bitter, neutral. Affinity: lungs, large intestine, kidneys. Effects: analgesic, antitussive, astringent to lungs and large intestine. Symptoms: persistent cough, diarrhoea, stomach ache. Treatments: dysentery, asthma, prolapse of rectum, opium withdrawal. It is important to note that there are strict legal restrictions on the use of opium and its derivatives. The opium poppy grows in both hot and temperate regions throughout the world, and is cultivated in gardens as a handsome ornamental plant. It is only the latex, or sap of milky appearance, contained in its stems and capsular fruits, which yields opium. Its seeds can be used for culinary purposes, for they do not contain opium. The relatives of the opium poppy, such as the corn, or common, poppy,

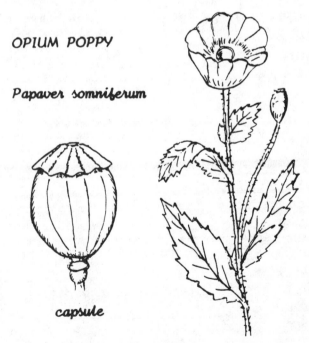

OPIUM POPPY

Papaver somniferum

capsule

Papaver rhoeas, and short-headed poppy, *Papaver dubium*, do not contain opium, and are used for culinary purposes. See **opium** and **poppy**.

opposing principles This was the term used by Shen Nong, one of the legendary emperors of China, to describe the yin-yang principle of complementary opposites, which accounts for all the causes and effects in nature, and explains all the thoughts and actions of mankind. See **Tai Chi**.

optical defects The eyes can suffer from a number of defects, the two commonest being myopia, or short-sightedness, and hypermetropia, or long-sightedness. A short-sighted person can see near objects but has difficulty in clearly seeing distant objects. The lenses of his eyes are too thick, and so images are brought to a focus in front of the retina. The retina contains light-sensitive nerve endings, and functions in much the same way as a photographic film. Opticians correct short-sightedness by providing spectacles with concave lenses. With a long-sighted person, the lenses are too thin, and so images are brought to a focus behind the retina. Convex lenses correct this defect. Astigmatism is a partial blurring of vision which is caused by an irregularity

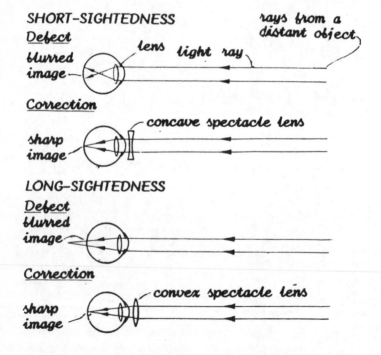

or other defect in the cornea. See **cornea**. Chinese physicians insist that the onset of these conditions can be deferred by regularly massaging the region above and below the eyes. This helps the ciliary muscles, which adjust the size of the lens, to retain their strength and elasticity. TSM has massage exercises designed for this purpose. There is a tendency for people to rub their eyes when they are tired, which suggests that nature knows best. It is interesting to note that the Chinese were the first to correct eye defects with glass lenses; and, in ancient times, Chinese scholars had a sound knowledge of the laws of optics. Even today, the Chinese optician tests eyes, and then grinds lenses to the appropiate size with considerable precision. See **eye** and **optical illusion**.

optical illusion Our eyes will sometimes play tricks on us, leading to a difference between reality and our perception of it. This deception is called an optical illusion. There are many examples of this. When travelling in a train, it sometimes appears that it is the countryside, and not the train, which is moving. Two optical illusions are shown in figures 1 and 2 below. In figure 1, both lines are of the same length, though A appears to be longer than B. In figure 2, the two lines are parallel, though they do not appear to be so. A common optical illusion is that produced by a reflection in a mirror. You will have noticed, when looking into a mirror, that the right-hand side of your body is on the left-hand side of your image in the mirror, and that the letters in printed or written words appear to go from right to left, and not from left to right. This phenomenon is called lateral inversion. It was well known to the sages and physicians of ancient China, for whom mirrors and lenses held a certain fascination. In some of the hexagrams of the *I Ching*, one trigram is the lateral inversion of

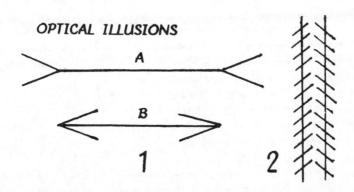

OPTICAL ILLUSIONS

A

B

1

2

the other. In some of their observations and discoveries in the realms of mathematics and optics, the Chinese were ahead of Sir Isaac Newton (1642–1727) by more than 3000 years. See **optical defects**, **mirrors** and **fung shui**.

optic nerve Second cranial nerve. See **eye**.

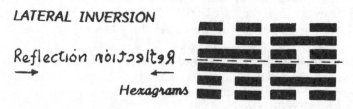

LATERAL INVERSION

Reflection ↔ noitɔɘ⁹ɘꓭ

Hexagrams

'oracle bones' See **prediction** and **Pa Kua**.

oral contraceptives There is some doubt about the reliability of oral contraceptives. They alter the level of oestrogen, the female sex hormone, which can produce some undesirable side-effects. Oral contraceptives are not popular in China, where condoms are favoured because they not only prevent conception, but also limit, though do not entirely prevent, the transmission of venereal diseases. See **birth control**, **oestrogen** and **nosebleed**.

oral hygiene Animals usually have perfectly sound teeth, despite the fact that they do not brush them. Why, then, should it be thought necessary for humans to clean their teeth and visit the dentist regularly? There are two main reasons, one hygienic, the other aesthetic. Unlike animals' diets, the human diet is unnatural, for it contains a wide range of substances, both cooked and uncooked – acids, sugars, food additives, etc – which penetrate the enamel on teeth and harbour micro-organisms that cause dental caries, or tooth decay. Also, humans regard discoloured teeth and a foul-smelling mouth as being unattractive. Obviously, in these respects, brushing the teeth with a suitable antiseptic and abrasive substance is helpful. For this, many Chinese will use a home-made toothpaste which is as effective as any of the proprietary brands that are so lavishly advertised. See **dentifrice** and **mouth infections**.

oral infections See **mouth infections**.

orange pith See **mandarin orange**.

organ A distinct part of the body with its own specialized function – heart, lungs, liver, etc. See **tissue**.

organic acid See **acid**.

organic farming This term applies essentially to the practice of growing fruit and vegetables without recourse to pesticides and artificial fertilizers, but it has been extended to cover all forms of farming, including animal husbandry, where natural conditions prevail. This means the non-use of chemical growth-regulators, hormone growth-stimulants, intensive rearing of chickens and pigs, chemical additives to give attractive flavours, colours and textures to meat and fish, and unnatural foodstuffs for animals. The incidence of 'mad-cow disease' in Britain must be due, at least in part, to feeding cattle on sheep offals. The charge of commercial greed is often levelled at farmers who use intensive farming methods, but, in fairness to them, it must be said that these methods are almost unavoidable in heavily populated regions. There would simply not be enough land available to produce sufficient eggs from free-range fowl to cater for the needs of the British population. What is more, eggs from battery-reared hens can be put on the market at a reasonable price. The Chinese have always had a distinct aversion to preserved foods and food additives, and so it follows that they favour organic farming. See **natural diet** and **green consumers**.

orgasm Climax. The peak of emotional excitement in sexual activity, and which, in the male, is usually accompanied by ejaculation. See **Yellow Emperor**.

oriental sore See **Leishmaniasis**.

ormer See **abalone**.

orthodox medicine See **conventional medicine**.

orthopaedics The treatment of fractures and deformities and other abnormalities in bones and joints.

ossicle See **ear**.

osteo-arthritis One of the three forms of arthritis, which mainly affects the weight-bearing joints. According to TCM, this condition is due to weakness of the liver and kidneys and blood stagnation. It is important to keep warm. The treatments are infusions or decoctions of the following, taken internally, using the parts and dosages indicated: angelica, *Angelica pubescens*, roots, 4–8 g; *fang feng*, *Ledebouriella seseloides*, roots, 4–6 g; cinnamon, *Cinnamomum cassia*, bark, 2–4 g; mulberry, *Morus alba*, leaves, 4–8 g. Mulberry warms the blood and meridians, improves the circulation and nourishes the joints. See **arthritis**.

osteo-arthrosis An alternative name for osteo-arthritis.

osteopathy A Western system of treatment and a form of alternative medicine based on the principle that many ailments can be cured or relieved by manipulation of the spine, bones and muscles. Osteopaths are of the opinion that standing upright imposes a great strain on the spine, which is a common cause of displaced vertebrae. Osteopathy is similar to chiropractic, but the latter makes more use of X-rays and other conventional techniques. The manipulative techniques of osteopathy are not unlike those used in the traditional Chinese healing exercises. See **chiropractic**.

osteoporosis Fragility and brittleness of the bones caused by a deficiency of minerals, particularly calcium, and which is common among women after the menopause. The spine becomes shorter and curved, and the bones at the hip and wrist are easily broken. The condition is aggravated by neglect of diet and exercise. This condition can only be effectively treated if it is caught in its early stages. One should take regular exercise, include calcium-rich foods – oily fish, yoghurt, milk, cheese, nuts and calcium-fortified white flour – and foods high in vitamin D – eggs, margarine and fatty-fish – in the diet, and reduce the intake of meat, salt and alcohol. Chinese physicians ascribe this condition to a kidney deficiency. For its treatment, they recommend the exercises of *tai chi chuan* and an infusion or decoction, taken internally, of 8–14 g bark of eucommia, *Eucommia ulmoides*.

otitis Inflammation of the ear. Otitis externa is of the outer ear, otitis media is of the middle ear, and otitis interna is of the inner ear. See **ear**.

Outlines and Branches of Herbal Medicine See **Ben Cao Gang Mu**.

outward-moving A term used in TCM to describe yang medicines, which ascend and stimulate, for they tend to move *qi* upwards and outwards, including perspiration and vomiting, which are indications that a disease is being ejected from the body.

ovaries The two female sex glands, which produce ova and secrete oestrogen and progesterone, the female sex hormones. See **reproductive systems** and **jing**.

overdoses See **dangers with medicines**.

overeating This is one of the main causes of illness among the people of the West. It is a healthy practice to end a meal feeling just a little unsatisfied. See **moderation** and **over-indulgence**.

over-exertion No one doubts the value of exercise, but over-strenuous exercise, and, in fact, over-exertion in all activities, both physical and mental, can cause stress and exhaustion, invalidate the immune system and even do irreparable physical damage. There is a Chinese saying, which originated in the *Nei Pien*: 'Life is the road along which you must travel, and death is your destination. Travel at a high speed, and you will reach your destination much quicker than you would wish.' See **exercise**.

over-indulgence Immoderate habits and over-indulgence of all kinds are damaging to the health. White rice porridge is a good treatment for those who are suffering from a surfeit of greasy or spicy food. See **white rice porridge** and **moderation**.

over-tiredness Tiredness has many causes, including anaemia and hormonal imbalances, some of which may be serious conditions. But a sudden bout of over-tiredness generally results from over-exertion or lack of sleep. This causes stress, which creates further tiredness and even insomnia. Over-tiredness of this kind can usually be prevented by moderate habits. See **exhaustion**, **insomnia** and **moderation**.

overweight See **obesity**.

oviduct See **reproductive systems**.

ovulation The monthly production and release of mature ova, which is manifested by menstruation, and which ceases at the menopause. See **reproductive systems** and **safe period**.

ovum Plural: **ova**. See **fertilization** and **safe period**.

oxygen An odourless and colourless gas which makes up about 20 per cent of the atmosphere. It is the most abundant of the chemical elements, but exists mainly in the combined state as oxides, nitrates, sulphates, silicates, etc. Water is a compound of oxygen and hydrogen. Oxygen is highly reactive and will combine with most other elements to form oxides, releasing energy in the process, as occurs in combustion. For example, in the burning of wood or coal, oxygen combines with carbon and hydrogen to form carbon dioxide and water. Sulphur burns in oxygen to form sulphur dioxide. Oxygen is essential to life. In respiration, which occurs in the tissues, it combines with sugar to form carbon dioxide and release energy. If there were no oxygen, there would be no life on the earth, at least not as we know it. See **air**, **breathing**, **respiration** and **qi**.

oxyhaemoglobin See **breathing** and **erythrocyte**.

oyster *Ostrea rivularis* Medicine. Distribution: global. Parts: powdered shells. Character: cool, sour-salt. Affinity: kidneys, liver, gall-bladder. Effects: sedative, astringent, suppresses liver yang, dissolves hard tumours. Symptoms: palpitations, insomnia, dizziness, headaches, blurred vision, spasms, cold sweats, diarrhoea. Treatments: hypertension, trauma, spermatorrhoea, menorrhagia, leucorrhoea, hard tumours, swollen lymph glands, calcium deficiency in pregnancy, osteoporosis. Dosage 5–8 g. Oysters are rich in zinc, iron, copper and retinol. Being rich in zinc, oysters are good for growth and assist in sexual maturation, but their great reputation as an aphrodisiac is ill-founded. See **zinc**.

ozone Ozone (O_3) is an allotrope, or polymorph, of oxygen (O_2). It is much more reactive than ordinary oxygen and occurs in the upper layers of the atmosphere, where it absorbs much of the sun's ultraviolet radiation, which would be harmful to animal life. The ozone layer, or ozonosphere, has been badly damaged by pollutants, and it is urgently important that measures should be taken to prevent further damage, which is an opinion with which all sensible people, including the Chinese, would wholeheartedly agree. See **pollution** and **chemicals**.

P

pacemaker This is the everyday term for an electronic device which, in Western medical practice, is inserted into the chest to stimulate or regulate the heartbeat where the natural pacemaker, the sino-auricular node, of the heart fails to function efficiently in initiating heartbeats by emitting rhythmic impulses. In TCM, the treatment for this defect would be a suitable cardiotonic to strengthen the heart as a whole. But this would need to be administered by a skilled physician. See **cardiotonic**.

pain Among its several functions, the nervous system is the body's alarm system, and the aches and pains which it manifests are nature's way of proclaiming that something is amiss. Therefore, pain often operates to our advantage, because, without it, we would often have no knowledge of a serious condition, which would go untreated and become progressively worse. Unfortunately, people are sometimes content to do no more than alleviate a pain without making any attempt to diagnose its cause. To treat, say, backache with a mild diuretic, such as barley water, instead of treating the dysfunction of which it is a symptom, and which may be far more serious than is realized, is just about as sensible as trying to extinguish a fire by switching off the fire-alarm. Of course, it is not unreasonable that a person will seek some form of alleviation of pain, particularly that of an an excruciating kind, but it is imperative that the cause of the pain should also be treated. It is obviously the case that, if the condition causing pain is effectively cured, the pain will depart. See **ache** and **painful disorders**.

painful disorders There are many disorders, minor and serious, chronic and short-lasting, which are accompanied by pain in varying degrees of intensity. One of the anomalies in this respect is that minor ailments are often much more painful than serious illnesses. For example, toothache and earache can be extremely painful whereas cancer and tuberculosis will eat away at the body, reducing it to its lowest ebb, yet the patient may feel no pain whatsoever, though he is likely to be considerably distressed.

The proper treatment for a painful disorder is to eradicate its cause wherever possible. Otherwise, pain-killing medicines can be used. In a hospital, physicians may suppress extreme pain by means of opium derivatives and other narcotic drugs. This is a case of desperate situations calling for desperate remedies. But, for minor ailments accompanied by pain, a wide range of analgesics is available. In the West, aspirin and paracetamol are widely used, but aspirin should not be taken for pains in the stomach or any other part of the alimentary canal, for it may cause bleeding. The analgesics used in TCM must be selected with care, for each one generally has an affinity for a particular vital organ, and so one must choose an analgesic which has an affinity for the organ wherein lies the cause of the pain. One should note that an analgesic which is effective with one organ may not be effective with another. Some pains, such as headaches and migraine, which are often due to tension, can be treated by acupuncture and acupressure techniques. But this should be done by a professional practitioner if the treatment is to be truly effective. See **pain, ache** and **analgesic**.

painful feet The two most common causes of painful and aching feet are the wearing of tight-fitting shoes and too much standing. The upright position of a human in walking puts an excessive pressure on his feet. There is something to be said for imitating the hoofed mammals by wearing shoes with high – but not too high – heels. See **corn** and **ingrowing toe-nails**.

painful urination See urinary disorders.

pain-killer A medicine to alleviate pain. See **analgesic**.

paired organs See **vital organs**.

Pa Kua Also spelt as *Ba Gua* or *Bhat Gwa*. This is a set of eight trigrams, usually arranged in a circle, which is the basis of the 64 hexagrams that the *I Ching* employs in making divinations. It is a component of the mystique of Taoism and symbolizes its Eight Pillars. According to tradition, it was invented by Wen, father of Wu (c. 1100 BC), the first Zhou king, though it is more likely that he developed it from the inscriptions on some 'oracle bones', which were the products of a much earlier age. In recent times, some of these 'oracle bones' have been unearthed by archaeologists. They are tortoise shells and oxen bones bearing crude inscriptions of the symbols used in making divinations, and which may have been devised by the legendary Fuxi, who is supposed to have lived about 7000 years ago. These days, the *Pa Kua* is commonly used as a decoration for porcelain, but it is also used as a charm to bring good luck. The Chinese hang it up in their houses to ward off unfriendly spirits and other evils, as British people might hang up a horseshoe. A common wall ornament in China consists of a flat piece of wood or some other material, octagonal in shape, with the Pa Kua painted on it, or in relief, and a mirror at its centre. The purpose of the mirror is to send away evil influences by reflection. If a building is badly sited so that it faces a graveyard or something else of an unpleasantly emotive nature, it is generally thought to be under evil influences, or it has bad *fung shui*, as the Chinese would say. But the Chinese belief in Pa Kua mirrors does indicate that the sages of ancient China were prepared to accept the existence of phenomena not visible to the naked eye. For instance, modern science has revealed the existence of micro-organisms and sound and electromagnetic waves. None of these can be directly observed by the senses, although we can detect their effects and manifestations. Perhaps in a roundabout way, the sages of ancient China had discovered some great scientific truths in regard to energy, as their preoccupation with *qi* might suggest. Over and over again, the discoveries made by modern science in the West confirm the validity of the opinions held by the wise men who served in the imperial courts of ancient China. There is a soft, or internal, style of kungfu, Taoist inspired, based on the trigrams of the Pa Kua. It lays stress on moral principles, meditation and harmonious relationships. See **fung shui**, **mirrors** and **optical illusion**.

pallor One of the symptoms of a yin ailment. See **ba gang**.

palpation In TCM, this is a form of diagnosis in which the condition of the internal organs is ascertained by touch or light massage. See **tactile diagnosis**.

palpitation An increased heartbeat due to exertion, tension or disease. One of the causes is the condition called Da Costa's syndrome, whereby a person imagines that he has a defective heart, which causes tension; and this, in turn, causes palpitation. According to TCM, palpitation may be indicative of a deficiency in the heart or blood, and the recommended treatment is a decoction, taken internally, of 6–14 g seeds of jujube, *Ziziphus jujuba*. Also effective is a suspension, taken internally, of 5–8 g powdered shells of oyster, *Ostrea rivularis*. Acupuncture may be an effective treatment where this condition is due to tension. See **nervous disorders**.

palsy An old-fashioned name for paralysis, especially with involuntary tremors. See **paralysis**.

panacea A dictionary would define a panacea as a universal remedy – something that will cure all ills and solve all problems. But it could be defined more narrowly as a medicine which will cure all illnesses. Such a medicine could not possibly exist, though the purveyors of pills and potions sometimes make exaggerated claims for their products. Perhaps the medicinal herb which deserves pride of place for being the one with the most wide-ranging medicinal benefits is garlic, but the Chinese would rate ginseng very highly. See **garlic** and **ginseng**.

pancreas This organ is a dual-function gland situated behind the stomach. It secretes digestive juices, which enter the duodenum via the pancreatic duct. A group of cells, called the islets of Langerhans, within the pancreas secrete insulin, which is a hormone that is necessary for the regulation of the level of sugar in the blood. In TCM, the pancreas is always associated with the spleen. It is quite remarkable that the Taoist physicians of ancient China were aware of the functions of the pancreas. See **insulin** and **endocrine glands**.

pancreatitis Inflammation of the pancreas. This is a serious abdominal condition. In TCM, it can be treated with herbal medicines, but the procedure is complex.

pangolin *Manis pentadactyla* Also called scaly ant-eater. Medicine. Distribution: South China, Taiwan, Vietnam, Africa. Parts: scales. Character: cold, salty. Affinity: stomach, liver. Effects: emmenagogue, reduces inflammation and pus, reduces swellings, increases circulation, galactagogue. Symptoms: stiff and painful joints and tendons, poor lactation. Treatments: skin infections and suppuration, amenorrhoea, wind-damp conditions. Dosage: 4–9 g. This medicine will strengthen the immune system. See **interferon**.

Pangu Also spelt as *P'an Ku* or *Pan Ku*. The Chinese have an old legend which explains how the world was created by Pangu. It is a charming story and, like the account of the creation in the Bible, it is allegorical. The main interest of this story to the student of Chinese medicine is its indication that the yin-yang principle of complementary opposites, or the Tai Chi, has strongly influenced Chinese thought from the earliest times. This is the story.

'Before the world came into existence, there was nothing except an egg-shaped primeval mass and the cosmic principle of yin and yang, which is both the origin and the essence of all matter and life. Pangu, the creator of the world, was fashioned out of yin and yang. Every day, during a period of 18,000 years, he underwent nine changes. He also laboured, with the assistance of a dragon, a unicorn, a phoenix and a tortoise, to mould the earth into its present shape. Eventually, the clear and pure elements condensed to form the stars, the sun and the moon, and the dark and impure elements condensed to form the earth. The earth, the heavens and Pangu himself gradually grew larger until, one thousand years later, he died. Then his body was remarkably transformed. His flesh became the soil, his blood the lakes and rivers, his hair the plants, his breath the wind, his sweat the rain, his left eye the sun, his right eye the moon, and his voice thunder. The parasites feeding on his body became the various members of the human race.'

In earlier ages, this story provided the Chinese peasantry with some sort of an explanation of the origin of the world and human life, and which, for them, was a naïve attempt at knowing the unknowable. But it is an explanation in very human terms, and which, apart from the yin-yang concept, was not taken seriously by the Chinese intellectuals, for whom deities in human form had no place in the scheme of things. See **Tai Chi** and **universe**.

panic Fright. One of the seven emotions of TCM. It is not related to any specific organ, being different from fear in that it arises unexpectedly and quickly, and is not easily controlled. At its outset, it mainly affects the heart, but if it persists, and so becomes a realized fear, it will affect the kidneys. See **fear** and **seven emotions**.

papilloma A benign growth, such as a wart or polyp, on the skin or a mucous membrane.

Paracelsus Philippus Paracelsus (*c.* 1493–1541) was a Swiss physician and alchemist. His real name was Theophrastus von Hohenheim, of which *Philippus Paracelsus* is a Latinized version. He wrote many medical and occult works. It is suspected that he derived some of his ideas from Chinese sources.

paracetamol An analgesic commonly used in Western medicine. It should be used with caution where the patient is suffering from a liver or kidney disease. See **painful disorders**.

paralysis This may be briefly defined as a condition where there is a loss of movement in a part of the body, often accompanied by a loss of sensation. The causes include strokes and diseases of the nervous system, where there is impairment of the motor or sensory nerves. Conditions where paralysis occurs include multiple sclerosis, paraplegia and Parkinson's disease. In TCM, the usual treatments are acupuncture, massage and remedial exercises, which are alleviative, often producing a return of sensation, but are rarely completely curative. See **stroke**.

paralysis agitans See **Parkinson's disease**.

paramedic A person who is trained to supplement and support the work of the physician. See **'barefoot doctors'**.

paranoia A mental disorder which is characterized by strong delusions of grandeur or persecution. This condition could arise from a complex or an obsession, and it may commence in childhood. It seems that the imagination gets out of hand, producing an attitude which cannot be reversed, and so the intelligence and the powers of accurate discernment are subjugated by the imagination. Thus, a sufferer may develop delusions about himself or irrational fears which he is unable to reject. Paranoids can be a danger to the community, for their delusion of persecution may lead to acts of violence. Here, the physician has a duty to the community as well as to the person who is sick in mind. He must take the appropriate legal measures to ensure that the paranoid can do no harm to others, and this is as true of the physician in China as it is of the physician in the West. But it is probably the case that the conditions which might give rise to this type of illness are less prevalent in China than in the West. To some extent, disordered minds are the products of a disorderly society. Paranoia is more common than is realized, but it may go unnoticed if the sufferers do nothing to draw attention to themselves. See **mental illness** and **nervous disorders**.

paraplegia Paralysis of the legs or a part or the whole of the lower half of the trunk, and which is due to a disease or injury of the spinal cord. In some cases, surgery is an effective form of treatment. The *Chinese Exercise Manual* contains a set of alleviative and healing exercises which are suitable for this condition.

parasite An animal or plant which lives on or in another animal or plant, drawing nutriment from it. There is a wide range of parasites which thrive on humans – fleas, mosquitoes, malarial parasites, fungi and viruses of various kinds, flukes, tapeworms, roundworms, hookworms, etc. – of which intestinal worms are particularly troublesome. It is important that all meat should be thoroughly cooked in order to destroy any parasitic worms it might contain. One of the problems with some parasites is that they not only feed on their human hosts but also transmit diseases, which are generally smaller parasitic organisms. The female mosquito, for example, not only feeds on human blood but also transmits the malarial parasite, *Plasmodium vivax*. See **anthelmintic**.

parathyroid glands Two of the four glands in the neck. Their hormone regulates the level of calcium in the blood. See **endocrine glands**.

paratyphoid fever A bacterial infection of the intestine which is similar to typhoid fever but is generally less severe. See **typhoid fever**.

Parkinson's disease *Paralysis agitans*. Shaking palsy. A slow and progressive degeneration of certain deep centres in the brain, and which adversely affects the muscles and some of the other organs. It is characterized by badly co-ordinated movements, stiffness of the muscles, tremors in the limbs, twitching of the thumbs, stooping, a shuffling gait or a short-stepping run, and a blank facial expression. In TCM, this condition is regarded as being due to liver and kidney weaknesses and a deficiency in the blood and of kidney-*qi*, which leads to a lack of nourishment to the brain. Here, one notices that both Chinese and Western physicians are aware that this condition is a defect in the brain, but the Chinese physicians go a stage further by trying to determine its cause. The condition is regarded as being generally incurable when it has reached an advanced stage, but young people with the condition in a mild form can be assisted by acupuncture and an infusion or decoction of one of the following, taken internally, using the parts and dosage indicated: wolfberry, *Licium chinense*, skin of roots, 10–14 g; morning star, *Uncaria rhynchophylla*, stems and spines, 5–8 g; peony, *Paeonia lactiflora*, roots, 4–9 g.

parotid gland The largest of the salivary glands. See **parotitis**.

parotitis Mumps. Inflammation of the parotid glands, which is characterized by fever and a painful swelling of the glands. The incubation period is 14–18 days, and the patient needs to be isolated until five days after the swellings have subsided. According to TCM, this condition is due to wind-damp-heat in the facial region. The treatment is an infusion of one of the following, taken internally, using the parts and dosage indicated: Japanese honeysuckle, *Locinera japonica*, flowers, 9–16 g; dandelion, *Taraxacum officinale*, all parts, 10–30 g; woad, *Isatis tinctoria*, leaves, 8–14 g; scullcap, *Scutellaria baicalensis*, roots, 4–7 g.

parsley *Petroselinum crispum* This herb is not indigenous to China but it is now cultivated throughout the world because of its value for both culinary and medicinal purposes. Its roots or leaves, in a dosage of 1–4 g, or its seeds, in a dosage of 1–2 g, taken internally as an infusion is useful as a diuretic, carminative, digestive tonic and antispasmodic. But it must NOT be administered to a pregnant woman.

parts of herbs With some medicinal herbs, such as the dandelion, *Taraxacum officinale*, and gulf seaweed, *Sargassum fusiforme*, the whole plant may be used in medicinal preparations; but, with most herbs, it is only a certain part of the plant which is used. Therefore, in preparing a herbal medicine, it is important to use the part indicated by the prescription, which may be the root, skin of the root, tuber, rhizome, leaves, stems, buds, floral buds, flowers, stalks, rootlets, seeds, kernels, fruits, fruit juice, root juice, leaf and stem sap, bark, and so on, for it is only that part which will contain the active ingredient in a sufficient quantity to be of medicinal value. Furthermore, it is sometimes the case that the various parts of a herb have different medicinal properties. For example, the skin of the roots of the wolfberry, *Lycium chinense*, is used as an antipyretic, whereas the fruits of the wolfberry are used as a tonic. With some plants, one part may be of medicinal benefit whilst some of the others are poisonous, and so the consequences could sometimes be fatal if a prescription is not correctly followed. For instance, the rhizomes of rhubarb, *Rheum officinale*, are used as a purgative, but its leaves contain toxic levels of oxalic acid. But an overdose of any medicine, toxic or otherwise, may have ill effects, such as diarrhoea, nausea and drowsiness. It is important in some medicines that the fresh herb, not the dried herb, should be used, but these are exceptions. One cannot be too careful in preparing medicines. See **dangers with medicines**.

parturition The correct medical term for childbirth.

passion flower *Passiflora incarnata* This herb is not indigenous to China but it is now cultivated in various parts of the world because of its value as a medicine. It is used as a sedative, antispasmodic and vasodilator. All parts of this herb, in a dosage of 1.5–3 g, taken internally as an infusion may be used as a treatment for irritability, depression, spasms and insomnia.

passive movements Involuntary movements of the body, that is, movements which occur without any exercise of the will, such as breathing and reflex actions. See **active movements** and **nervous system**.

'pass-water medicine' This is a literal translation of the Chinese term for a diuretic, which is a medicine which increases urination. Diuretics are commonly used to treat conditions arising from oedema, or water retention, and poor circulation. See **diuretic**.

paste In TCM, pastes are prepared as medicines for both internal and external use. The procedure for preparing a paste for internal use is that the herbal ingredients are first boiled in water until a concentrated liquid is formed, and then more water is continuously added and boiled away as steam until the liquid is smooth and viscous. This is filtered to remove debris and heated until all the water has evaporated to leave a dense, smooth paste. Rock sugar or honey is added for flavour and to disguise any unpleasant taste. The paste is then put into jars, which are sealed and stored in a cool, dry place. See **ointment** and **paste-medicine**.

paste-medicine In TCM, paste-medicines are prepared for external use, generally in poultices. They must NOT be taken internally, for they contain toxic substances; nor should they be confused with medicinal pastes, or 'medicine-pastes', as the Chinese describe them, which are ointments. A paste-medicine is prepared by boiling the herbal ingredients in water until nearly all the water has been lost as steam, removing the sediment from the bottom and the impurities on the surface, and adding petroleum jelly and mercury or lead oxide to make a sticky paste. This paste is spread on cloth or paper and applied to an injured or diseased region for about 10 hours. This type of poultice is used to relieve spinal disorders, arthritis, rheumatism, sprains and aches and pains in joints, muscles and tendons. Chinese physicians would claim that this treatment is very effective, and perhaps it is in certain circumstances; but, by the standards of Western medicine, the use of lead or mercury compounds in medicines is an extremely dangerous practice, and one for which there is no justification since there are alternative procedures which are just as effective but also much safer. See **paste** and **ointment**.

paste pills To make paste pills, the herbal ingredients are powdered and mixed with water and rice or wheat flour to form a thick paste, which is then rolled between the thumb and forefinger to make pills. These pills are used chiefly in the treatment of stomach and intestinal disorders, such as ulcers and colitis, where direct contact with potent herbal medicines might have an adverse effect. The flour acts as a buffer so that the active ingredients are slowly and beneficially absorbed. See **pills** and **buffer**.

past history The Chinese physician will require some knowledge of a patient's past history, which will assist him considerably in making an accurate diagnosis of the patient's present condition, and determining the most suitable treatment to be applied. For example, the knowledge that, in the past, the patient has suffered from nephritis will prompt the physician to look for the symptoms of a recurrence of this condition or the onset of some other renal disorder. It is often the case that the physician's knowledge of a patient's past enables him to beneficially provide for the patient's future, and perhaps make some predictions. In this regard, the Chinese physician behaves no differently from any other physician in any other part of the world, but his behaviour is much in accord with the Confucian dictum: 'Study the past, if you would divine the future.' Most Chinese people take an active interest in their country's history. A feature of that history has been a tendency for advances in medicine to go hand in hand with advances in other aspects of Chinese culture. For instance, Chinese literature is riddled with references to traditional medicine. Similarly, Chinese rulers have always fostered Taoism, Confucianism, sound agricultural methods and preventive medicine.

pastille Lozenge. A tablet of medicine, sugar and flavouring intended to be slowly dissolved in the mouth. It is not one of the main features of TCM, but proprietary brands of Chinese herbal medicines are often made in tablet form with rice flour, gelatin or beeswax used as a binder. See **pills**.

patella Kneecap. See **skeleton**.

patent medicine A proprietary brand of medicine that is protected by a patent, which is a legal document conferring the sole right to the use of an invention or manufacturing process. Nowadays, in China, the manufacture of patent herbal medicines is quite a big industry. These medicines do away with the need for physicians or patients to prepare their own medicines, which can be a tedious business. But many physicians practising TCM still prefer to prepare their own medicines, using the traditional methods, and they would argue that, as the ingredients in patent medicines are refined from extracts of the crude herbs, they are unreliable in treating serious conditions, and cannot be applied with precision to those conditions which have been determined by differential diagnosis. However, patent medicines are effective in the continual treatment of minor and chronic ailments, and they are often manufactured in the Western style, as pills, tablets, capsules, powders, extracts, essences, lotions, liniments, etc. The Western-style techniques for refining medicinal extracts do have one outstanding advantage, which is that a pure and highly concentrated essence can be obtained. This may be put into an organ or its meridian by injection, where it will take immediate effect. See **herbal prescriptions** and **ba gang**.

TIME-SCALE OF CHINESE HISTORY

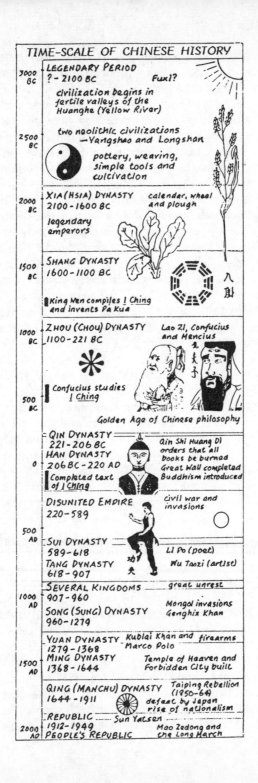

3000 BC

LEGENDARY PERIOD
? – 2100 BC   Fuxi?

civilization begins in
fertile valleys of the
Huanghe (Yellow River)

2500 BC

two neolithic civilizations
—Yangshao and Longshan

pottery, weaving,
simple tools and
cultivation

2000 BC

XIA (HSIA) DYNASTY   calendar, wheel
2100 – 1600 BC   and plough

legendary
emperors

1500 BC

SHANG DYNASTY
1600 – 1100 BC

King Wen compiles I Ching
and invents Pa Kua

1000 BC

ZHOU (CHOU) DYNASTY   Lao Zi, Confucius
1100 – 221 BC   and Mencius

500 BC

Confucius studies
I Ching

Golden Age of Chinese philosophy

QIN DYNASTY
221 – 206 BC   Qin Shi Huang DI
HAN DYNASTY   orders that all
0 206 BC – 220 AD   books be burned
                            Great Wall completed
Completed text   Buddhism introduced
of I Ching

DISUNITED EMPIRE   civil war and
220 – 589   invasions

500 AD

SUI DYNASTY
589 – 618   Li Po (poet)
TANG DYNASTY   Wu Taozi (artist)
618 – 907

SEVERAL KINGDOMS   great unrest
1000 AD 907 – 960
                            Mongol invasions
SONG (SUNG) DYNASTY   Genghiz Khan
960 – 1279

YUAN DYNASTY   Kublai Khan and firearms
1279 – 1368   Marco Polo
MING DYNASTY   Temple of Heaven and
1500 AD 1368 – 1644   Forbidden City built

QING (MANCHU) DYNASTY Taiping Rebellion
1644 – 1911   (1850–64)
                            defeat by Japan
                            rise of nationalism
REPUBLIC   Sun Yatsen
2000 AD 1912 – 1949
PEOPLE'S REPUBLIC   Mao Zedong and
                            the Long March

481

pathogen A disease-causing agent. See **micro-organism**.

patience One of the most important qualities in a Chinese physician is his capacity for patience and perseverance. He regards no illness as being incurable, though some conditions certainly are, and he is prepared to persevere in trying out remedy after remedy – and there are about 2000 medicinal herbs in TCM – until he achieves a total cure or some degree of alleviation. It must be a great consolation for a patient to know that there is a physician striving so avidly on his behalf. With some conditions, particularly mental and nervous disorders, this knowledge could be regarded as a part of the treatment since it breeds self-confidence. See **physician** and **medical education**.

pa tuan chin 'The eight sets of embroidery'. This is a Chinese fitness exercise, believed to be more than 800 years old, which consists of eight sets of movement designed to exercise the arms, trunk, head and neck, but with the main emphasis on the arms. The exercise can be performed in either the standing or the bent-knee position. Its purpose is to strengthen the joints and muscles, and so make invasion by disease less possible. It is fully described in the *Chinese Exercise Manual*.

p.c. The abbreviation for the Latin words *post cibum*, meaning 'after food', and used in prescriptions.

peace of mind In its importance, this ranks with diet and exercise because without it, the health suffers and the chances of a long life are greatly diminished. Problems are sometimes created for us, but it is also the case that we create many problems for ourselves by being over-ambitious and not knowing our own limitations, by failing to take good advice, or by not organizing our lives in such a way that stressful situations can be avoided. Peace of mind together, with the sound state of health which is its accompaniment, results from a wise philosophy of living. Peace of mind is as much a matter of morality as of medicine. Recklessness, selfishness, dishonesty and impropriety may produce pleasure or profit in the short term; but, in the long term, they lead only to confusion and despair. See **morality**, **mental illness**, **nervous disorders** and **Confucianism**.

peach *Prunus persica* Herbal medicine. Distribution: China, Japan, Europe, North America. Parts: kernels. Character: neutral, bitter-sweet. Affinity: liver, heart, large intestine. Effects: laxative, emollient, antitussive, improves circulation, prevents clotting. Symptoms: constipation, pain and fullness in rib-cage, postnatal abdominal pain. Treatments: dysmenorrhoea, amenorrhoea, blood clots, traumatic injuries, hypertension, chronic appendicitis. Dosage: 4–8 g. High doses of this medicine are poisonous.

Peach of Immortality See **Lao Zi**.

peanut *Arachis hypogaea* Also called a ground-nut, monkey-nut or earth-nut. It is not a nut but the seed of a small leguminous plant which is native to tropical South America, but is now grown in other regions where the climate is suitable. Peanuts are highly nutritious and, weight for weight, they contain more protein than beefsteak. They are also high in fat, of which the greater part consists of monounsaturated fatty acid, and so it does not lead to the formation of cholesterol. They also contain sugars, starch and dietary fibre, and they have a high energy value of 570 kcal/100g. Peanuts contain a wide variety of minerals, including calcium, magnesium, potassium, sulphur, manganese, zinc and molybdenum, and the vitamins niacin, thiamin and folic acid. The Chinese value peanuts as an item of diet, and they cook them as a vegetable, generally with pork or in stews. Peanut butter is a thick, oily paste derived from crushed peanuts.

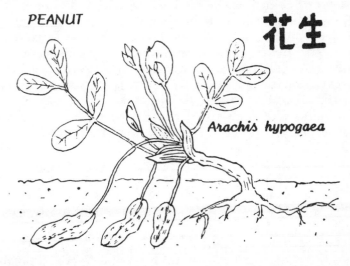

PEANUT

花生

Arachis hypogaea

peanut oil This oil, which is rich in unsaturated fatty acids, is used extensively by the Chinese for frying food. See **oil** and **peanut**.

pearl A white or bluish-grey concretion formed inside the shell of an oyster. At one time, pearls were used in Chinese medicine as a source of calcium. See **nacre** and **Nei Pien**.

pearl barley Barley grains from which the outer layers have been removed by attrition. See **barley water**.

Pediculus humanus See **head lice**.

pellagra A disease due to a deficiency of niacin. It is characterized by inflammation of the mouth, rashes, diarrhoea and anaemia. It may lead to mental and nervous disorders or even death. See **fish** and **nervous disorders**.

pelvis A girdle of bones at the base of the vertebral column. See **skeleton**.

penicillin See **antibiotic** and **moulds**.

penis The male organ of copulation. See **reproductive organs**.

peony *Paeonia lactiflora* Herbal medicine. Distribution: China. Japan, Siberia. Parts: roots. Character: cool, bitter. Affinity: liver. Effects: antipyretic, emmenagogue, haemostatic, antiseptic, blood tonic, promotes yin-*qi*. Symptoms: heat rash, amenorrhoea. Treatments: ulcers, intestinal infections, conditions of heat excess. Dosage: 5–9 g. There are two varieties of this plant – white and red. The one described here is the white variety, which is sometimes called the Chinese white peony. The red variety has slightly different medicinal properties, and it is effective in improving the circulation.

peony tree *Paeonia moutan* Herbal medicine. Distribution: North China. Parts: skin of roots. Character: cool, pungent-bitter. Affinity: liver, heart, kidneys. Effects: antipyretic, refrigerant, antiseptic, diuretic, emmenagogue, anticoagulant, improves the circulation. Symptoms: nosebleeds, amenorrhoea, irritability, blood in urine or sputum. Treatments: ulcers, intestinal infections, conditions of heat excess, deficiency of yin-*qi*. Dosage: 5–9 g. The properties of this herb are similar to those of a related species, *Paeonia lactiflora*. It has a powerful antiseptic action. See **peony**.

People's Republic of China Founded in 1949 by Mao Zedong, the People's Republic of China brought about great political and economic changes which improved the standard of living of the Chinese peasants whom Mao had always regarded as being the backbone of Chinese society, and who had been his main supporters in a revolution which was to give China a new direction. But the revolution was not so much the realization of a new China as a revival of the old China. Traditional cultural values and institutions were not suppressed but encouraged, and traditional Chinese medicine received full support from the new government. See **'barefoot doctors'**.

peppermint *Mentha piperita* Herbal medicine. Distribution: China, Europe. Parts: whole plant. Affinity: lungs, liver, stomach, large intestine. Effects: carminative, antispasmodic, vasodilator, diaphoretic, antipyretic. Symptoms: indigestion, flatulence, diarrhoea, fever. Treatments: nervous bowel, colic. Dosage: 3–12 g. Peppermint is in popular use in Western medicine, but mainly as a flavouring.

peppermint tea This is a popular medicinal drink in the West, but it is no different from a Chinese-style infusion of the dried leaves of *Mentha piperita*. It is used as a carminative, breath-sweetener and a remedy for tiredness. It is also a refreshing drink. See **peppermint**.

pepsin An enzyme in the stomach which breaks down proteins to form peptones, which are soluble in water.

peptic ulcer An ulcer in the stomach or duodenum. See **ulcer**.

peptone See **pepsin**.

percussion A TCM diagnostic technique. The middle finger of one hand is placed over the region of the organ under examination. Then this finger is struck on its middle joint with the middle finger of the other hand. The resonance so produced indicates the condition of the organ below. This technique is also used in Western medicine. *Percussion* is also the name of a massage technique, variously described as drumming, cupping, chopping, hacking or pounding, in which short, sharp blows are delivered with the sides of the hands. See **massage**.

pericarditis Inflammation of the pericardium, which is a serious condition requiring expert medical attention.

pericardium The membraneous sac which encloses the heart. In Western medicine, the pericardium is not a vital organ, but only a part of a vital organ, namely the heart; but, in TCM, it is regarded as one of the solid vital organs. Chinese physicians, with their great love of harmony, introduced the pericardium, which they describe as the heart-constrictor, as a kind of afterthought to correspond with the triple-warmer, which is one of the hollow organs. An uneven number of solid organs and an uneven number of hollow organs would offend against the yin-yang principle. See **vital organs**.

period Menstrual period, or time of menstruation. See **menstruation**.

period pains Painful menstruation. This is sometimes a cramp-like pain which could be due to over-activity of the uterus. Chinese physicians sometimes recommend massage with an oil derived from soya beans or wheat. An acupressure treatment is to firmly massage the acupoint which is four fingers' width below the kneecap and just outside the shinbone. See **dysmenorrhoea** and **menstruation**.

peristalsis See **exercise**.

ACUPRESSURE FOR PERIOD PAINS

peritoneum A double membrane lining the abdominal cavity and covering the abdominal organs.

peritonitis Inflammation of the peritoneum, which sometimes results from untreated appendicitis. This is a serious condition requiring urgent and skilled medical attention.

permitted additive See **additives**.

pernicious anaemia This condition is characterized by a decrease in the number of red blood cells, as in the case with most forms of anaemia. But, with pernicious anaemia, the stomach cannot provide the secretions which are necessary to enable the intestine to assimilate cobalamin (vitamin B_{12}), which is essential to the formation of red blood cells. In the West, the treatment is to provide cobalamin by regular injections, which must be carried out for the rest of the patient's life. But Chinese physicians would claim that the inclusion of chopped raw liver and winter mushrooms in the diet could help to alleviate this condition. See **anaemia** and **winter mushrooms**.

perseverance See **patience**.

persimmon *Diospyros kaki* Herbal medicine. Distribution: China, Japan, Vietnam, India, North America. Parts: peduncles (flower-bearing stems). Character: neutral, bitter. Affinity: stomach. Effects: reduces hiccups and coughs, controls stomach-*qi* and spleen-*qi*. Symptoms: hiccups. Treatment: hiccups. Dosage: 4–6 g. As a treatment for hiccups, this medicine is most effective when it is combined with cloves, *Eugenia caryophyllus*, and fresh ginger, *Zingiber officinale*. Parts: ripe fruits. Character: neutral, sweet. Affinity: stomach, liver, spleen. Effects: stomachic, astringent. Symptoms: diarrhoea, colicky pains. Treatments:

gastritis, peptic ulcers, colitis, diverticulosis. Dosage: 3–6 g. The unripe fruits are a remedy for hypertension. This plant is sometimes called the Japanese persimmon to distinguish it from other species in the same genus.

persimmon wine The fruits of the persimmon, *Diopyros kaki*, have medicinal properties. Here is a simple recipe for persimmon wine. Ingredients: 6 dried persimmons, 575 ml rice wine, 45 g refined sugar. Quarter, but do not wash, the persimmons. Put all the ingredients into a large clean jar, cover, seal and store where cool, dry, dark and undisturbed. After nine months, strain and put into a clean bottle. The Chinese drink this wine as an appetizer and to prevent colds and flu, increase virility and counter exhaustion. Two small glasses a day is the maximum dosage. See **medicinal wine**.

personal hygiene The Chinese attach much importance to personal hygiene, which is necessary to prevent unpleasant odours, an unkempt appearance, infection and contamination by poisonous substances. It includes regular baths, washing the hands before and after meals or using the toilet, keeping the hair clean and tidy and the finger-nails clean and trimmed, brushing the teeth, avoiding coughing, breathing or sneezing on food, covering the mouth with the hand when coughing, changing into clean clothes quite regularly, avoiding walking barefooted in a changing room, abstaining from casual sexual relationships, and so on, and it should be extended to include cleanliness in the handling of food. On the other hand, the Chinese would be of the opinion that the washing and cleaning processes should not be overdone, for they destroy the natural oils in the skin, which nature provides as a lubricant and a protection against infection; and, unless the skin is rinsed well in hot water, the fats in soap will block up the pores. Cosmetic creams and powders are not to be recommended, for they also block up the skin pores, and are sometimes mildly toxic. The application of perfume is often just a matter of using one smell to cover up another. It is as well to remember that the benefits of cleanliness are sometimes more aesthetic than medical. White is traditionally symbolic of purity; but, though the white coats worn by doctors and dispensers do have the advantage that they show up the dirt, they are no more germ-free than the blue overalls worn by plumbers and mechanics. The daily-bath enthusiast who believes that he is seven times cleaner than the individual who takes a bath only once a week is surely deceiving himself. In any case, a little dirt is necessary to induce the body to strengthen its defences, so conferring a natural immunity to infection. See **hygiene**, **athlete's foot** and **immune system**.

personality What has the personality to do with health? A great deal, Chinese physicians would say. A person's attitude and behaviour – whether he is carefree or cautious, sociable or morose, good-tempered or ill-tempered, calm or fidgety, bold or timid, courageous or cowardly, sincere or deceitful, generous or selfish, extroverted or introverted, etc. – provide some indication of his state of health, both mental and physical. For example, a person who laughs too much may have a heart condition, and a person who is fearful may have a kidney defect. The emotions are registered and may be initiated by the brain, but the hormones, which are secreted by the endocrine glands, and which are related to the vital organs, are the means by which they are carried out. It seems that the romantic poets who associate the emotions with the heart rather than the brain were not entirely mistaken. Chinese physicians attach so much importance to the emotions that they give full consideration to a patient's personality and emotional state when making a diagnosis. See **endocrine glands**, **emotion**, and **personology**.

personology This is a study of a person's current attitudes and abilities, together with his personal qualities in relation to his state of health. It is a Taoist concept and a component of the *tao* of supremacy, which is one of the Eight Pillars of Taoism. See **personality** and **supremacy**.

perspiration Perspiration is generally not harmful even when it appears to be excessive. It is a self-regulating device which helps to remove excess water from the body, and also keep it cool. In a hot, dry climate, more water is lost from the body by perspiration than by urination. Moisture on the skin evaporates; in so doing, it takes heat from the body. There are two kinds of perspiration: that from the occrine glands, which cover the whole body and are stimulated by heat, and that from the apocrine glands, which are situated mainly in the armpits and genital areas and are stimulated by emotional changes and nervous activity. Excessive perspiration, particularly of the hands, feet and armpits, is traditionally regarded as a symptom of debility, though it is more likely to be due to anxiety or stress. It can be an embarrassment if it produces an unpleasant body odour. It is best to avoid stimulants, such as coffee and colas. Antiperspirants are not to be recommended, for they block up the skin pores, which makes matters worse by eliminating perspiration altogether, which is certainly not desirable. Chinese physicians sometimes recommend a simple acupressure treatment. On both hands, firmly press or massage the acupoint which is three fingers' width from the wrist crease and in line with the thumb. Herbal treatments include infusions, taken internally, of 15–30 g unripe grains of wheat, *Triticum aestivum*, and 2–6 g leaves of sage, *Salvia officinalis*. In TCM, the beneficial effects of perspiration are used as a form of treatment. See **sweats** and **diaphoretic treatment**.

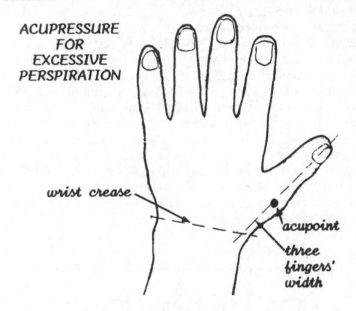

ACUPRESSURE
FOR
EXCESSIVE
PERSPIRATION

wrist crease

acupoint

three fingers' width

perspiration diagnosis In TCM, the quantity and degree of stickiness of perspiration, and when and where it occurs, are among the symptoms used in diagnosis. See **sweats**.

pertussis Whooping cough. This condition, which is due to a bacterium spread by water droplets, is a disease of childhood. Its symptoms are a mild fever, runny nose, vomiting, loss of appetite and a cough which begins mildly but worsens to spasms followed by a noisy inspiration – the whooping. The incubation period is 7–14 days, and the sufferer is infectious for 21 days, but the illness may linger for up to four months, and eczema may develop. But one attack should give immunity for life. In Western medicine, a whooping-cough vaccine is available, and it should certainly be administered to whooping-cough victims who are epileptics. In TCM, whooping cough is regarded as a damp-cold condition which can be prevented to some extent by the avoidance of damp and stuffy rooms and by containing colds as soon as they arise. Herbal remedies are a combination of relaxants and expectorants, which include infusions of the following, taken internally, using the parts and dosages indicated: liquorice, *Glycyrrhiza uralensis*, roots, 2–8 g; mullein, *Verbascum thapsus*, 6–20 g leaves, 3–6 g flowers; thyme, *Thymus vulgare*, leaves, 2–4 g; *bai bu*, *Stemona tuberosa*, tubers, 5–9 g.

pesticide See **chemicals** and **organic farming**.

petit mal See **epilepsy**.

petrisage See **compression**.

pets We do love our pets, but cats and dogs can be a source of infection and contamination, and so they are not allowed in catering establishments. In this respect, the Chinese have no problems. In the rural areas of China, cats and dogs are kept as working animals: cats as mousers, and dogs as guards – or as items of diet. In the towns and cities, the keeping of dogs is forbidden by law, and so there is little possibility of rabies. See **food hygiene**.

pH This symbol expresses the degree of acidity or alkalinity of a solution. pH7 is neutral, pH1–6 are acid, and pH8–14 are alkaline. The liquids in the human body are normally alkaline.

pharmacopoeia See **herbal**.

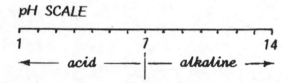

pH SCALE

'Pharmacopoeia of Shen Nong' See **Shen Nong Ben Cao Jing**.

pharyngitis Inflammation of the pharynx. In TCM, the usual treatment is an infusion, slowly sipped, of 2–8 g roots of liquorice, *Glycyrrhiza uralensis*, or 4–10 g leaves and stems of Japanese catnip, *Schizonepeta tenuifolia*.

pharynx The rear wall of the throat. See **epiglottis**.

philosophy The *tao* of philosophy is concerned with the meaning and purpose of life, spiritual evaluation and human destiny, the laws of nature, social development, and the health and well-being of the individual. See **Eight Pillars of Taoism**.

philosophy of health In the West, philosophy is an academic study. In China, it is put into practice. But, then, the Chinese are philosophical and practical by temperament. The Chinese value health above all else, which is a sure indication of their wisdom. It follows that their philosophy of living is to do with the benefits of health, longevity and peace of mind, and how they may be attained by a sound diet, adequate exercise, moderate habits and respect for one's ancestors. See **Hei Jing** and **Nei Pien**.

phlebitis Inflammation of a vein. It is helpful to take exercise and avoid the use of oral contraceptives. According to TCM, this condition is due to heat, poison or a blockage in a vein. The treatment requires that the blockage be removed and the blood cooled and the poison counteracted. The usual treatment is one of the following, taken internally, using the parts and dosage indicated: peony tree, *Paeonia moutan*, skin of roots, 4–5 g; safflower, *Carthamus tinctorius*, golden rod, *Solidago virgaurea*, all parts, 1.5–5 g. This treatment is essentially alleviative, but occasionally it proves to be curative.

phlegm Viscous liquid discharged by the lungs. See **humour**.

phobia Unnatural fear or aversion. See **anxiety state**.

phosphorus See **mineral**.

photophobia Abnormal sensitivity to, or fear of, light. See **migraine**.

photosynthesis See **survival**.

phrenic nerve See **hiccups**.

physical strength See **stamina**.

physician See **medical education** and **patience**.

physiology The study of the functions of the parts of an animal or plant, as opposed to anatomy, which is the study of its structure. See **anatomy**.

physiotherapy The treatment of diseases and deformities by physical methods, such as massage, water and sunshine. This is a term used in Western medicine, but it can be applied to massage, remedial and breathing exercises, acupressure and many of the other techniques used in Chinese medicine. See **nature's treatment**.

phytotherapy Herbal medicine.

pigeon breast A condition in which the breastbone sticks out and the sides of the chest are slightly sunken, and which begins in early childhood as a consequence of chronic tonsillitis or rickets. Pigeon-breasted people are susceptible to pneumonia and bronchitis. The treatments include fresh air, sunshine, foods containing vitamin D, such as eggs, margarine, oily fish and cod-liver oil, swimming, games and breathing and remedial exercises of the kind contained in the *Chinese Exercise Manual*.

pigeon pea *Sophora subprostrata*. Herbal medicine. Distribution:

South China, Vietnam, India. Parts: roots. Character: cold, bitter. Affinity: heart, lungs. Effects: antipyretic, antiphlogistic, antidote. Symptoms: sore throat, fever. Treatments: pharyngitis, laryngitis, heat-excess conditions. Dosage: 3–8 g.

pig's bladder Steamed with dried hops, a pig's bladder is a traditional Chinese remedy for hernia, incontinence and diseases of the urinary tract.

pig's feet Pig's trotters. Cooked in black rice vinegar, pig's feet are a traditional remedy for mothers during the postnatal period. It increases lactation, relieves tension and is a medicine for a wide variety of ailments, which include aches and pains, impoverished blood, poor circulation, blood clots, windiness and irregular bowel movements. Here is a recipe for pig's feet in black rice vinegar. Ingredients: 4 pigs' feet, 4 eggs, 575 ml black rice vinegar (from a Chinese grocer), 375 g green ginger, 1 teaspoon salt, 90 g sugar. Boil the eggs hard and shell them. Wash the feet, removing the bristles. Immerse the ginger in boiling water, scrape off the skin, crush slightly and fry without oil in a pan/wok until slightly dry and fragrant. Put the vinegar into an earthenware pot, add the salt, sugar and ginger, bring to the boil, cover and simmer for 40 minutes. Add the feet, bring to the boil, cover and simmer very gently for 3 hours. Add the eggs, marinate for 8 hours and then serve at room temperature. Note: the bristles on the feet may be easily burnt off with a candle flame. Then the feet are scrubbed and rinsed.

pig's gall-bladder In TCM, a refined extract from the fluid in a pig's gall-bladder is used as an antipyretic, diuretic, sedative, tonic for the heart and treatment for spasms and skin infections.

pig's heart It is traditional in China for a pig's heart to be cooked as an ingredient in a soup which is consumed as a mild sedative.

pig's liver See **anaemia**.

pig's tail Medicinally, these are used in the same way as pig's feet. See **pig's feet**.

pigtail This hair-style, which was imposed on Chinese males as a badge of servitude by the emperors of China, was quickly abandoned when China became a republic in 1912. At the same time, the practice of bandaging girls' feet, producing painful deformities, was also abandoned.

piles See **haemorrhoids**.

pills In TCM, pills are made by grinding the herbal ingredients to make a fine powder, adding a binder, such as honey, maltose, water, flour-paste or beeswax, and then hand-rolling the mixture to produce spherical pills, which vary in size from pellets to large marbles, according to the potency of the medicine indicated by the prescription. Herbal pills are gentle and slow in action, and so are effective in treating chronic ailments. It is because the absorption rate of herbal pills is slow and gentle that they are used to administer potent or poisonous medicines which, otherwise, would not be tolerated by the body. Generally, pill prescriptions require the patient to take 15–20 small pills three or four times daily. This ensures that the medicine is slowly and evenly absorbed and constantly present. Herbal pills are in four classes: honey, water, flour-paste and wax.

pimples and spots At puberty, it is quite normal for pimples and spots to appear on the skin, but they can be embarrassingly ugly. The body's metabolism is undergoing changes which result in toxins occurring in the skin. According to TCM, this condition is caused by heat in the blood and stomach, and cooling medicines must be applied. For mild cases, the treatments are herbal teas as follows: chrysanthemum, *Chrysanthemum morifolium*, flowers, 4–8 g; honeysuckle, *Lonicera japonica*, flowers, 8–15 g; dandelion, *Taraxacum officinale*, all parts, 10–15 g. For severe cases, the treatments are infusions of the following, taken internally, using the parts and dosages indicated: scullcap, *Scutellaria baicalensis*, roots, 4–7 g; rhubarb, *Rheum officinale*, rhizomes, 0.3–1 g. It is helpful to avoid sugary and fatty foods and keep free of constipation. In China, there are proprietary brands of herbal creams which are most effective in treating this condition, but they are not readily available in the West. As an alternative, the skin can be cleansed with fresh water-melon or cucumber.

pineal gland See **endocrine glands**.

'pink eye' See **conjunctivitis**.

'pins and needles' Sensation felt in recovery from the numbness caused by a temporary decrease in circulation in a surface area of the body. See **menopause**.

pin-worm Threadworm. A small parasitic worm which commonly infects the large intestine, causing inflammation and itchiness around the anus. Pin-worms are one of the oldest infections known to humans, and are mainly spread by contaminated food. They are not dangerous, and can be eliminated by clean habits and an intake of garlic and raw carrots. See **garlic**.

pistil The female sexual organ of a flowering plant, and the part used in some herbal medicines.

pituitary gland See **endocrine glands**.

placebo Hypochondriacs generally feel that they have need of medicines, though their ailments are imaginary; and there are

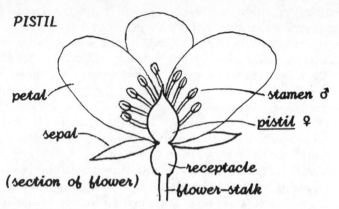

PISTIL

petal

sepal

(section of flower)

stamen ♂

pistil ♀

receptacle

flower-stalk

those who believe that no kind of medical treatment can be regarded as being entirely satisfactory unless a bottle of medicine or a box of pills is provided. For these people, the physician may prescribe a dummy medicine, that is, one with inactive ingredients. But placebos are not to be despised, for they sometimes have a good psychological effect, especially in giving the patient some degree of confidence in himself or his future, though his future could be bleak. But, perhaps, as a means of reassurance, the *I Ching* has more to offer than placebos. See **medicine** and **I Ching**.

placenta Afterbirth. An organ which develops in the uterus during pregnancy, and which conveys nutriment from the mother's blood to that of the foetus. Normally, the placenta and foetal membrane are discharged immediately after the birth of the baby, but the placenta is sometimes retained, creating a condition which requires treatment under proper medical supervision. In TCM, one of the treatments is a decoction, administered internally, of the preputial follicles of the musk-deer, *Moschus moschiferus*.

plague See **flea**.

plain flavour See **taste**.

planets See **element** and **symbolism**.

plant-derived medicines Most of the medicines used by the Chinese are herbal, that is, derived from plants, and they are considered to be safer and gentler in their effects than those derived from animals or minerals. Most of the tonic medicines, such as ginseng, wolfberry and garlic, are plant-derived. However, a few are derived from animals, for plants cannot supply such things as male hormones, albumins, amino acids and interferon. See **animal-derived medicines** and **virility**.

plasma The fluid part of blood. See **blood**.

Plasmodium vivax See **malaria**.

plastic surgery Traditionally, Chinese physicians are opposed to surgery, which they regard as often being an unnecessary mutilation of the body, and so the surgeon is expected to apply his skills as a last resort – when all other methods of treatment – herbal medicines, diet, remedial exercises, acupuncture, etc. – have failed. Therefore, to employ surgery for purely cosmetic purposes, and for someone to suffer pain and mutilation in the cause of vanity, might seem to be the height of folly. On the other hand, there is every justification for plastic surgery where a person has received appalling injuries which could be damaging to his health either physically or psychologically. See **surgery**.

plastron The lower part of the shell of a turtle or tortoise. In TCM, the former is employed as a medicine. See **turtle**.

platelet See **thrombocyte**.

pleasure Philosophers cannot agree on a definition of pleasure. Yet it seems obvious that one can have no real pleasure unless one is in a good state of health, whereby one will eat well, sleep well and generally feel well, and will probably live to a great age. 'Be healthy, and pleasure will surely follow,' says the *I Ching*. Too much pleasure not only jades one's appetite for pleasure; it is unhealthy and can be as causative of stress as is worry. What is more, a treat ceases to be treat if it is experienced too often. With many of our pleasures, there is more enjoyment in the anticipation than in the realization.

pleura The double membrane inside the chest, and which covers the lungs.

pleuritis Inflammation of the pleura. Complications can develop, and so this condition requires professional medical attention, though it is easily treatable by means of antibiotics. In TCM, the usual treatment is a combination of expectorant and warming medicines, which include decoctions of the following, taken internally, using the parts and dosages indicated: comfrey, *Symphytum officinale*, roots or leaves, 3–10 g; liquorice, *Glycyrrhiza uralensis*, roots, 2–8 g; thyme, *Thymus vulgare*, leaves, 1.5–9 g; mullein, *Verbascum thapsus*, leaves or flowers, 5–20 g; garlic, *Allium sativum*, 2–3 cloves; ginger, *Zingiber officinale*, rhizomes, 3–7 g.

plexus See **solar plexus**.

PMT The abbreviation for *premenstrual tension*.

pneumonia Pneumonitis. An inflamed and congested condition of the lungs due to exposure to pneumococcal bacteria and cold and wet conditions, which lower the ability of the lungs to extract oxygen from inhaled air. At one time, pneumonia had a high mortality rate, but it now responds very favourably to treatment with modern antibiotics, which are supplemented by expectorants and 7–28 days rest in bed. One of the perils of pneumonia is that it can leave the sufferer with emphysema. When pneumonia is suspected, medical advice must be sought immediately. According to TCM, pneumonia is a condition of heat and phlegm in the lungs caused by wind-heat or wind-cold. In the initial stages, where there is coughing, fever and chest pain, the treatment can be as for bronchitis, with an infusion of one of the following, taken internally, using the parts and dosage indicated: garlic, *Allium sativum*, 2–3 cloves; ginger, *Zingiber officinale*, rhizomes, 3–7 g; thyme, *Thymus vulgare*, leaves, 3–10 g. A traditional remedy among the country people of China is to slowly swallow a crushed garlic clove in a spoonful of honey, which functions as a diaphoretic, antibiotic and expectorant. It is also helpful to apply a poultice of the crushed seeds of black mustard, *Brassica nigra*. It is imperative that the patient should have a good supply of fresh air, and this must NOT be allowed to become dry, as can occur in an overheated bedroom. If the condition worsens, and particularly where there is blood in the sputum, the treatment is a decoction of one of the following, taken internally, using the parts and dosages indicated: scullcap, *Scutellaria baicalensis*, roots, 4–7 g; fritillary, *Fritillaria verticillata*, corms, 4–8 g; lepidium, *Lepidium apetalum*, seeds, 4–8 g; peach, *Prunus persica*, kernels, 6–9 g; yarrow, *Achillea millefolium*, flowers, 3–10 g.

pneumonitis Inflammation of the lungs. See **pneumonia**.

podogra Gout. This is a type of arthritis in which faulty metabolism causes deposition of uric acid crystals in the joints, especially those of the big toe, which become inflamed and very painful. It is helpful to keep the affected foot elevated and at rest, apply a pack of crushed ice for a few minutes, soak the foot in hot water for 5–10 minutes, drink plenty of water to eliminate uric acid salts, drink yarrow or peppermint tea to increase the circulation, avoid drugs which increase uric acid levels, avoid alcohol and keep the intake of the following foods at a minimum: herrings, sardines, kidneys, liver, gravy and meat extracts, shellfish, asparagus, cauliflower, spinach, wholegrain bread and cereals, mushrooms and pulses. According to TCM, podogra is due to heat and damp in the blood and liver meridian and a deficiency of kidney-*qi*. The treatment is the same as for kidney-stones and arthritis, and includes acupuncture and moxibustion to relieve pain, and decoctions of the following, taken internally, using the parts and dosages indicated: akebia, *Akebia quinata*, stems, 4–6 g; quince, *Chaenomeles lagenaria*, fruit, 3–9 g; nettle, *Urtica dioica*, leaves, 6–12 g.

point massage This is a system of treatment, used as an alternative to acupuncture and acupressure, in which the acupoints are massaged instead of being needled or pressed. But it is only effective with a few simple treatments. See **pressure-point therapy**.

poisonous plants Some of the plants used in both Western and Chinese medicine, such as mistletoe, *Viscum album*, deadly nightshade, or belladonna, *Atropa belladonna*, and aconite, *Aconitum napelus*, are very poisonous, but are beneficial, generally as stimulants or relaxants, when taken in small amounts. See **nux vomica** and **Medicines Act 1968**.

poliomyelitis Infantile paralysis. A viral disease which affects the nervous system, so producing paralysis of the muscles. Vaccines are now available for this condition, and so it is far less common now than it was 40 years ago. It is spread by sewage, contaminated water and poor personal hygiene. Fortunately, most cases are mild, with symptoms of fever, headaches and a sore throat, and so they go largely unnoticed. Only in a few cases does the sufferer develop encephalitis, or inflammation of the brain, with symptoms of drowsiness, stiff neck muscles, cramp-like pains in the muscles and paralysis. However, the disease should not be regarded as being inevitably incapacitating or fatal, and the patient may be able to live a normal life if he employs remedial exercises and takes good care of his general health. In TCM, the recommended treatments to alleviate the after-effects of poliomyelitis are acupuncture and the remedial exercises of the *tai chi chuan*, together with tonic medicines to strengthen *qi* and the nerves and blood.

pollen Some people are allergic to pollen, to which hay-fever is often attributed. Pollen grains are the male reproductive structures of flowering plants, and Chinese physicians would claim that the traces of pollen in honey and royal jelly have a beneficial effect on the health by increasing virility. See **royal jelly**.

pollution Pollution is now recognised by most countries, including China, as a serious threat to the health and safety of mankind. See **chemicals, ozone, environment** and **air pollution**.

polyneuritis See **beriberi**.

polyp A small growth on a mucous membrane. See **papilloma**.

polysaccharide See **sugar**.

polyunsaturated fat See **fatty acid**.

pomegranate *Punica granatum* Indigenous to the subtropical regions of Asia, an infusion of the peel of its fruit, taken internally, is a Chinese folklore remedy for intestinal worms.

pomelo Grapefruit or shaddock. Native to South-east Asia, and of various species, including *Citrus grandis* and *Citrus paradisi*, the pomelo is a reliable source of ascorbic acid (vitamin C).

poppy There are several species of poppy. The corn poppy, *Papaver rhoeas*, grows in temperate regions throughout the world. For centuries, its juice has been used as a mild sedative and to alleviate whooping cough and bronchitis. See **opium poppy**.

porcelain spoon See **eating utensils**.

pork offal In the West, pork offal – heart, kidneys, feet, tails, bladder, etc. – are regarded as butcher's waste, and so are rather despised as items of diet, but the Chinese value them for their medicinal properties. See **pig's feet** and **pig's heart**.

positive cycle See **element**.

postmenstrual syndrome This term describes the combination of conditions – depression, headaches, aggressiveness, fullness of the abdomen, pain in the abdomen and limbs and water retention – which a woman may experience immediately after menstruation. In TCM, this syndrome is ascribed to an imbalance of the liver, kidneys and spleen, and the stagnation which has interfered with the monthly release of blood. The recommended treatments are a more wholesome diet, acupuncture and an infusion or decoction of one of the following, taken internally, using the parts and dosage indicated: scullcap, *Scutellaria baicalensis*, roots, 4–7 g; peony, *Paeonia lactiflora*, roots, 6–8 g; Indian bread, *Poria cocos*, all parts, 4–8 g; angelica, *Angelica sinensis*, roots, 9–4 g; mandarin orange, *Citrus reticulata*, peel of fresh green fruits, 4–8 g. Sage, *Salvia officinalis*, is mildly effective in regulating feminine hormonal levels, and it is used for that purpose in the West.

post-mortem See **autopsy**.

postnatal problems After giving birth, a woman will experience vaginal bleeding, which could last for several weeks. Also, there could be pains due to the uterus shrinking back to its normal size, piles, fatigue, depression, difficulties with lactation and 'postnatal drop', or a dripping nose, which is caused by dryness of the mucous membranes in the nose, throat and sinuses. Birth is a natural process, and these conditions should disappear automatically after a few weeks, but if they persist, medical advice should be sought. For postnatal abdominal pains, Chinese physicians would probably recommend an infusion or decoction of 6–12 g fruits (haws) of the hawthorn, *Crataegus pinnatifida*, to be taken internally; and for weakness, they would recommend 10–14 g fruits of longan, *Euphoria longan*, also to be taken internally. *Tienchi, Panax pseudo-ginseng*, is a good general tonic. See **tienchi** and **pig's feet**.

posture Bad posture in standing or sitting, and which may be due to bone defects, congenital deformities and a psychological condition which encourages laziness and lolling, can give rise to backache, spinal curvature, poor breathing, strained ligaments and severe fatigue. The *Chinese Exercise Manual* contains a wide range of exercises which will help to correct defects in posture.

potassium See **mineral**.

poultice A hot and dense medicated dressing applied to counter inflammation and irritation. In TCM, a poultice is prepared by mixing powdered herbs with hot water to make a dense paste which is spread over a piece of cloth or paper and applied to the inflamed or injured area and kept tied in place for 8–14 hours. The moisture of the herbs combined with the heat of the body produces healing vapours and draws out evil-*qi*. Herbal poultices are commonly used as a treatment for sprains, arthritic joints, bruises, swellings, abscesses and blocked meridians. See **paste-medicine**.

pounding See **percussion**.

powdered herbs In TCM, medicinal herbs are generally ground into powders, which breaks down their fibres, exposes the active ingredients and creates more surfaces, and so increases their solubility when boiling water is added to make an infusion or decoction. But it is only very rarely that medicinal herbs are administered in the dry powdered form, for they would then be difficult to swallow and could have a choking effect.

praying mantis *Paratenodera sinensis*. Medicine. Distribution: global. Parts: egg-cases. Character: neutral, salty-sweet. Affinity: kidneys, liver. Symptoms: enuresis, urinary incontinence, premature ejaculation. Treatments: spermatorrhoea, impotence, conditions due to kidney-yang deficiency. Dosage: 3–9 g.

'Precious Prescriptions' See **Sun Simiao**.

prediction A physician often needs to make a prediction about a patient's state of health. For example, if a patient is terminally ill, the physician may predict how long he has to live. Such predictions can never be in the nature of certainties, but they are highly accurate if they are based upon known facts, past history and logical reasoning. The Chinese have always had an interest in divination, or prediction-making, using various methods, including astrology, geomancy, automatic writing and the *I Ching*. In ancient times, they used the so-called 'oracle bones', which were probably the forerunners of the hexagrams used in the *I Ching*. When predictions are on an intellectual level, as are those made by philosophers, scientists, politicians and economists, they are extremely valuable. But when they are based on blind guesswork or wishful thinking, they are no more than superstition or a source of entertainment, though even fortune-tellers sometimes take the trouble to express their predictions in such general terms that they cannot possibly be wrong. For example, to be told that one will have some good news next year is a prediction which could be applied to almost any person at any time or in any place. The *I Ching* owes its accuracy to the fact that many of its so-called predictions are really no more than snippets of sound advice, though that does not detract from their usefulness, for they often indicate how to best deal with a difficult situation if it should arise. See **divination**, **I Ching** and **prognosis**.

pregnancy This is a natural process, but as we tend to live unnaturally, it presents more problems for women than it does for the females of the lower animals. Most pregnancies progress smoothly, but it is imperative that a pregnant woman should have regular check-ups with a physician in order to ensure that nothing is seriously amiss. It is also important to understand that a disease caught in the first three months of pregnancy can adversely affect the baby's eyesight, hearing, heart and mental development. Rubella, or German measles, can do much damage in this respect. A healthy diet, regular but not strenuous exercise and the avoidance of alcohol will help to ensure a satisfactory pregnancy. Pregnant women are subject to minor health problems, such as constipation, backache, indigestion, headaches, haemorrhoids, oedema, morning sickness and a level of hypertension which, if not treated, could assume dangerous proportions. All of these conditions can be treated by means of herbal medicines, but one should be aware that some herbal medicines, such as parsley and celery seeds, cannot be safely administered to pregnant women. In TCM, pregnant women are advised to eat foods rich in calcium, which will help in the bone-formation of the baby, and dietary fibre, which will prevent constipation, and to take exercise or even do work to prevent stagnation of *qi* and the blood, which could lead to oedema or hypertension. Labour is easier if the pregnancy is active. The *Chinese Exercise Manual*

contains some exercises which are designed to promote suppleness of the abdominal muscles and the general health during
pregnancy. The Chinese have various methods by which they
are able to determine the sex of an unborn baby, or so some of
them would claim. One of these is dietary. If the diet of both
parents during the seven-day period prior to intercourse is
essentially yin – consisting of vegetables, mushrooms, pasta,
bean curd and non-citrus fruits but no pickles – they will have a
son. But if it is essentially yan – consisting of meat, chicken, fish,
citrus fruits and pickles – they will have a daughter. Another
method is to use numbers, starting with 49, which is the product
(7×7) of the seven seven-year periods in a woman's maturity
cycle, to which is added the number of the month in which she
conceived, and from which her age is subtracted. If the final
number is odd, the baby will be a boy; and if it is even, the baby
will be a girl. Thus, if a pregnant woman is aged 22 and she
conceived during April, a simple calculation – 49 + 4 − 22 = 31
– will reveal that the baby will be a boy. But it would be
impossible to accurately predict the sex of an unborn child by
this technique, which really does no more than indicate that, in
China, as elsewhere, boys and girls are born in approximately
equal numbers. They will certainly not be distributed in a way
which will suit the wishes of all Chinese parents, who generally
have a preference for boys. See **morning sickness** and
postnatal problems.

premature ageing The causes of premature ageing have been
variously listed as inadequate diet, stress, lack of exercise,
over-strenuous exercise, a breakdown in the immune system,
hormonal underactivity and immoderate habits, including sexual
over-activity and a weakness for alcohol. It often occurs in a
severe form in middle age or even earlier. See **Alzheimer's
disease** and **ageing**.

premature ejaculation In TCM, there are a number of yang
tonics which are suitable for treating this condition, which is
mainly due to nervousness and over-excitement. An infusion or
decoction of any of the following, taken internally, would be
suitable as a yang tonic to treat this condition: horny goat weed,
Epimedium sagittatum, leaves, 10–12 g; caltrop, *Tribulus terristes*,
mature fruits, 10–14 g; dodder, *Cuscuta japonica*, 10–14 g;
broomrape, *Cistanche salsa*, stems, 8–12 g. See **impotence**.

premature greying This condition has various causes, and a
hereditary factor is generally involved, but there is certainly no
cause for alarm, for the disadvantages are purely cosmetic. The

BROOMRAPE

Cistanche salsa

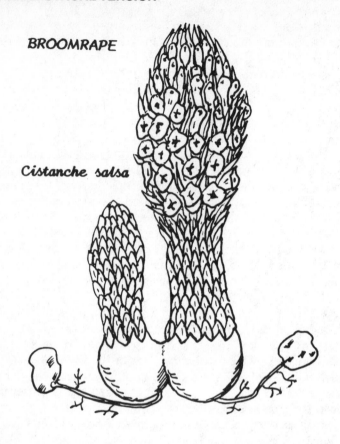

usual TCM treatment is a decoction of 8–15 g leaves and stems of *han lian cao*, *Eclipta prostrata*, taken internally. A useful tonic for the hair is an infusion, taken internally, of 8–14 g fruits of longan, *Euphoria longan*. See **hair loss**.

premenstrual tension Most women suffer from this condition to a greater or lesser degree. It occurs during the days leading up to a period, and is characterized by such symptoms and ailments as skin problems, weight gain, weakness, headaches, cravings for food or alcohol, swollen ankles, oedema, irritability, insomnia, loss of interest in sex, inability to concentrate, weepiness and depression. The causes are changes in hormonal levels and a deficiency of progesterone, one of the female sex hormones, and unsaturated fatty acids, and an accumulation of salt and water in the body. The suffering due to these conditions can range from mild discomfort to utter misery, and the sufferer may behave irresponsibly and in a way which is quite out of character. However, the condition is generally harmless, for it is a part of a natural, though troublesome, process. It is helpful to avoid stress by relaxing with gentle exercise or a warm bath, and to reduce the intake of salt, sugar, tea, coffee, alcohol and animal fats. In the West, a dietary supplement of pyridoxine (vitamin B_6) has been found to have some merit as a treatment, and oil of evening primrose, *Oenochera biennis*, has become popular. In TCM, the recommended treatments are light massage and acupuncture or moxibustion applied to the meridians related to the kidneys, liver and conception- and governor-vessels. Royal jelly is helpful, as is an infusion, taken internally, of 3–10 g flowers of camomile, *Matricaria chamomilla*. Chinese women seem to suffer less from premenstrual tension than do their counterparts in the West. Perhaps this is due to their natural stamina, their tenacity in matters of health and their matter-of-fact attitude towards sexual reproduction.

preparation of herbs In China, the large-scale preparation of herbs so that they are ready for use by the pharmacist involves a large number of processes which will ensure maximum efficacy in treatments. The collected herbs are first cleaned, the dirt and other impurities being removed and the parts of no medicinal value being discarded, and then sorted according to their uses. The flowers are removed and set aside to dry separately, and the other items are thoroughly washed to remove all the remaining traces of dirt. However, a few of the very delicate herbs are not washed, for this may destroy their natural ingredients. The various items are then dried in the sun, or by a fire indoors when the weather is wet, dull or cold. When dry, they are cut into suitable sizes and shapes for convenient storage. Roots, rhizomes and woody stems are cut into thin slices, leaves and barks are cut into long thin strips, and whole plants are separated into their parts – seeds, fruits, etc. They are then put into labelled containers, such as ceramic jars, glass bottles and wooden drawers, and stored in a cool, dry, dark and well-ventilated place. They are occasionally exposed to the sunshine to prevent dampness and the development of moulds and mildews. Some medicinal plants are of great value, especially the rarer, slow-growing perennials, and it is important that they should be kept alive, and so, in gathering herbs, these plants are not entirely stripped of their leaves and bark, and only the small roots and rhizomes are removed, the larger ones being left in the ground.

preputial follicle The small sac, containing an odour-producing substance, which is situated within the prepuce, or foreskin, of certain mammals, such as deer. See **musk-deer**.

prescription A physician's directions, usually written, for the composition and application of a medicine. See **herbal prescriptions.**

'Prescriptions of the Golden Chamber' See **treatment principles**.

preserved food Foodstuffs are preserved mainly by smoking, pickling, dehydration, canning, bottling, refrigeration, deep-freezing and pasteurization. These preservation methods have the same basic function, which is to prevent food from being contaminated by bacteria, such as staphylococci, but they achieve this purpose in different ways. Smoking produces a hard layer containing substances which are poisonous to bacteria. Pickling is done in vinegar or brine, in which bacteria cannot live. Bacteria cannot live without moisture, and so they have less chance of survival in dry foods. Nor can they grow and multiply at low temperatures. Also, they cannot enter sealed containers. With the exception of pasteurization, which is used for preserving milk, these methods are also used in China, but not on a wide scale, for the Chinese have a distinct preference for fresh food. See **frozen food**, **fresh food** and **food poisoning**.

pre-senile dementia Senility at an early age. See **Alzheimer's disease**.

pressure massage A diagnostic technique employed in kinesology, or pressure-point therapy. The manner of response of a muscle when a pressure-point is massaged is supposed to be an indication of the state of health of certain organs. See **pressure-point therapy**.

pressure-point One of the points on the body which is believed to be ultra-sensitive and which is massaged as a means of diagnosis in kinesology. A pressure-point may be quite remote from the organ to which it is said to be related. Thus, one of the pressure-points related to the nose is on the hand. The term *pressure-point* is sometimes used to describe an acupoint, but this is misleading because the points used in acupuncture and acupressure are not necessarily the same as those used in kinesology. See **acupoints**.

pressure-point therapy Point massage. Kinesology. This is a Western-world system of alternative medicine based on the principle that each set of muscles is related to one of the organs of the body, and so, if some muscles are massaged to maintain them in a sound state of health, the related organs will also be maintained in a sound state of health. This would seem to be an altogether over-simplistic view of physiology, but the practitioners of kinesology claim that it is effective in treating such conditions as backache, neck pain, headaches, colds, influenza, catarrh, fatigue, tension and depression, and that it will strengthen the immune system. It is sometimes likened to acupuncture, but the resemblance is purely superficial, for acupuncture is based on an entirely different principle, it is much more sophisticated, and its practitioners require a much longer period of training. Most orthodox practitioners are suspicious of kinesology, which they regard as being so simple as to be dangerous. It could deceive people into thinking that they are receiving an effective medical treatment when, in fact, they are not, and so serious conditions could go untreated. Its benefits are probably no greater than those of any other form of massage. It does have the merit of being easy to apply, but that could really be a demerit if no worthwhile results are achieved. See **pressure-point**.

pressure sore An ulcer of the skin caused by persistent pressure. Bed sores are of this nature. See **ulcer**.

preventive diet Prophylactic diet. The Chinese have a wide range of health foods which may be used as alternatives to medicines in preventing illnesses and inhibiting the ageing process. In this connection, it is interesting to note that many of the foodstuffs which we, in the West, are inclined to despise, such as pig's feet and sprats, simply because they are inexpensive or are derived from an unglamorous source, have health-giving properties, and so are highly esteemed in China. But the Chinese are pragmatic people and they recognise that good health is invaluable. China has an economy which is basically agricultural, and, in the south, a climate which is hot and wet, but not unpleasantly so, and so there is no shortage of exotic foodstuffs, which means an ordinary Chinese family can partake of meals of many nutritious, health-giving and mouth-watering courses whose components of fish, fruits and fungi would be the envy of the very rich in the West. As far as the Chinese are concerned, food is medicine, and medicine should be essentially preventive. See **health foods**.

preventive medicine Prophylaxis. Prevention is one of the cardinal principles of traditional Chinese medicine, and it is based on the very sound principle that some of the illnesses which are virtually incurable can easily be prevented by the application of a little forethought in matters of diet, exercise and personal habits, and a judicious application of herbal medicines. This explains why there is a low incidence of cancer, sugar diabetes and heart and circulatory complaints in China. What is more, it must be the case that, no matter how effective a cure may be, it cannot undo all the damage which the illness has already caused, and so the body will never be quite the same again. With the human body, as with a machine, regular maintenance may prevent a disaster. And so, in TCM, the emphasis is more on the preventive than the curative or alleviative, but this does not mean that the Chinese do not have any efficacious alleviative or curative medicines. On the contrary, Chinese physicians have a vast repertoire of herbal remedies at their disposal, but they realize that people can be spared a great deal of pain and anxiety and even permanent injury if an illness is prevented from arising in the first place. In the West, there is a tendency for people to put off visits to the doctor and to shut illness completely out of their minds until the situation is so critical that something simply has to be done – and then it may be too late. See **curative medicine**.

prickly heat Milaria. Heat rash. A condition in which the sweat glands become blocked, so causing the formation of a rash and small blisters. See **heat rash**.

primary This term is applied to an illness or abnormal condition which later causes another, or secondary, illness or condition. Thus, primary amenorrhoea is a condition where menstrual periods have never occurred, but secondary amenorrhoea is where they cease after having been in existence previously.

primary sex characteristics These are the characteristics which determine a person's sexuality. Essentially, they are the sex glands and the hormonal secretions which they produce. They determine the secondary sex characteristics, which include the genitalia, degree of hairiness, pitch of voice, etc. In the male, they are the testes and the hormone testosterone; and, in the female, they are the ovaries and the hormones oestrogen and progesterone. Chinese physicians have long known of the existence of these characteristics, which they describe as semen-essence. See **jing**.

'Principles of Longevity' See **essence**.

principles of traditional Chinese medicine TCM is not only the oldest and finest system of preventive medicine in the world; it is also one of the most complex, and to describe its principles in a few well-chosen words would be a particularly daunting task. But perhaps one could say that its principles, briefly expressed, are prophylaxis, herbal medicines, a sound diet, adequate exercises, peace of mind, moderate habits, a wise philosophy of living, minimal surgery, dedicated physicians, acupuncture, moxibustion, meditation, treatments to ensure longevity and an approach which is both allopathic and naturopathic, all expressed in terms of yin and yang, and based on the philosophies of Taoism and Confucianism.

p.r.n. The abbreviation for the Latin words *pro re nata*, meaning 'as and when required', and used in prescriptions.

processed foods See **natural foods**, **organic farming**, **food poisoning** and **foods to avoid**.

procidentia See **prolapse of womb**.

procreation See **sex**.

proctitis Inflammation of the rectum, which is aggravated by faeces, particularly if they are of an acidic content, and which can be causative of haemorrhoids. The usual TCM treatment is a wholesome and non-spicy diet and the external application of a suitable antiseptic ointment. There are several proprietary brands of Chinese medications which are very suitable for this purpose. See **haemorrhoids**.

progesterone A hormone secreted by the ovaries and placenta, and which partly regulates the menstrual cycle and the normality of the pregnancy process. See **hormone** and **primary sex characteristics**.

prognosis A forecast of the probable course and outcome of a disease. A prognosis made by a Chinese physician is always based on a thorough diagnosis. See **prediction**.

prolapse The lowering or displacement of an organ or one of the larger structures of the body, as with a prolapsed rectum or womb. According to TCM, this condition is due to a deficiency of *qi* in the central part of the body, which is a weakness often associated with elderly people. The spleen needs to be toned, and there is a proprietary brand of Chinese pills which are intended specifically for this purpose. Herbal treatments include infusions or decoctions of the following, taken internally, using the parts and dosages indicated: astralagus, *Astralagus membranaceus*, roots, 8–14 g; hare's ear, *Bupleurum falcatum*, roots, 2–4 g; *dang shen*, *Codonopsis tangshen*, roots, 9–14 g. The *Chinese Exercise Manual* contains remedial exercises to treat prolapse of the rectum or womb. Of course, the precise nature of the treatment will be determined by the character of the organ involved, and it must be carried out under proper medical supervision.

prolapsed disc See **intervertebral disc**.

prolapse of rectum This is quite a common condition. In TCM, there is a wide range of herbal treatments, which include infusions or decoctions of the following, taken internally, using the parts and dosages indicated: astralagus, *Astralagus membranaceus*, roots, 8–14 g; ginseng, *Panax ginseng*, roots, 2–8 g; hare's ear, *Bupleurum falcatum*, roots, 2–4 g. A suspension of 6–10 g powdered magnetite (magnetic iron oxide) could also be used, but this is a treatment which would hardly meet with the approval of the physicians of the West. See **prolapse**.

prolapse of uterus See **prolapse of womb**.

prolapse of womb Procidentia. Prolapse of the womb, or uterus, is quite a common condition. TCM herbal remedies include infusions or decoctions of the following, taken internally, using the parts and dosages indicated: hare's ear, *Bupleurum falcatum*, roots, 2–4 g; astralagus, *Astralagus membranaceus*, roots, 8–14 g. Prolapse of the womb is sometimes associated with urinary disorders. See **prolapse** and **urinary incontinence**.

promiscuity See **sex**.

prophylactic diet See **preventive diet**.

prophylaxis See **preventive medicine**.

proprietary medicines In China, a wide range of proprietary brands of herbal medicines are manufactured as lotions, pills and ointments. They are very efficacious and convenient to use, and they are soundly based on many centuries of herbal wisdom and expertise. See **patent medicine**.

propriety Correct moral behaviour and one of the Confucian virtues. The Chinese place great value on this, since they regard it as essential to social harmony. See **Confucianism**, **sex** and **AIDS**.

prostate gland This gland, which occurs only in men, is situated around the neck of the bladder and the body end of the urethra. It secretes one of the components of semen. See **reproductive systems**.

prostate problems There are three common disorders of the prostate gland: prostatitis, which is inflammation and infection of the prostate gland, sometimes by venereal disease; enlargement, or benign prostatic hypertrophy, which is common in older men; and prostatic cancer, which is generally caused by the other two disorders. In the West, infection is treated with antibiotics, and the patient must drink much water for several days in order to clean out the urethra. In TCM, the treatment requires that the dampness of the body be eliminated and that *qi* be made active. This treatment is complex, and it must be carried out by a physician, but it involves the administering of such herbal medicines as seeds of plantain, *Plantago asiatica*, tubers of water plantain, *Alisma plantago-aquatica*, and bark of cinnamon, *Cinnamomum cassia*. See **prostate gland** and **urinary disorders**.

prostatitis See **prostate problems**.

protective-qi See **qi**.

protein This substance is an essential component of all living material, and consists of amino acids. Protein is contained in all the body tissues and the blood, enzymes and hormones. There are about 20 amino acids, eight of which are called essential amino acids because they cannot be made within the body and so must be derived from food. High-quality proteins, found in eggs, fish and milk, are those which contain all of these essential amino acids. High-quality proteins available to the Chinese are those contained in eggs, fish, pork, soya beans, doufu (soya-bean curd), peas, peanuts, wheatgerm and yeast. Protein is needed for growth, and so it is imperative that the diet of children be high in protein. In adults, a deficiency of protein causes poor condition of the skin, hair and nails, hair loss and wasting of muscles. Too much animal protein is thought to be causative of constipation and a possible cause of cancer. Centuries ago, Chinese physicians did not think in terms of proteins, for they were not aware of their existence as such, but they were aware of those foods which are necessary for growth and the healthy formation of bones and muscles, and long before the medical scientists of the West regaled us with so much information about the chemistry of food. See **food**, **nitrates** and **amino acids**.

protozoa See **micro-organisms**.

pruritis This is the medicinal name for violent itchiness of the skin, which can be symptomatic of a wide variety of skin disorders, including eczema, acne, hives, lice and scabies. It can also be symptomatic of psychological disorders and an accompaniment of jaundice. Pruritis ani, or itchiness of the anus, can be caused by anxiety, pin-worms or haemorrhoids, and itchiness of the scalp by lice or nits. Persistent itchiness may be symptomatic of a liver or kidney disorder, and so medical advice should be sought. According to TCM, itchiness is due to external wind-damp or wind-cold, and the recommended treatment is snake skin, applied externally, but this treatment would not have much appeal for people in the West. Where the cause of itchiness is an allergy or nervousness, and there is no serious underlying cause, fresh chickweed, *Stellaria media*, is an effective and soothing treatment if applied externally in a compress. Another helpful treatment is the external application of a lotion made by mixing powdered fresh root of salad burnet, *Sanguisorba officinalis*, with sesame oil. As a blood cleanser, an infusion of 2–10 g roots or leaves of burdock, *Arctium lappa*, or 6–10 g leaves of stinging nettle, *Urtica dioica*, can be taken internally. See **eczema, hives** and **pin-worm**.

prussic acid Hydrocyanic acid (hydrogen cyanide). This acid is highly poisonous, and is contained in small quantities in bitter almonds, which must NOT be consumed to excess. See **foods to avoid**.

psoriasis This is a skin disease which is characterized by red, scaly patches that generally occur on the knees and elbows, though other parts of the skin may be affected, with the finger-nails and toe-nails becoming pitted. There is some doubt about the cause of this condition, but it sometimes occurs after a throat infection, and is triggered off or exacerbated by anxiety or some other condition. In both China and the West, blood cleansers are considered to be the best form of treatment, and an infusion of 10–30 g leaves, flowers and roots of dandelion, *Taraxacum officinale*, is certainly worth a trial.

psyche 'Soul' or 'mind'. Psyche is not now in common use as a word, but it does appear as a prefix in many words whose use is now widespread. For example: psychology, psychedelic, psycho-therapy, psycho-analysis, psychometric, psycho-kinesis, psychosis. See **mental health** and **psychology**.

psychedelic A hallucinogenic drug which increases the mind's awareness. Mescaline, which is an alkaloid contained in certain plants, such as the peyote cactus, is a drug of this kind. See **drug**.

psychiatry A dictionary might define this term as the study and treatment of mental disorders. One could say that it is the sum total of the medical applications of psychology. During the past hundred years or so, this branch of medicine has developed rapidly. However, it is not an exact science and some of its theories and systems are contradictory and confusing, and so some people regard its value as being questionable. Psychiatry exists in a variety of systems – for which great claims have been made, but none of which have achieved much more than has been achieved by the meditation exercises and common-sense approach to mental health which Chinese physicians have been prescribing for their patients since ancient times. See **meditation** and **mental health**.

A neurotic is a man who builds castles in the air. A psychotic is a man who lives in them. A psychiatrist is the man who collects the rent.

Jerome Lawrence

psychoanalysis Devised by the Austrian psychiatrist Sigmund Freud, 1856–1939, psychoanalysis is a system of treatment by which mentally-sick people are encouraged to discover for themselves those unconscious fears and repressed yearnings which may be the cause of their current frustrations and inability to cope with the complications of human existence, and thereby escape from the mental prison which may be largely of their own making. Freud's attitude towards the influence of sex on human conduct might have been a bit overdone, and it certainly shocked some of the inhabitants of Victorian England, but he surely had a point, for sex, like food, keeps many people thoroughly preoccupied, and it has a far greater effect on our lives than many of us would have the honesty to admit. Even Confucius, whose moral values are quite unassailable, was prepared to concede that sex cannot be ignored, though some suppression of sexual activity would be necessary to protect society against the worst excesses of its enthusiasts. However, Freud's approach was a case of putting old wine in new bottles, for Chinese physicians have always believed that there is much to be gained by self-awareness, which can be achieved by meditation exercises, and which can lead to a proper understanding and full mastery of one's situation, and thereby become healthy in both mind and body, and also successful in all endeavours. The *tao* of supremacy, which is one of the Eight Pillars of Taoism, indicates how we may gain some insight into our own behaviour and that of others, and so it would seem, that in some respects, psycho-analysis is much older than Freud – as old as Taoism, in fact. See **meditation** and **supremacy**.

psychology This is the science, or systematic study, of the mind and behaviour – and of animals as well as of humans. But it is not a very exact science, for there are many imponderables, and since the mind and behaviour are manifestations of the bodily functions, it is as much a matter of physiology as it is of anything else. The belief that the body has a soul which can be studied as if it could exist separately from the body has been largely discredited, and so the term *psychophysiology* is more meaningful than *psychology* in some respects. Psychology is certainly not a new discovery: man has always employed his wits to gain an advantage over his opponents, and psychology has been used effectively by medicine-men, priests and law-givers, sometimes to their own advantage, and sometimes in the interest of the community. In modern society, psychology is used with devastating effect by advertisers and politicians. At an intellectual level, psychology is an offshoot of philosophy. But the Chinese are philosophers by temperament, and so who could have been better qualified than the Taoist sages of ancient China to make a deep study of human thought, behaviour and aspirations. They were aware of some of the influences of the endocrine glands, which they described as 'houses', and the benefits of sound diet and adequate exercise in maintaining 'a healthy mind in a healthy body'. They also understood binary numbers, which they used to compile the computer-like arrangement of hexagrams in the *I Ching*, and so reduce all human thoughts and forms of behaviour to 64 emotive or emotional situations, for each of which they were able to forecast the likely outcome. It is significant that the Swiss psychiatrist C.J. Jung regularly consulted the *I Ching* and adapted it to suit the needs of his patients. The Taoist philosophers understood the scientific principle of cause and effect, and they embraced the doctrine of predestination, but rejected the doctrine of self-determination, or free will, which they believed to be an illusion. See **cause and effect**. In this and other respects, the sages of ancient China had anticipated some of the modern scientific research in the West by thousands of years. An interesting adaptation of psychology is in the Chinese years, which are arranged as a 12-year sequential cycle, each year being named after one of the animals that, according to an old legend, had found great favour with Buddha. At one time, it was the common belief that a person would have the good qualities of the animal after which the year of his birth had been named. Thus, a person born in a Rat Year would be astute and have a great capacity for survival, a person born in a Tiger Year would be courageous and have nobility of character, a person born in a Dragon Year would be charming and ingenious, and so on. This may be regarded as mere superstition; but, in so far as a person would try to emulate the example set by the animal governing his year of birth, which he would regard as being in the nature of a prophecy, he would improve his own character, so increasing his worth to himself and to society as a whole. This is surely social psychology at its best. See **I Ching**, **Chinese years** and **psychotherapy**.

psychoneurosis An illness which is both mental and nervous, combining the conditions of psychosis and neurosis. See **psychosis** and **neurosis**.

psychopathy An abnormal condition of the mind, and a mental illness rather than a nervous disorder, but not one in which organic changes are involved. See **psychopath**.

psychopath A person who is suffering from a chronic mental illness, and who is both mentally and emotionally unstable. He may also be a danger to society. His condition can be likened to that of a telephone exchange in which the lines have not merely become crossed but have been irretrievably damaged. See **psychosis**, **mental illness** and **neuropath**.

psychosis An abnormal mental condition involving a change in behaviour and beliefs, and also a loss of a sense of reality. The sufferer is likely to be unaware of the seriousness of his condition. See **neurosis**, **insight** and **mental illness**.

psychosomatic This term describes those physical illnesses which are mental or emotional in origin or are exacerbated by mental or emotional influences. The liver, for example, can be severely damaged by repeated bouts of anger. There is a tendency for the physicians of the West to be more concerned about the psychological aspects of such illnesses, whereas Chinese physicians are more concerned with the pathological aspects, that is, the severe damage done to the vital organs by emotional upheavals. Chinese physicians would contend that meditation, with its content of self-hypnosis, could be very effective in treating some psychosomatic conditions. This would be a case of controlling the emotions in order to remedy physical defects. See **emotion**, **nervous disorders** and **meditation**.

psychotherapy This is the treatment of illnesses, whatever their nature or causes, by psychological methods as opposed to the use of drugs and other physical methods. In TCM, this is regarded as a very valuable form of treatment, and sometimes the only safe and effective treatment for psychosomatic ailments, where the emotions can be regulated in ways that will eradicate an unwanted physical condition, though TCM physicians will not use the term *psychotherapy*, but will use such terms as *meditation*, *self-hypnosis* and 'suppressing evil-*qi*' which amounts to the same thing, more or less. Psychotherapy, for example, can be effective in the treatment of hysteria and bed-wetting, where sedatives would merely suppress the symptoms but not eliminate the cause. One type of emotion may be used to counter the ill-effects of another emotion. In some respects, a penal system could be regarded as an extension of psychotherapy in which the fear of deprivation, discomfort or pain is used to discourage wrongdoing and control those persons whose emotional needs are damaging to themselves or society. See **meditation**, **psychosomatic** and **morality**.

ptisan See **infusion**.

ptomaine poisoning See **food poisoning**.

ptyalin See **maltose**.

puberty The stage in life when sexual maturity begins. See **maturity cycle** and **jing**.

puff ball *Lycoperdon perlatum* Herbal medicine. Distribution: global. Parts: spores (dust). Character: neutral, pungent. Affinity: lungs. Effects: antipyretic, antiphlogistic, antitussive, haemostatic, antidote. Symptoms: coughs, wheezing. Treatments: heat-excess respiratory problems, bronchitis. Dosage: 0.5–2 g. This medicine may be applied externally to stop bleeding.

pulled muscles and tendons The usual TCM treatments are acupuncture, acupressure, moxibustion or a cold-water compress to relieve pain. Massage, rest and time should effect a cure.

pulmonary Of the lungs.

pulmonary artery The artery which conveys blood from the heart to the lungs, though it contains venous, or de-oxygenated, blood. See **circulation**.

pulmonary embolism A blockage of one of the main arteries of the lungs. See **embolism**.

pulmonary emphysema See **emphysema**.

pulse Heartbeat. The rhythmic throbbing of the arteries as blood is pumped through them by the action of the heart, and which can be clearly felt on the wrists and temples. The heart beats about 72 times per minute in a healthy person at rest. See **pacemaker**.

pulse diagnosis In TCM, this is one of the techniques by which the Chinese physician makes a diagnosis and decides upon an appropriate course of treatment. He may ascertain a patient's pulse rate and intensity by applying a stethoscope to his chest, but it is more likely that he will feel the radial artery, which is on the wrist. A similar technique is used by the physicians of the West, but the Chinese technique is much more complicated, for the Chinese physician may not have a cardiograph and other devices to aid him. In TCM, the physician places his first three fingers on the radial artery and feels for three separate points. Light pressure reveals three separate pulses, and heavy pressure reveals another three, making a total of six. This process is repeated with the other wrist, and so there are 12 pulses in all. Each of these pulses indicate the state of one of the 12 vital organs or the presence of some disease. For example, a rapid pulse is one of the symptoms of hyperglycaemia. The state of the pulse is indicated by such terms as 'weak', 'fluttering', 'galloping', 'chaotic', 'rhythmic', and 'sunken', but they are qualitative, not quantitative, and so they may not mean quite the same to one physician as they do to another. The table shows how the state of the pulse relates to the general conditions of the body. However, this kind of pulse diagnosis requires a great deal of skill, and it takes many years for a Chinese physician to thoroughly master the art, which provides information about past as well as present illnesses. In fact, it may indicate weaknesses in one of a person's vital organs a long time before the condition could become serious, and so the appropriate preventive treatments could then be applied. See **hearing**, **murmur** and **tactile diagnosis**.

PULSE DIAGNOSIS

Condition	Pulse
yin	slow, weak, sunken
yang	rapid, heavy, floating
internal	weak, sunken
external	rapid, floating
empty	slow, weak
full	galloping
cold	slow, weak
hot	rapid, galloping

pumpkin *Cucurbita moschata* Herbal medicine. Distribution: global. Parts: seeds. Character: warm, sweet. Affinity: stomach, large intestine. Effect: anthelmintic. Symptoms: swollen and painful abdomen. Treatment: intestinal worms. Dosage: 35–45 g. This herb has a reputation, probably quite unfounded, as an aphrodisiac. When used as an anthelmintic, it will need to be followed by cathartic treatment in order to eliminate dead worms from the bowel.

pungent See **odour** and **taste**.

pupil See **iris**.

pure-qi See **qi**.

pure water See **water**.

purgative A powerful cathartic. The purgatives used in TCM include the following: Glauber's salt (sodium sulphate crystals), 8–16 g; rhubarb, *Rheum officinale*, rhizomes, 2–4 g; Barbados aloe, *Aloe vera*, juice of leaves, 0.3–0.9 g; Tinnevelly senna, *Cassia augustifolia*, 4–12 pods. The most powerful of the TCM purgatives is purging croton, *Croton tiglium*, but it is highly poisonous, and so it is NOT to be recommended, not even in small doses. Purgatives must NOT be administered to patients who are elderly or frail or have cancer or a heart condition. See **cathartic**.

purpura This is a disease in which blood escapes into the skin, subcutaneous tissues and mucous membranes, so causing purple or red bruiselike patches on the skin. There are three types of this disease, of which two are incurable, but one can be alleviated by calisthenics or such exercises as the *tai chi chuan*.

pus The body fluid and remains of dead micro-organisms and leucocytes which accumulate at a seat of infection. See **interferon**.

pustule A pus-filled blister or pimple.

putrid See **odour** and **taste**.

'putting on the overcoat' A quaint colloquial Chinese term which refers to the practice of coating pills with a substance which will keep out dampness and small organisms or provide a pleasant flavour to disguise the taste of bitter ingredients. Or it may be that the outer coat is an active ingredient which, for some reason or other, the physician wants to be assimilated first.

pyorrhoea A discharge of pus from infected tooth-sockets. The usual treatment is an antiseptic mouthwash. The Chinese would use a saline solution. See **salt**.

pyridoxine See **vitamin**.

Q

qi Also written as *chi* or *ch'i*. 'Vital energy'. 'Life-force'. One of the basic assumptions of TCM is that all living organisms, whether plant or animal, are motivated by *qi*, or 'vital energy'. This is a reasonable assumption since one of the differences between living and dead organisms is that the former are capable of movement, in which energy is bound to be involved. *Qi* is invisible, odourless, tasteless and without shape, but it exists in all parts of the universe, including food, water and air, and it can move from one place to another, and be changed from one form into another. The *qi* from food, which is extracted by digestion, combines with the *qi* from air, which is extracted by the lungs, to form human-*qi* that is then circulated throughout the meridians, blood vessels and tissues of the body, and so, by its quantity, quality and level of balance, determines a person's state of health and life-span. *Qi* also means *'air'*, *'breath'* and *'spirit'*, and it is likely that the people of ancient China believed, as did other peoples in the ancient world, that, when a person 'draws his last breath', he is giving up his spirit, or what the Chinese might describe as residual-*qi*, without which he could not survive, though he is, in fact, struggling to obtain oxygen. They also believed that water is a source of *qi* for the body, which was another reasonable assumption because, though water may have no value as a source of available energy, it is necessary for the transport of nutrients containing *qi*. Moreover, they believed that medicinal herbs are an immediate source of *qi* because, as they have an affinity for certain organs, *qi* is transferred directly to the organs where it is required. In the West, *qi* has been likened to *élan vital*, or 'life-force', a concept postulated by the French philosopher Henri Bergson, 1859–1941, but this is only a philosophical notion, and since Bergson's time, it has been repudiated by other French philosophers, but they could well be wrong. Modern Western science probably provides the best explanation of the nature of *qi*, which is that it is probably the energy released by oxidation within the body when air-*qi*, or oxygen from the lungs, combines with food-*qi*, or the carbon in nutrients from the intestine, to form carbon dioxide. *Qi* can be either yin or yang, and so there is yin-*qi* and yang-*qi*. It is also associated with the organs and other parts of the body. Thus, there is kidney-*qi*, liver-*qi*, heart-*qi*, lung-*qi* and *xue-qi*, or 'blood-*qi*'. One suspects that these forms of *qi* are essentially one and the same thing – energy released by oxidation – and differ only in location, though there may be some apparent differences which are due to the action of hormones. For example, kidney-*qi* may be influenced by adrenalin, or, as Chinese physicians would say, one becomes fearful if kidney-*qi* is weak. *Qi* may be hot or cold and dry or moist, and so there is hot-*qi*, cold-*qi*, dry-*qi* and moist-*qi*. Evil-*qi* is believed to emanate from swamps and other unhealthy locations, and it causes diseases, which may explain the evil influences which are attributed to bad *fung shui*, though the malaria-carrying mosquito, which inhabits swampy regions, may have something to do with this. Pure-*qi*, on the other hand, which occurs in clean air and mountain mists, promotes health and prolongs the life-span. The lungs will not function effectively if they become dry, and so, perhaps, pure-*qi* could be regarded as a combination of oxygen and moisture. This explains why the Chinese attach so much importance to breathing exercises, for they help to ensure a supply of pure-*qi*, which could, in fact, be additional oxygen. Human-*qi* takes two forms: *ying-qi*, or 'nourishing-*qi*', and *wei-qi*, or 'protective-*qi*'. Nourishing-*qi* is derived from the purest components of food, and it nourishes the organs and tissues. Protective-*qi* is derived from the inferior elements in food, but, as it cannot enter the blood vessels, it circulates around the meridians and subcutaneous tissues, so controlling the opening and closing of pores and protecting the body against attack by evil-*qi*. Where there is a deficiency of nourishing-*qi*, the body is weak; and where there is a deficiency of protective-*qi*, the body is liable to attack by cold, damp, wind and other excesses in the environment. Stagnant-*qi* is sluggishness of *qi*, and it can be a manifestation of the dysfunction of an organ. Leukaemia is thought to be due to an excess of stagnant-*qi* in the blood. Ligament sprains are also thought to be due to stagnant-*qi*. Stagnant-*qi* could be an accumulation of carbon dioxide or toxins. Rebellious-*qi* is *qi* in rapid motion or not behaving as it should, as with a fever, when the body temperature rises to a harmful level because of an excess of heat energy. One should note that such items as evil-*qi*, pure-*qi* and rebellious-*qi* are concerned with the functions of *qi* rather than any differences in its actual nature. *Qi* is affected by the emotions. Where there is anxiety or grief, lung-*qi* becomes sluggish; and where there is anger, liver-*qi* becomes uncontrollable, and so the liver is injured. Lack of exercise or over-strenuous exercise will cause *qi* to deteriorate, as will excess or unsuitable food. Breathing will rejuvenate *qi*, but foul air will cause its deterioration. *Jing*, or 'vital essence', is formed by the action of *qi* on food, as is *jin ye*, or 'body fluid'. *Yuan qi*, or 'primeval vital energy', which is the *qi* with which a person is born, is the initial 'staying power' derived from the nutrients and oxygen supplied to a foetus by its mother. But all the foregoing comments can be briefly summarized by saying that the condition of the body, and the regulation of its health and stamina, and its chances of attaining a great age, are dependent on the fine yin-yang balance achieved by the constant conflict between evil-*qi*, or the collective undesirable forms of *qi*, and pure-*qi*, or the collective desirable forms of *qi*. In this, the *Nei Jing*, or 'The Classic of Internal Medicine', says: 'The origin and governance of life, of birth and of growth and change is *qi*, which is the law obeyed by all myriad things of both heaven and earth. *Qi*, on the exterior, envelops both heaven and earth; and, in the interior, it stimulates them. It is the source from which the sun, moon and stars derive their light, the thunder, wind and rain derive their existence, and the four seasons and the myriad animals and plants derive their birth, growth, gathering and storage. All this is brought about by *qi*, on which all myriad things depend, as does mankind.' See **six excesses**, **fung shui**, **jing**, **jin ye**, **Nei Jing** and **yuan qi**.

que mai A Chinese term, which means 'pulse-taking'. See **pulse diagnosis**.

qi gong Also written as *ch'i kung* or *chi kung*. A system of meditative exercises intended to cultivate physical and mental perfection. Since its emphasis is on *qi*, or 'vital energy' or 'subtle breath', it is generally regarded as being the forerunner of traditional Chinese medicine. It achieves its purpose by conditioning the body so that it is able to resist disease, adapt to the environment and be restored to its correct internal functioning. This is done by adjusting the posture, the breathing cycle and the mind and nervous system. As a method of remedial treatment, it is considered to be superior to acupuncture and chemotherapy, and it is used to treat a wide variety of chronic conditions, which include diabetes, anxiety, depression, hypertension, coronary heart disease and ulcers. See **healing exercises** and **movement**.

Qin dynasty Although the study of medicine with a systematic approach was established at the time of the Zhou dynasty, it became consolidated during the period of the Qin dynasty (221–206 BC), which lasted for only 15 years, but which instituted a system of language, culture and centralized bureaucracy within an autocratic and feudal state that was to be the basis of the system of government in later dynasties. Its ruler, Qin Shi Huang Di (259–206 BC), or 'First Sovereign Emperor of Qin', is regarded as the first emperor of China. He introduced standardized weights and measures and a calendar, unified the various systems of coinage and writing, built roads for carriages of standardized width, and conquered and subjugated the other states. But he was a tyrant, and he was so afraid that his power might be undermined by freedom of expression that he issued a decree that all books be burnt. However, he exempted books on divination, agriculture and medicine from this order, and so the practice of medicine did not suffer as a consequence of this fiery holocaust.

Qing dynasty Also called the Manchu dynasty because its first emperor, Fu Lin, was a prince of the Manchu tribe, who had established the Jin dynasty in northern China (c. 1150). During the first 40 years of the Qing dynasty (1644–1912), the whole of China was conquered, and by the middle of the eighteenth century, China was larger and more powerful than it had ever been before. Under the Qing rulers, Confucianism was adopted as the doctrine of the state, which helped in creating a long and settled period, in which the Chinese lived peacefully, though isolated from the rest of the world until European merchants and military adventurers entered China, introducing Western medicine, science and technology. In medicine, there was a two-way process of exchange, and many Chinese herbs became components of European pharmacology. However, relations between the Chinese and the Europeans were often strained, and more so after Britain and France had used military intervention to compel China to open its doors to free trade. As a consequence of this intervention, some of the European nations benefited by one-sided agreements which robbed China of much of its wealth and destroyed the livelihoods and health of millions of peasants. The final years of the Qing dynasty were beset with weak and corrupt government, which came to a close, rather ignominiously, with the Sino-Japanese War (1894–5), the Empress Dowager Ci Xi yielding to foreign pressure, the abdication of Pu Yi, the young emperor, in 1911, and the founding of the republic in

1912. See **Chinese history**.

ginghao *Artemisia apacia* An extract of this Chinese herb has been shown to be effective in treating pernicious and cerebral malaria.

qing lo Also written as *ching lo* or *jing luo*. Meridians. Pathways. Channels. See **meridian**.

Qin Shi Huang Di In 246 BC, Lord Zheng became the king of Qin. In 221 BC, he founded the first Chinese feudal state, and became its first emperor, as Qin Shi Huang Di. See **Qin dynasty**.

quail grass *Celosa argentea* Herbal medicine. Distribution: South China, India, Africa, America. Parts: seeds. Character: cool, bitter. Affinity: liver. Effects: antipyretic and antiphlogistic to liver. Astringent to conjunctivitis. Symptoms: red eyes. Treatments: hypertension, conjunctivitis and other eye conditions. Dosage: 5–14 g.

quarantine See **isolation**.

quicksilver See **mercury**.

quince See **Chinese quince**.

quinine An alkaloid derived from the bark of the cinchona tree. It is used as a tonic and antipyretic. See **malaria**.

quinsy Inflammation of the throat with an abscess in the tissues around the tonsils. It is an uncommon condition, the symptoms being pain on one side of the throat, and sometimes in the ear, together with difficulty in swallowing and speaking. One side of the inside of the throat will be red and swollen. If the condition is severe, a surgeon will lance the abscess to release the pus, which will give immediate relief. In TCM, the treatment is to drink plenty of liquids, especially fruit juices, apply a cold compress around the neck to relieve the pain, and gargle with an infusion of one of the following, using the parts and dosage indicated: dandelion, *Taraxacum officinale*, all parts, 10–30 g; scullcap, *Scutellaria barbata*, 8–28 g; honeysuckle, *Lonicera japonica*, flowers, 8–16 g; golden bell, *Forsythia suspensa*, fruit, 4–8 g, pigeon pea, *Sophora subprostrata*, roots, 3–7 g.

R

R The abbreviation for the Latin word *recipere*, which means 'take' or 'receive', and is used to introduce a prescription.

rabies Hydrophobia. A virus disease transmitted by the bite or lick of an infected animal, which could be a dog, cat, fox or bat. In animals, the condition is called rabies; in humans, it is called hydrophobia. After an incubation period which varies from ten days to many weeks, the virus attacks the brain and spinal cord, so causing fever, paralysis of the breathing muscles, painful constriction of the throat, difficulty in swallowing, delirium, convulsions and coma – and death if it is not treated early enough. The French chemist Louis Pasteur (1823–95) developed a vaccine for the treatment of rabies. The Chinese, with their usual wisdom in matters of health, prevent the spread of rabies by prohibiting the keeping of dogs and cats in populous areas. See **pets**.

race A person's state of health is determined in some degree by genetic factors, a few of which must inevitably be racial characteristics. But there are so many factors involved in health and inheritance that it would be difficult to make a quantitative assessment of the extent to which people's health is determined by their racial characteristics. For example, two of the characteristics of the Chinese are stamina and longevity, but are these due to heredity or a sound diet and an adequate amount of exercise? See **Mongoloid races**.

rachitis See **rickets**.

radiation sickness Illness caused by exposure to ionizing radiation from a nuclear explosion or leakage, or even X-rays if the exposure is for a long period. It causes hair loss, bleeding, nausea, vomiting, diarrhoea, cancer, leukaemia, failure of the immune system and adverse genetic effects. Natural radiation results from radioactivity which is the spontaneous disintegration of certain elements, such as radium, uranium and thorium, and is accompanied by the emission of alpha and beta particles and gamma rays. But elements which are not naturally radioactive can be made radioactive by bombarding their neutrons in a nuclear reactor. Some natural radiation is due to radon, which is a radioactive gaseous element produced by the disintegration of the radium occurring in granite. The inhabitants of properties situated above granite formations are liable to exposure to radon, which can cause lung cancer. This is one of the possible explanations of *fung shui*, which is the Chinese belief that some locations are healthier than others. In some quarters, there is a belief that radiation from electromagnetic equipment and the earth's magnetic field cause geopathic stress, which could produce migraine, insomnia and rheumatism. This is another possible explanation of *fung shui*, and why the Chinese erect their buildings so that they benefit from the lines of natural harmony, and so avoid bad *fung shui*. Many people are disquieted about the radiation from nuclear-energy installations and the destruction of the ozone layer, which prevents harmful solar radiation reaching the earth. Radiation is undoubtedly productive of free radicals. See **fung shui**, **ozone**, **free radical** and **tea**.

radiology The diagnosis and treatment of diseases by radioactive materials and radiographs. See **X-rays**.

radius See **skeleton**.

ramsons *Allium ursinum* Also called wood garlic. A species of wild garlic with broad leaves and medicinal properties similar to those of cultivated garlic, *Allium sativum*.

rancid See **odour** and **taste**.

rank See **odour** and **taste**.

rash There are several causes of a rash – heat, hives, measles, shingles, etc. – and one must establish the cause before one can decide upon a suitable treatment. But, for a rash due to a poor condition of the blood, an infusion of 6–12 g leaves of stinging nettle, *Urtica dioica*, to be taken internally, is often helpful.

raspberry *Rubus idaeus* Herbal medicine. Distribution: Europe, Northern Asia. Parts: leaves. Character: warm, sweet-sour. Affinity: liver, kidneys. Effects: antiseptic, astringent, tonic. Symptoms: sore throat. Treatments: difficult and painful labour, gravid uterus. Dosage: 6–24 g. An infusion can be used as a gargle and mouthwash to treat infections and inflammations of the throat, and as a lotion to treat conjunctivitis.

raw See **odour** and **taste**.

Raynaud's disease This is a common condition in which the blood vessels in the toes, fingers, nose or ears become constricted, which causes them to become cold, numb and pale. In severe cases, they become blue and there is a very painful burning sensation. There is some doubt about the cause of this condition, but a deficiency of iron is suspected, and hypersensitivity to drugs for nervous disorders could also be a cause. It affects women more than men. If it is caught in its early stages, the prognosis is good; but, in advanced stages, which are rare, gangrene may develop. The treatment, which is generally more alleviative than curative, is to try to improve the blood supply to the extremities by swinging the arms in a circular motion, consuming iron-rich foods and hot meals rather than cold meals, wearing warm clothing and mittens rather than gloves, occasionally immersing the hands in warm water, maintaining a calm attitude so that tension does not cause blood to flow away from the extremities towards the brain, and taking vasodilators, such as yarrow, sage, feverfew, peppermint, hawthorn, camomile, garlic, ginger and Siberian ginseng. In TCM, the usual treatment is a decoction, taken internally, of 1-5 g twigs of cinnamon, *Cinnamomum cassia*, or 8–14 g roots of Chinese angelica, *Angelica sinensis*.

rebellious-qi Uncontrolled ascending vital energy, as with fever, sweating and vomiting. See **qi**.

recessive characteristics See **hereditary defects**.

recreational exercises See **games** and **sports**.

rectum See **intestine**.

red dates Green dates, or jujubes, which have been dried in the sun until they become red. They may also be boiled, wind dried and heat dried until they become black. Both forms are used as a treatment for insomnia and anaemia, and also as a tonic for women in childbirth or at the menopause. See **jujube**.

red date wine See **medicinal wine**.

'red eye' See **conjunctivitis**.

red meat Beef, mutton, lamb, venison, etc., and which, in the Chinese view, is damaging to the health if consumed in large quantities. See **meat** and **white meat**.

red sage See **sage**.

'red tea fungus', or *hongcha jun*, as the Chinese call it, is made by growing yeast in an infusion of red tea with sugar added. In Chinese folk medicine, it is used as a treatment for constipation and as a means of strengthening the liver and kidneys and inhibiting the ageing process. But there is some evidence that it could reduce blood pressure by lowering the level of cholesterol in the blood, increase resistance to toxins and be preventive of cancer. See **tea**.

reed grass *Phragmites communis* Herbal medicine. Distribution:

global. Parts: roots, stems. Character: cold, sweet. Affinity: lungs, stomach. Effects: antipyretic, refrigerant, demulcent. Symptoms: heat, thirst, dry throat, vomiting, coughing, expectoration of dark thick phlegm. Treatments: conditions due to excess heat, especially lung heat, seafood poisoning. Dosage: 18–36 g.

reedmace *Typha latifolia* Also called bulrush and cat's tail. Herbal medicine. Distribution: North China, Northern Europe, North America. Parts: pollen. Character: neutral, sweet. Affinity: liver, pericardium. Effects: astringent, haemostatic, diuretic, improves circulation, anti-coagulant. Symptoms: blood in vomit, sputum, urine or stools, nosebleeds, pressure and pain in heart region, postnatal abdominal pain. Treatments: menorrhagia, dysmenorrhoea, traumatic injuries. Dosage: 3–7 g.

refined sugar See **sugar**.

reflex See **involuntary movement**, **hiccups** and **nervous system**.

reflexology Foot massage. Although reflexology is believed to have originated in China about 5000 years ago, when massage and similar techniques were used to control energies within the body, as with acupressure and *shiatsu*, it is now very much a Western treatment, and is not regarded as one of the prominent features of TCM. This system of therapy was, in fact, introduced into Britain from America in 1960, where it had been evolved from zone therapy. Its essential principle is that by massaging certain parts of the feet, which are called reflex areas, there will be a curative or alleviative response in those parts of the body that correspond with the stimulated areas on the feet. However, these so-called reflexes are not the same as the reflexes, or involuntary movements, effected by the nervous system, nor are the energy-carrying channels the same as the meridians and acupoints used in acupuncture and acupressure. The soles of the feet could be regarded as 'maps' of the body, with the left foot representing the right-hand side of the body, and the right foot representing the left-hand side of the body. Reflexologists claim that illness is caused by blockages in the energy channels, and that by removing these blockages by massaging the appropriate reflex areas there can be effective treatment for a number of ailments. The diagrams show the reflex areas on the soles of the feet. To treat headaches, one massages the head reflexes on the big toes; to treat tension, one massages the solar plexus reflex at the centre of the foot; and so on. The conditions which are thought to benefit from this treatment include migraine, stress, stroke, back pain, multiple sclerosis and period, sinus and digestive problems. But it must be used with great care or NOT at all in the treatment of diabetes, arthritis, thyroid complaints and where there is a condition of pregnancy. See **zone therapy** and **shiatsu**.

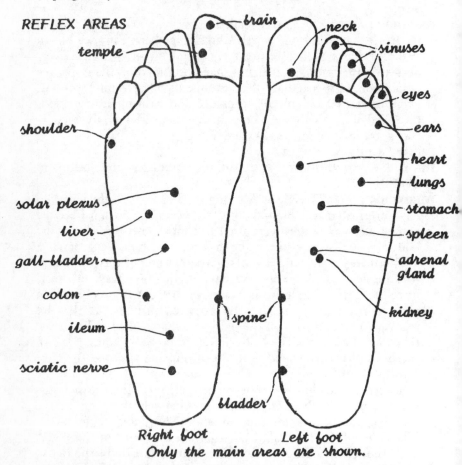

REFLEX AREAS

brain — temple — neck — sinuses — eyes — ears — shoulder — heart — lungs — solar plexus — stomach — liver — spleen — gall-bladder — adrenal gland — colon — ileum — kidney — sciatic nerve — spine — bladder

Right foot   Left foot
Only the main areas are shown.

refrigerant Antipyretic. Febrifuge. The three terms are generally regarded as being interchangeable; but, strictly, an antipyretic, or febrifuge, is a medicine to allay a fever, whereas a refrigerant is a medicine to both allay a fever and reduce a temperature. Some refrigerants commonly used in TCM are gardenia, *Gardenia jasminoides*, reed grass, *Phragmites communis*, lotus, *Nelumbo nucifera*, honeysuckle, *Lonicera japonica*, and kudzu vine, *Pueraria lobela*.

regulated sex See **sex** and **moderation**.

rejuvenation See **revitalization**.

relapse A deterioration in a patient's condition after an apparent improvement.

relationships of vital organs See **meridian** and **vital organs**.

relaxation breathing See **fang sung kung**.

religion The three main religions of China are Taoism, Confucianism and Buddhism, and all three have played a part in the development of TCM. In matters of doctrine, Taoism and Confucianism are opposed to each other, and there was a time when the Taoists completely condemned the social philosophy of Confucianism; but, in matters of practice, these two religions complement each other, with Taoism placing emphasis on harmony with nature, and Confucianism emphasising harmony in society, and both are beneficial to the Chinese in that they encourage natural living, moderate habits and a regulated life-style, which are necessary if a sound state of health and a youthful old age are to be attained. The Buddhist contribution to the health of the Chinese is a matter of diet. Buddhists are opposed to the slaughter of animals, and so they have evolved a wide range of delectable and nutritious vegetarian dishes. It is important to note that Confucianism and Taoism are not religions in the Western sense of the term, but are philosophies or ways of living, which are humanist and much concerned with ethics but very little with mysticism. Of course, there are a few superstitions in China, as elsewhere, and some of the peasants may still believe in ghosts; and, in the past, there were local deities and strange forms of worship and beliefs, including animism. But the educated Chinese have always leaned towards Taoism or Confucianism, which speak vaguely of Heaven as a representation of a god – or gods – which may or may not exist, and attribute most of the occurrences in the universe to the Tai Chi, or 'Supreme Absolute', an inanimate deity which is more of a philosophical concept than a reality. Chinese philosophers would probably go along with a well-known verse by Pope: 'Know then thyself, presume not God to scan, the proper study of Mankind is Man.' See **Taoism**, **Confucianism** and **Buddhism**.

remedial exercises See **healing exercises**.

remedy See **medicine**.

'remove-cold medicine' See **warming medicines**.

renal Of the kidneys.

renal disorders Kidney stones, pyelonephritis and nephritis are the three main problems associated with the kidneys. Pyelone-phritis is infection of the kidneys by bacteria, but may also be due to other conditions, such as cystitis and prostate disorders. The symptoms are pain over the kidneys and in the waist and abdomen, fever, blood and protein in the urine, and frequent urination. In TCM, the treatment is to drink large amounts of boiled water and take an infusion of 4–8 g seeds of plantain, *Plantago asiatica*. A traditional remedy is to add 60 g red kidney beans and 250 g watercress to 1 litre water, bring to the boil, simmer for one hour and then drink as a soup. Kidney stones are concentrations of calcium and uric acid which crystallize in the kidneys. They are due to an infection or urine that is too concentrated. They cause no pain while in the kidney, but they certainly do when they enter the ureter. They may block the urethra, so preventing urination. For a person who is susceptible to this condition, certain preventive measures can be taken. One should drink plenty of water, reduce the intake of protein foods, dairy products and other calcium-rich foods, salt and foods high in vitamin C, add a magnesium supplement to the diet, and take regular and strenuous exercise. A daily intake of 1 g Epsom salt (magnesium sulphate) should supply the body's magnesium requirement as well as keeping the bowel open. According to TCM, kidney problems are often due to a yang deficiency, and acupuncture, acupressure and moxibustion are thought to be helpful, as are the exercises of *tai chi chuan*. But these treatments must be carried out by a professional. Infusions, taken internally, of the following are also advised: Indian bread, *Poria cocos*, whole plant, 4–8 g; water plantain, *Alisma plantago-aquatica*, tubers, 4–12 g; Indian corn, *Zea mays*, pistils, stamens and silk, 14–28 g. However, kidney complaints can be very serious if incorrectly treated or left untreated, and so, where a kidney condition is suspected, professional medical advice should be sought, for correct diagnosis and treatment are imperative. Do-it-yourself treatments for renal disorders are NOT to be recommended. See **nephritis**, **nephrosis** and **urinary disorders**.

ren yi 'Benevolent physician'. A term which came into being at the time of the Song dynasty (960–1279), and which indicates that physicians were beginning to be highly respected.

'repair emptiness' A literal translation of the Chinese term for a tonic medicine. It is an apt term, for the purpose of a tonic medicine is to increase the body's resistance to disease where it has been impaired, and to restore energy where it has become deficient. After all, fatigue and 'run-down' conditions are characterized by a feeling of emptiness. See **tonic**.

repression A term used by psychiatrists and psychologists in the West to describe the rejection of unpleasant and unwelcome thoughts and memories from the conscious mind, and which may then lie latent in the subconscious mind, but which may be manifested by stress and occasional outbursts of antisocial activity. The Chinese, who have a great capacity for compromise, would argue that no society can exist satisfactorily without discipline, but this is better achieved by culture than by rigid laws, for the individual will not be resentful of the discipline which he imposes upon himself, as he would be of discipline imposed by legislation, particularly if it is harsh and without apparent purpose. Laws and a social code which cannot be equated with natural living are likely to be productive of undesirable repressions. See **morality** and **mental health**.

reproductive systems The two illustrations show, in diagrammatic form, the main parts of the reproductive systems of a man and a woman. In the male system, spermatozoa, which are the male sex cells, are produced by the testis (there are two testes), whence they enter the vas deferens, combine with fluid from the seminal vesicle, and are then discharged from the penis, via the urethra, when ejaculation occurs. The ureters, which are not a part of the reproductive system, convey urine from the kidneys to the bladder, and the urethra provides a common oulet for the testes and the bladder. In the female system, ova, which are the female sex cells, are produced by the ovaries, whence they enter the fallopian tubes, or oviducts, where it is usual for no more than one of them to unite with one of the spermatozoa which will have migrated to the fallopian tubes if coitus, or mating, has occurred. This process is called fertilization, or conception, and it is the beginning of a new life. The egg so formed then enters the uterus and attaches itself to the wall and begins to develop. A placenta grows over the inner membrane of the uterus, and an umbilical cord connects the placenta to the embryo ensuring that it will receive oxygen and nutrients from its mother's blood, though the blood of the mother and that of the baby do not have blood vessels in common. Immediately after birth, the umbilical cord is severed, the remains of which are to be seen in the umbilicus, or navel, which is a depression at the centre of the abdomen. See **embryo** and **foetus**.

resistance to disease Chinese physicians regard the human body as being largely self-regulating, self-healing and resilient, and resistance to disease as not so much a matter of providing this or

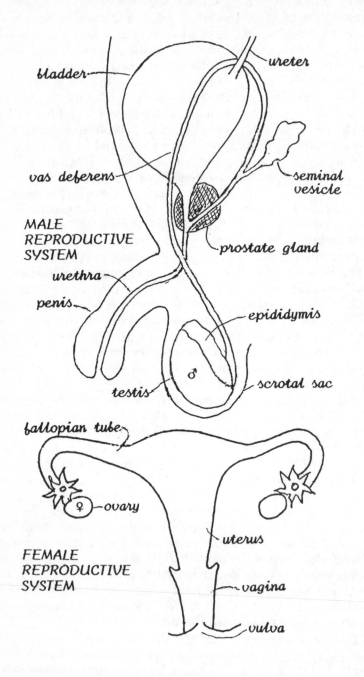

bladder

ureter

vas deferens

seminal vesicle

MALE REPRODUCTIVE SYSTEM

prostate gland

urethra

penis

epididymis

testis

scrotal sac

fallopian tube

ovary

uterus

FEMALE REPRODUCTIVE SYSTEM

vagina

vulva

that medicine for this or that disease but as that of maintaining the vital organs in a healthy state so that they are able to cope with infections when they arise. Apart from this, the body does have its own immune system, but tonic medicines are available if this should become impaired. See **immune system**, **immunity** and **tonic medicine**.

respiration This is an oxidation process which is vital to life and which occurs in the body tissues, where carbon combines with oxygen to form carbon dioxide and release energy. It should not be confused with breathing, which is the mere intake of oxygen and discharge of carbon dioxide. Respiration does not occur in the lungs. See **breathing**, **air** and **qi**.

restless foetus In TCM, the usual treatment for this condition and some of the others associated with pregnancy, such as dizziness, weakness and back pain, is an infusion or decoction, taken internally, of 8–14 g bark of eucommia, *Eucommia ulmoides*. See **pregnancy** and **morning sickness**.

restlessness According to TCM, this symptom, which is often associated with premenstrual tension, anxiety or the menopause, or may follow an illness, indicates heat in the heart due to a blood or yin deficiency. Some temporary relief may be obtained by administering an infusion of 2–4 g seeds of lotus, *Nelumbo nucifera*, but it is important that the underlying cause should be ascertained and treated accordingly.

resuscitation See **'open spirit-gate'**.

retching Ineffectual vomiting, usually involuntary.

retention of urine The inability to urinate, which is generally due to an enlarged prostate gland or a kidney stone in the urethra. It should not be confused with retention of water, or oedema. See **prostate problems** and **renal disorders**.

retina See **eye**.

retinol See **vitamin**.

revitalization Rejuvenation. The *tao* of revitalization is concerned with the promotion of health and longevity by means of internal exercises, which fall into three categories: those to promote healing by correct posture and movement, those to elevate the energy levels by meridian meditation, and those to promote healing by breathing techniques. Acupuncture and acupressure are offshoots of meridian meditation. See **Eight Pillars of Taoism**, **internal exercises**, **meridian meditation** and **movement**.

rheumatic fever A condition which is believed to be due to an allergic reaction to a throat infection caused by streptococci. It is accompanied by fever, and the larger joints become swollen and inflamed, and the heart valves may become permanently damaged. See **rheumatism**.

rheumatism This is a vague term used to describe aches and pains and inflammation of the joints and muscles, which could be due to one or more of a wide variety of different conditions, including fibrositis, rheumatic fever, myalgic encephalomyelitis and the various forms of arthritis. The condition is generally worse when the weather is cold and windy. TCM attributes this condition to damp and wind-heat in the body, and chronic rheumatism to excessive *qi* stagnation, and recommends acupuncture and moxibustion to be applied to the meridians of the kidneys, gallbladder, stomach, large intestine and governor-vessel. It also recommends an infusion, to be taken internally, of 8–28 g seeds of Job's tears, *Coix lacryma-jobi*. A wide variety of other treatments are available, including liniments, poultices and cupping, but it is surely the sensible approach to determine the cause of this condition before attempting a treatment.

rheumatoid arthritis This is one of the three main kinds of arthritis. The TCM treatment is more or less the same as for rheumatism, and includes acupuncture; but, as there is more coldness, more potent herbs are likely to be required. The powdered rhizome of rhubarb, *Rheum officinale*, mixed with sesame oil may be applied as a lotion to reduce swellings. See **rheumatism** and **arthritis**.

rhinitis Inflammation of the mucous membrane of the nose, as with a cold or hay fever.

rhinoceros *Rhinoceros unicornis* Medicine. Distribution: Africa, India. Parts: horn. Character: cold, bitter-sour, salty. Affinity: liver, heart, stomach. Effects: cardiotonic, antispasmodic, antipyretic, haemostatic, antidote. Symptoms: nosebleeds, blood in sputum, giddiness, delirium, convulsions, rash, scanty and murky urine. Treatments: serious conditions due to persistent heat excess. Dosage: 1–2 g. This medicine is now expensive but water-buffalo horn may be used as a cheaper alternative. See **water-buffalo**.

rhizome Some of the herbal medicines described as roots, such as ginger root and rhubarb root, are really rhizomes. A rhizome is a creeping underground stem. See **tuber**.

rhubarb *Rheum officinale* Herbal medicine. Distribution: Tibet, West China. Parts: rhizomes. Character: cold, bitter. Affinity: stomach, spleen, pericardium, liver, large intestine. Effects: cathartic, emmenagogue, refrigerant, astringent. Symptoms:

constipation, sore eyes. Treatments: inflamed liver, amenorrhoea, stagnation of blood or *qi*. Dosage: aperient 0.2 g, laxative 1–1.5 g, purgative 2–4 g, astringent 0.3 g. The powdered rhizome may be applied externally to relieve burns and rheumatoid arthritis. One should note that the leaves of rhubarb are poisonous to humans. See **mastitis**.

rhythm A Chinese term for the pulse. See **pulse diagnosis**.

riboflavin See **vitamin**.

rice *Oryza sativa* The grains of this cereal plant are the staple food in China and many other Asiatic countries. Rice is a good source of B-complex vitamins, but when consumed as polished rice, it lacks these micronutrients and dietary fibre. See **beriberi**.

rickets Rachitis. A disease of childhood due to a deficiency of vitamin D and characterized by deformity of the ribs and legs as a consequence of defective bone formation. This condition is uncommon in China, where the diet has always been sound, but it was once very common in the slum areas of the West, where the diet was inadequate. See **sunlight**.

ringing in the ears See **tinnitus**.

ringworm This is not a worm but a highly contagious infection due to a fungus of the genus *Tinea*. It is so called because, as the infection spreads outwards, a ring-shaped inflamed region is formed. It can occur on any part of the body, but the armpits, groin and feet are particularly vulnerable. Ringworm of the scalp, *Tinea capitis*, is common among children. The treatment can be the same as for athlete's foot, *Tinea pedis*. The consumption of one garlic clove per day is a good preventive measure. See **athlete's foot**.

rodents These are mammals such as rats, mice, squirrels and beavers, which have strong incisor teeth but no canine teeth. They do much damage to our foodstuffs and carry diseases which are harmful to humans. In Chinese mythology, the rat is admired, for he has a great capacity for survival. Despite his bad reputation, he makes an intelligent and affectionate pet if he is properly fed and kept under clean conditions. See **vector**.

rose A common species is the dog, or hedge, rose, *Rosa canina*, which is not a typical TCM herb, though it is indigenous to Northern Asia as well as Europe, but the medicinal properties of its fruits (hips) are somewhat similar to those of the fruits (haws) of the hawthorn, *Crataegus pinnatifida*. See **hawthorn**.

rotten See **odour** and **taste**.

roughage See **dietary fibre**.

roundworm See **anthelmintic** and **parasite**.

royal jelly Obtained from bees, royal jelly functions as a quick-acting pick-me-up. Whether one regards it as a magic medicine or a mere health food, it does have valuable medicinal properties; and, for many centuries, the Chinese have used it as a general tonic and a regular dietary supplement. Unlike the various kinds of pep pills, usually containing caffeine, which are on the market, it is a natural medicine, more in the nature of a food, and without any undesirable side-effects. It is a treatment for stress, tiredness, run-down conditions, headaches, tired eyes, arthritis, acne, premenstrual tension, varicose veins and other conditions. As prepared for pharmacies, royal jelly contains vitamin C, B-complex vitamins, many amino acids, traces of honey and pollen and other health-giving substances. It is stocked by Chinese herbalists and grocers and quite a few British pharmacies, and is supplied in liquid form in small 10-ml glass vials or in concentrated form in 100 mg capsules. In using the jelly, one should follow the instructions on the container. But what is royal jelly? If a queen bee should die, the worker bees – females that do not lay eggs – provide a replacement by selecting a grub which, in the normal course of things, is destined to be a worker and feeding it on a special liquid from their mouths. This special saliva is royal jelly. The selected grub then develops into a new queen.

rubefacient A medicine or similar agent which is applied to the skin to induce local vasodilation with an effect that may range from a mild reddening to blistering. This acts as a counter-irritant, so producing an additional inflammatory response which cleans damaged or toxic tissue. Such substances as cayenne pepper, mustard and ginger are used as rubefacients in TCM, and are effective in the treatment of arthritis when applied in poultices or hot baths.

rubella German measles. This is an infectious disease of childhood which is characterized by a slight fever, a sore throat, swollen glands in the neck and a rash of small pink spots which first appear on the face and neck. The incubation period is 14–21 days, and the patient should be isolated for about seven days. According to TCM, this condition is due to external wind-cold or wind-heat. An infusion of 4–6 g roots of *fang feng*, *Ledebouriella seseloides*, or 4–10 g leaves and floral buds of Japanese catnip, *Schizonepeta tenuifolia*, taken internally, clears the wind-cold. An infusion of 9–16 g flowers of honeysuckle, *Lonicera japonica*, or 4–8 g flowers of chrysanthemum, *Chrysanthemum morifolium*, taken internally, clears the wind-heat.

rubeola See **morbilli**.

rules for health The basic guidelines of Chinese-style health care can be briefly summarized as follows: adopt the Chinese diet, consume one fresh garlic clove daily, take a large drink of boiled water before breakfast each day, take an adequate but not over-strenuous amount of exercise, be clean personally and in handling food, be of moderate and regular habits in all you do – diet, tobacco, alcohol, sex, work and play – avoid the vices of casual sex and drug-taking, avoid social friction and other stressful situations, worry less, laugh more, do not miss out on sleep, and consult a physician if you have doubts about your health, for prevention is better than cure.

run-down condition See **debility** and **tonic**.

rupture See **hernia**.

S

saccharin See **sweetener**.

safe food See food hygiene and preserved food.

safe period In some quarters, there is a mistaken belief that, during the menstrual cycle, there is a so-called safe period when ovulation temporarily ceases, and so sexual intercourse can take place at that time without incurring the risk of conception. See **birth control**.

safety See **moderation**.

safety with medicines See **dangers with medicines** and **Medicines Act 1968**.

safflower *Carthamus tinctorius* Herbal medicine. Distribution: China, Tibet, Vietnam. Parts: flowers. Character: warm, pungent. Affinity: heart, liver. Effects: emmennagogue, astringent, anticoagulant, aids circulation. Symptoms: stiffness and pain in joints, postnatal abdominal pain. Treatments: dysmenorrhoea, amenorrhoea, abdominal, haemorrhages, traumatic injuries. Dosage: 2–4 g. This medicine must NOT be administered to pregnant women.

safflower oil This oil is used in *tui na* massage.

sage *Salvia officinalis* There are many different species and varieties of sage, but the ones mainly used in the West are the common sage, *Salvia officinalis*, and red sage, *Salvia officinalis purpurea*, which is a variety of the common sage. In TCM, the most commonly used species of sage is *dan shen*, *Salvia miltiorrhiza*. See **dan shen**.

salad burnet *Sanguisorba officinalis* Also called garden burnet and great burnet. Herbal medicine. Distribution: China, Northern Asia, Northern Europe. Parts: roots. Character: cool, bitter-sour. Affinity: liver, large intestine. Effects: haemostatic, astringent, refrigerant. Symptoms: blood in stools or urine. Treatments: menorrhagia, haemorrhoids, dysentery. Dosage: 3–8 g. For external use, the powdered fresh roots are added to sesame oil to make a lotion, or to lard to make an ointment, which may be applied to burns, eczema and some rashes. This species of burnet should not be confused with lesser burnet, *Sanguisorba minor*, which, also, is called salad burnet.

saline See **salt**.

saliva The secretion of the salivary glands, which are in the cheeks. Salivation increases as a response to food tastes and odours. Saliva is mildly antiseptic, and some scientists have suggested that it may contain a factor which promotes the rapid healing of wounds. And so, when a cat licks its wounds or cleans its fur by licking, it is achieving by instinct what humans achieve by intelligence. Saliva moistens food, and contains ptyalin, which is a digestive enzyme that converts starch into sugar. See **maltose** and **jin ye**.

salivary glands See **saliva**.

salmon See **fish liver**.

salmonella See **food poisoning**.

salt Sodium chloride (NaCl). Also called table salt and common salt. The salt used as a condiment is not pure sodium chloride, and contains traces of other mineral salts. The salt derived from sea water contains iodine salts, which are beneficial to the health in helping to prevent hyperthyroidism. The body needs some salt if it is to be in a healthy condition, and the salt lost from the body by perspiration or diarrhoea needs to be replaced, though this is generally no problem, for salt occurs naturally in many foods. However, an excessive intake of salt can be conducive to strokes, hypertension and stomach cancer, and so people with renal or circulatory disorders are advised to reduce their salt intake. Salt substitutes are available, but they usually contain potassium chloride (KCl), which can be harmful to people with a heart condition. Where there is doubt, medical advice should be sought. Salt has mildly antiseptic properties, and in TCM, a saline solution, made by dissolving 6 g salt in 1 litre warm water, is used as a mouthwash and gargle and for cleaning small wounds. Bathing in salt water, such as sea water, provides some relief for stiff and painful muscles and joints. See **hyperthyroidism** and **dentifrice**.

saltpetre Potassium nitrate (KNO_3). Also commonly known as nitre. An ingredient of gunpowder and used in curing bacon, saltpetre was used in ancient China as a treatment for extreme cases of fever in the blood.

salty See **taste**.

salve See **ointment**.

sandfly See **Leishmaniasis**.

san jiao Also written as *san chiu*. 'Three-points.' See **liu fu**.

san qi *Panax notoginseng* Also commonly known as notoginseng. Herbal medicine. Distribution: Sichuan and Yunnan provinces of China, Japan. Parts: roots. Character: warm, bitter-sweet. Affinity: stomach, liver. Effects: analgesic, haemostatic. Symptoms: nosebleeds, blood in stools or sputum. Treatments: traumatic injuries, severe haemorrhages. Dosage: powder 0.5–2 g, infusion or decoction 4–8 g. This medicine is a most effective styptic when applied directly to severe wounds, either internal or external. In taking this medicine, one should avoid beans, seafood and cold drinks, for they neutralize the styptic effect.

sarcoma See **cancer**.

satori See **Zen Buddhism**.

saturated fatty acid. See **fatty acid**.

savour See **taste**.

sa za fu pei 'Knocking on the door of life'. A Taoist term which refers to the attainment of health and longevity by a system of breathing and physical exercises. See **Chinese Exercise Manual**.

scabies Itchiness of the skin due to the presence of the parasitic insect *Acarus scabiei*, which thrives on dirty skin, where it lays its eggs. The armpits, nipples and genitals are particularly vulnerable. Scabies is prevented by strict personal hygiene, but where it is present, toilets must be disinfected and bedclothes boiled. Daily baths with disinfectants added to the water should destroy the insects on the body. TCM recommends the external application of a strong infusion of garlic. The consumption of one garlic clove each day could be helpful.

scalds Treat as for burns. See **burns**.

scallion *Allium ascalonicum* Shallot. See **onion**.

scapula Shoulder blade. See **skeleton**.

scarlatina Scarlet fever. An acute infection and a disease of childhood, which is caused by a strain of streptococcus. Its symptoms are fever, a sore throat, a rash of tiny bright-red spots and a peeling skin. The incubation period is 4–5 days, and the isolation period is seven days, at the end of which time, the condition should have cleared up. Scarlatina is a notifiable disease.

scarlet fever See **scarlatina**.

scars After wounds have healed, scars are usually left behind. But this need not be the case if wounds are treated with *san qi*, *Panax notoginseng*. See **Yunnan bai yao**.

schizophrenia *Dementia praecox* A form of psychosis in which a person becomes lethargic and withdrawn from some aspects of reality. He may have delusions and become paranoid, and he may also behave as if he has more than one personality. This condition may begin in childhood as withdrawal and morbid fantasizing, which is called autism. According to TCM, this condition is due to heat in the heart, which causes the sufferer to be excitable and aggressive. An infusion, taken internally, of 2–4 g sprouted seeds of lotus, *Nelumbo nucifera*, is the recommended treatment. Acupuncture is also helpful. See **mental illness**.

sciatica Neuralgia of the back of the thigh and leg. This has several causes, including an inflamed sciatic nerve or a strained intervertebral disc. In TCM, this condition is attributed to damp-heat stagnation in the bladder or gall-bladder meridian. Coldness and blood stagnation are also involved if the condition is chronic. Acupuncture and massage are effective treatments.

sclerosis Abnormal hardening of an organ or tissue. See **multiple sclerosis**.

scorched See **odour**.

scorpion *Buthus martensi* Medicine. Distribution: global. Parts: entire animal. Character: neutral, pungent. Affinity: liver. Effects: nerve tonic, antispasmodic, sedative, analgesic, antidote. Symptoms: spasms, convulsions, headaches, abscesses. Treatments: boils, tetanus, pains due to wind-damp conditions. Dosage: powder 0.05–0.8 g, infusion 1.5–2.5 g. This medicine is poisonous, and so the dosage should not be exceeded. But, in any case, this is not a remedy which would be favoured by the physicians of the West.

scratch See **cuts**.

scrofula An archaic name for tuberculosis of the lymph glands in the neck. In TCM, this condition is attributed to a combination of yin deficiency in the kidneys and liver with heat and phlegm stagnation. The treatment is to nourish yin with infusions, taken internally, of the following, using the parts and dosages indicated: gardenia, *Gardenia jasminoides*, mature fruit, 4–9 g; *han lian cao*, *Eclipta prostrata*, entire plant, 8–14 g; self-heal, *Prunella vulgaris*, flowers, 4–6 g; fritillary, *Fritillaria verticillata*, corms, 5–9 g.

scrotal pain See **hawthorn**.

scullcap *Scutellaria baicalensis* Herbal medicine. Distribution: North China, Siberia. Parts: roots. Character: cold, bitter. Affinity: lungs, heart, gall-bladder, large intestine, small intestine. Effects: antipyretic, refrigerant, styptic, antidote, sedative. Symptoms: heated body, thirst but not wanting to drink, diarrhoea, blood in stools and sputum, nosebleeds, irritability.

Treatments: jaundice, dysentery, conditions of fullness and heat excess, oppression in the chest, restless foetus, hypertension, various infections, insomnia. Dosage: 4–7 g. This herb must NOT be confused with some of the other species of scullcap, such as blue scullcap, or mad-dog weed, *Scutellaria laterifolia*, which is indigenous to North America, and the common scullcap, *Scutellaria galericulata*, and lesser scullcap, *Scutellaria minor*, which are indigenous to all northern temperate zones and are used in Western medicine.

scurvy A condition due to a deficiency of vitamin C, and which is characterized by debility, bleeding gums, patchy skin and pain in the bone membranes. This disease is not likely to trouble the Chinese, whose diet contains an abundance of citrus fruits, which are the best source of vitamin C.

sea cucumber Also known as *bêche-de-mer*, sea slug and trepang. It is not a plant but a mollusc, and it is greatly esteemed by the Chinese as a highly nutritious seafood, which is rich in minerals, and a health food for treating tuberculosis, arteriosclerosis and nervous debility. It also promotes male virility.

sea-ear See **abalone**.

seafood See **shellfish**.

seafood poisoning This is one of the worst forms of food poisoning, and medical advice should be sought when it occurs. TCM treatments are infusions, taken internally, of the following, using the parts and dosages indicated: ginger, *Zingiber officinale*, rhizomes, 3–7 g; reed grass, *Phragmites communis*, roots and stems, 18–38 g; Chinese olive, *Canarium album*, fruits, 5–8 g.

seasickness See **travel sickness**.

seasons See **six excesses**.

seaweeds Marine algae, which are a good source of iodine. Agar, which is a protein derived from seaweeds, is a useful alternative to gelatin, which is derived from animals, in preparing vegetarian dishes.

sebaceous glands See **acne** and **jin ye**.

seborrhoeic eczema See **eczema**.

sebum See **acne** and **jin ye**.

secondary sex characteristics. See **genitalia**.

sedative Tranquillizer. Relaxant. This is a medicine which has a calming effect, so reducing excitement, nervousness and irritation, and may promote a restful sleep. Some nervines, which are medicines to strengthen the nervous system, have a relaxing effect, but others have a stimulating effect. In TCM, there is a wide range of what the Chinese aptly describe as 'calm the spirit medicines', which include *dan shen*, *Salvia miltiorrhiza*, longan, *Euphoria longan*, chrysanthemum, *Chrysanthemum morifolium*, nut grass, *Cyperus rotundus*, and Indian bread, *Poria cocos*. But many of these sedatives are specific in their effects, and to use them correctly, one must know the organs for which they have an affinity. For example, jimson weed, *Datura metel*, which has an affinity for the lungs, can be used a sedative in treating asthma, but it would not be effective with other conditions. The seeds of jujube, *Ziziphus jujuba*, are specifically sedative for liver conditions. Chinese physicians regard sedatives as energy-regulators which are required to treat full conditions, where there is evil-*qi*, which is energy in excess, in the wrong place or behaving improperly. In this, they heed one of the dicta of *The Internal Book of Huang Di*: 'Where there is fullness, sedate it, and where there is emptiness, tone it.' See **pig's heart** and **qi**.

sedentary habits See **exercise**.

seizures See **stroke**.

selective breeding See **genetics**.

self-diagnosis See **self-treatment**.

self-heal *Prunella vulgaris* Also called heal-all. Herbal medicine. Distribution: North China, North America, Northern Europe. Parts: flowers. Character: cold, bitter-pungent. Affinity: liver, gall-bladder. Effects: antipyretic, refrigerant, diuretic. Symptoms: headaches, dizziness, sore eyes, swollen eyeballs, over-sensitivity to light, jaundice. Treatments: gout, hypertension, tuberculosis of the lymph glands in the neck. Dosage: 4–6 g.

self-hypnosis Auto-suggestion. This is a system of therapy by which a person empties his mind of conscious thoughts, and then, by repeating certain words and phrases, he implants instructions in his subconscious mind so that the unconscious processes in his behaviour become desirably directed. He has conditioned his subconscious mind in such a way that he might benefit his health and general well-being. A system of self-hypnosis, or auto-suggestion, which became known as Couéism, was devised by Emile Coué, 1857–1926, a French apothecary. In fact, Couéism was not so very original, for its techniques are similar to those of the meditation exercises in TCM. Self-hypnosis can alleviate pain, stress, anxiety, depression, asthma, allergies and some psychosomatic illnesses, and also help to eradicate certain addictions, such as smoking, alcoholism and drug addiction. See **hypnotherapy** and **meditation**.

self-immunity See **immunity**.

self-massage See **massage**.

self-treatment Do-it-yourself medicine might be satisfactory for minor ailments or with those long-standing chronic ailments whose causes have been accurately diagnosed, and whose treatments have become well established. But, generally, it is not a practice to be recommended, for mistakes can easily be made with dosages and other procedures, and self-diagnosis can be misleading, which can result in symptoms being repressed and the real causes of illness going untreated. It could be the case that what appears to be a trifling ailment is really a symptom of a much more serious condition which only a qualified medical practitioner can accurately diagnose. It could be said that no one could know a person's body better than he knows it himself; but it is doubtful if this could always be the case, for it must sometimes be very difficult for a person to make a totally objective judgment in what is an essentially subjective situation. The self-diagnosis made by a hypochondriac, who will imagine that every little ache or pain heralds the onset of a terminal illness, is likely to be very different from that of the super-optimist taking the nonchalant view that 'whatever it is, it will soon wear off'. See **diagnosis** and **symptom**.

semen-essence See **jing, interferon** and **sperm problems**.

semicircular canals. See **ear**.

seminal vesicle See **reproductive systems**.

senile dementia See **Alzheimer's disease**.

senile keratosis See **complexion**.

senility See **Alzheimer's disease**.

senna *Casia tora* Herbal medicine. Distribution: South China, India, Vietnam. Parts: seeds. Character: cool, bitter-sweet, salty. Affinity: liver, gall-bladder. Effects: antipyretic, cathartic, improves vision. Symptoms: sore and swollen eyes, constipation. Treatments: eye problems due to liver conditions. Dosage: 5–7 g. As a cathartic, this medicine is a safe, natural and effective treatment for chronic constipation. It is sometimes called sickle senna, and it must NOT be confused with tinnevelly senna, *Cassia augustifolia*, or Alexandrian senna, *Cassia senna*, which are not indigenous to countries in the Far East, and are much more potent in their effects.

sensitivity See **allergy, hypersensitivity** and **intolerance**.

sensory nerve See **nerve**.

septicaemia Blood poisoning. This is due to the rapid multiplication of bacteria which have entered the bloodstream, usually via an external wound, and is sometimes the sequel to a failure to treat a wound with an antiseptic. This condition can spread very quickly and so become serious. Therefore, professional medical aid should be sought immediately. See **antiseptic** and **tetanus**.

septum The part of the nose which serves as a partition between the nostrils. See **nosebleed**.

serenity Calmness. Peace of mind. It is only in death that we can be completely free of troubles, as the Buddhists inform us. But most people do not crave for death, for they have an instinctive desire to live. They are prepared to accept that pains and problems are natural to our existence, that appreciation of pleasure derives from the awareness or even the experience of pain, and that dealing with problems is a component of the learning process on which a person's survival largely depends. However, although a trouble-free existence is hardly possible, a virtually stress-free existence could be within the grasp of most people, which is a most desirable state of affairs in view of the damage done to both mind and body by stress and its associated psychosomatic illnesses. Serenity of mind and the avoidance of stressful situations is largely a matter of having a healthy and wholesome attitude of mind. One is reminded of an Indian proverb: 'I complained because I had no shoes: and then I met a man who had no feet, and so I complained no more.' It is certainly clear to the Chinese that a wise philosophy of living, as formulated by Confucius, can produce an untroubled and benevolently masterful attitude of mind. There is certainly much truth in the aphorism that the giver receives more than the taker. Achieving serenity is largely a matter of appreciating the true value of health and knowing how to be content without constantly seeking material wealth. See **peace of mind**.

'serum hepatitis' See **hepatitis**.

sesame *Sesamum indicum* Both the seeds and oil of this plant are regular features of the Chinese diet. They flavour food, assist digestion, prevent constipation and tone the hair. Pork and chicken fried in sesame oil are given to women in the postnatal condition in order to prevent constipation.

seven emotions TCM recognizes seven emotions: joy, anger, anxiety, concentration, sorrow, fear and panic. Some of them are associated with certain organs, on which they have a deleterious effect if in excess: joy, heart; anger, liver; anxiety, lungs; concentration, spleen. Sorrow can affect several organs, namely the lungs, heart, pericardium and triple-warmer. Excess fear injures the kidneys, and also the bladder if it becomes very intense. Panic can affect both the heart and the kidneys.

seven glands theory The Taoist physicians in ancient China based some of their practices on the seven glands theory, which is the notion that the body contains seven glands, or houses, which regulate the flow of energy within the various organs and systems of the body. It says much for their perspicacity that modern medical science has shown that the body contains a number of glands which are ductless and secrete hormones that regulate its activities. These endocrine glands, as they are called, approximately correspond in their functions with the glands as described in Taoist medical theory. See **endocrine glands**.

sewage See **water**.

sex The Chinese have always maintained a moderate, matter-of-fact attitude towards sex, regarding it as being as natural and normal as eating, drinking or any other bodily function. Too much or too little sex is considered harmful. Practices such as homosexuality, bisexuality, promiscuity, prostitution and voyeurism tend to be heavily discouraged in China. There is a contrast here with attitudes in the West, where a shift has taken place from Victorian times, when sex was surrounded by taboos, to the present, where restrictions on sexual freedom are fast disappearing. The Chinese attitude is informed by the *I Ching*, which says 'Men and women are meant to love and complement each other.' The Chinese advocate marriage on a secular basis – not as a religious institution – as a way of preventing the spread of disease and providing the security of good parenthood for their children. Procreation is taken seriously in recognition of the fact that important characteristics are passed on from parents to their children. As far as contraception is concerned, it is regarded as an unnatural but necessary compromise to restrain population growth. In ancient times, the Taoists thought that a man should regulate his sexual activity and, as far as is possible, conserve his semen in order to prolong his life. See **moderation, homosexual, Yellow Emperor, food and sex, marriage** and **sperm problems**.

sex symbols ♂ (male), ♀ (female) These symbols, which have an international currency, are used in biological diagrams as a kind of shorthand to indicate *male* and *female*.

sexual arousal See **impotence**.

sexual-jing. Sexual vital essence, which matures at different ages in males and females. See **jing** and **maturity cycle**.

sexual maturity See **maturity cycle**.

sexual problems See **menstruation, menopause, pregnancy, impotence** and **infertility**.

sexual therapy In the West, sex has always been associated with youth, and so regarded as an activity which would be quite unseemly if it were performed by elderly people. But this attitude is now changing, and some physicians regard sex as a suitable therapy for rheumatism and similar conditions because it helps the blood to circulate and stimulates the secretion of cortisone by the adrenal glands. This is in line with the thinking of Chinese physicians, who regard virility as one of the indications of a sound state of health. See **sex wisdom**.

sex wisdom The *tao* of sex wisdom is concerned with human sexuality and how it may be used as a form of therapy and to strengthen the ties of love. It is also concerned with eugenics and birth control. See **Eight Pillars of Taoism**.

shaking palsy See **Parkinson's disease**.

shallot *Allium escalonicum* Scallion. See **onion**.

shaman Priest-cum-medicine man who, in China, was the forerunner of the true physician. Shamans flourished during the time of the Han dynasty (206 BC–AD 220). See **xian**.

shampoo See **chemicals** and **soap**.

Shan Hai Jing See **acupuncture needles**.

Shang Han Lun See **Zhang Zhongjing**.

Shangri-La An imaginary paradise depicted in James Hilton's novel *Lost Horizon*. It is in a hidden valley in Tibet, and its inhabitants age only very slowly. This is fiction based on fact, for the Tibetans, as with the Chinese, do try to attain a long life. See **longevity** and **life-span**.

shan qi See **Yunnan bai yao**.

shaojiu See **wine**.

Shaolin kungfu This is a popular hard style of the martial arts, which is named after the Buddhist temple at Shaolin, in the Sung mountains of Honan province, where it originated. See **martial arts**.

sheep dung See **antibiotics**.

shellfish Seafood. Edible crustaceans and molluscs. They are a good source of protein, zinc and iodine. They are much esteemed by the Chinese because they contain no fat. Shellfish poisoning can be very serious, and so it is important that they be bought fresh and thoroughly cleaned. See **crustaceans**, **mollusc** and **seafood poisoning**.

Shen Nong Also written as *Shen Nung*. One of the legendary emperors of China, and to whom the discovery of herbal medicines and sound agricultural methods is attributed. As far as can be ascertained – or conjectured – he lived about 3500 BC. According to the Han historian Sima Qian, Shen Nong tested many herbs in order to decide which of them had medicinal properties. Seemingly, there were about 365 such herbs. See **legendary emperors**.

Shen Nong Ben Cao Jing 'The Pharmacopoeia of Shen Nong'. In this book, scholars of the period of the Han dynasty (206 BC–AD 220) recorded all herbal knowledge which had been in existence since the time of the legendary emperor Shen Nong. It contains the dictum: 'Treat cold illnesses with warming medicines, and hot illnesses with cooling medicines.' And so it seems that Shen Nong's approach was essentially allopathic. See **Shen Nong**, **allopathy** and **classification of herbs**.

shiatsu This is a Japanese system of massage and manipulation whereby ailments are treated by balancing or releasing *ki*, or 'vital energy', which is called *qi* by the Chinese. It is similar to acupressure in that stimulation is applied to hundreds of acupoints, or *tsubos*, as the Japanese call them, but it differs in that, whereas only the fingertips are used in acupressure, the fingers, thumbs, knuckles, palms, elbows and even feet are used in *shiatsu*. In common with TCM, *shiatsu* is based on the belief that all energies are either yin, which is negative, or yang, which is positive, and so are complementary, and that illnessses are either *jitsu*, meaning 'external', or *kyo*, meaning 'internal'. But it is as well to understand that both *shiatsu* and acupressure have been developed from *amna*, which is an ancient system of massage that originated in China. But, despite its ancient origin and long history, *shiatsu* was not developed as a complete therapy until the beginning of this century, when it was introduced and popularized by Tokujiro Namikoshi.

shigella The bacterium, in the genus *Shigella*, which causes dysentery. See **dysentery**.

shih erh tuan chin 'Twelve sets of embroidery'. A set of self-massage and fitness exercises which has been popular with the Chinese for many centuries. These exercises have the advantage that they can be performed by both the elderly and the infirm, including those who are suffering from chronic diseases. The full details of these exercises will be found in the *Chinese Exercise Manual*.

Shi Ji Also written as *Xi Ji*. 'Historical Records'. Written by Szuma Chien, a historian of the period of the Han dynasty (206 BC–AD 220), these records contain the earliest written account of the success of the physician Bian Que in giving the first effective acupuncture treatment. See **Bian Que**.

Shijing See **Book of Odes**.

shin do See **acupressure**.

shingles Herpes zoster. This condition is caused when the chicken pox virus, after lying dormant in nerve roots for many years since childhood, becomes reactivated in adulthood, sometimes as a consequence of stress or contact with someone who has chicken pox. It is characterized initially by inflamed nerves and a severe pain in the chest or one side of the body, and then by a painful, blistering rash with spots which become encrusted. The rash normally departs after several weeks, but it may leave scars, and the pain, known as post-herpetic neuralgia, may persist for months or even years. In TCM, shingles is attributed to heat and damp in the liver and gall-bladder meridians. The treatment is an infusion, taken internally, of 3–7 g roots of Chinese gentian, *Gentiana scabra*, or 4–8 g leaves and stems of sweet wormwood. *Artemisia annua*. After the rash has cleared, the pain can be treated by acupuncture to the stomach, intestine and governor-vessel meridians. See **varicella**.

shin tao See **acupressure**.

shock This condition may be emotional or physical. Emotional, or psychological, shock can be caused by sudden bad news or minor injuries. Physical, or clinical, shock is due to lack of blood to the vital organs, especially the brain and kidneys, and can be caused by severe burns or bruises, accidents where there is heavy bleeding, severe fractures, intense pain or distress, severe allergy or a blood infection, and it is characterized by pallor, intense perspiration and a weak and rapid or irregular pulse. Gentle massage, comfort and a few friendly words are good remedies for emotional shock unless it happens to be very severe, and then it may lead to physical shock. Intense fear sometimes causes involuntary urination, which is a clear indication that there is an association between the kidneys and the emotion of fear. The initial treatment for physical shock is one which is well known to first-aiders: 'Lay the patient down, turn the head to one side, raise the legs, loosen the clothing at the neck, chest and waist, give no drinks but moisten the lips, cover with a blanket and seek medical aid.' These simple procedures, which are the same in China as they are in the West, are intended to ensure that the patient has air, warmth and a supply of blood to the vital organs. Of course, the condition causing the physical shock – diarrhoea, allergy, blood infection, etc. – will also need to be treated. See **trauma**.

short-sightedness See **optical defects**.

shu di huang *Rehmannia glutinosa* Herbal medicine. Distribution:

North China. Parts: steamed roots. Character: warm, sweet. Affinity: liver, heart, kidneys. Effects: haemostatic, blood tonic, promotes yin. Symptoms: dizziness, palpitations, insomnia, debility, night sweats. Treatments: dysmenorrhoea, menorrhagia, spermatorrhoea, blood deficiency, diabetes, deficiency of kidney-yin. Dosage: 8–28 g. The fresh root is used as a refrigerant for the blood. The unsteamed dried root, which is then called *gan di huang*, has an affinity for the small intestine also, and is a demulcent, diuretic, cardiotonic and treatment for conditions due to internal heat excess. Its dosage is 5–7 g. *Gan di huang* is a safe cardiotonic for people with a weak heart, and is effective in lowering the level of blood sugar.

Siberian ginseng *Eleutherococcus senticosus* Herbal medicine. Distribution: Siberia, Korea, north China. Parts: roots. Character: neutral, sweet. Affinity: spleen, lungs. Effects: tones *qi*, lungs, spleen and *jin ye*, aphrodisiac. Symptoms: debility, tiredness, loss of appetite, insomnia. Treatments: diabetes, cardiovascular disturbances, arthritis. Dosage: 0.6–3 g. The precautions which apply to the use of Asiatic ginseng must surely apply to this herb, for it is more potent than the other forms of ginseng. See **Asiatic ginseng**.

sickle-cell anaemia See **anaemia**.

sickle senna See **senna**.

side-effects One of the advantages of herbal medicines is that they generally do not have any unpleasant side-effects, which is certainly not the case with synthetic medicines. See **active ingredient** and **buffer**.

silicosis See **occupational disease**.

silver wood ears *Wunyi*. Also called cloud ears or 'jelly fungus'. This fungus, which grows on the trunks of old pine trees, is much esteemed by the Chinese as an item of diet and for its medicinal properties. It is a tonic for the blood, brain and heart, it strengthens the lungs and digestive system, alleviates coughs, revitalizes the skin and benefits the spleen and kidneys. See **mukyi**.

Sima Qian See **Shen Nong**.

simples Seee **culinary herbs and spices**.

sinew See **tendon**.

sinus A cavity in the body, especially one of those around the nose.

sinusitis Inflammation of the sinuses. In TCM, this condition is attributed to lung-*qi* deficiency and damp-heat. An effective remedy is a decoction, taken internally, of 6–8 g corms of fritillary, *Fritillaria verticillata*, or 5–7 g floral buds of magnolia, *Magnolia liliflora*. See **catarrh**.

si qa luo *Luffa cylindrica* Herbal medicine. Distribution: China, Japan, Vietnam, Philippines. Parts: fibres of mature fruits. Character: neutral, sweet. Affinity: stomach, lungs, liver. Effects: analgesic, haemostatic, antirheumatic, tonic to the meridians. Symptoms: rheumatic aches and pains. Treatments: fibrositis, breast tumours. Dosage: 4–8 g. The flesh of the fruit is used as a refrigerant.

si qi 'Four energies'. See **four energies** and **energy**.

six excesses The Chinese recognize, as we do in the West, that the general climatic conditions and the weather changes associated with the seasons have an effect on health, and for a variety of reasons. In TCM, climatic and weather conditions are described as excesses, which are broadly categorized as wind, cold, summer-heat, damp, dryness and fire. Of course, these excesses can be in various combinations. Thus, in the winter season, the weather could be cold-dry, and in the summer, it could be hot-damp. The influences of the six excesses on health are fully explained in a modern work, *The Art of Acupuncture*, by Cheng Mingchi. See **climate** and **excess combinations**.

si zhen The Chinese term for the four basic diagnostic techniques. See **diagnosis**.

skeleton The human skeleton is a framework of 208 bones of various sizes and shapes. It supports the soft parts of the body, protects the internal organs and provides attachments for the muscles. The part of the skull which encloses and protects the brain is called the cranium. The rib-cage, which contains 12 pairs of ribs, protects the heart and lungs. The pelvis, which is a solid ring of bone, encloses and protects some of the organs in the lower abdomen. Two pairs of ribs are not attached to the rib-cage and sternum, and so they are commonly known as 'floating ribs'. Knowing the names and positions of the bones is sometimes an aid to diagnosis and treatments in that it helps one to locate the organs and other parts of the body. In the diagram, the bones are labelled with their medical names, but their common names – where they have a common name – are as follows: mandible *jaw-bone*, cervical vertebrae *neck-bones*, clavicle *collar-bone*, scapula *shoulder-blade*, sternum *breastbone*, humerus *upper arm-bone*, vertebral column *backbone*, pelvis *hip-bone*, radius and ulna *lower arm-bones*, carpals *wrist-bones*, phalanges *toe-bones* and *finger-bones*, femur *thigh-bone*, patella *kneecap*, tibia *shin-bone*, fibula *calf-bone*, tarsals *ankle-bones*. The bones which are the most

SKELETON

likely to be fractured are the skull, clavicle, scapula, humerus, vertebral column, radius, ulna, pelvis, carpals, femur, patella, fibula and tibia. See **fracture**.

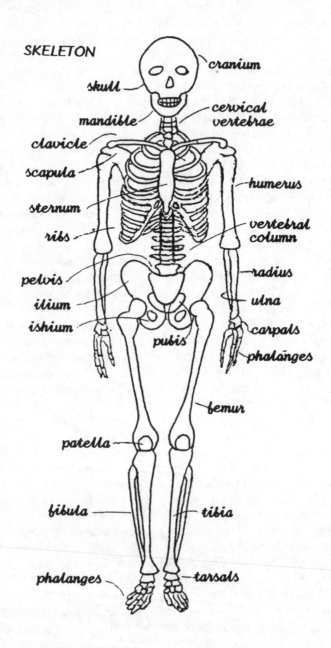

SKELETON

cranium
skull
mandible
cervical vertebrae
clavicle
scapula
humerus
sternum
ribs
vertebral column
pelvis
radius
ilium
ulna
ishium
carpals
pubis
phalanges
femur
patella
fibula
tibia
phalanges
tarsals

skin care See **complexion, personal hygiene, hair care** and **lecithin**.

skin problems See **personal hygiene, complexion** and **pimples and spots**.

skin scrape This TCM technique is used to alleviate hot and full ailments, such as fevers, influenza, colds, headaches, heat exhaustion, heat-stroke, arthritic joints, colic and indigestion. A metal object without sharp edges, such as a coin or knife handle, is sterilized by dipping it into wine or a saline solution, and then scraped rapidly and without cessation over the patient's skin with forceful massage-like strokes until bright-red stripes appear. Excess heat is drawn to the scraped region on the skin. The usual places for scraping are the regions along each side of the spine and between the eyebrows, and on the upper chest, the bridge of the nose and the back and sides of the neck. A skin scrape is generally supplemented with cooling yin medicines.

skull See **occipital bone**.

skull-cap Alternative spelling of *scullcap*. See **scullcap**.

sleep diagnosis In TCM, sleeping habits are used in diagnosis. Over-sleeping is a symptom of a deficiency of yang, insomnia of anxiety, poor circulation or a deficiency of spleen-*qi*, early rising of an over-active heart or tension, and restless sleep of emotional disturbance or over-indulgence in food or drink. Sleep apnoea may be a symptom of obesity or a heart condition. See **sleep disorders**.

sleep disorders The most common disorders and problems to do with sleep are insomnia, hypersomnia, nightmares, restlessness, snoring, sleep apnoea and jet lag. Insomnia is the sheer inability to sleep. It is a chronic condition and not a temporary bout of sleeplessness. Hypersomnia is constant oversleeping and yet always feeling tired, as if the additional sleep has not brought any benefit. Nightmares may be due to anxiety, but they are not a problem unless they continue for long periods. Restlessness has many causes, which range from a serious illness to something as simple as an uncomfortable bed. Sleepwalking is a rare condition which generally only affects children. The cause may be anxiety, but no harm is done if the sleepwalker is guided, unawakened if possible, back to bed. Snoring is a problem only when it is due to sleep apnoea, which is a condition whereby a sleeper may stop breathing altogether, and for as long as 90 seconds, and then awake gasping for breath. It could be a symptom of obesity or a heart disorder. Jet lag is no more than an interruption of the normal pattern of sleep. Chinese physicians would argue that, if a person is in a sound state of physical health and without anxieties of any kind, he should rarely fall victim to any of these disorders. But, where these disorders do occur, acupuncture is often helpful, although it is also important to diagnose and treat the conditions of which these disorders are merely symptoms. Normal sleep is a good medicine. See **insomnia**, **hypersomnia**, **sleep diagnosis** and **jet lag**.

slipped disc See **intervertebral disc**.

small intestine One of the hollow organs of TCM. It is paired with the heart, and its associated element is fire. See **liu fu** and **intestine**.

smallpox See **immunology** and **Jesuits**.

smell See **odour** and **hearing**.

smoking Few people would argue that smoking is a healthy activity. Yet, in moderation, it is regarded tolerantly by the Chinese. It is interesting that one of the traditional Chinese remedies for asthma is to smoke a mixture of tobacco and coltsfoot leaves. See **addiction**, **tobacco**, **infertility** and **ear acupuncture**.

snake bite The TCM remedy for a venomous snake bite is to directly apply the juice squeezed from the leaves and stems of dandelion, *Taraxacum officinale*, Chinese violet, *Viola yedoensis*, or *ban zhi lian*, *Scutellaria barbata*.

snake gourd *Trichsanthes kirilowii* Herbal medicine. Distribution: South China, Vietnam. Parts: seed kernels. Character: cold, sweet. Affinity: stomach, lungs, large intestine. Effects: emollient, expectorant, bronchi-dilator, laxative. Symptoms: coughs, thick yellow phlegm, chest pains, constipation. Treatments: lung tumours, breast tumours, excess heat in lungs. Dosage: 8–14 g. The root is an antipyretic and galactogogue.

sneezing An involuntary ejection of air from the mouth and nose, and which is due to irritation or inflammation of the nasal membranes. Its common causes are colds, influenza, hay fever and accidentally breathing in a powdery substance, such as dust, soot or pepper. Emotional stress is sometimes a cause of sneezing. This condition is not an illness but a symptom, which can be prevented by obviating its cause.

snoring See **sleep disorders**.

soap It is as well to remember that soap, shampoo and other cleaning agents can be damaging to the skin in a variety of ways. They may contain chemicals that are irritants, and they may wash away sebum, which is a natural oil that protects the skin. Also, some soaps are greasy, and the grease blocks up the skin pores, which is no help to those who have acne. Actually, many cosmetic products are best avoided. A non-irritant soap can be made by mixing oatmeal with water. See **chemicals**.

social evils A social evil may be defined as any agency which causes disharmony in society. Many people would regard excess consumption of tobacco, alcohol and drugs, and gambling and promiscuity as the main social evils, although by definition crime and other disruptive influences should also be included. It is the view of Chinese physicians that bad social habits can contribute to ill health, both physical and mental. See **morality** and **moderation**.

social harmony It is the Chinese view that social harmony is necessary for the health of the individual. Social unrest causes disquiet in the individual, which may lead to the development of psychosomatic illnesses. See **harmony** and **morality**.

sodium See **mineral**.

solar plexus A ganglion, or assemblage of nerve cells, which lies behind the stomach. See **ulcer**.

solid organs *Wu zang* is the Chinese name for the solid organs, which TCM designates as the heart, liver, lungs, kidneys, spleen and heart-constrictor. The heart-constrictor is the pericardium, which is not an organ in our sense of the term, and it has more significance in acupuncture than it has in herbal medicine. The solid organs are yin, and each is paired with one of the hollow organs, which are yang, as follows: heart and small intestine, liver and gall-bladder, lungs and large intestine, kidneys and bladder, and spleen and stomach. Illnesses which affect a solid organ will generally affect its corresponding hollow organ. Similarly those herbal medicines which have an affinity for a solid organ will generally also have an affinity for its corresponding hollow organ. Each solid organ and its corresponding hollow organ are associated with the same element. See **herbal prescriptions**, **vital organs**, **element** and **pericardium**.

soluble See **solution**.

solute See **solution**.

solution Herbal medicines are mainly administered as infusions and decoctions, which are solutions. To make a solution, a substance is dissolved in water or some other liquid. The liquid part of a solution is called the solvent, and the dissolved substance is called the solute. Those substances which will dissolve in water are said to be soluble in water. In medical work, solutions in which the solvent is water are called aqueous solutions. Some substances are insoluble in water, but this creates no problems for the pharmacist, for some of the substances that will not dissolve in water will dissolve in other liquids. Iodine, for example, will dissolve in alcohol. A solution in which the solvent is alcohol or glycerine is called a tincture. Some solids can be ground into a fine powder and shaken or stirred in water, where the tiny particles float about, so forming a suspension. Similarly, an oil can be shaken in water to make an emulsion. See **emulsion**, **concentrated** and **dilute**.

Song dynasty The period of the Song (or Sung) dynasty (960–1279) was one of great advance in administration, trade, agriculture and technology in China. The irrigation systems were re-established, iron, tin, copper, gold and silver were being mined, coal was used as a fuel in the smelting of iron, the magnetic compass was being used in navigation, and gunpowder, paper money and movable type for printing were invented. Pastes, poultices and pills were introduced into medicine, and herbal prescriptions were standardized.

soporific Hypnotic. A medicine to induce sleep. Many of the sedative medicines can be used for this purpose. See **insomnia** and **sedative**.

sore eyes In TCM, bathing the eyes with an infusion of 4–8 g seeds of plantain, *Plantago asiatica*, is the treatment usually recommended. See **conjunctivitis**.

sore throat A rather vague term which could mean pharyngitis, laryngitis or tonsillitis. The main causes of a sore throat are viral or bacterial infections and a low-humidity atmosphere, as occurs in centrally heated rooms. In TCM, the recommended treatment is to gargle with a saline solution, made by dissolving 7 g salt in 1 litre water, an infusion of 3–12 g leaves of blackberry, *Rubus coreanus*, or an infusion of 10–15 g flowers of honeysuckle, *Lonicera japonica*. A solid-fuel or gas fire is the healthiest form of heating in one's own home, for it not only heats a room but also draws in a supply of cool and fresh air, which helps to prevent the sore throats that are the consequence of a dry atmosphere.

sorrow Grief. This is one of the seven emotions of TCM. It is not associated with only one organ, as are the other emotions, but may reside in the heart, lungs, heart-constrictor or triple-warmer. It has a debilitating effect and seriously depletes the body's *qi*. See **seven emotions**.

soul See **spirit**.

sound On a limited scale, sound has a therapeutic value, as when it is combined with dancing and rhythmic breathing. The pleasant sounds of music can relieve tension. The Buddhists have evolved meditative and spiritual exercises based on sound. See **noise**.

south See **direction**.

soya bean *Glycine max* This legume is a good source of protein, polyunsaturated fatty acids, starch, sugars and dietary fibre. It also contains some valuable minerals and vitamins. Untreated soya beans, whether cooked or uncooked, are not easily digested, but this is not the case with soya bean products, of which there are many. Soya beans are used as a meat substitute throughout the world. Soya-bean sprouts contain vitamin C and are easily digested, which are two of the culinary advantages of bean sprouts, and of which the cooks of the West have been totally unaware until recent years.

Spanish fly See **aphrodisiac**.

spasms See **cramp**.

spastic A person suffering from cerebral palsy, which is due to lack of development or injury in some part of the brain, and which is characterized by retarded activity, abnormal movements and defective vision, hearing, speech or tactile sense. As this condition is to do with the brain, and not the musculature, there is little to be gained substantially by remedial exercises. But the Chinese have made attempts at acupuncture treatments with some patients.

spastic colon See **irritable bowel syndrome**.

spa water See **water**.

spectacles See **optical defects**.

sperm An abbreviation for **spermatozoon**.

spermatorrhoea Abnormally excessive discharge of semen. See **sperm problems**.

spermatozoon Plural: *spermatozoa*. The male reproductive cell. See **fertilization**.

sperm count See **jing**, **interferon** and **sperm problems**.

sperm problems The problems associated with sperm include infections of the testes, a low sperm count, spermatorrhoea and abnormal sperm which cannot fertilize an ovum. The last condition may be due to stress, obesity, varicose veins near the testicles, hormone imbalances, retrogade ejaculation, when semen enters the bladder instead of the penis, and premature ejaculation, when semen fails to enter the vagina. According to TCM, most of these conditions are due to a deficiency of kidney-*qi*, kidney-essence, kidney-yang, or kidney-yin. The recommended treatments are tonic herbs to strengthen the kidneys and acupuncture or moxibustion to strengthen the bladder, kidney, stomach and conception-vessel meridians. The treatments for spermatorrhoea are infusions or decoctions, taken internally, of the following, using the parts and dosages indicated: *han lian cao*, *Eclipta prostrata*, entire plant, 8–14 g; foxnut, *Euryale ferox*, seeds, 10–28 g; blackberry, *Rubus coreanus*, unripe berries, 6–8 g. A suspension of 5–8 g powdered shells of oyster, *Ostrea rivularis*, taken internally, is also helpful. See **jing** and **interferon**.

spice A plant or part of a plant which contains aromatic oils or pungent substances and is used to flavour food. Many spices, such as ginger and cinnamon, have medicinal properties. See **culinary herbs and spices**.

spiders See **bites**.

spinach See **health foods**.

spine See **vertebral column**.

spinal canal The cavity at the centre of the vertebrae, and which contains the spinal cord. See **intervertebral discs**.

spinal cord See **involuntary movement** and **intervertebral discs**.

spirit This word, which derives from the Greek word *spiritus*, meaning 'breath', has a variety of meanings, but all are connected in one way or another. *Spirit* is used as an everyday name for alcohol and some other volatile liquids. Alcohol will vaporize and escape into the atmosphere, and so it is understandable that, in ancient times, when language was much more limited than it is today, *spirit* was also used to mean 'air', or 'what we breathe out', for it was once the common belief that air is a product of breathing. *Spirit* was also used to mean 'soul', which escapes like air from the body at the time of death, or even during dreaming, which is a belief that was once held by many of the Chinese peasantry. It can be used to mean 'personality' or 'psyche' in a psychological and non-spiritual sense. It is in this sense that the Taoist philosophers in ancient China regarded the pineal gland as being the 'house of the spirit'. They would have equated it with *qi*, or 'life-force', and air and breath because, in the Chinese language, *qi* also means 'air' and 'breath'. The heart, also, was associated with the spirit, which makes much sense if *spirit* is taken to mean a person's emotional nature, for the heart is certainly affected by the emotions. Some Chinese – in common with some other peoples all over the world – also believed in the literal (not just symbolic) existence of a soul separate from the rest of the body. One of their beliefs was that the human body possesses two souls, one being of a spiritual nature, or the 'higher self', which is called *hun* or *shen*, and the other being a person's unsophisticated animal nature, which is called *po*. In their meanings, these terms are very similar to *super-ego*, meaning, 'conscience-motivated personality', and *id*, meaning 'primitive personality', which are expressions used in psychology in the West. It was believed that, at the time of death or in dreaming, *hun* escapes from the body through a hole in the top of the cranium. In fact, this belief was so strongly held in ancient times that it was the common practice to make a hole in the top of the cranium of a deceased person to ensure that his soul would have an adequate escape route. In fairly recent years, archaeologists unearthed some pierced skulls at a site near Beijing, and came to the erroneous conclusion that they had found evidence that the surgeons in ancient China had engaged in a form of brain surgery known as trepanning. However, all this should not be lightly dismissed as superstition, for the people of ancient China had at least realized in a roundabout way that a person's animal nature, or emotional make-up, is influenced not only by his brain but also by his body, as our knowledge of hormones indicates to be the case. See **air**, **dreams**, **endocrine glands**, **hormone**, **heart** and **qi**.

spleen The spleen, which is yin, is one of the *wu zang*, or 'solid organs', of the body. Its element is earth, and the hollow organ with which it is paired is the stomach, which is yang. It assists in developing immunity and the formation of red blood cells. According to TCM, the spleen houses the mind, and so is damaged by intense over-concentration. It regulates the movement of the vital essence derived from food, and distributes nutrients and *qi* to all parts of the body. It operates in conjunction with the stomach, and neither organ could function effectively without the other. But TCM uses the term *spleen* to include the pancreas, which secretes digestive juices, and so the connection between the spleen and the stomach is not surprising. The symptoms of a spleen dysfunction are weakness, emaciation and inner-coldness, which can lead to oedema and nephritis. The spleen is associated with the production of saliva, but perhaps for no better reason than that, according to TCM theory, the spleen, stomach and saliva are all involved in digestion. See **solid organs**, **concentration** and **jin ye**.

spleen disorders A traditional remedy for spleen disorders, and one much favoured in the rural areas of China, is to steam 250 g chicken, 30 g dates, 60 g dried mushrooms, 4 slices ginger, 3 chopped spring onions (*cong bai*), 10 g white sugar, 10 g soy sauce and 0.5 g salt in rice wine for 15–20 minutes. The mixture must then be consumed with a dressing of sesame oil.

spotted deer *Cervus nippon* In TCM, powders, decoctions and other extracts from the velvet antlers of this animal are considered to be excellent nutrient tonics for the treatment of anaemia, weight loss and weak sinews, cartilage and bone marrow. The blood and secretions from the cut antlers are highly esteemed as an aphrodisiac. However, this is not the type of medicine which would meet with the approval of the people of the West.

spotted fever See **meningitis**.

sports Confucius taught that the body should be well cared for so that there is a full development of its inner strength and complete harmony among the forces and elements within the body and mind. Accordingly, over the centuries, the Chinese have participated in sporting activities of many kinds, including the martial arts, using feet, fists, poles, flails, swords and other devices, calasthenics involving breathing exercises, bending and stretching, and acrobatics. At the time of the Han dynasty (206 BC–AD 220), a ball game similar to football was played in China, but habits have changed since then, perhaps because, since then, the Chinese have learned that over-strenuous exercise does more harm than good. Every day in China, in the coolness of the early morning, both the young and the elderly congregate in the parks and other open places, where they practise the martial arts movements and other exercises, which are partly remedial and partly recreational. Many of the remedial exercises are of ancient origin and are components of the Eight Pillars of Taoism. Some of these exercises require a great deal of skill, and so they exercise the mind as well as the body. They are supplemented with games which require only mental effort, such as chess, dominoes, draughts and spillikins. Diabolo, which requires both physical and mental skill, is a popular game in China. Unfortunately, the Chinese are inveterate gamblers, which seems to be rather out of character for a race which, in other respects, is remarkably practical and level-headed. During recent years, and with official approval, the Chinese have shown much interest in the sporting activities and games which are characteristic of the West, probably as a matter of national pride – 'anything that the others can do, the Chinese can do better!'. For example, table tennis is now a very popular game in China. See **games**.

spots See **pimples and spots**.

sprain Injury to a joint caused by violent twisting, and which involves some damage to the ligaments. It should not be confused with a strain, which is a stretched muscle. The TCM treatment is the same for both conditions. Keep the injured part at rest and apply a cold compress. A clean cloth soaked in cold water is quite adequate. Follow this up by gently massaging the injured part with a liniment made by steeping 10 g garlic cloves in 250 ml olive oil, or by applying a poultice made of hot water and crushed capsules of the corn poppy, *Papaver rhoeas*. A paste of flour, rice wine and the crushed fruits of gardenia, *Gardenia jasminoides*, also makes an effective poultice. If there is much pain, an analgesic or sedative can be administered.

spring onion An onion which has been taken from the ground before a bulb has formed. See **onion** and **cong bai**.

spring wine In TCM, spring wine is a tonic wine which is intended to be drunk at the beginning of the spring season, when the blood and *qi* may be stagnant as a consequence of the inactivity of the winter season, and when the libido may be in need of a boost. Recipes vary from region to region, but a spring wine is basically a strong spirit, such as *gao liang*, in which a wide variety of medicinal herbs have been steeped. Brandy or vodka makes an excellent substitute for the Chinese spirit. The ingredients in spring wine are eliminatives, blood-cleansers, aperients, ageing-inhibitors, powerful nutrients and aphrodisiacs, and will include such items as glue and powdered horn from the spotted deer, *Cervus nippon*, roots of angelica, *Angelica sinensis*, fruits of blackberry, *Rubus coreanus*, fruits of wolfberry, *Lycium chinense*, roots of *huang qi*, *Astralagus membranaceus*, roots of *shu di huang*, *Rehmannia glutinosa*, roots of Asiatic ginseng, *Panax ginseng*, and leaves of horny goat weed, *Epimedium sagittatum*. The horny goat weed functions as a vasodilator, which aids the circulation of the other ingredients. The wine may be flavoured with honey or sugar. However, the preparation of a spring wine is a complicated and long-winded business, and so those in the West who wish to sample this wine are advised to obtain it from a Chinese grocery store. See **wine**.

sputum Expectorated matter, which will contain saliva, and may also contain phlegm and pus if there is an infection of the throat or lungs.

staggers See **bovine spongiform encephalopathy**.

stagnant blood See **stagnation**.

stagnant qi See **qi**.

stagnation A somewhat vague term used in TCM to indicate emptiness, a poor condition of an organ, lack of vitality, debility, or sluggishly circulated blood or *qi*. A yang tonic medicine is the usual treatment. See **qi**.

stag's genitals See **lu chong**.

stamen One of the male sexual organs of a flowering plant, which usually has more than one flower, each containing several stamens. The anther, which is at the head of a stamen, contains pollen. Stamens are used in some herbal medicines. See **pistil** and **pollen**.

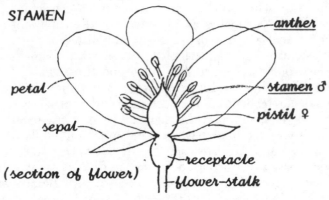

STAMEN

petal

sepal

(section of flower)

anther

stamen ♂

pistil ♀

receptacle

flower-stalk

stamina In TCM, there are many herbs suitable for the treatment of debility and lack of stamina. There are also some invigorating and revitalizing exercises. For athletes who wish to increase their stamina and improve their performance, there are tonic medicines which can be used safely. See **debility**, **tonic**, **steroids**, **caterpillar fungus**, **royal jelly** and **li shou**.

stammering This is a very common speech defect, for which there is a variety of causes, including an emotional shock in childhood, a fault in the brain mechanism which controls speech, slow development of the ability to methodize the movements of the lips, palate and tongue used in speech, and partial paralysis of the face or mouth as a result of a stroke. Anxious parents who display their concern about a young child's speech problems make the child even more nervous, which is no help. There are many possible treatments, such as breathing exercises, speech therapy and self-hypnosis, but none of them are effective in every case. In TCM, the usual treatments for voice problems are relaxation exercises to build confidence, which are described in the *Chinese Exercise Manual*, and acupressure applied at the bottom of the outside edge of the thumbnail.

staphylococcus See **food poisoning**.

stapling This is an ear-acupuncture technique whereby small needles are inserted into the ear and left in place for up to two weeks. It is effective in alleviating the withdrawal symptoms

ACUPRESSURE FOR
STAMMERING

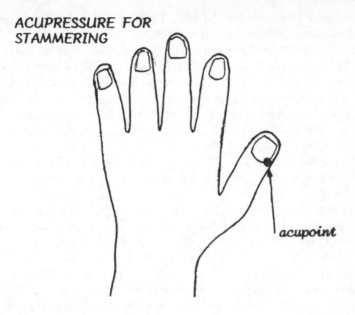

acupoint

which arise from all types of addiction. See **ear acupuncture**.

starch See **sugar**.

starwort *Inula britannica* Herbal medicine. Distribution: China, Japan, Europe. Parts: flowers. Character: warm, bitter-pungent, salty. Affinity: lungs, stomach, spleen, large intestine. Effects: antitussive, expectorant, antiemetic. Symptoms: coughs, eructation, nausea, vomiting. Treatments: excess phlegm, bronchitis. Dosage: 4–9 g.

steeping Impregnating with liquid. Thus, in making medicinal wines, herbs are steeped in rice wine.

sterilization The various techniques by which food, tissues, surgical instruments, etc. are kept free of micro-organisms. Traditionally, in China, all water intended for drinking is boiled, and fresh food ingredients are used as far as is possible. In TCM, surgical instruments are immersed in boiling water, the points of needles are held in a flame for a few seconds, and wounds are treated with antiseptics. See **antiseptic** and **autoclave**.

sternum Breastbone. See **skeleton**.

steroids A large group of organic compounds which includes bile acids, some hormones and vitamin D. This term is often used to describe the hormones secreted by the adrenal glands, but which, strictly, should be called corticosteroids. In the West, steroids are sometimes taken by body-builders and athletes in order to get some kind of 'lift'. They are not to be recommended. See **corticosteroids** and **stamina**.

stethoscope An instrument for auscultation, that is, listening to the sounds made by the heart, lungs, intestines and other organs. By tradition, a Chinese stethoscope is a bamboo tube. One end is held against the physician's ear, and the other on the patient's body. The advantage of this simple instrument is that the wood, as well as the column of air within it, conducts sound. See **hearing** and **pulse diagnosis**.

stimulant This is a medicine which increases the activity of the body or a part of the body. But a stimulant can make greater demands on the body than the body is able to give, and so its effects can be exhausting, if not damaging. This is the case with alcohol, caffeine and some aphrodisiacs if they are used too frequently. Therefore, a stimulant should be used only as a temporary measure or in conjunction with some other medicine which is genuinely restorative. The stimulants used in Western medicine are usually of a general nature, and so tend to affect the body as a whole, whereas those used in TCM have an affinity for certain organs, and they will generally have an effect only on those same organs. Most of the stimulants used in TCM are better regarded as tonics, and they must be taken over a long period of time if they are to be truly effective. See **tonic**.

stimulation treatment This is one of the eight methods of herbal treatment in TCM. It is sometimes called warming treatment, for it requires the use of medicines which will remove coldness from the interior of the body, stimulate the circulation of the blood and *qi*, tone yang-energy, and eliminate cold-*qi* or *qi* deficiency in any of the organs.

stinging nettle *Urtica dioica* Herbal medicine. Distribution: temperate regions worldwide. Parts: leaves. Character: cold, sweet. Affinity: liver, kidneys. Effects: haemostatic, astringent, diuretic, galactogogue, circulatory stimulant. Symptoms: poor skin condition, eczema, acne, rheumatic pains, low lactation. Treatments: anaemia, eczema, arthritis, gout, diabetes mellitus, oedema. Dosage: 6–12 g. The seeds are reputed to have aphrodisiac properties. The small, or garden, nettle, *Urtica urens*, a related species, has the same medicinal properties.

stings One should not confuse stings with bites. Snakes, spiders and mosquitoes do not sting: they bite. The scorpion, which is a member of the spider family, is an exception. It has a sting at the end of its tail. Some creatures, such as bees, wasps and jellyfish, defend themselves by means of venom-filled organs. If a person is stung, the skin at the site of the sting becomes inflamed, itchy and painful. Sometimes, though rarely, a sting can cause an allergic reaction called anaphylactic shock. The victim becomes delirious and breathless, and his blood pressure falls, his pulse becomes rapid and weak, and he develops a widespread rash. Immediate medical attention is then required. Otherwise, simple remedies are effective, and they are much the same in TCM as they are in the West. The venom from a wasp is alkaline, which can be neutralized by applying a mild acid, such as lemon juice or vinegar. A bee's sting has a serrated edge, which breaks off and becomes embedded in the skin when a bee stings someone. Therefore, the first procedure in treating a bee sting is to remove the sting, but carefully so that the venom sac is not broken, for that would release more poison. An alkaline substance, such as bicarbonate of soda, is then applied because bee venom is acidic. The application of crushed leaves of plantain, *Plantago asiatica*, or marigold, *Calendula officinalis*, is also effective. This treatment can also be applied to stings from nettles and other plants. In the West, dock (genus *Rumex*) leaves would be used for this purpose. See **bites**.

stomach The stomach, which is yang, is one of the *liu fu*, or 'hollow organs', of the body. Its element is earth, and the solid organ with which it is paired is the spleen, which is yin. The cells of the stomach secrete gastric fluid, which contains hydrochloric acid and the enzymes pepsin and rennin. Pepsin converts proteins into peptones and proteoses which, when they enter the duodenum, will be converted into peptides by the enzyme trypsin, which is secreted by the pancreas. Rennin coagulates casein, which is the protein in milk. See **spleen** and **liu fu**.

stomach-ache See **stomach upsets**.

stomachic Generally, *stomachic* and *digestive* are regarded as being interchangeable terms, but the former is often taken to mean a medicine which is a tonic for the stomach, and the latter as an appetizer, or digestive stimulant. For example, an aperitif, which is an alcoholic drink, could be described as a digestive, but it is hardly a medicine. The Chinese regard wolfberry wine as both a stomachic and a digestive. See **digestive**.

stomach ulcer See **ulcer**.

stomach upsets For nausea, vomiting and stomach upsets due to eating too much of the wrong things, and providing there is no serious underlying cause, there is much to be said for a decoction, taken internally, of 6–14 g fruits of hawthorn,

Crataegus pinnatifida, to be followed later by white rice porridge. For stomach-ache, which TCM attributes to inner cold, a decoction, taken internally, of 4–10 g *cong bai*, *Allium fistulosum*, is usually effective. See **flatulence**, **indigestion** and **white rice porridge**.

stomatitis Inflammation of the inside of the mouth, and not of the stomach, as this term seems to suggest, though an overheated stomach could be causative of this condition.

stools Evacuated faeces. The condition of a patient's stools provides the physician with some information that will help him in making a diagnosis. Constipation, together with hard stools, is symptomatic of a hot and full condition. Diarrhoea or loose stools containing incompletely digested food is symptomatic of a cold and empty condition. Blood or mucus in the stools indicates that further investigation is certainly necessary. See **consultation**.

'stop the wind' This is the Chinese term which describes liver sedatives. Here, the word *wind* is suggestive of hurried activity, as are giddiness, delirium, quick temper, convulsions, spasms and excitability, which can be symptoms of a diseased liver. Obviously, for Chinese physicians, 'stop the wind' is just another way of saying 'sedate the liver'. See **liver sedation** and **sedative**.

storing herbs See **collecting herbs**.

strain See **sprain**.

streptococcus This bacterium is a common cause of infections. See **scarlatina**.

stress Chinese physicians do not underestimate stress as a source of ill health, both in the mind and the body, which is why they attach so much importance to moderate habits and a wise philosophy of living. The symptoms of stress are not only depression, anxiety, sleeplessness and tension but also certain physical conditions, such as fatigue, fainting, dizziness, palpitations, hyperventilation, headaches, neck pains, hives, loss of appetite, digestive problems and incontinence, which can be extremely distressing and also increase the risk of heart disorders and cancer. The TCM treatment for stress is to first find its source, which may be a complex, a phobia, grieving over the death of a loved one, failure to fulfil an ambition, the sheer inability to cope within one's emotional or professional territory, and so on, and eradicate it, though this is often easier said than done; and then to eat wholesome food, obtain plenty of sleep and participate in relaxing activities. Meditation and acupuncture are sometimes helpful, as are sedative medicines. But stimulants should be avoided, for they usually exacerbate the condition, and one can become too dependent on them, which inevitably results in a disguised, but uncured, state of chronic stress, which could lead to a complete nervous collapse. Some sedatives for stress are infusions or decoctions of the following, taken internally, using the parts and dosages indicated: peony tree, *Paeonia moutan*, skin of roots, 4–9 g; scullcap, *Scutellaria baicalensis*, roots, 4–7 g; Asiatic ginseng, *Panax ginseng*, roots, 2–8 g; *dang shen*, *Codonopsis tangshen*, roots, 8–14 g; schisandra, *Schisandra chinensis*, fruits, 2–4 g; motherwort, *Leonurus cardiaca*, entire plant, 3–10 g. There are those who say that stress can be healthy when it is a product of that creative pressure which fulfils worthwhile ambitions or raises living standards. But stress is stress, and it imposes burdens on the body even when it is involved with pleasure or profit. Pleasure is sometimes as demanding as duty. See **mental health**, **nervous disorders**, **serenity**, **peace of mind** and **anxiety state**.

stress and fatigue Stress produces fatigue which, if it continues, can become chronic and perhaps culminate in sheer exhaustion. However, one should not assume that continual fatigue and feelings of exhaustion are due to stress, for they could have other causes, such as anaemia and a deficiency of *qi*, as TCM physicians would say. See **exhaustion** and **fatigue**.

stress and the environment In TCM, the cardinal principle in the treatment of stress is to advise the sufferer to eliminate its cause. This is sound advice, but only practicable within certain limits because, though a person may be able to do something about the problems he creates for himself, there is often little he can do about the problems which derive from his environment, and his social environment in particular. In an uncaring society, individuals tend to live in-isolation, and the individual without collective support feels powerless. He may in fact be powerless if his burdens are not of his own making but derive from wider social problems or from the large institutions of society. Since the time of Confucius, the Chinese have been aware that a sound state of both mental and physical health is largely dependent on a wise philosophy of living. Se **mental health**.

stroke Apoplexy. Seizure. Cerebral haemorrhage. This condition is generally defined as a rupture or blockage of one of the blood vessels in the brain, resulting in a sudden disturbance of some brain functions, together with paralysis or loss of sensation in some parts of the body. There may be loss of memory and difficulty in speaking or swallowing. It could even be fatal.

However, paralysis has many different causes, and so, no doubt, in earlier times, the term *stroke* would have been applied to those conditions where there is some loss of movement or which arise quite suddenly, and which we variously describe as coronary thrombosis, a heart attack, Bell's palsy, etc. TCM recognizes two types of stroke: of the head and of the heart. A head stroke is attributed to wind, and the treatment, which is complicated, requires herbs to nourish the liver and kidneys, activate the blood and unblock the meridians. An infusion or decoction, taken internally, of 1.5–6 g roots of lovage, *Levisticum officinale*, is effective in dissolving or preventing blood clots. Acupuncture and massage are sometimes effective in providing some measure of alleviation of the paralysis. Blood-letting sometimes gives relief. Heart stroke is coronary thrombosis or angina pectoris. Both forms of stroke are more easily prevented than cured, and a wholesome diet, an adequate amount of exercise, moderate habits and avoidance of unnatural habits and stressful situations are the keys to success in this direction. See **coronary thrombosis, qi gong** and **angina**.

strychnine See **nux vomica**.

stupor Torpidity. Semi-consciousness.

stye Hordeleum. Infection and inflammation in a sebaceous gland on an eyelid, and with the formation of a small boil, or abscess. The TCM treatment is to bathe the eye with a decoction of 4–9 g flowers of chrysanthemum, *Chrysanthemum morifolium*, or 5–6 g bark of northern ash, *Fraxinus bungeana*. As a blood-cleanser, an infusion of one of the following is taken internally: burdock, *Arctium lappa*, roots, 3–8 g; marigold, *Calendula officinalis*, flowers, 2–4 g; garlic, *Allium sativum*, 2 cloves.

styptic See **astringent**.

success Chinese views about success are certainly very different from those held by many of the people of the West. Respect for one's family and ancestors features prominently in the social code of the Chinese, and Chinese philosophers are of the opinion that it is this love for one's family and respect for one's ancestors, together with the sense of continuity they bring, that is the only kind of immortality which humans can ever hope to achieve. Therefore, the wise man will make the most of his condition by being as healthy as he can for as long as he can and as contentedly as he can, for therein lies the key to success, and he will not put his faith in illusions. The *tao* of achievement, which is one of the components of Taoist philosophy, explains how success can be achieved. It reveals the exact mechanisms of human existence and analyses the influences which create events and shape their ends. It also reveals stratagems by which an individual may adjust his thoughts and deeds so that they will comply with the laws of nature, which are universal laws, and so make his life fuller and more rewarding. Surprisingly, although this *tao* was formulated more than 5000 years ago, its approach is practical and analytical and has much in common wih modern scientific thought. It involves a complete study of the phenomena and laws of nature which, in this modern age, are clearly defined by chemistry, physics, biology, astronomy, mathematics and the other branches of science. It also involves a study of social philosophy and psychology, which is sometimes called the *tao* of change, and which is based on the 64 hexagrams of the *I Ching*. It is by understanding the patterns of social change that one may develop safeguards against adversity. Is this not being done all the time, but not always successfully, by such people as economists and politicians? If to be forewarned is to be forearmed, it must surely be a wise practice to predict events by means of the *I Ching*, which operates on the principle that no event is unique, and that what has occurred before can occur again. What is abundantly clear to the students of Taoism is that its earliest contributors, who were philosophers-cum-physicians, were very much aware of the need for the right kind of climate for the promotion of sound mental health, and to this end, and with the later collaboration of the Confucians, they introduced a social code which would obviate many of the conditions and mistaken beliefs which give rise to stress and psychosomatic illnesses. They clearly perceived that, though everyone cannot be rich, powerful or talented, nor would that be desirable, everyone can aspire to a sound state of health and a long life, together with the peace of mind which derives from integrity and respect for one's family. It is surely the case that the man who attends to the needs of his family will have a non-illusory sense of purpose, and will, inevitably, be far happier than the man who gives first priority to material gain or equates ambition with power. Respect for one's ancestors does have a stabilizing and health-giving effect on society. In China, neither the young nor the elderly are neglected. The Taoists have never had any objection to commercial practices, for they are realists, and they recognize that commerce is vital to people's needs. Here, it is interesting to note that the Chinese were the first to invent coinage and paper money; and, at the time of the Song dynasty (960–1279), bills of exchange were being used. The dangers arise when money ceases to be a means to an end, and becomes an end in itself. See **I Ching**, **mental health** and **Eight Pillars of Taoism**.

sucrase See **sucrose**.

sucrose As used in TCM, sucrose is a type of sugar obtained from the sugar-cane. In the West, it is also obtained from sugar-beet and the sugar-maple, which is a tree closely related to the sycamore. It is a disaccharide, or 'double-sugar'. In the small intestine, the enzyme sucrase converts sucrose into glucose and fructose, which are monosaccharides, or simple sugars, so that they can be easily assimilated by the small intestine. See **sugar**.

suction cup See **cupping**.

Su Dongpo A poet of the period of the Song dynasty (960–1279), Su Dongpo (1036–1101) made many references to diet, health and medicine, so reflecting the Chinese preoccupation with longevity and the means of survival. See **survival**.

sudorific See **diaphoretic**.

sugar This substance, which exists in so many different forms, and which is called a carbohydrate because it is a compound of the elements carbon, hydrogen and oxygen, is an energy food. It plays an important part in the metabolism of plants and animals. By photosynthesis, plants convert carbon dioxide, water and the energy in sunlight into glucose, which is a simple sugar, and which, in turn, is converted into starch. The starch is stored in the organs of plants, but mainly in their roots, as an energy reserve, from which animals derive energy when they consume plants. In the body of an animal, by a reversal of the metabolic process, starch is converted into sugar which, in turn, is broken down into carbon dioxide and water, and energy is released and so, indirectly, animals derive their energy from sunlight.

carbon + water + sunlight energy → sugar

Clearly, the Taoists in ancient China were not thinking erroneously when they concluded that some qi, or 'vital energy', is contained in the plants and animals which are consumed as food. They had come to the important conclusion that energy has a ubiquitous quality and is manifested in different forms – light, heat, movement, etc. Sugars and starches may be conveniently classified as monosaccharides, disaccharides and polysaccharides. Monosaccharides, which are also called hexoses, are the simplest forms of sugar, and they have the chemical formula $C_6H_{12}O_6$. The commonest monosaccharide is glucose, which is also called dextrose, grape sugar and blood sugar, and it is contained in honey, grapes and some other fruits. During digestion, glucose is directly assimilated by the small intestine and carried to the liver, whence it is distributed to the tissues as a source of energy, or is converted into fat and glycogen, or animal starch, which can be stored by the body. Fructose is another monosaccharide. It is contained in honey and many fruits. Disaccharides are sometimes called 'double-sugars', because a molecule of a disaccharide, which has the chemical formula $C_{12}H_{22}O_{11}$ consists of a molecule of glucose and a molecule of fructose, which students of chemistry remember as 'one molecule of a disaccharide equals two molecules of monosaccharide less one molecule of water'.

sugar → carbon dioxide + water + energy

The most common disaccharides are lactose, from milk, maltose, from sprouting grain, and sucrose, from sugar-cane, sugar-maple and sugar-beet. Enzymes in the digestive system convert disaccharides into glucose so that they can be assimilated by the small intestine. Polysaccharides are the starches and other more complex forms of sugar. A molecule of starch may be regarded as an aggregation of many glucose molecules. Starches are tasteless and insoluble. In the digestive system, the enzymes ptyalin and amylase convert starch into glucose. The physicians of ancient China certainly did not have a detailed knowledge of the chemistry of sugar, but they were aware that it was a source of energy and could be converted into fatty tissue. They also realized that sugar could be damaging to the health if consumed to excess or of the wrong kind, and their opinions in this respect are just as valid today as they were 2,000 years ago. Whether it is used for sweetening or as a source of energy, the Chinese have a preference for brown sugar, the raw sugar-cane and honey. They are suspicious of refined sugar because it has been subjected to treatment with chemicals to make it look white and clean, but which may have also removed all the minute traces of natural substances with health-giving properties. But, in any case, the Chinese are of the opinion that the fruits and vegetables which are the normal items of diet should contain sufficient sugar for the body's needs. There is a low incidence of both diabetes and cancer in China, and it is likely that the consumption of unrefined sugar, coupled with the fact that the Chinese are not sweet-toothed, and so consume very little sugar of any kind –

they do not take sugar in tea – is one of the contributory factors in this fortunate state of affairs. See **food, cellulose, cell, survival, lactose, maltose, sucrose, sweetener** and **diabetes mellitus**.

$$C_{12} H_{22} O_{11} = 2 (C_6 H_{12} O_6) - H_2O$$

suicide See **mental illness**.

Sui dynasty The period of the Sui dynasty (581–618) was short, but it was one of great reforms and consolidation. Standard systems of money and weights and measures were introduced, the Great Wall was enlarged, the construction of the Grand Canal to link Beijing (Peking) with Hangzhou was commenced, and the empire was united under a centralized authority, which created stability, so paving the way for the Tang dynasty, which was one of immense cultural advance, including many improvements in medicine.

sulphur See **brimstone and treacle** and **mineral**.

summer food During the summer season, the Chinese will tend to consume more cooling foods, such as salads and melons and other fruits. See **cold food** and **classification of foods**.

summer-heat This is one of the six excesses of TCM. It is associated with the element fire, and it is prevalent at the height of the summer season. Its characteristic effects are a high body temperature, profuse perspiration, a dry mouth and throat, palpitations, dizziness, headaches, exhaustion and constipation. Where there is a combination of summer-heat and dampness, there will be abdominal pains, nausea and vomiting. It is important to drink plenty of liquids to replace the water lost by dehydration. See **excess combinations**.

sunburn Sunlight has some health benefits, it is true, but overexposure to fierce rays of sunshine will lead to sunburn or even skin cancer. Sunburn will heal of its own accord, but if there is severe itchiness or pain, the affected areas can be bathed or sponged with a weak infusion of any of the following: nettle leaves, camomile flowers, lettuce leaves, green tea, slices of cucumber. See **sunlight**.

sunflower *Helianthus annuus* The Chinese value this plant as a health food. Its seeds are one of the richest plant sources of protein, and they are high in polyunsaturated fatty acids and contain a wide range of minerals – iron, potassium, magnesium, manganese, copper, calcium, and phosphorus – and vitamins A, D and E and some B-complex vitamins. Sunflower oil has a high energy value – 900 kcal/100g – and it is widely used for culinary purposes in China.

Sung dynasty See **Song dynasty**.

Sun Simiao A renowned physician of the period of the Tang dynasty, Sun Simiao (618–707) perceived that there was a strong connection between diet and health, and he specialized in the treatment of deficiency diseases, which are those due to malnutrition. He found cures for hyperthyroidism and beriberi. He treated beriberi with almonds, calf's and lamb's liver, wheat germ and Sichuan pepper, all of which are rich in vitamin A and B-complex vitamins. In his 'Precious Prescriptions', he points out that longevity may be attained by wholesome food and regulated sexual habits. Liu Ching, another seventh-century physician, gave similar advice. Sun Simiao died at the age of 101, and so it is apparent that he successfully practised what he so fervently preached. His methods were essentially holistic. See **goitre, hyperthyroidism, beriberi, food and sex, essence** and **holistic medicine**.

sunlight Our survival depends on sunlight, which provides heat energy and light energy. It also forms vitamin D in the skin, which is preventive of rickets. But sunlight in excess can be damaging to the health. See **sunburn, rickets** and **survival**.

sun therapy This type of therapy can be beneficial to the health, but only to a limited degree. See **sunlight, sunburn** and **nature's treatment**.

super-ego A term used in Western psychology to denote the part of the personality which is concerned with conscience and moral issues. See **spirit** and **ego**.

superiority complex Over-valuation of one's own worth, often affected to cover a sense of inferiority. This is generally manifested as arrogant or antisocial behaviour. Chinese physicians perceive quite clearly that there is a strong connection between the health of society and the health of its individuals. On these grounds, they would discourage such behaviour since it is socially destructive and therefore likely to disturb the peace of mind and physical health of individuals.

superstitions There have always been superstitions associated with health and the practice of medicine. However, in considering some of their beliefs in Chinese folklore, one should not jump to conclusions, for many of these seemingly superstitious beliefs have a basis in fact. A good example of this is *fung shui*, which is the belief that a person's fortune is influenced by the position in which his home is situated. It is certainly the case that he will be likely to meet misfortune in the form of radiation sickness if his home has been erected above granite formations which are emanating radon. The people of ancient China knew nothing of radon, but they did know that some locations were less healthy than others. In Chinese mythology, a dragon is likened to a slumbering mountain. But when the dragon is disturbed, he awakes and then breathes fire as a sign of his anger, just as a volcano will emit burning gases and vapours when it becomes active. At one time, it was a common belief that diseases are caused by demons. In fact, the French chemist Louis Pasteur (1822–95) had great difficulty in convincing the French Medical Academy that it might be otherwise. But little demons are destructive and not to be seen. Is this not the case with pathogenic micro-organisms? See **fung shui, radiation sickness** and **micro-organisms**.

suppression This is the technique by which yin medicines are used to suppress external illnesses, which are yang. But an external illness is likely to be also hot and full, and these conditions will require cooling and sedative medicines. A yin medicine which suppresses is sometimes called a suppressor. See **herbal prescriptions**.

suppressive cycle See **element**.

suppressor See **suppression**.

suppuration The production or discharge of pus. See **pus** and **pangolin**.

supremacy The *tao* of supremacy, or mastery, is concerned with providing those devices by which a person may understand himself and others, and thereby become master of himself and his situation. To assist a person to gain this supremacy, the Taoists in ancient China provided a set of divinatory devices, which include numerology, astrology, personology, fingerprinting, directionology and symbolism. Fingerprints are taken to be an indication of a person's character, weaknesses and tendencies. The Taoists were aware that, just as no two persons are exactly alike, no two sets of fingerprints are exactly alike. Most people are surprised to learn that the art of fingerprinting originated in China, and not in India, as is the popular belief. Directionology involves electro-magnetism and the other physical influences of nature. In Japanese factories, it is used to promote harmonious relationships among the workers. See **astrology, personology** and **symbolism**.

Supreme Absolute See **Tai Chi**.

Supreme Ultimate See **Tai Chi**.

surgery A Chinese surgeon is not 'quick on the draw' with his knife, for he would argue that, as far as is possible, patients should be spared the misery of post-operative shock and pain, and that, in any case, crude surgery could do damage to tissues and organs which is almost as destructive as the condition that it is intended to cure or alleviate. Surgery is regarded as the last resort, and to be used only when other methods are ineffective. Fractures are treated with herbs, and the application of such medicines as *Yunnan bai yao* ensures that healing proceeds speedily. The *qi gong* exercises, which are described in the *Chinese Exercise Manual*, are considered to be superior to surgery for the treatment of some conditions. Be that as it may, in ancient times, the Chinese made considerable advances in surgery. At the time of the Han dynasty (206 BC–AD 220), anaesthetics were being used in the excision of tumours. See **fracture**, **Yunnan bai yao**, **qi gong**, **anaesthesia**, **Guan Yu** and **trepanning**.

survival All living organisms have six basic needs: air, water, food, warmth, light and some means of defence. If they could not satisfy these needs, they would simply not survive. The need for light is not so obvious until one comes to understand that sunlight is the main source of energy – and some would say, the only source of energy – for all organisms. Green plants trap the energy of sunlight by photosynthesis, and this energy also becomes available to animals when they feed on plants. The carnivores, or flesh-eating animals, feed on herbivores, or plant-eating animals, and so, directly or indirectly, all animals derive their energy from plants, which means that, indirectly, it is derived from sunlight. Fungi thrive in the dark, and so it could appear that they can survive without light. But that is not the case. They derive their energy from sunlight via the decaying green plants on which they feed. Means of defence take many different forms. Some plants have thorns or contain toxic substances which deter animals from feeding on them. Many animals defend themselves by camouflage, speed, flight, strength, venom, fangs, talons, keen senses of sight, hearing or smell, etc. But, for most plants and the lower animals, the main means of defence is the reproductive process. They produce large numbers of offspring, so that, even if many perish, a few will survive, which ensures the continuance of the race. Man's main means of defence is his intelligence. As the consequences of his ingenuity and inventiveness, he can outdo the large animals in strength, the birds in flight, the fish in flotation, the deer in speed, and the serpents in producing poisons; and, by speech and writing, he passes on his ideas to future generations, which provides means of defence for his offspring as yet unborn. But the greatest advantage which man's intelligence brings to him is that he can anticipate death, illness and other disasters, and so take the necessary precautions by adopting a wise philosophy of living, which surely will include a sound system of preventive medicine. But the term *preventive medicine*, as it is used here, can be misleading, for the practise of medicine in China is largely about those measures which must be taken in order to make medicine unnecessary. In this, the Chinese could claim to be masters of the arts of survival. It has been said that, if the Chinese are adept at survival, it is because they need to be, for China has many mouths to feed. Most of the arable land of China, together with the greater part of its population, is located in the valleys and on the plains which are drained by four great rivers and their tributaries. The Huanghe, or Yellow River, is subject to the most destructive floods, in which it changes its course and the banks are washed away, resulting in a great loss of crops, homes and lives. This is why it is sometimes called China's Sorrow. It is not surprising that, after many centuries of combating the destructive forces of nature exhibited by the quixotic Huanghe, the Chinese have become expert at survival. This is one of the several reasons why the Chinese manage to live together in social harmony, for they consider that they have more than enough to do in battling against nature without battling with each other. This desire has spread and become a restraining force in all the activities of the Chinese. See **cell**, **sunlight** and **life**.

suspension See **solution**.

sweat gland See **perspiration**.

sweats Diaphoresis. A term commonly used for excessive sweating, which is occasionally a symptom of thyroid disorders, and is often associated with the menopause. Night sweats are often symptomatic of nervous debility. According to TCM, sweats are caused by a deficiency of defensive-*qi*, and are common with elderly people and invalids. Night sweats are due to a yin deficiency. The treatment for the *qi*-deficiency sweating is an infusion or decoction, taken internally, of 3–6 g roots of *fang feng*, *Ledebouriella seseloides*, or 7–14 g roots of *huang qi*, *Astralagus menbranaceus*. For the yin-deficiency condition, the treatment is an infusion or decoction, taken internally, of 4–8 g roots of peony, *Paeonia lactiflora*, or 4–9 g tubers of lily turf, *Liriope spicata*. A treatment for cold sweats is an infusion or decoction, taken internally, of 5–14 g seeds of jujube, *Ziziphus jujuba*, or a suspension of 4–8 g powdered shells of oyster, *Ostrea rivularis*. A treatment for night sweats is a decoction of 12–28 g roots of *shu di huang*, *Rehmannia glutinosa*. See **perspiration** and **diaphoretic**.

sweet-and-sour dishes A Chinese meal of any size usually has at least one sweet-and-sour dish. The sauce contains vinegar, which has four advantages: it is appetizing; it provides an acid medium, which is necessary for the functioning of the enzyme pepsin; it dissolves minerals; and it destroys some of the harmful bacteria which enter the stomach. See **hydrochloric acid**.

sweet corn A variety of Indian corn, or maize, which has sweet-flavoured grains. See **maize**.

sweetener Sweetening-agent. The most commonly used sweeteners in China are honey, brown sugar and the raw sugar-cane. Artificial sweeteners, such as saccharin, aspartame and cyclamate, are avoided altogether, for they are thought to have a deleterious effect and to be possible causes of cancer. Saccharin has 300 times the sweetening power of cane sugar, but it has no energy value whatsoever. See **additives** and **sugar**.

sweet flag *Acorus gramineus* Herbal medicine. Distribution: South China, Japan, Tibet, India. Parts: rhizomes. Character: warm, pungent. Affinity: heart, liver. Effects: stomachic, digestive, resuscitive, expectorant, demulcent, soporific. Symptoms: fainting, hysteria, deafness, fullness in the chest. Treatments: tinnitus, chronic dysentery, conditions due to heat excess, excess of phlegm. Dosage: 3–7 g. There is a European species of sweet flag, *Acorus calamus*, which has similar medicinal properties.

sweet potato *Ipomoea batatas* This vegetable is a popular item of diet in China. It is a rich source of starch and easily digested. Its starch is converted into maltose on a commercial basis. See **maltose** and **yam**.

sweet wormwood *Artemisia annua* Herbal medicine. Distribution: China, India, Vietnam. Parts: stems and leaves. Character: cold, bitter. Affinity: liver, gall-bladder. Effects: antipyretic, refrigerant. Symptoms: non-sweaty fever, summer colds, nocturnal sweating. Treatments: malaria, all conditions of heat excess. Dosage: 4–9 g.

swellings A TCM remedy of a general nature for most swellings is an infusion or decoction, taken internally, of 14–28 g pistils, stamens and 'corn-silk' of maize, *Zea mays*. See **lumps** and **contusion**.

swollen eyes A TCM remedy for swollen eyes due to tiredness or a minor infection where there is no serious underlying cause is to bathe them with an infusion of 4–9 g flowers of chrysanthemum, *Chrysanthemum morifolium*, or 4–8 g leaves of mulberry, *Morus* *alba*. See **eyestrain**, **conjunctivitis** and **stye**.

swollen feet According to TCM, swollen feet are caused by tiredness, tight-fitting shoes, excessive walking and renal conditions. For tired feet, it is usually enough to remove the footwear, immerse the feet in warm water for a few minutes, apply a gentle massage, and then rest. For swollen feet due to renal conditions, a yin diuretic should be taken until the swelling departs. For cold arthritic feet, steep 60 g sage, *Salvia officinalis*, in 1 litre strong gin or some other strong spirit for 14 days, and then drink a small glass each day until the swelling subsides. For hot arthritic feet, drink an infusion of 4–5 g bark of cork tree, *Phellodendron amurense*.

symbolism In past ages, Chinese philosophers had a fondness for the use of symbols, probably because they were convenient labels and a means of identification for those concepts and entities which, otherwise, might require much tortuous explanation, particularly when conveying information to the masses. Also, the Chinese seek harmonious relationships in both the animate and inanimate world, and these symbols are convenient indications of relationships in a totally integrated world. But it is important to understand that the symbols themselves are not always realities, but forces and influences which sometimes defy definition. Thus, the element water is not real water, though it might have some of its qualities – motivity and coldness, for example. The relationships of some of these symbols are obvious, as with the element fire and Mars, the Red Planet, or with the element water and the kidneys, but the origins of some of the others are lost in the mists of antiquity and are shrouded in mystery. Many of these symbols are associated with TCM, astrology and the arts of divination. Thus, in medicine, there are relationships between the solid vital organs and tastes, climate, odours, emotions, sounds, fruits, cereal grains and animals, for some are symptoms of illness and others are medicinal ingredients or items of diet. The table below shows some symbolic dietary items. A simple colour-coding system is used with medicines and the organs for which they have an affinity. The directions – north, south, east, west, etc. – have an obvious association with astrology. Symbolism, or symbology, is a component of the *tao* of supremacy, and it employs signs, as we, in the West, employ mathematical formulae to express the laws which underlie natural events, and which may sometimes be extended to explain commercial and social trends. See **element**, **direction**, **colour** and **meridian**.

SYMBOL	HEART	LIVER	LUNGS	KIDNEYS	SPLEEN
element	fire	wood	metal	water	earth
fruit	apricot	plum	pear	chestnut	date
grain	glutinous rice	wheat	rice	pea	millet
animal	horse	chicken	dog	pig	cow

sympathetic nervous system See **nervous system**.

symptom This could be defined as one of the signs which a patient feels or notices about his condition. It could be extended to include any one of the signs which the physician finds when he makes a methodical examination. Two of the weaknesses of the practice of medicine in all parts of the world, including China, are misreading symptoms, and the tendency to suppress symptoms, that is, to treat the symptoms, and not the causes of illness. But it is fair to say that many ailments have similar symptoms, which can be very misleading; and, as one condition may lead to another, what is regarded as a symptom may also be an illness in its own right. For example, oedema is regarded as an illness, and there are treatments available, but it may also be a symptom of renal dysfunction. Therefore, *indications*, which covers both symptoms and illnesses, is a term which is preferable to *symptoms*. As far as TCM is concerned, a good rule to remember is that symptoms of conditions involving stimulation of the vital organs are yang, and those involving suppression of the vital organs are yin. See **diagnosis**, **yin-yang diagnosis**, **medicine**, **consultation** and **consultative discussion**.

syncope See **fainting**.

syndrome A characteristic combination of the signs and symptoms of a disease.

synergy A condition where the combined effects of medicines exceeds the sum total of their individual effects. This may sometimes be an advantage, but it could also produce effects which are the equivalent of an overdose. The reverse situation may also obtain, as where drugs are incompatible or mutually negating in their effects, so that their combined effects are less than the sum total of their individual effects. See **dangers with medicines** and **buffer**.

synthesis The processes by which complex chemical compounds are formed from simpler compounds, as occurs in the metabolism of plants and animals or in the artificial production of drugs (as opposed to extracting them from plants or animals). Thus, plants synthesize starch from sugar, and chemists can synthesize rayon from cellulose.

synthetic medicines See **synthesis** and **herbal medicines**.

syphilis See **venereal disease**.

systematic Of the body as a whole, and referring to treatments which affect the whole of the body, as opposed to localized treatments.

Szuma Chien See **Shi Ji**.

T

tablet See **pastille**.

tactile diagnosis This is diagnosis by feeling or touch, and as employed in TCM, it involves palpation, acupressure, percussion and pulse diagnosis. The acupoints on the meridians will be tender and painful under acupressure if the associated organs are defective. Light massage reveals swellings and the temperature of the skin. See **touch**, **palpation**, **percussion** and **pulse diagnosis**.

Tai Chi Also written as *T'ai Chi* or *Tai Ji*. The Tai Chi, which is usually translated as 'Supreme Absolute' or 'Supreme Ultimate', but which more literally means 'Great Energy' or 'Great Spirit', is the Taoist concept of a deity – and an inanimate one! – and the First Cause of the universe and the origin of life. Taoist intellectuals have always tried to understand the universe in terms of philosophy rather than religion, and they have never conceived of gods in human-like form – or, worse still, humans in godlike form – nor have they ever been ready to subscribe to naïve beliefs or accept facile explanations about the origin of the universe and man's place in the scheme of things. No doubt, the Tai Chi was first evolved as a philosophical concept which might tentatively provide a basis for discussion and evaluation of the cosmos; but, as time and time again, it has been shown to satisfactorily account for all the causes and effects in nature and all the motivations of mankind, it has come to be regarded as a reality, and one for which the ordinary Chinese have a respect which borders on reverence. The Tai Chi embodies the yin, which are negative (−) poles or forces, and the yang, which are positive (+) poles or forces. According to Taoist philosophy, order and harmony throughout the universe and within the human body are maintained by keeping these opposing and complementary forces in a constant state of delicate balance. Without this fine balance, there would be chaos. A yin force and a yang force attract each other, but two yin forces or two yang forces repel each other. 'Like poles repel: unlike poles attract.'

TAI CHI

This same rule may be applied to magnetism and many other physical phenomena. Clearly, if the yin-yang balance within the body is disturbed, ill health will result. Of course, this kind of thinking is the essential principle of allopathic medicine. The yin-yang principle of complementary opposites is quite consistent with modern scientific ideas about the structure of matter and the nature of energy. Modern science has provided us with many examples of complementary opposites in nature: light and shadow, acceleration and deceleration, the north and south poles of magnets, positive and negative charges of electricity, evaporation and condensation, etc. It is awesome to realize that the sages of ancient China anticipated Newton's Third Law of Motion – 'Action and reaction are equal and opposite' – by over 3,000 years. And the atom itself, which is the fundamental unit of matter, is a finely balanced assemblage of particles among which the protons are positive (+), or yang, and the electrons are negative (−), or yin. An atomic bomb is a spectacular example of what happens if there is a shift in the fine balance between yin and yang. The Swedish physicist Neils Bohr (1885–1962) perceived concurrence between the yin-yang principle and the theories of atomic science. The Tai Chi is the key to understanding the hexagrams of the *I Ching*, binary numbers and the electronic computer. On the Tai Chi symbol, which is shown below, the black segment, which is yin, contains a small white circle, which is yang; and the white segment, which is yang, contains a small black circle, which is yin. This is a symbolic

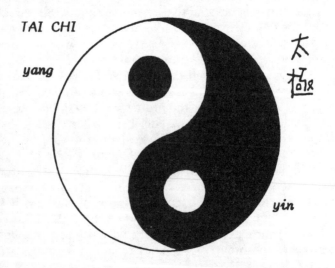

way of indicating that yin contains a little yang, and yang contains a little yin, and so neither yin nor yang can ever be entirely predominant. It also indicates that there are degrees of positivity and degrees of negativity, which is one of the principles of modern chemistry and physics. It further indicates that the universe is a finely balanced and integrated whole, as also is the human body – and, because of the influence of Confucius, so is Chinese society and its institutions. The Chinese physician regards his purpose as being that of preventing disharmony within the body; and that, by and large, is a scientific procedure as inspired by the Tai Chi. See **symbolism**, **harmony**, **allopathy** and **Taoism**.

tai chi chuan Also written as *t'ai-chi ch'uan* or *tai ji quan*. This is a system of slow-moving and gentle exercises which is suitable for the young and old alike, and which is intended to promote mental and emotional awareness as well as physical health by correcting imbalances of *qi*, or 'vital energy', within the body. Although its movements are gentle, it has been derived from kungfu, or the martial arts, and as is the case with the martial arts, it must be done skilfully if it is to be effective. It requires patience and perseverance and the ability to relate mental states to physical patterns. It is a treatment for anxiety and stress, and it stimulates the circulation and tones the muscles and other organs. It is also helpful as a therapy for diabetes, osteoporosis and poliomyelitis. According to legend, *tai chi chuan* was instituted during the eleventh century by Chang San Feng, a Taoist philosopher who sought a gentler form of the martial arts. It was further developed during the fourteenth century, when it incorporated the movements of five animals – the tiger, monkey, bear, deer and crane – which had been developed much earlier, during the time of the Han dynasty (206 BC–AD 220), by the celebrated physician Hua Tuo (141–208), but with emphasis on yin, the passive and peaceful feminine force, and yang, the active and creative masculine force. It is now a recreational and healing procedure in which everyone can participate. Some of its exercises are performed as a kind of dancing or shadow-boxing. *Tai chi chuan* is fully explained in the *Chinese Exercise Manual*. See **Tai Chi**, **Hua Tuo** and **healing exercises**.

Tai Ji See **Tai Chi**.

tai qi quan See **tai chi chuan**.

tainted and stale food See **food hygiene**.

talc Magnesium silicate. Medicine. Distribution: global. Parts: powdered salt. Character: cold, sweet. Effects: antiphlogistic, refrigerant, diuretic. Symptoms: difficulty in urination, diarrhoea, fullness in chest, summer chills, mild fever. Treatments: urethritis, damp-heat conditions. Dosage: 4–10 g. Talc has a dehumidifying effect, and it can be applied externally as a treatment for excessive perspiration, prickly heat and boils.

ta na See **healing exercises**.

Tang dynasty The period of the Tang dynasty (618–907) was one of great advance in all directions. The Grand Canal between Beijing (Peking) and Hangzhou was completed, and stage-coaches and messenger services promoted trade. Agriculture was vastly improved by irrigation systems, and the cities and large towns became manufacturing centres for silk, dyes and metal goods. The first emperor instituted professional training and formal examinations for physicians, the pharmacopoeias were brought up to date and contained illustrations of herbs, and a school of medicine was founded in the capital city in AD 629. This was the time of the physician and pharmacist Tao Hongjing, who wrote two valuable books about the development of herbal medicine since the time of the legendary emperor Shen Nong. It was also the time of Hua Tuo (141–208), who was the first Chinese physician to practise anaesthesia, and who did much research into the causes and treatments of goitre and other deficiency diseases. See **Tao Hongjing** and **Hua Tuo**.

Tao Also written as *Dao*. See **Taoism**.

tao Also written as *dao*. A Chinese word which is usually translated as 'way', but it can also be rendered as 'path', 'method', 'technique', 'mind', 'philosophy', 'principle', 'science', 'art' or 'system'. Each of the Eight Pillars of Taoism is described as a *tao*. Thus, the *tao*, or 'technique', of success, the *tao*, or 'way', of healing art, etc. See **Taoism** and **Eight Pillars of Taoism**.

Tao Hongjing A Tang-period physician and pharmacist who contributed two valuable books to Chinese medical literature: 'The Herbs of Shen Nong' and 'Anecdotes of Celebrated Physicians'. See **Tang dynasty**.

Taoism In some quarters, it has been said that Taoism is a Chinese philosophy-cum-religion which emphasizes the virtues of inactivity and the avoidance of all effort. But this could hardly be the case when one considers the enormous contribution made by the Taoists to the development of the medical arts in China. Perhaps it would be nearer the truth to say that Taoism teaches people to value their health and be inactive in the pursuit of wealth and its attendant illusions. It has also been said that Taoism and Confucianism were opposed to each other, but that, too, could hardly be the case, for Taoism, with its emphasis on harmony with nature, and Confucianism with its emphasis on harmony in society, complement each other perfectly, and they have been a twin blessing to the Chinese. What is more, Confucius had an overwhelming and respectful interest in the *I Ching*, which would not have been the case if he had had any antipathy towards Taoism, for the *I Ching* is essentially a by-product of Taoist philosophy. In fact, such was the respect which Confucius had for this Taoist-inspired work that some of his students contributed an appendix. It is generally assumed that Taoism was founded by Lao Zi, who lived at about the same time as Confucius, during the period of the Zhou dynasty (1122–245 BC), which was the Golden Age of Chinese philosophy, when Chinese society took on the form that it still retains today. But some of the tenets of Taoism preceded Lao Zi by hundreds of years, and there is uncertainty about their origins, although it is apparent that Taoism is probably the oldest religion in the world. However, there is an enigma, for people are enjoined to seek Tao, or 'the Way', but there is no clear indication of how this might be attained. Lao Zi said: 'Those who say they can explain Tao do not understand it, and those who understand it do not say.' This could make one wonder if Taoism once functioned as a brotherhood, or tong, as it would be called in China, similar to some of the secret societies in the West, whose members do their good works with stealth. But, whatever else Taoism might be, it is certainly the main source of the ever-present desire for harmony which enters into each and every thought and action of the Chinese. It is their *raison d'être*. In its purest form, Taoism contains much that is highly commendable, but in its debased forms, it often contains elements of superstition and local polytheistic religions, and in the past, it has had associations with alchemy, witchcraft, elixirs of immortality and other such practices, which are all very different from the scholarly quietism preached by Lao Zi himself. But, perhaps, the greatest debasement of Taoism was due to the influences of Mahayana Buddhism during the sixth century, and whereby, in some measure, it took on the character of a religious system, which had never been the intention of its founder. Undoubtedly, Lao Zi was a person of academic detachment because, in his advice to the peasants, he advised them to accept the status quo: 'Man can only achieve personal harmony by accepting nature and the inevitable.' See **Lao Zi**, **Tai Chi**, **I Ching**, **Tao Te Ching** and **Eight Pillars of Taoism**.

Taoist Patrology See **Lao Zi**.

Tao Te Ching Also written as *Tao-Teh-King*. 'The Classic of the Way and Power of Virtue and Nature'. This is a book of poems, proverbs and sayings which collectively represent the doctrines of classical Taoist philosophy. Its compilation is attributed to Lao Zi, who lived during the sixth century BC, but it was probably compiled during the third century BC. See **Lao Zi** and **Taoism**.

tao yin This is a version of the *tao* of revitalization, and its purpose is to utilize thoughts, body movements and instruments to control the flow of *qi*, or 'vital energy', in order to heal various ailments. See **qi** and **revitalization**.

tapeworm In TCM, the usual treatment for tapeworms is to kill them with a decoction, taken internally, of 23–50 g seeds of pumpkin, *Curcubita moschata*, and then to expel the dead worms with a strong purgative, such as 2–4.5 g rhizomes of rhubarb, *Rheum officinale*. A decoction of 5–9 g betel nuts, which are the fruits of the betel palm, *Areca catechu*, could be used as an alternative to pumpkin seeds. After treatment, it may be necessary to tone the spleen.

taro *Colocasia esculenta* The so-called root of this plant, which is, in fact, a tuber, was once the staple food in the south of China, exceeding rice in popularity. It is cultivated as a useful supplement to the cereals, and it is a valuable crop in times of famine, for it withstands floods and the depredations of locusts and other pests much better than cereals, and it is very versatile in its culinary uses. Taro, or *yutay*, which is its Chinese name, is high in carbohydrate, and so it is a good source of energy. It is also easily digested. It must not be confused with arrowroot, *Maranta arundinacea*, which is an entirely different species of plant. However, taro must be used with care. Uncooked taro tubers, stems and leaves are acrid in taste and poisonous because of the presence of crystals of calcium oxalate. If raw peeled taro tubers are handled too much, they will cause skin rashes, and if they are insufficiently cooked, they will irritate the tongue and throat. But the calcium oxalate crystals are destroyed by strong heat, so taro must be thoroughly cooked before it is eaten. As a safety precaution, the Chinese generally pre-cook taro tubers in boiling water before they peel and slice them in readiness for further cooking. See **taro starch jelly**.

taro starch jelly The starch extracted from taro tubers, which can usually be purchased from high-class grocers, can be made into a most nutritious and delicious jelly suitable for invalids and

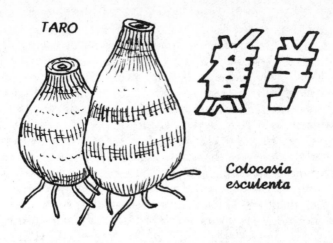

TARO

Colocasia esculenta

elderly people with an impaired digestion. Here is a recipe: put 4 tablespoons of taro starch and 6 tablespoons sugar into a large heat-proof dish, add 1 litre boiling water, stir vigorously and then set aside to cool. Consume when a cold jelly has formed. It can be consumed when hot, but it is less appetizing that way. See **taro**.

tarragon *Artemisia dranunculus* This herb, which probably originated in Central Asia, and which is used extensively in Europe for culinary purposes and as a digestive to prevent indigestion, flatulence and colic, belongs to the same plant family as mugwort, *Artemisia vulgaris*, moxa weed, *Artemisia capillaris*, and sweet wormwood, *Artemisia annua*, all of which are used in TCM.

taste The tongue is the organ of taste, or flavour. The nerves in the tongue end in taste-buds, producing four sensations of taste, which Western medicine describes as sweet, salty, sour and bitter. The illustration shows how the taste-buds are grouped and the specific areas of the tongue which produce the various sensations of taste. But, in TCM, there are five tastes, or *wu wei*: sweet, salty, sour, bitter and hot. This difference arises because Western science defines a taste as a sensation produced by a group of taste-buds on the tongue. But this definition cannot be applied to the sensation of hotness, which is produced by parts of the body other than the tongue. This is a fine distinction, and whether the Chinese or Western system of classification is better is a matter of opinion. But it is certainly the case that substances such as pepper and mustard do have a hot taste, and by no stretch of the imagination could their taste be said to be sweet, salty, sour or bitter. It so happens that hot, or hotness, is also one of the four energies of TCM, and so, to avoid confusion, substances of a hot taste are better described as having a pungent taste. Substances which have no taste are said to be insipid, tasteless or of neutral, flat or plain taste. But systems and conditions where there is little or no energy are said to be of neutral energy, and so, again, to avoid confusion, substances with neutral taste are better described as being of plain taste. The tastes are a means of classifying herbs, for the taste of a herb is a guide to the organs for which it has an affinity. Sour, salty and bitter herbs are yin; and sweet, pungent and plain-tasting herbs are yang. The taste of a herb is associated with the same element as the organs for which the herb has an affinity. Some examples are shown in the table below. The taste of a herb is also a guide to

TASTE	ORGANS	YIN-YANG	ELEMENT	HERBS
sweet	spleen, stomach	yang	earth	liquorice, hemp
pungent (hot)	lungs, large intestine	yang	metal	corn mint, ginger
sour	liver, gall-bladder	yin	wood	quince, oyster
bitter	heart, small intestine	yin	fire	rhubarb, aloe
salty	kidneys, bladder	yin	water	pangolin, cuttlefish

its medicinal properties. A few examples of the effects of medicines as indicated by their tastes are as follows. Sweet: stomach, digestive. Pungent: induce perspiration, balance *qi*, unblock meridians. Plain: diuretic, increase circulation. Sour: astringent, antipyretic, refrigerant. Bitter: astringent, anti-dysenteric. Salty: emollient, cathartic, diuretic. The table shows, in outline, the properties of medicines in terms of yin-yang, energy and direction in relation to their tastes. There can be much complexity because there is some overlapping and exceptions to the general rules. Thus, some medicines may be alike in taste but different in energy, and some may be alike in energy but different in taste. This means that, unless the physician proceeds with great care, he may treat a yin illness

PROPERTIES OF MEDICINES

YANG	YIN
Energy: hot, warm	Energy: cold, cool
Direction: ascending – moving upwards, strengthening *qi*; elevating – moving outwards, scattering	Direction: descending – moving downwards, sedating *qi*; suppressing – moving inwards, intensifying
Tastes: sweet, pungent (hot), plain	Tastes: sour, bitter, salty

with a medicine that is yang in energy, which would be satisfactory, but yin in taste, which would be unsatisfactory, for it would be contrary to allopathic principles. Furthermore, a herb may have several tastes, as is the case with cinnamon, *Cinnamomum cassia*, which is both pungent and sweet, and burdock, *Arctium lappa*, which is both pungent and bitter. This is due to the fact that a herb may contain several chemical constituents, each having its own individual properties in taste and energy. The Chinese physician is sufficiently experienced to be able to deal with these complexities, and he should generally have few difficulties, for his pharmacopoeia contains thousands of herbs, from which he should be able to select those which are suitable for the needs of his patients. Sometimes, he makes a compromise by using a medicine which is, say, appropriate in energy but inappropriate in taste, but he will know from experience that the desirable property of the medicine is potent enough to more than offset the adverse or negating effect of the undesirable property. But, in any case, there are no hard-and-

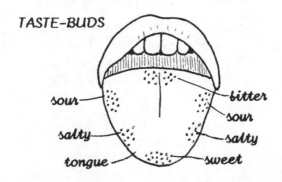

TASTE-BUDS

sour — bitter
— sour
salty — salty
tongue — sweet

fast rules, and the Chinese physician is dealing with tendencies rather than rigid situations. There are degrees of potency with the properties of a medicine, and so a medicine which is, say, predominantly cold but only slightly bitter could probably be used quite safely as a treatment where a cold medicine is required but a bitter medicine could have an adverse effect. Of course, appearances can be deceptive, and a medicine of a certain taste may have none of the properties which are regarded as being characteristic of medicines of that same taste. There are many commonly used words which are descriptive of tastes – rancid, rotten, putrid, burnt, scorched, sugary, etc. – but most of them are misleading, for they are more applicable to odour than taste. When someone says that something has a rotten taste, he means that it has a disagreeable taste – too bitter or too sour, perhaps – for putrefaction is more likely to be detected by the sense of smell than the sense of taste. The sense of taste is sometimes masked by the sense of smell. If a person is blindfolded and a slice of potato is put into his mouth, and then a slice of apple is held under his nose, he is likely to believe that his mouth contains a slice of apple. See **odour**, **energy**, **element** and **herbal prescriptions**.

taste diagnosis To a small degree, the sense of taste can be indicative of illness, and so, if a patient has an insipid, bitter, sour, sweet or unusual taste in his mouth for no apparent reason, he should inform his physician. See **taste** and **consultation**.

taste powder See **monosodium glutamate**.

TB The abbreviation for *tuberculosis*.

TCM This is now the generally accepted abbreviation for *traditional Chinese medicine*.

t.d.s. An abbreviation for the Latin words *ter in die sumendus*, meaning 'three times a day', and which is used in prescriptions.

t'e A Fujianese word which means 'tea'. See **tea**.

tea *Camellia sinensis* An infusion of this herb is commonly drunk in China as a stimulant, an aid to digestion and a refreshing beverage. But the biggest tea-drinkers in the world are not the Chinese but the Irish, who average four cups per person per day. The Chinese prefer quality to quantity, for they know that, though tea has some medicinal benefits, it can be damaging to the health if it is too strong or consumed to excess. The English word *tea*, which was once written as 'tay' or 'tey', derives from the Dutch word *tee*, and *tee* derives from the Fujianese word *t'e*. The colloquial word *char* derives from the Mandarin word *cha*, which is also written as *tcha*. Tea as a beverage is an infusion of the leaves of the tea plant, which is an evergreen shrub with shiny, laurel-like leaves and white flowers of waxy appearance. But, in the West, the word *tea* is also used loosely as the name of an infusion of any of the parts of other plants – leaves, stems, roots or flowers – or some other substances, and so, in Britain, we have camomile tea, beef tea and mint tea; and, in China, there are those fragrant flower teas, such as jasmine, honeysuckle, chrysanthemum and rose. But a tea should not be confused with a tisane, or ptisan. The Chinese insist on tea being correctly made so that it will be of the maximum benefit to the health. For this purpose, they have six rules:

1. For general purposes as a beverage, use green tea.
2. Do not use water which is stale from standing or previous boiling.
3. If you can, use soft water, but not artificially softened water. Hard water makes the tea cloudy, and water that has been artificially softened makes it muddy. Naturally soft water, filtered water or peaty water makes a good cup of tea.
4. Use a teapot of the right size. One cannot make a large amount of tea – enough for six persons, say – in a small teapot; and to put a large amount of tea – enough for six persons, say – into a small teapot will result in an infusion which is far too strong.
5. Do not allow the tea to stand too long. Over-infusion produces tannin, which is astringent and unpleasant in taste.
6. Do NOT add milk or sugar. Milk destroys the fine flavour of green tea, and large amounts of sugar especially, refined sugar, are not good for the health.

Tea contains caffeine, theophylline and theobromine, which stimulate the nervous system and assist in relaxing muscles, and polyphenols and a few of the B-complex vitamins. Polyphenols, or tannin, give tea its flavour, but an excess of them, which forms when tea is over-infused, is not beneficial. The Chinese have always valued tea for its medicinal properties, and they claim that it brings a wide range of health benefits. Apart from its function as a beverage, it is used as a soporific. A pillow or pomander is filled with black tea and other herbs as a device to improve the vision or alleviate insomnia. Tea-drinking originated in China during the time of the Qin dynasty (209–247 BC), becoming widespread in the north of China and the valley of the Yangtze at the time of the Han empire (202 BC–AD 220), and assuming great importance in the Tang period (618–907). After the end of the Han dynasty (206–AD 220), the Buddhist monks did much to popularize tea, which they cultivated on the vast estates attached to their monasteries. They claimed that tea kept them awake during their meditations. They instituted tea-drinking ceremonies as part of their religious rituals. Their example was quickly followed. Tea-houses were established all over China, and tea-drinking developed into a fashionable cult which was avidly fostered by scholars, poets and the nobility. Now, of course, the tea-drinking habit is well established world-wide. Six kinds of tea are consumed in China, and they are as follows:

Green: unfermented green leaves producing a pale yellow and slightly astringent infusion. This is the kind generally served with a meal, always being drunk plain and sipped at any stage.
Red: a fermented tea producing a strong infusion, but much less popular than green tea.
Black: fermented black leaves producing a reddish infusion with a rich and strong flavour.
Oolong: a semi-fermented tea with the fine flavour of green tea and the strength of red.
Brick: mixed teas pressed into a block. This is popular with the Tibetans and nomadic tribes in the north of China.
Flower-scented: good-quality green tea mixed with dried fragrant flowers.

The two most valued – and most expensive – teas grown in China, and which are not only of exquisite flavour but also revive the flagging spirits, are *Lung Ching*, or 'Dragon's Well Tea', which is a green tea from the province of Fujian, and *Ti Kuan Yin*, or 'Iron Goddess of Mercy Tea', which is a green tea from the countryside around Hangzhou. An interesting fact about tea is that modern scientific research supports all the seemingly exaggerated claims made for the health-giving properties of tea. It contains about 20 amino acids and about 30 polypeptides. Recent research in China and Japan has revealed that regular tea-drinkers are less likely to be affected by radioactivity. See **green tea**, **infusion**, **sugar**, **flower tea**, **herbal teas**, **Cha Ching**, **'red tea fungus'** and **tea legends**.

tea legends By tradition, tea is one of the seven essentials in a Chinese household. The others are firewood, rice, salt, oil, soy sauce and vinegar. If tea has such importance in Chinese tradition, it is not surprising that it is the subject of many legends. Some of the legends are a bit far-fetched, but they are very entertaining when told in an elaborate story-form, and some, no doubt, contain some elements of fact. According to one of these legends, the emperor Shen Nong, who is said to have taught the Chinese the arts of agriculture and medicine, was possessed of a transparent abdomen, and so he was able to follow the movements and observe the effects of the food and drink which had entered his body. He noticed that tea cleaned out his bowels, and so he recommended it as a medicine. According to another legend, there was an occasion when some leaves blown by the wind fell into the pot in which the emperor's drinking water was being boiled. The emperor was so pleased with the fine flavour which the leaves had imparted to the water that he ordered that the tree whence the leaves came should be cultivated. This tree was the wild tea plant. Another legend tells us that Buddha cut off his eyelids so that he would not fall asleep during his meditations. A tea plant sprang up from each spot where an eyelid had fallen. See **tea** and **Cha Ching**.

tears Normally, the lacrimal glands, which are situated in the upper outer corner of the eye, secrete just enough fluid to keep the eyeball moist. This tear fluid contains lysozyme, which is mildly antiseptic. According to TCM, the liver converts some of the *jin ye*, or 'body fluid', into tear fluid. See **jin ye**.

teasel *Dipsacus asper* Herbal medicine. Distribution: Central China. Parts: roots. Character: warm, bitter. Affinity: kidneys, liver. Effects: haemostatic, nutrient to bone and connective tissue, stimulates and tones the liver and kidneys. Symptoms: backache, coldness of the extremities, bleeding in pregnancy. Treatments: deficiency in liver-*qi* and kidney-*qi*, traumatic injuries to bones and sinews, menorrhagia, menstrual disorders, abscesses, pus-filled wounds. Dosage: 9–14 g.

teat Nipple. The pigmented protuberance at the centre of the breast. It contains the ducts through which the baby sucks milk from the mammary gland. See **mammary glands** and **mastitis**.

teeth The mouth of an adult human contains 32 teeth – 16 in the upper jaw, or upper dental arcade, and 16 in the lower jaw, or lower dental arcade. Of these, eight are incisors, which are for biting and chewing, four are canines, which are for tearing, eight are premolars, which are for grinding, and 12 are molars which are also for grinding. The milk teeth of an infant begin to erupt at about six months after birth, and they are fully developed by the end of the second year. There are 20 milk teeth – 10 in each jaw. Of these, eight are incisors, four are canines, and eight are

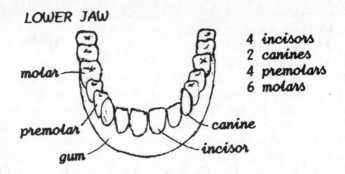

LOWER JAW

4 *incisors*
2 *canines*
4 *premolars*
6 *molars*

molar

premolar

gum

canine

incisor

molars. The milk teeth are shed when the permanent teeth erupt. The shape of a tooth indicates its purpose. An incisor is chisel-shaped for cutting, a canine is pointed for tearing, and a molar is flat-topped for grinding. See **dentistry**, **dentifrice** and **tooth-ache**.

telling fortunes See **prediction**.

temperature It is important to distinguish between temperature and heat. For example, a teaspoonful of boiling water is at a much higher temperature than a bucket of cold water; but, if the teaspoonful of boiling water is poured into the bucket of cold water, the water in the bucket will still be at a much lower temperature than boiling water even though it contains at least as much heat as a teaspoonful of boiling water. This is because the heat in the teaspoonful of boiling water is 'concentrated' into a small volume, whereas that in the bucket of water is dispersed throughout a much larger volume. Heat is a quantity of energy, but temperature is a degree of energy – hotter or colder. Heat is measured in calories or joules, and temperature is measured in degrees Celsius (centigrade), which is abbreviated as °C. The temperature of boiling water is 100°C, and that of melting ice is 0°C. The normal temperature of the human body is stated as 36.9°C (or 98.4°F on the older Fahrenheit scale, which is now obsolete). A physician may determine a patient's temperature by placing his hand on the patient's brow, but this is not an accurate way of measuring temperature, and so, these days, physicians

CLINICAL THERMOMETER

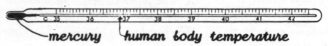

mercury   human body temperature

and nurses, including those practising TCM, will use a clinical thermometer, which is specifically designed to measure body temperatures. See **calorie**.

tender points In acupressure, these are the points where there is the most discomfort and sensitivity in a painful area. The Chinese aptly describe them as *ah shi*, which means 'ouch points'. They often correspond with the acupoints, or vital-energy points. See **acupoints**.

tendinitis Inflammation of a tendon. See **tendon disorders**.

tendon Commonly known as a sinew, a tendon is a short length of tissue which attaches the end of a muscle to the bone on which it acts. A tendon should not be confused with a ligament. See **tendon disorders** and **ligament**.

tendon disorders According to TCM, the liver controls the tendons, and so, if the liver is fully nourished, the tendons will be strengthened. However, even strong tendons can be damaged by injuries sustained in sporting activities. It would then be necessary to administer medicines to improve the circulation and *qi* in order to prevent internal bleeding and clear bruises. *Yunnan bai yao* is usually effective here. Sometimes, the tendon becomes completely detached from the muscle. This will heal in time, but some temporary relief can be provided by acupuncture and massage. The cold and damp associated with chronic arthritis may cause tender and swollen tendons. See **contusion**, **Yunnan bai yao** and **arthritis**.

tennis elbow This is a form of bursitis. One of the TCM treatments is an infusion or decoction, taken internally, of one of the following, using the parts and dosages indicated: cinnamon, *Cinnamomum cassia*, bark, 2–4 g; mulberry, *Morus alba*, leaves, 4–8 g; angelica, *Angelica anomala*, 3–6 g. See **bursitis** and **whiplash injury**.

tension The natural purpose of tension is to prepare the muscles for immediate emergency action. But, more often than not, the tension is not released, and then it could build up, and the subsequent stress could cause headaches, neck and back pains, digestive disorders, hypertension and other problems. See **stress** and **nervous disorders**.

testicle See **testis**.

testis Plural: *testes*. Testicle. Male reproductive organ. See **genitalia** and **reproductive systems**.

testosterone The male sex hormone, which is produced within the testis. See **primary sex characteristics** and **jing**.

'test-tube baby' See **artificial insemination**.

tetanus An infection caused by a bacterium present in soil, dust and the intestines of animals. It affects the nerves and spinal cord, and is characterized initially by muscular stiffness and difficulty in moving the jaw, and then by severe spasms, convulsions and difficulty with breathing. Immunization is the only effective form of prevention or treatment. See **viper**.

thalidomide In 1961, it was found that if this sedative drug is taken early in pregnancy it can cause deformity of the limbs of the foetus. This certainly indicates that laboratory-tested medicines are not always safe. See **herbal medicines**.

theobromine A white, bitter-tasting alkaloid contained in the seeds of the cacao tree, *Theobroma cacao*, and which is similar to caffeine in its stimulant effects. Cacao seeds, or cocoa beans, as they are better known, are ground to make cocoa, which is one of the ingredients of chocolate. The Aztecs valued chocolate as an aphrodisiac, which says something for the theobromine – and chocolate! The Chinese, however, are of the opinion that chocolate should not be consumed to excess. For the same reason, they do not drink large quantities of strong tea, which also contains theobromine – in addition to caffeine. Stimulants should not be overdone. See **tea**.

therapeutic athletics See **healing exercises**.

therapy Medical treatment of a disease. See **treatment**.

thermometer See **temperature**.

thiamin Aneurin. See **vitamin**.

thirst One of the symptoms of hot ailments. See **ba gang**.

thorn apple See **jimson weed**.

'Thoughts of Eminent Doctors' Also translated as 'Anecdotes of Celebrated Physicians' See **Tao Hongjing**.

threadworm See **pin-worm**.

three-points See **liu fu**.

three-stage diagnosis See **diagnosis**.

throat infections See **sore throat**, **pharyngitis**, **laryngitis** and **tonsillitis**.

thrombo-angiitis obliterans Buerger's disease. This condition, which mainly affects men, is characterized by narrowing and inflammation of the blood vessels, a tendency to blood clots and painfulness in walking. There is also the possibility of gangrene. In TCM, acupuncture and moxibustion are tried occasionally, as are medicines to improve the circulation, such as angelica, *Angelica sinensis*, notoginseng, *Panax notoginseng*, and hawthorn, *Crataegus pinnatifida*. But this condition must be treated under proper medical supervision.

thrombocyte Platelet. A small rounded body in the blood which plays a significant part in inducing coagulation, or clotting, of blood. See **blood**.

thrombosis The formation of a thrombus, or blood clot. A thrombus can occur in any part of the body, but the condition is serious when it blocks a blood vessel or interferes with the functioning of a vital organ. In TCM, a regular intake of garlic, *Allium sativum*, say, one clove per day, is considered to be effective in preventing this condition. It is significant that there is a lower incidence of thrombosis in such countries as Italy, Spain and Greece where garlic features prominently in the diet. A diet rich in tocopherol, or vitamin E, is also preventive of this condition. Sunflower seeds, soya beans, green and leafy vegetables, vegetable oils and wholegrain cereals are good sources of tocopherol. See **blood clot**, **coronary thrombosis**, **heart failure** and **vitamin**.

thrombus See **thrombosis**.

thrush Yeast infection. According to TCM, this condition is due to internal damp in the body, which is caused by an infection or a fungus. The usual treatment is an infusion or decoction, taken internally, of 4–8 g leaves of sweet wormwood, *Artemisia annua*, or 3–7 g roots of gentian, *Gentiana scabra*. Sweet and creamy foods should be avoided. There is also much to be said for strict personal cleanliness and the avoidance of casual sex, dusting powders, deodorants, perfumed tampons and foods and beverages which employ yeasts and moulds in their manufacture – beer, wine, pickles, bread, etc. – until the infection is cured. See **Candida albicans**.

thymus gland The exact function of the thymus gland, which is situated behind the upper part of the sternum, is uncertain, but it is known that it produces lymphocytes, and it is believed to have a role in the body's immune system. In TCM and Taoist philosophy, it is associated with the heart and circulatory system. Its condition can be determined by applying finger pressure to the point between the nipples. If this point is tender, the thymus gland is not functioning normally. The treatment is a more wholesome diet, the avoidance of fatty foods, and adequate, but not over-strenuous, exercise. See **endocrine glands**.

thyroid gland An endocrine gland which is situated across the trachea in the base of the neck. It consists, in fact, of four ductless glands, two of which are called parathyroids. The thyroid contains a high concentration of iodine, without which it

TESTING THE THYMUS
GLAND

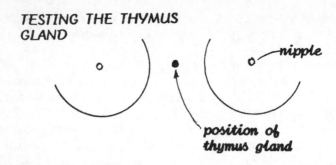

would not be able to secrete the thyroid hormone. This hormone, which contains two amino acids, regulates metabolism, thereby influencing growth and oxidation. In TCM and Taoist philosophy, the thyroid gland is associated with growth, which clearly indicates that the physicians in ancient China became aware of the function and significance of the thyroid gland long before the physicians in the West. Its two most common defects are over-activity and underactivity. See **hyperthyroidism**, **hypothyroidism**, **goitre** and **endocrine glands**.

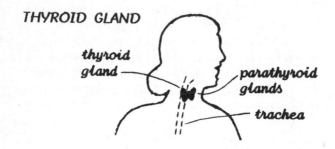

thyroiditis Inflammation of the thyroid gland, and which may be one of the causes of hypothyroidism. Its symptoms are simimilar to those of a sore throat, and the gland becomes swollen and tender. See **hypothyroidism**.

thyrotoxicosis Toxic goitre. Basedow's disease. Grave's disease. This condition, which is due to over-activity of the thyroid gland, is characterized by rapid metabolism and heart action, loss of weight, irritability and a goitre. It may also produce exophthalmus, or protruding eyeballs. TCM physicians have treated this condition successfully for thousands of years. See **hyperthyroidism** and **goitre**.

thyroxine The two main thyroid hormones. Their production is indirectly regulated by the pituitary gland, situated at the base of the skull, which secretes a thyroid-stimulating hormone.

tian ma *Gastroda elata* Herbal medicine. Distribution: China, Japan, Korea, Tibet. Parts: rhizomes. Character: warm, sweet. Affinity: liver. Effects: unblocks the meridians, liver sedative. Symptoms: dizziness, fainting, headaches, loss of feeling. Treatments: convulsions caused by excess heat, inflamed liver. Dosage: 4–9 g.

tic A habitual spasm, such as twitching the mouth, blinking the eyes and nodding the head, for which there is no apparent reason. It is often of psychological origin. It will generally clear up without treatment after a month or so. But if the condition persists, medical advice should be sought, though there is rarely any cause for alarm. According to TCM, this condition is due to wind in the liver, which may be caused by heat in the liver or blood deficiency. A helpful treatment is an infusion or decoction, taken internally, of 4–9 g rhizomes of *tian ma*, *Gastroda elata*.

tic doleureux See **neuralgia**.

tienchi *Panax pseudo-ginseng*. Despite all the great claims that are made for Asiatic ginseng, and not without justification, it seems that ginseng has a rival. It is *tienchi*, which grows abundantly in Yunnan province, as do many other efficacious medicinal herbs. When steamed, it becomes an effective blood tonic, giving strength to the body, promoting growth and bringing about an increase in vitality. It is used as a treatment for a wide variety of ailments and conditions: debility, anaemia, insomnia, fatigue, postnatal weakness and arteriosclerosis. Whether one regards it as a health food or a medicine, it is generally administered as a powder in a soup or a chicken stew. No doubt, we shall be hearing more of this remarkable substance, for it is very likely that it will soon be introduced into the pharmacies of the West. There are some proprietary brands of this medicine; and, in using these, one should comply with the dosage and instructions indicated on or in its container.

tightness of chest See **hyperventilation**.

tincture See **solution**.

Tinea The generic name for a number of fungi which infect the skin, as, for example, *Tinea pedis* (athlete's foot) and *Tinea capitis* (ringworm of the scalp). See **athlete's foot** and **ringworm**.

tinnevelly senna *Cassia augustifolia* Herbal medicine. Distribution: India, Middle East, Africa. Parts: leaves. Character: cold, bitter-sweet. Affinity: large intestine. Effect: cathartic. Symptom:

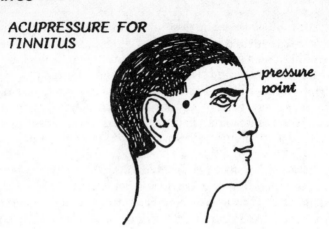

ACUPRESSURE FOR
TINNITUS

pressure
point

constipation. Treatment: constipation due to heat excess. Dosage: aperient 0.25–0.75 g, laxative 1–2.5 g, purgative 3–7 g. These dosages must NOT be exceeded, for overdoses are likely to produce nausea, stomach-ache and other unpleasant effects. See **senna**.

tinnitus A ringing or buzzing noise in the ears, and which has a wide variety of causes, including blockage by wax, hypertension and a tumour of the auditory nerve. This condition may be exacerbated by anxiety or depression. If a serious cause is suspected or the sufferer is greatly distressed, medical advice should be sought. In TCM, this condition is attributed to a deficiency of kidney-*qi*. Some recommended treatments are acupuncture to the liver, gall-bladder and governor meridians, together with moxibustion to the kidney and bladder meridians. It can sometimes be alleviated by applying acupressure at the point which is about 2 cm in front of the ear and at the top of the cheekbone. Where the condition is due to age, effective herbal remedies are eucommia bark, eclipta leaves and mulberry fruits. Haematite and magnetite are also recommended. See **deafness**.

tired eyes See **eyestrain**.

tiredness One expects to feel tired after taking strenuous exercise or working hard, but when one constantly feels tired and is easily fatigued for no apparent reason, some kind of treatment is obviously required. Persistent tiredness has many possible causes, and the obvious procedure is to identify and then treat the underlying condition. The cause could be anaemia, hypoglycaemia, premenstrual tension, menopausal difficulties, hypothyroidism, stress or hyperventilation. In its most chronic form, this condition is known as myalgic encephalomyelitis. See

exhaustion, **fatigue**, **insomnia**, **hyperinsomnia** and **myalgic encephalomyelitis**.

tisane See **infusion**.

tissue Organic matter which is homogeneous in that it consists of cells of a similar structure, and which has a particular function – fatty tissue, muscle tissue, connective tissue, etc. A tissue must not be confused with an organ, which may contain more than one type of tissue. See **organ**.

TNS The abbreviation for *transcutaneous electrical nerve stimulation*.

tobacco A narcotic-yielding plant of the genus *Nicotiana*. Tobacco is rich in nicotine, which is a poisonous alkaloid. Recent research has indicated that there is a possible link between smoking tobacco and lung cancer, but it is the tars formed by burning tobacco which are likely to be the carcinogenic agents. Tobacco addiction can constrict the arteries and increase blood pressure, irritate the throat and lungs, depress the action of the heart and cause stomach discomfort. It may lead to emphysema, and it has been known to cause loss of memory. See **smoking** and **ear acupuncture**.

tocopherol See **thrombosis** and **vitamin**.

toe-nails In TCM, brittle and fragile toe-nails are regarded as being symptomatic of a liver disorder. See **ingrowing toe-nails**.

tofu Also written as *doufu*. Said to have been discovered by Lui An in *c*.164 BC, tofu is a soya-bean curd. It is white in colour, soft in texture, low in fat and high in calcium and protein. It can be fried, grilled, boiled or steamed, and it is a good source of protein for those who cannot take lactose or milk protein.

toiletries See **cosmetics**, **chemicals** and **soap**.

Tong Sing See **Chinese Almanac**.

tongue diagnosis One of the most important parts of diagnosis by observation is examination of the tongue, and this is just as true of Western medicine as it is of TCM. The physician needs to consider the colour and texture of the tongue, the colour and texture of the fur, and the moistness and overall shape, size and muscularity of the tongue, which indicate the full/empty character of disease, together with its degree of severity. But, in making his observations, the physician must ensure that they are not obscured by temporary appearances, particularly in colour, which are due to the presence of traces of food or drink in the mouth. In a normal state of health, the tongue is pale pink in colour, soft, moist and of normal size, and the fur is thin, white and clear and neither too dry nor too moist. Generally, a swollen tongue indicates an excess of moist-heat within the body; a tender, thick and porous tongue indicates an empty ailment; a tongue of a strained and contracted appearance indicates a full ailment; a pale tongue indicates a *qi*-empty or blood-empty condition; and a bright-red tongue indicates a hot and full condition. Disease generally causes the fur to thicken. If it is also white, the ailment is cold and moist; if it is also yellow, the ailment is hot and full. As one would expect, these symptoms occur in various combinations, and the physician needs to be very observant and skilful if he is to make an accurate diagnosis. The table shows a few examples of these combinations of tongue and fur conditions. According to TCM, the tongue connects with every meridian in the body. See **observation**.

TONGUE DIAGNOSIS

Tongue appearance	Fur	Conclusion
pink, tender and lumpy	none	*qi*-empty, weak yin
white, contracted	white, thin	*qi*-empty, blood-empty
pink	white, thick, greasy	indigestion, internal inflammation
bright-red	white, very thin	yin-empty, excess heat
red	yellow, thin	ascending heat
red	yellow, greasy	excess moist-heat
red	black, dry	yin damaged by heat excess

tonic A medicine which is intended to increase resistance to disease and restore *bu yuan qi*, or 'vital primeval energies', or, as the Chinese would aptly say, 'to repair emptiness'. Tonics are used to treat debility and run-down conditions generally, and sometimes to increase virility and improve the libido. In the Chinese view, weakness is due to empty kidney glands (adrenal glands), and some tonic medicines are needed to strengthen these glands, particularly with older people, who cannot rely on food and sex alone to maintain their vigour, and so increase their chances of a long life. The most effective tonics are plant derived, and they include ginseng, tienchi, wolfberries, longans and *dang* *shen*. Horny goat weed, broomrape and a number of animal-derived tonics are effective in improving the libido. It is important to understand that tonics are either yin or yang, and a yin tonic is administered for a yin-deficiency condition, and a yang tonic for a yang-deficiency condition. See **yang tonics**, **yin tonics**, **spring wine** and **tonic treatment**.

tonic foods The Chinese have a wide range of tonic foods, which are substances that are basically nutritious but also have health-giving properties. But, apart from the medicinal effects, nutritious food of any kind can only have a beneficial effect on the body. Some of the tonic foods much esteemed by the Chinese are caterpillar fungus, longans, figs, knotty yam, hairweed, jujubes, silver wood ears and sea cucumbers. Some of these tonic foods are specific in their action: silver wood ears for the blood, jujubes for anaemia, knotty yam for loss of appetite, and so on. See **health foods**.

tonic soups In China, packeted soup mixtures, containing dried fruits, nuts, vegetables and medicinal herbs, are in common use. Some have a tonic effect, and they are usually steamed with meat and consumed during the winter months when fresh fruit and vegetables are not available. One of the more popular of these tonic soup mixtures contains cabbage, mushrooms, potatoes and carrots. Watercress, which is a high-fibre food, is a common ingredient in Chinese tonic soups. Here is the recipe for an all-purpose tonic soup which can be easily prepared from ingredients available in the West. Ingredients: 2 litres chicken stock, ½ teaspoon honey/brown sugar, 2 spring onions, 2 large carrots, 30 g Chinese wolfberries, ½ teaspoon sesame oil, 2 slices fresh ginger, 2 sticks celery, 4 cloves garlic, 1 tablespoon pearl barley. Slice the carrots, crush the garlic and wolfberries and chop the onions and celery. Put the stock into an earthenware pot, add all the other ingredients except the sesame oil, bring to the boil, cover and simmer gently for 3–4 hours, replacing the water lost as steam. Strain so that all the solids are removed, add the sesame oil, and serve the clear liquid immediately while it is still hot. Chinese wolfberries can be purchased from a Chinese herbalist and a few Chinese grocery stores, but if one knows where to look, and what to look for, they may be obtained free of charge. See **wolfberry** and **tonic foods**.

tonic treatment This is one of the eight herbal treatments of TCM. It is employed to treat those conditions described as empty because there is a deficiency of some kind, which lowers energy and resistance to disease. The deficiency is usually due to an imbalance between yin and yang in *qi*, or 'vital energy', and the blood. Tonics are broadly classified as four main types for the purposes of this treatment: those which nourish yin, those which nourish yang, those which nourish *qi* and those which nourish the blood. Yin tonics are used to treat a deficiency of yin-energy or injury to yin-energy due to yang excesses, such as fever, hotness and dryness. Yang tonics are used to treat cold-empty ailments, which are yin. *Qi*-nourishing tonics are used to treat debility and general weakness. Blood-nourishing tonics are used to treat anaemia, malnutrition, menorrhagia and other blood-deficiency conditions. See **qi**, **tonic**, **yin tonics** and **yang tonics**.

tone The yin-yang principles of complementary opposites pervades all aspects of TCM, and so it is helpful to remember this simple rule: 'Tone empty illnesses, and sedate full illnesses.' See **empty illness** and **full illness**.

tonsils Two areas of lymphatic tissue at the back of the throat, one on each side.

tonsillectomy Surgical removal of the tonsils. Tonsils seem to serve no useful purpose, and they can easily become infected, and so this operation was widely undertaken in the thirties. But it was surely a very drastic way of dealing with a condition which is not serious, and which can be so easily treated with medicine. See **tonsillitis**.

tonsillitis An infection and inflammation of the tonsils, which is characterized by a sore throat, fever, a headache, a dry cough and swollen neck glands. The condition in children, which is highly infectious, is generally due to a virus, but it can be caused by streptococcal bacteria, when the condition is then known as scarlatina, or scarlet fever. Unless the condition is serious, plenty of liquids and rest is the usual treatment. This condition rarely lasts for more than 48 hours, but if it does persist, medical advice should be sought. In TCM, tonsillitis is attributed to wind-heat and even fire-poison. The recommended treatments are an infusion, taken internally, of 8–15 g flowers of honeysuckle, *Lonicera japonica*, and a gargle with a saline solution. See **salt** and **tonsillectomy**.

tooth See **teeth**.

toothache Most people in the West would say that the only effective treatment for toothache is to visit a dentist for a filling or an extraction. But one may wonder why people are so ready to lose teeth, which are very useful tools if we wish to enjoy our food – and false teeth do have certain disadvantages. According

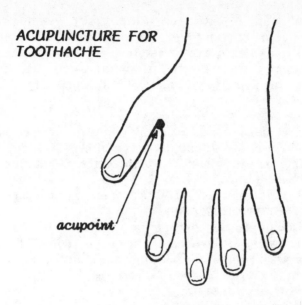

ACUPUNCTURE FOR
TOOTHACHE

acupoint

to TCM, toothache is of two kinds. One is due to heat in the stomach, and is often accompanied by an abscess or some other swelling near or under the tooth. Generally, dentists will not extract teeth from a mouth in that condition, and so the extraction has to be postponed until the abscess has cleared. However, the pain is not postponed, and so a misunderstanding sufferer might feel that his dentist has failed him at a time when he needs him most. The other kind of toothache has little to do with the condition of the mouth, and it is similar to a headache in that it is caused by a liver disorder. The treatment for the former kind of toothache is an infusion, taken internally, of 0.3 g rhizomes of rhubarb, *Rheum officinale*, or 10–30 g crystals of gypsum (calcium sulphate). The treatment for the latter kind is acupuncture applied to the point between the thumb and forefinger, but an infusion, taken internally, of 2–5 g roots of *xi xin*, *Asarum sieboldii*, 4–9 g flowers of chrysanthemum, *Chrysan-themum morifolium*, or 4–8 g roots of Asiatic ginseng, *Panax ginseng*, could be helpful. Where there is a tooth cavity exposing a nerve, chewing a clove (*Eugenia coryophyllus*) or cumin (*Cuminum cyninum*) seeds, or inserting a drop of oil of cloves into the cavity could bring temporary relief. See **dentistry** and **teeth**.

toothpaste See **dentifrice**.

tortoise *Trionyx sinensis* Medicine. Distribution: global. Parts:

powdered carapace. Character: neutral, salty. Affinity: liver, kidneys, spleen. Effects: antipyretic, tones yin, dissolves tumours and blockages. Symptoms: overheating, night sweats, amenorrhoea, pains in ribs. Treatments: heat excess, yang excess, deficiency of kidney-yin, infected and inflamed pancreas, tumours. Dosage: 8–18 g.

touch Feeling. This is one of the five senses. The body is made aware of external conditions, as indicated by mechanical, thermal and electrical stimuli, by means of nerve endings in the skin and internal membranes. See **taste** and **tactile diagnosis**.

tourniquet See **ligature**.

toxaemia A condition where there are toxins in the bloodstream.

toxic goitre See **thyrotoxicosis**.

toxin A poison of plant or animal origin, as distinct from a poison of mineral origin. Bacteria are a common source of toxins. Disease is often a case of the body or some of its functions being damaged by the toxins produced by bacteria.

trace elements See **mineral**.

trachea Windpipe. See **epiglottis**.

traditional medicine Herbal remedies are components of the folklore of people of all cultures; and, though many of these traditional remedies have been lost, a few have survived as items of conventional medicine. Some of these traditional remedies were ineffective and no more than superstition, although they might have inspired some self-confidence in the faint-hearted. On the other hand, some were extremely effective, which is as one would expect, for they were the fruits of many centuries of experience. In recent years, the medical scientists of the West have come to realize that these traditional medicines, and not only those of Chinese origin, but also those from other cultures, are worthy of study, for some of them could prove to be of immense value. For example, for hundreds of years, the juice from willow leaves has been used as a remedy for headaches and fever, but modern scientific analysis has shown that its active ingredient is acetylsalicylic acid, which is the main constituent of aspirin. Onions have always featured prominently among traditional remedies, and here, again, modern scientific analysis has shown that they contain some valuable medicinal substances. Some of the medicinal herbs used by the American Indians, such as the evening primrose, *Oenocheroa biennis*, American ginseng, *Panax quinquefolium*, and saw palmetto, *Serenoa serrulata*, have found their way into the pharmacopoeias of the West. Kola, *Cola vera*, comes from Africa. These traditional remedies have the advantages of being natural and generally without side-effects. Also, they are usually inexpensive. The Chinese have a special benefit here in that their traditional remedies have not been lost or discarded, and this, eventually, will surely prove to be a boon to the whole of mankind. See **herbal medicines**, **conventional medicine** and **aspirin**.

tranquillizer See **sedative**.

transcutaneous electrical nerve stimulation A treatment similar to acupuncture in which the nerve endings and the points on the meridians are stimulated electrically. See **acupuncture** and **meridian**.

trauma A serious external injury. In psychology, this term refers to emotional shock in its severest form. In TCM, the treatments for traumatic injury include a suspension, taken internally, of 6– 14 g powdered magnetite (magnetic iron oxide) and infusions, taken internally, of the following, using the parts and dosages indicated: centipede, *Scolopendra subspinipes*, entire animal, 1–3 g; safflower, *Carthamus tinctorius*, flowers, 2–4 g; turmeric, *Curcuma aromatica*, roots, 4–9 g; notoginseng, *Panax notoginseng*. See **shock**.

travel sickness Motion sickness. TCM recommends acupuncture and an infusion, taken internally, of 3–7 g rhizomes of ginger, *Zingiber officinale*, as preventive treatments. But it is difficult to conceive how a passenger in flight could obtain acupuncture treatment. A person travelling in a road vehicle should look to the front and not to the side, for the apparent motion of what is seen may cause dizziness and nausea which, in turn, may cause vomiting. When travelling or just before setting out on a journey, alcohol and greasy, spicy or sugary foods should be avoided. If one can prevent airsickness, one is less likely to experience severe jet lag. See **jet lag**.

'Treatise on Fevers' See **Zhang Zhongjing**.

treatment Therapy. With all forms of treatment, herbal or otherwise, TCM emphasizes the importance of finding the real cause of an illness, of not confusing symptoms with causes, and of recognizing that internal conditions are often masked by external conditions. For example, with skin blemishes, more is generally achieved by treating the blood and internal organs than by applying lotions and ointments. See **symptom** and **herbal treatments**.

treatment principles According to the ancient texts, all TCM treatments are categorized as 12 broad principles, which are as follows:

1. Treat cold illnesses with hot or warming medicines.
2. Treat hot illnesses with cold or cooling medicines.
3. Treat dry conditions with moistening agents.
4. Remove dampness with hot or drying medicines or some eliminative technique.
5. Treat elevating and outward-moving conditions with suppressive medicines.
6. Treat conditions of excess and fullness with purgatives, emetics or other eliminative medicines.
7. Treat deficiencies with stimulants or tonics.
8. Remove external causes of illness, such as climatic influences.
9. Treat sluggish or stagnant *qi* or blood with stimulants.
10. Where there is prolapse or ptosis, such as a drooping eyelid, apply a lifting technique.
11. Treat looseness, such as diarrhoea or nocturnal emissions, with a consolidating medicine.
12. Treat debility and exhaustion with warm tonics.

One should notice the allopathic nature of these principles. There is some overlapping of these principles, which is to be expected, for illnesses often occur as a combination of causes with a combination of symptoms and requiring a combination of treatments. The methods of treatments can be reduced to eight main forms. But the patient's condition is constantly changing, and so the physician must be prepared to constantly revise his diagnosis and modify the treatments and prescriptions. In this connection, Zhang Zhongjing, the author of 'Treatise on Fevers' and 'Prescriptions of the Golden Chamber', said: 'Individual treatments require not only a special consultation for each patient, as provided by the physician's own opinions and experience, but also treatments and prescriptions which will be constantly modified in accordance with the pathological changes, and several times daily if necessary'. See **herbal treatments**, **herbal prescriptions** and **Zhang Zhongjing**.

tree peony See **peony tree**.

tremor A quivering or shaking in any part of the body, and which is symptomatic of a wide variety of conditions – fear, coldness, intense excitement, etc.

trepanning A surgical technique by which a hole is made in the skull. Some archaeologists claim to have found evidence which indicates that this kind of operation was being performed in ancient China. See **spirit**.

trifoliate orange *Poncirus trifoliata* Herbal medicine. Distribution:

China, Japan. Parts: unripe fruits. Character: cool, bitter. Affinity: stomach, spleen. Effects: stomachic, digestive, anti-diarrhoeic, expectorant, controls *qi*. Symptoms: indigestion, fullness and pain in the abdomen, diarrhoea, constipation, excess phlegm in the lungs. Treatments: undigested food in the alimentary canal, stomach distension, prolapse of the rectum or womb. Dosage: 4–9 g. With constipation, this medicine has a cathartic effect. With diarrhoea, it also has the same effect, which removes the remaining toxic substances causing the diarrhoea.

trigeminal nerve See **neuralgia**.

trigeminal neuralgia. See **neuralgia**.

trigger point Trigger spot. Western medical science recognizes that there are small areas of skin which, if made tender by massage, heat, injection or some other influence, can be used to alleviate pain. Most of these small areas of skin, which are called trigger points, correspond with the acupoints of TCM. See **acupoints** and **electro-acupuncture**.

trigger spot See **trigger point**.

trigram See **Pa Kua**, **I Ching** and **Eight Pillars of Taoism**.

triple-heater See **triple-warmer**.

triple-warmer Also called the triple-heater or three-points. This is one of the Chinese hollow organs, and it is associated with the emotion of sorrow and an excess of fire. One of the three parts of this organ is the opening to the stomach, and this, when heated, as is the case with a disordered stomach, causes unpleasant effects in the mouth, and so the TCM association of the triple-warmer with fire can be understood. See **liu fu**.

tropical sore See **Leishmaniasis**.

tsa fu pei Also written as *za fu pei*. Literally translated, *tsa fu pei* means 'knocking on the door of life'. It is an easy-to-do system of exercises involving massage and waist exercises which improve the digestion and the circulation of the blood. Full details of this technique are to be found in the *Chinese Exercise Manual*.

Tsien Chin Fang Also written as *Xien Qin Fang*. 'The Thousand Prescriptions'. This remarkable work, which enjoys immense popularity in China, chronicles the history and explains the methods of all the healing exercises. See **healing exercises**.

tsubo See **shiatsu**.

tuber This the swollen tip of a root or underground stem (rhizome). The potato, *Solanum tuberosum*, is a good example of a stem tuber. Sometimes, the stem tubers of some medicinal herbs are mistakenly described as roots. See **rhizome**.

tubercle See **tuberculosis**.

tuberculosis Infection by the tubercle bacillus. There are two main kinds of tuberculosis which affect man: the bovine type, which is transmitted to man through milk from infected cows; and the human type, which is transmitted by the droplets of moisture produced by the sneezing or coughing of an infected person. At one time, this condition, was called a decline or consumption, presumably because of the emaciated appearance of the sufferer. Also, before the introduction of powerful antibiotics, and when living standards were very low, tuberculosis often had fatal consequences, for which reason it was known as the 'white plague'. Pulmonary tuberculosis is the name given to this condition when it mainly affects the lungs. Scrofula is the old-fashioned name for tuberculosis of the lymph glands in the neck. A tubercle is a mass of dense pus within an area of inflammation and destroyed tissue. The infection may proceed swiftly with a result which could be fatal. Hence, the term 'galloping consumption'. Alternatively, the tubercle may heal – or have its development arrested – by becoming encased in calcified fibrous tissue, but this can affect the functions of the surrounding tissues and adjacent organs. Primary tuberculosis is a comparatively mild condition, and may go undiagnosed. If it is contracted by a young and healthy person, it will generally heal, conferring some degree of immunity. Post-primary tuberculosis is a reactivation of the original primary tuberculosis. This can be serious, and professional medical aid will need to be sought. Tuberculosis is very much a disease of poverty and unhealthy living or working conditions. During the nineteenth century, it was very prevalent in the industrial areas and populous cities of the West, where living standards were very low. The TCM attitude is that this disease is more easily prevented than cured, and people who have a varied and wholesome diet, take regular exercise and breathe clean air, and so are in a robust state of health, should generally be able to throw off this condition quite easily. A regular intake of garlic, which has mildly antibiotic properties, could do a little towards reinforcing the body's defences against this condition. The TCM treatment is an infusion, taken internally, of 5–10 g roots of *bai bu*, *Stemona tuberosa*. Recent research in the West has shown that this is an effective remedy for tuberculosis. Traditionally, abalone, *Haliotis gigantea*, boiled with lean pork and consumed as a soup is regarded as a valuable food supplement in the treatment of this condition. Chinese physicians do not recommend rest as a therapy for tuberculosis, for this merely gives the condition a chance to develop unhindered. It is important to restore the patient's stamina and peace of mind. This can often be achieved by exercises and gymnastic activities of the type contained in *qi gong* and *tai chi chuan*. But, initially, the exercises must not be too strenuous if the patient is in a weakened state. It needs hardly to be said that one should refrain from consuming cow's milk. In this respect, the Chinese display their usual wisdom in dietary matters, and so cow's milk does not feature prominently in their diet. See **qi gong** and **tai chi chuan**.

tui na See **massage** and **healing**.

tuo mo The Chinese name for the meridian of the governor-vessel. See **meridian**.

tumour Neoplasm. Popularly described as a growth, a tumour is often named according to its position within the body, but *neoplasm* is the general medical name. It is a growth of cells of a single tissue, and which forms a swelling which has no functional purpose within the body. Tumours may be broadly classified as two main types: benign and malignant. A benign tumour does not spread throughout the body, and so it is harmless unless it exerts pressure or creates an obstruction which prevents the normal functioning of the adjacent tissues and organs. A malignant tumour spreads throughout the body or invades adjacent tissues and organs, and then expert medical aid will be required. A brain tumour is one of the causes of epilepsy. A tumour must not be confused with a cyst, though they may have a similar external appearance. TCM treatments include a suspension of 4–10 g powdered shells of oyster, *Ostia rivularis*, and an infusion of 10–30 g leaves, stems and flowers of dandelion, *Taraxacum officinale*, to be taken internally. Oyster shell is considered to be very effective in softening hard tumours. The leaves of mistletoe, *Viscum album*, are reputed to have antitumour properties, but they must be used with caution, for the berries of this herb are poisonous, and they cannot be prescribed by anyone other than a registered medical practitioner. See **cyst**, **lumps** and **cancer**.

turmeric *Curcuma aromatica* Herbal medicine. Distribution: India, Taiwan, Vietnam. Parts: roots. Character: cold, pungent-bitter. Affinity: lungs, heart, liver. Effects: haemostatic, anticoagulant, refrigerant, stimulates and tones the gall-bladder. Symptoms: fullness and pain in the chest, semi-consciousness, fainting, nosebleeds, blood in vomit or urine. Treatments: traumatic shock, hysteria, dysmenorrhoea, amenorrhoea, jaundice. Dosage:

4–9 g. Note that the turmeric described here is the wild species, which is somewhat more potent that the cultivated species, *Curcuma longa.*

turtle *Chinemys reevesii* Medicine. Distribution: global. Parts: powdered plastron (underside shell). Character: neutral, salty-sweet. Affinity: heart, liver, kidneys. Effects: tonic to kidneys and yin, nourishes bones and connective tissue. Symptoms: heat bouts, night sweats, weakness of voice, weakness of limbs, backache. Treatments: deficiency of kidney-yin, injuries to bones and connective tissue, deficiency of yin caused by heat injuries, menorrhagia, lack of contractions associated with difficult or delayed childbirth, poor growth in bone and cartilage in infants. Dosage: 9–24 g.

twelve pulses See **pulse diagnosis**.

tympanum Ear-drum. See **ear**.

typhoid fever An infectious bacterial disease characterized by fever, diarrhoea, pain in the intestines, red spots on the chest and abdomen, and bloodstained stools, sometimes with a heavy loss of blood. The disease is severe; and, in past ages, it took many lives. The typhoid bacteria, which occur in unclean food and water and the stools and urine of man, are spread by flies and poor sanitation. Improved sanitation and powerful antibiotics have made this disease much less of a killer. In the Chinese view, typhoid is more easily prevented than cured – and the preventive treatment must surely be cleanliness. At one time, in the West, wells to provide drinking water were commonly sunk near to graveyards, and with consequences which were often disastrous. Such wells certainly had a great deal of very bad *fung shui*! See **paratyphoid fever** and **fung shui**.

typhus A group of infectious diseases caused by parasitic micro-organisms of the genus *Rickettsia*, and which are transmitted by lice, fleas, mites and ticks. The condition is characterized by fever, purple spots and other rashes, aching limbs and back, severe prostration, delirium and sometimes a mild form of pneumonia. See **vector**.

U

ulcer An ulcer may be briefly defined as an open sore resulting from a break or defect in the skin or a membrane, and which exposes the underlying tissues. An ulcer may lead to the formation of a fistula, which is a tubelike structure connecting two hollow organs or a hollow organ and the skin. Ulcers are internal or external, and they are usually named after the part of the body where they occur: a gastric ulcer in the stomach, a duodenal ulcer in the small intestine, an oesophageal ulcer in the oesophagus, and so on. Gastric, duodenal and oesophageal ulcers are collectively described as peptic ulcers. Small ulcers in the mouth, and which often result from an over-heated stomach, are generally easily treated by gargling with an antiseptic fluid. There are many kinds of skin ulcers, which generally result from some kind of irritation or infection, and they include bed, or pressure, sores, leprosy sores and those due to varicose veins and other circulatory disorders. Peptic ulcers are caused by an excess of acid or the enzyme pepsin. The small ones may occur without symptoms and heal without treatment. But some, which generally occur among men in the upper age group, are much more serious, and are characterized by flatulence, indigestion, vomiting, abdominal pain, tenderness below the breastbone and, occasionally, bloody vomit and black stools. They are aggravated by stress, alcohol, smoking and spicy or greasy food. With these ulcers, medical advice must be sought because, if a peptic ulcer ruptures, some of the infected contents of the intestine may enter the abdominal cavities, so causing peritonitis, or inflammation of the peritoneum, which is a dangerous condition. Stress, including the effects of anxiety or noise, is often the cause of duodenal ulcers in young men, but these are generally not incapacitating, and the only symptoms are indigestion and a dull pain in the abdomen. Until recent years, troublesome peptic ulcers were removed by surgery; but, nowadays, the preference is for the use of medicines and other less drastic methods. In TCM, peptic ulcers are attributed to stagnation of stomach-*qi* and liver-*qi* and

CUTTLEFISH

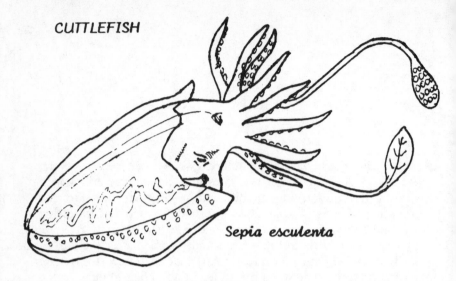

Sepia esculenta

weakness of the spleen. Liver stagnation causes anxiety and depression, which introduces further complications. With mild cases, the treatment involves medicines to clear the heat, remove stagnation and assist digestion. Some beneficial effects are derived from the application of acupuncture to the meridians of the stomach, liver, spleen, bladder, conception-vessel and governor-vessel. In chronic cases, where there is likely to be internal bleeding and spleen weakness, astringent medicines will need to be applied. Also, the patient must relax and take care with his diet, avoiding tea, coffee, alcohol, milk and spicy, greasy and cold foods, such as salads and duck meat. The TCM herbal treatments are infusions or decoctions, taken internally, of the following, using the parts and dosages indicated. Dandelion, *Taraxacum officinale*, stems and leaves, 10–30 g; notoginseng, *Panax notoginseng*, roots, 4–8 g; peony tree, *Paeona moutan*, skin of roots, 4–9 g; honeysuckle, *Lonicera japonica*, flowers, 9–16 g; liquorice, *Glycerrhiza uralensis*, roots, 2–8 g. Also helpful is a suspension, taken internally, of 4–8 g powdered bone of cuttlefish, *Sepa esculenta*. Some of these herbs could be administered as paste pills, which ensure that the potent ingredients are absorbed without any adverse effects. Medicines for the treatment of stress may also be required, but it is important that they should not have an irritant effect on sensitive membranes. Peony tree, as listed above, is useful here. An effective treatment for minor ulcers on the skin is an ointment or cold compress of the flowers of marigold, *Calendula officinalis*. Peptic ulcers may cause severe pain and discomfort in the solar plexus, where there is a network of nerves which relate to the stomach and intestines. In the West, it is sometimes the practice to eliminate this pain by severing the vagus nerve. But this really is a case of treating the symptoms and not the cause. See **sedative**, **stress**, **paste pills**, **mouth ulcers**, **olive oil**, **colitis** and **vagus nerve**.

ulcerative colitis This is a condition in which the large intestine is ulcerated, and accompanied by diarrhoea and blood and mucus in the stools. TCM attributes it to dampness and internal burning heat injuring the blood vessels and poisoning the intestine. The treatment is an infusion or decoction, taken internally, of 10–30 g leaves and stems of dandelion, *Taraxacum officinale*. Where the condition is chronic, there may be a spleen deficiency, which is treated with an infusion or decoction, taken internally, of 7–14 g roots of *huang qi*, *Astralagus membranaceus*. See **colitis**.

ulna See **skeleton**.

ultraviolet rays Electromagnetic radiation of short wavelength which converts a cholesterol derivative in the skin into vitamin D. This is beneficial to the health, and so the Taoist philosophers were not mistaken when they perceived that sunlight is a source of *qi*, or 'vital energy', though they could not have been aware of its full range of benefits. But, then, primitive man was not entirely mistaken when he regarded the sun as an object of worship. See **sunlight** and **rickets**.

umbilical cord See **reproductive systems**.

umbilicus Navel. See **reproductive systems**.

umbilical pulse There are several places on the body, other than the wrist, where the pulse of the heart can be felt. From the beginning of the third month of pregnancy, a pregnant woman should be able to feel her pulse, which she shares with her unborn baby, at her navel. See **pulse**.

unconsciousness This condition is generally due to a fall in the blood supply to the brain, which can be caused by shock, severe haemorrhage or heart failure. But it can also be caused by a blow to the head, a brain tumour or an overdose of a sedative, soporific or narcotic drug. Depending on the cause, unconsciousness can lead to death. Providing that there is no serious underlying cause, a semi-conscious state due to traumatic shock or loss of blood can be treated with an infusion or decoction of 4–9 g roots of turmeric, *Curcuma aromatica*. See **fainting** and **coma**.

undulant fever See **brucellosis**.

unguent See **ointment**.

universe In ancient China, as in medieval Europe, ideas about the
structure and nature of the universe were vague and sometimes
based upon the wildest of conjectures. The Chinese believed that
the earth is in the shape of a square, and that China is at its
centre. The Chinese word for *China* literally means 'centre-land'.
In Chinese astrology, there are four directions – perhaps *positions*
would be a more accurate term – which are used symbolically in
Chinese medicine to denote the vital organs and their relationship
to other influences. Fevers and hot illnesses are said to be
ascending, or north-moving, and fainting and traumatic injuries
are said to be descending, or south-moving. No doubt, inward-
moving and outward-moving conditions could be related to
movements between east or west and the centre. The condition
of a person in a normal state of health is symbolized by the point
which is midway between the complementary opposites of north
and south and east and west, that is, the centre. In TCM theory,
the heart, which is south and hot, is complemented by the
kidneys, which are north and cold. The liver, which is east and
windy, is complemented by the lungs, which are west and dry.
The spleen is at the centre, for it is the TCM opinion that it is the
spleen, and not the heart or the brain, which is the most
important organ in the body. The Chinese also assumed that
heaven is circular. But, here, they were not using the word
heaven in a religious sense, but as we in the West use the words
firmament and *hemisphere*; and, indeed, the sky does have the

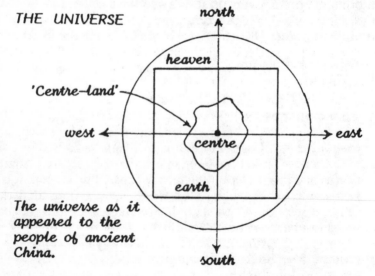

THE UNIVERSE

The universe as it
appeared to the
people of ancient
China.

appearance of an inverted dome. 'And that inverted Bowl we call The Sky, whereunder crawling coop't we live and die,' wrote the eleventh-century Persian poet Omar Khayyám. The appearance of the night sky, with its array of stars, does create an impression of solidity. It is not altogether surprising that the people of medieval Europe believed that the stars are holes in the floor of heaven. Of course, the philosophers in ancient China were totally wrong in some of their assumptions. Nevertheless, here and there, their reasoning had the quality of logic. See **heaven**, **element**, **vital organs** and **Pangu**.

uraemia An abnormally excessive amount of urea in the blood, which is associated with renal failure. See **urea** and **urinary disorders**.

urea A soluble and colourless crystalline nitrogeneous substance which is one of the main products of the breakdown of protein within the body. See **urine**.

ureter The tube which conveys urine from the kidneys to the bladder. See **reproductive systems**.

urethra The part of the urinary tract which conveys urine from the urinary bladder to the outside of the body. See **reproductive systems**.

urethritis Inflammation of the urethra. See **urinary disorders**.

uric acid One of the main products of the breakdown of proteins within the body. See **urine**.

urinary bladder The sac that holds urine, which is conveyed to it from the kidneys by two ureters. It is commonly called the bladder, and it is only referred to as the urinary bladder when it is necessary to distinguish it from the gall-bladder. See **urinary tract** and **reproductive systems**.

urinary disorders Two of the main infections of the urinary tract are cystitis and urethritis. Cystitis, which rarely affects men, is characterized by a burning sensation in urination, frequent trips to the toilet and pain in the back and abdomen, and is generally due to bacteria from the anus entering the bladder, where they infect and inflame the membrane. But there are other causes, such as food allergies, sensitivity to chemicals and certain drugs, vaginal thrush and bruising due to violent sexual intercourse. If there is blood in the urine, medical advice should be sought. TCM ascribes this condition to damp-heat, and its recommended treatment is an infusion, drunk as a tea, of 4–10 g seeds of plantain, *Plantago asiatica*, or 4–5 g bark of cork tree, *Phellodendron amurense*, which will ease the discomfort. A remedy from Chinese folklore is a tea, to be drunk frequently, made by infusing a mixture of 5 g leaves of bamboo, 5 g tubers of water plantain, *Alisma plantago-aquatica*, and 4 g corn silk of maize, *Zea mays*. The TCM treatments for urethritis are infusions or decoctions, taken internally, of the following, using the parts and dosages indicated: burdock, *Arctium lappa*, seeds or roots, 4–10 g; long yam, *Discorea hypoglauca*, roots, 9–14 g; talc (magnesium silicate), powder, 4–10 g. Other disorders of the urinary tract are bladder stones and bladder cancer, but these conditions are rare. The normal functioning of the urinary tract can be affected by a diseased prostate gland or kidney stones, which may block the urethra. As items of diet, maize, celery and a pig's bladder have a soothing effect with urinary disorders. Uraemia is associated with urinary disorders, but it is almost always caused by a renal disorder. The *Chinese Exercise Manual* contains healing exercises for the treatment of cystitis and to strengthen the pelvic muscles. See **urinary incontinence**, **prostate problems**, **uraemia**, **pig's bladder** and **renal disorders**.

urinary incontinence This very common condition among elderly people is characterized by frequent and uncontrolled urination. The sufferer may dribble and not be aware of it. The causes include cystitis, stroke and spinal injury, together with prostate problems in men, and prolapse of the womb, bladder or rectum in women. TCM treatments to provide some relief include acupressure applied upwards to the hollow between the inner ankle bone and the Achilles tendon. See **urinary disorders**, **incontinence**, **enuresis** and **prolapse**.

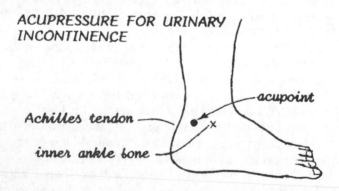

ACUPRESSURE FOR URINARY
INCONTINENCE

acupoint

Achilles tendon

inner ankle bone

urinary stone Bladder stone. Urinary stones generally form only when the mucous membrane of the bladder is damaged by an infection. Therefore, treatment for a bladder infection may assist in preventing the formation of bladder stones. Larger stones are removed surgically, but the smaller stones will pass out with the urine, a process which can be assisted by administering suitable diuretics. TCM recommends infusions, taken internally, of the following, using the parts and dosages indicated. Chinese plum, *Prunus japonica*, kernels, 4–6 g; dandelion, *Taraxacum officinale*, leaves and stems, 10–30 g; Indian bread, *Poria cocos*, whole plant, 4–9 g; plantain, *Plantago asiatica*, seeds, 4–9 g; akebia, *Akebia quinata*, stems, 4–6 g. See **calculus** and **urinary disorders**.

urinary tract This comprises the ureters, bladder and urethra. See **reproductive systems**.

urination Micturition. There are problems which can affect the normal passage of urine from the body. See **urinary disorders** and **urinary incontinence**.

urine This liquid, which is derived from blood by the filtering mechanism of the kidneys, is the means by which the body excretes its nitrogeneous wastes, which are mainly urea and uric acid, together with excess water and excess mineral salts. See **urination**.

urine diagnosis In TCM, as with other systems of medicine, the condition of the urine is an aid to diagnosis. Its colour, hotness and scantiness are usually the tell-tale signs of some diseases and defects of the body. In TCM, clear and abundant urine may be a symptom of a cold and empty ailment, whereas dark and scanty urine is usually a symptom of an excess of heat. Cloudy urine generally indicates an excess of damp-heat. If there is blood in the urine, there may be cause for alarm. Understandably, the condition of the urine is taken to be an indication of the state of the kidneys and bladder, but other organs may be involved. See **observation, jin ye** and **ba gang**.

urino-genital organs See **urogenital organs**.

urogenital organs Urino-genital organs. The urinary and genital organs are generally studied together because they are in close proximity and their separate functions may be carried out by the same organ or part of an organ. For example, both semen and urine are discharged from the body via the urethra. Furthermore, they are often susceptible to the same diseases. Sexually transmitted diseases are likely to affect the bladder and ureters, which are urinary organs. A disease of the prostate gland may affect the bladder, and weakness of the pelvic muscles may lead to prolapse of the rectum, which can affect both urination and sexual performance. The *Chinese Exercise Manual* contains exercises to strengthen the pelvic muscles. See **urinary disorders**.

urticaria See **hives**.

uterine disorders Among the various conditions which produce infertility or cause a miscarriage are those which directly affect the uterus. They include failure to ovulate, which may be due to hormonal imbalance, stress or anxiety, a sudden weight loss or a condition affecting the ovaries. Also, a deficiency of the hormone progesterone can lead to failure of the embryo to implant itself in the lining of the wall of the uterus, the uterine tubes may become blocked by an infection, too much cervical mucus may prevent the spermatozoa from reaching the ova, and certain abnormalities, such as fibroids or the shape of the uterus, may prevent implantation of the embryo. Fibroids are non-malignant tumours. TCM attributes most uterine disorders to fibroids, colic and infections. The Chinese physician will use a wide range of herbs which both enlarge the uterus and contract the fibroids, thus eliminating the need for surgery. But do-it-yourself medicine should be avoided with these conditions, for there are risks involved. Where uterine disorders are suspected, medical advice should be sought. See **infertility** and **reproductive systems**.

uterus Womb. A hollow organ which is situated in the pelvis in females, and in which a fertilized ovum, or egg, becomes implanted and then develops during the period of pregnancy. See **fertility**, **reproductive systems** and **ear acupuncture**.

V

vaccination See **immunology** and **Jesuits**.

vaccinia See **immunology**.

vagina The 'passage', in a female, which connects the vulva to the uterus. See **reproductive systems**.

vaginal bleeding See **postnatal problems**.

vaginal disorders The most common disorder of the vagina is an excessive discharge accompanied by itchiness, inflammation and an unpleasant odour. This condition is generally due to an infection, which has a variety of causes: *Candida albicans*, a small micro-organism called *Trichomonas*, gonorrhoea or pin-worms. The vagina may become dry and sore after the menopause, and it may also be painful during sexual intercourse. A regular intake of garlic, say, one clove per day, helps to prevent all vaginal disorders. See **Candida albicans** and **pin-worm**.

vaginal thrush See **Candida albicans**.

vaginitis Inflammation of the vagina. See **vaginal disorders**.

vagotomy Surgical severance of the vagus nerve as a treatment for a severe peptic ulcer. TCM physicians would probably regard this as an example of surgery at its unenlightened worst. See **ulcer**.

vagus nerve Pneumogastric nerve. Tenth cranial nerve. Its branches are connected with the muscles of the throat, and also regulate the secretions and tonicity of the organs in the chest and abdomen. See **ulcer**.

varicella Chicken-pox. This highly infectious viral disease, which generally only affects children, is characterized by an irritating rash of small pink spots on the trunk and upper thighs, which turn to blisters. The incubation period is 14–21 days, and the isolation period is about 14 days, though enforced isolation is not always helpful, for catching chicken-pox in childhood confers immunity to the disease in later life, when it can be far more serious in its effects. Adults who fall victim to chicken-pox will feel very ill for a few days, and the blisters will turn into scabs. In TCM, chicken-pox is attributed to invasion by wind and heat, and the treatment is an infusion, taken internally, of 9–15 g flowers of safflower, *Carthamus tinctorius*. Duck meat and raw garlic, say three cloves per day, are also helpful. See **shingles**.

varicose veins According to the medical scientists of the West, varicose veins are an inherited condition which affects about one-fifth of the population, who are mainly women. Its sufferers have weakened veins which are ineffective in returning blood to the heart, and so the blood becomes sluggish and the veins become lengthened and distended and form tortuous networks with persistent itchiness and aches in the affected areas. Varicose veins occur mainly in the legs because their veins are at the greatest distance below the heart, and therefore in positions where the blood is likely to accumulate and cause distension. It is helpful to lose weight to reduce pressure on the legs, wear loose-fitting clothes which do not restrict the circulation, avoid standing for long periods and take exercise to keep the blood on the move. In TCM, and as one would expect, poor circulation of the blood is regarded as being the major cause of this condition. And again as one would expect, the TCM treatment requires that *qi*, or 'vital energy', and the blood should be kept on the move. For this purpose, infusions or decoctions, taken internally, of the following, using the parts and dosages indicated, are recommended: angelica, *Angelica sinensis*, roots, 9–14 g; *huang qi*, *Astralagus membranaceus*, roots, 7–14 g; cinnamon, *Cinnamomum cassia*, bark, 1–4 g. If the veins become ulcerated, honey or a wet compress of flowers of marigold, *Calendula officinalis*, could be applied. They have a sterilizing and healing effect. See **ulcer**.

varied diet See **dietetics**.

variola Smallpox. See **immunology** and **Jesuits**.

vasodilator A medicine to dilate blood vessels, and so inhibit coagulation and the formation of thrombi, thereby preventing strokes, hypertension and heart failure. Vasodilators commonly used in TCM are garlic, *Allium sativum*, hawthorn, *Crataegus pinnatifida*, and corn mint, *Mentha arvensis*.

vas deferens The tube which conveys spermatozoa from the testis to the urethra. See **reproductive systems**.

vasectomy The surgical severance of the vas deferens as a method of sterilizing the male. This is not a surgical procedure which would meet with the wholehearted approval of TCM physicians. It is rather on a par with severing the gullet to inhibit gluttony.

vector An animal which carries an infection or a source of infection. Rats, mice, fleas, lice, ticks, mites, cockroaches, houseflies and mosquitoes are some well-known vectors. They all carry micro-organisms of one kind or another, some of which infect humans. For example, mosquitoes carry the malarial parasite, *Plasmodium vivax*, the tsetse fly carries the sleeping-sickness parasite, *Trypanosoma gambiense*, and the housefly carries the typhoid fever bacterium. Sometimes, the vector is the carrier of a carrier. This is the case with the rat, which carries a species of flea that harbours the micro-organism causing bubonic plague. For the health-conscious Chinese, pest control is as much a priority as it is for the people of the West. See **parasite**, **flea**, **malaria** and **Weil's disease**.

vegan A person who consumes no animal produce of any kind, not even milk, eggs or cheese. See **vegetarian diet**.

vegetable oil See **oil**.

vegetables In general, vegetables have low energy values because most of their content is water; and, with the exception of the pulses and certain cereals, they contain very little protein or fat. But they are high in dietary fibre, and contain varying amounts of starch and sugar, together with a wide range of minerals and vitamins, though some of the vitamins are destroyed when the vegetables are cooked. Some medical experts in the West are of the view that regular consumption of green leafy vegetables is preventive of cancer, and that lack of dietary fibre can cause cancer of the large intestine. The causes of cancer are complex and so it is difficult to make simple statements about single items of diet. A healthy diet does NOT make a person cancer-proof, but it will certainly increase the odds against developing cancer. But there is tremendous variety in the nutritive and medicinal contents of vegetables, and so they must be consumed in a wide variety if the fullest benefit is to be derived from them, as the Chinese well know. See **dieting**, **vegetarian diet** and **cancer**.

vegetarian diet The Chinese diet is essentially vegetarian, but it is certainly not a vegan diet, for the Chinese recognize that some nutrients and health-giving substances are more readily available in meat, fish and eggs than they are in plant produce. But, with the Chinese, this is a matter of sensible compromise. They arrange their diet in such a way that the ill-effects of consuming red meat and animal fats are considerably outweighed by the beneficial effects of consuming plant produce. See **vegan**, **dieting** and **Buddhism**.

venereal disease A disease that is transmitted by sexual activity, and which is rarely transmitted in any other way. The three most common forms are gonorrhoea, syphilis and chancroid. The other forms occur mainly in the tropical regions. Syphilis is due to infection by the bacterium *Treponoma pallidum*, and develops in three stages. At the first stage, a chancre, or sore, appears about three weeks after the infection at the point where the infection entered the body, which is likely to be the genitals, anus or mouth. The secondary stage develops about six weeks after the chancre has healed, when the bacteria begin to spread throughout the body, and the skin and membranes are affected by the development of sores, rashes and swollen lymph glands. The third stage may appear many years later, and is characterized by injuries to the brain, spinal cord, heart, eyes, bones and other organs. Chancroid is due to infection by the bacterium *Haemophilus ducrey*, and is characterized by an open soft sore on the genitals, but it is not related to syphilis. In the West, the development of powerful antibiotics has done much towards the effective treatment of these conditions, but Chinese physicians have always taken the view that they are easily prevented by the exercise of self-control. See **gonorrhoea**, **AIDS**, **morality**, **mercury** and **general paralysis of the insane**.

venereal herpes See **herpes**.

venom A toxic fluid secreted by scorpions and certain spiders, snakes and insects, and introduced into the victim by a bite or sting. See **toxin**, **bites** and **stings**.

ventilation Breathing. See **hyperventilation**.

vermicide A medicine to kill parasitic worms in the intestine. See **vermifuge** and **anthelmintic**.

vermiform appendix See **intestine**.

vermifuge A medicine to expel parasitic worms from the stomach. See **vermicide** and **anthelmintic**.

verruca See **wart**.

vertebra Plural: *vertebrae*. One of the 33 small bones which make up the vertebral column. See **intervertebral discs**.

vertebral column Backbone. Spine. Spinal column. See **intervertebral discs**, **skeleton**, **osteopathy** and **chiropractic**.

vertigo Giddiness and loss of balance accompanied by the sensation that the head or the surroundings are in motion. It has a variety of causes, which include nausea, travel sickness, tinnitus, inflammation of the semicircular canals in the middle ear, hypertension and arteriosclerosis. If this condition persists, medical advice should be sought. TCM regards this condition as a symptom of hypertension, which it attributes to one of three possible causes: a deficiency in *qi* or in the blood, liver-wind or excess phlegm. A TCM treatment for hypertension is an infusion, taken internally, of 5–9 g flowers of chrysanthemum,

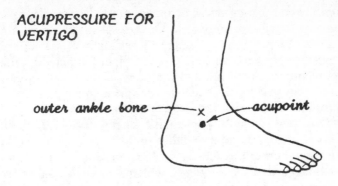

ACUPRESSURE FOR
VERTIGO

outer ankle bone —— x —— acupoint

Chrysanthemum morifolium. Some relief is achieved by acupuncture or moxibustion applied to the meridians of the governor-vessel, gall-bladder and bladder. Acupressure can be helpful. It is applied to a point which is about two centimetres below the outer ankle bone. See **ear** and **hypertension**.

veterinary medicine In recent years, a few of the veterinary surgeons in the West have adopted acupuncture as a technique for treating certain conditions in animals. But, at the time of the Han dynasty (206 BC–AD 220), the Chinese were developing veterinary medicine, for one of the Gansu books contains a remedy for the treatment of a sick horse. See **Gansu books**.

vibrio See **bacterium**.

victor-vanquished rule See **element**.

victory-subjugation rule An alternative name for the victor-vanquished relationship of elements. See **element**.

vinegar Briefly defined, vinegar is an impure and dilute – about 3–6% – solution of ethanoic acid, which is obtained by the action of bacteria on wine, beer or cider. At one time, vinegar was made by standing wine with its surface exposed to the atmosphere. Bacteria entered it and decomposed the alcohol to form sour-tasting vegetable acids. Malt vinegar, as its name suggests, is made from beer. Vinegar is also made synthetically. In China, vinegar is derived from rice wine, and that made from black rice wine is considered to be the best for medicinal purposes. Vinegar is commonly used as a condiment and for preserving foodstuffs, but it also has medicinal properties. See **ethanoic acid**, **Candida albicans** and **sweet-and-sour dishes**.

viper *Agkistrodon acutus* Medicine. Distribution: East China, Vietnam. Parts: Whole animal except the head. Character: warm, sweet-salty. Affinity: liver. Effects: sedative, anthelmintic, antirheumatic. Symptoms: paralysis, rheumatic aches and pains, convulsions. Treatments: arthritis, gout, Bell's palsy, paralysis, leprosy, tetanus, ringworm. Dosage: 4–10 g. There are many species of viper, and it is likely that some have similar medicinal properties, but it is unwise to use a viper medicinally unless one is certain that it is suitable for that purpose. Also, one should remember that the flesh of a viper is poisonous.

Virginia truffle See **Indian bread**.

virility Sexual strength, particularly of the male. Where there is a loss of virility, an improved diet could be helpful. In TCM, there are some herbal medicines, such as ginseng, *Panax ginseng*, and wolfberry, *Lycium chinense*, which could be taken for this condition. There are also some animal-derived medicines which are thought to be effective in this respect. But some of them are reputed to be aphrodisiacs, and so they should be regarded with suspicion, for they take more out of the body than it can safely give. They provide a temporary boost, but, after that, there is more likely to be a state of exhaustion than any increase in virility. Traditionally, in China, persimmon wine is regarded as being an aid to the libido. But improving the quality of the sperm by natural methods is probably the only reliable way of increasing virility. See **animal-derived medicines**, **libido**, **impotence** and **jing**.

virus This is the simplest form of life. Viruses are parasites and are completely dependent upon their host organisms. It seems that they represent a stage which is intermediate between the living and the non-living, for they can exist as crystals but can multiply only in living cells. Of course, the physicians in ancient China were not aware of the existence of viruses, but they certainly knew how to treat those ailments, such as hepatitis, influenza and the common cold, which are viral infections. Recent research in China has shown that some of the herbs of TCM are effective in destroying viruses. It could well be that some of those conditions of the body which TCM variously describes as wind-heat, *qi*-deficiency, blood stagnation, and so forth, are caused by viruses. It is to be hoped that further research, in both China and the West, will provide some elucidation. See **micro-organisms**.

visceral spasms Abdominal cramp. This condition should not be confused with menstrual pains, which are sometimes called cramps. See **cramp**.

viscus Plural: *viscera*. Entrails. Any of the soft internal organs of the body, as distinct from components of the nervous, muscular and skeletal systems. The vital organs are viscera, as are the urogenital organs. See **vital organs**.

vision See **eye**, **eyesight**, **eyestrain** and **optical defects**.

vital energy See **qi**.

vital essence See **hormone** and **jing**.

vital organs In TCM, there are 12 vital organs – six solid and six hollow. The six solid organs are the heart, lungs, liver, spleen, kidneys and pericardium. The six hollow, or bladder, organs are the small intestine, large intestine, gall-bladder, stomach, bladder and triple-warmer. Originally, there were only five solid organs, which are called *wu zang* by the Chinese. (*Wu* means 'five'.) The heart-constrictor, or pericardium, was added later to correspond with the triple-warmer, such is the Chinese desire for harmony. The six hollow organs are called *liu fu* by the Chinese. (*Liu* means 'six'.) The triple-warmer, which is also called the triple-heater or three-points, is the entrances to the stomach, small intestine and bladder; and the heart-constrictor, or pericardium, is the membranous sac which encloses the heart. Neither of these is an organ in the Western sense of the term, and neither has much significance in herbal medicine, though they are of some importance in acupuncture and acupressure. The other solid and hollow organs are arranged in corresponding pairs – each of which is associated with an element, emotion, climate, season, direction, taste and sound – as follows. *Heart and small intestine*: fire, joy, hot, summer, south, bitter and laughter. *Lungs and large intestine*: metal, anxiety, dry, autumn, west, pungent and weeping. *Liver and gall-bladder*: wood, anger, windy, spring, east, sour and shouting. *Spleen and stomach*: earth, concentration, moist, midsummer, centre, sweet and singing. *Kidneys and bladder*: water, fear, cold, winter, north, salty and moaning. In order to create harmonious relationships, the Chinese have 'invented' midsummer as an additional season to correspond with the element earth and the spleen and stomach. It is not difficult to understand these relationships. There is an obvious relationship between fire, hot, summer and south (at least in the Northern Hemisphere), and where there is joy there is likely to be laughter. And, in the spring, winds blow from the east. These relationships are used quite successfully in diagnosis and treatments. Thus, the child who is a bed-wetter is likely to be fearful, and so there is an obvious connection between fear, water and the kidneys. To eliminate this kind of fear, the kidneys need to be strengthened with tonic herbs or by acupuncture. Similarly, a person who is anxious will be inclined to weep and perhaps be prone to the condition of the lungs which is called hyperventilation. The vital organs are also associated with colours, odours, animals, numbers, fruits, cereals and the planets, but these have less significance in diagnosis and treatments. Each of the other parts of the body, such as the eyes, ears, nose, skin and muscles, are associated with one of the pairs of vital organs and its related element, and TCM physicians believe that treating these parts is largely a matter of keeping the vital organs in a healthy state. Thus, the person who suffers from anxiety and those ailments that are productive of anxiety can usually be cured by treating his lungs; and the person who is always joyful and suffers from the ailments associated with joy – such as hysteria and a florid complexion – may be cured by treating his liver. Treatments may involve the victor-and-vanquished relationships of the elements. For example, a heart condition could be treated by strengthening the kidneys, for the heart is associated with the fire, and the kidneys with water, and water extinguishes fire. Similarly, a liver condition could be treated by strengthening the heart, for the liver is associated with wood, the heart is associated with fire, and fire destroys wood. TCM physicians also believe that the tongue is connected directly or indirectly to the meridians of the vital organs, and this, they would claim, is what makes the tongue so important in diagnosis. The Taoists used the generative cycle of the elements as a symbolic device to show the relationships of the solid organs. Thus, fire generates earth (ash), earth generates metal (mineral), metal generates water (liquid), water generates wood (vegetation), and wood generates fire (fuel); and so the heart (fire) supports the spleen (earth), the spleen supports the lungs (metal), the lungs support the kidneys (water), and the kidneys support the liver (wood). Obviously, to treat an organ fully, its supporting organ must also be treated. Each of the hollow organs has the same relationship as its paired solid organ. Similarly, the Taoists used the victor-and-vanquished rule to show the adverse effect that one organ can have on another. Thus, where *qi* is imbalanced, the heart (fire) is destructive to the lungs (metal), the lungs are destructive to the liver (wood), the liver is destructive to the spleen (earth), the spleen is destructive to the kidneys (water), and the kidneys are destructive to the heart (fire). A study of the TCM theories about the vital organs reveals that the Taoist physicians in ancient times attached far more importance to the physical causes of the emotions than do the physicians of the West. See **solid organs, liu fu, element** and **psychosomatic**.

vital-energy points See **acupoints**.

vitamin A vitamin may be defined as one of a number of

substances which, in the tiniest amounts, are essential to the body to assist in growth, metabolism and the promotion of health. A vitamin differs from a trace element in that the former is an organic compound, and generally complex, whereas the latter is a simple inorganic mineral salt. The body makes some of its own vitamins from food or other vitamins, but some vitamins cannot be made by the body, and these must be derived from food. If the body does not obtain all these vitamins, the symptoms of a vitamin-deficiency disease will develop. But the body requires only certain quantities of the vitamins, and so where they are consumed to excess, those that are water-soluble will pass out of the body via the urine, but the others will accumulate until they attain toxic levels, and so, with vitamins, as with many other things, one can have too much as well as too little of a good thing. Some vitamins are destroyed by cooking, which indicates the importance of salad-type meals. The physicians in ancient China were unaware of the existence of vitamins as such, but they did believe that foodstuffs contain qi and essences which are beneficial to the health. They were also aware of the adverse effects – what we, in the West, call deficiency diseases – which could result from a lack of certain kinds of food in the diet. In this respect, they were many centuries ahead of the physicians of the West in their thinking. Our knowledge of vitamins has been in existence for less than 100 years. Vitamins were first designated by letters, but those which have been analysed now have chemical names. Vitamin B was once thought to be a single vitamin, but is now known to have several components, each of which is named as B_1, B_2, B_3, etc. Some of the better-known vitamins are as follows: vitamin A, or retinol; vitamin B, or thiamin (also called aneurin); vitamin B_2, or riboflavin; vitamin B_3, or niacin (also called nicotinic acid); vitamin B_6, or pyridoxine; vitamin B_{12}, or cobalamin; vitamin C, or ascorbic acid; vitamin D; vitamin E, or tocopherol; vitamin H, or biotin; and vitamin K. Vitamin A occurs in fish liver, egg yolk, dairy products, green and yellow vegetables and yellow fruits, and is necessary for growth and a healthy skin and membranes. A deficiency of vitamin A causes night-blindness and poor vision. Vitamin B_1 occurs in cereals, yeast, pork, pulses and nuts, and is necessary for growth, metabolism and releasing energy from glucose. A deficiency of vitamin B, can lead to loss of weight, insomnia, depression and beriberi. Vitamin B_2 occurs in yeast, liver, soya beans and eggs, and is necessary for growth. Vitamin B_6 is necessary for the formation of proteins, but its absence from the diet does not seem to cause any pronounced ill-effects. Vitamin B_{12} occurs in liver, shellfish, fish, meat, eggs, milk and cheese, and is necessary for growth and the formation of red blood cells. Vegans will develop deficiency unless they consume food which has been enriched with vitamin B_{12}. Whilst the above information is of interest to nutritionists, it is quite enough for the average person to know that if his diet is balanced and varied, there should be no risk of vitamin deficiency or toxicity. In this respect, the Chinese-style diet would be excellent. See **vitamin supplements**.

vitamin-deficiency diseases See **vitamin**.

vitamin-enriched foods These are foods to which the manufacturers have added vitamins to supplement or increase those they contain naturally. Sometimes, the enrichment of food is required by law. This is the case with margarine, which is enriched, or fortified, by adding vitamins A and D, and the flour for making white bread, which is enriched by adding vitamins B_1 and B_3 and calcium. However, the Chinese are suspicious of food additives of any kind, and prefer to rely on those health benefits which derive from a natural diet. See **vitamin**.

vitamin supplements In the West, it is a fairly common practice for a condition due to a vitamin deficiency to be treated with a vitamin supplement. For example, one form of anaemia is due to a deficiency of folic acid, which is a B-complex vitamin, and which can be taken as a supplement. Similarly, vitamin B_{12}, or cyanocobalamin, can be taken for weak blood and nerve conditions due to an entirely non-meat diet. But, generally, vitamin supplements should be administered under proper medical supervision because of the risk of toxicity from excessive amounts of vitamins. TCM physicians prefer the dietary methods of treatment which have been in successful use for many centuries. See **vitamin**.

vocal cords Folds of the membrane of the larynx, and whose vibrations by an air-stream produce voice sounds. See **epiglottis**.

vodka This alcoholic drink, which is of Russian origin, is made from cereals or potatoes. It is one of the purer spirits, and is sometimes used as a substitute for medicinal alcohol. The Chinese will use it as an alternative to rice wine in making medicinal wines.

voluntary action See **voluntary movement**.

voluntary movement Voluntary action. Voluntary reaction. Active movement. See **active movements** and **nervous system**.

voluntary reaction See **voluntary movement**.

vomiting Generally, one inhibits vomiting by preventing nausea, which may lead to vomiting, and which has a wide variety of causes, such as travel sickness, morning sickness, migraine, vertigo, a surfeit of rich food and untreated diabetes. On the other hand, vomiting is a symptom, not an illness, and it may not be helpful to prevent vomiting, which is nature's way of ridding the stomach of harmful substances. However, after vomiting, the stomach can be settled down with an infusion, taken internally, of one of the following, using the parts and dosage indicated: ginger, *Zingiber officinale*, rhizomes, 3–7 g; mandarin orange, *Citrus reticulata*, peel, 3–7 g; cinnamon, *Cinnamomum cassia*, young stems, 1–4 g. White rice porridge is particularly helpful in this respect. Acupressure is sometimes also helpful. Pressure is applied to the point which is midway between the navel and the breastbone. Excessive vomiting can lead to dehydration, and so it is important to take plenty of liquids, such as water and diluted fruit juices, but not alcohol, tea or coffee. If vomiting persists for no apparent reason, there may be something seriously amiss, and so medical advice should be sought. See **nausea**, **emetic** and **white rice porridge**.

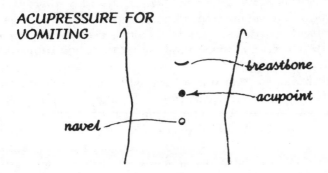

ACUPRESSURE FOR VOMITING

voyeurism Obtaining sexual gratification by watching the sexual activities of others. See **sex**.

vulva The entrance to the vagina, and the external genital organ of the female. See **reproductive systems**.

vulvitis Inflammation of the vulva. The treatment is the same as for vaginitis. See **vaginal disorders**.

W

walnut A tree of the genus *Juglans*. An infusion of its leaves has antiseptic properties. See **head lice**.

Wang Chi Also written as *Huang Qi*. Wang Chi was one of the Song dynasty (960–1279) scholars who devised the system of *fung shui* as it is known today, but which is based on the ancient classics and the notion that the first cause of all that exists is an abstract principle – the Supreme Absolute – whose first breath in movement was yang, the great male principle of life, and whose first breath at rest was yin, the great female principle of life. See **fung shui** and **Tai Chi**.

Wang Shou See **diabetes mellitus**.

warm See **energy**.

warming medicines These medicines are aptly described as 'remove-cold medicines' by the Chinese. They are generally pungent and dehydrating, and so should be used with care where there is a deficiency of yin or fluid. See **stimulation treatment**.

warmth See **survival**.

wart This is a small skin tumour caused by the papilloma virus. Warts are regarded as being harmless, but they are infectious and can spread very quickly, and so they should not be ignored. They are usually classified as two main types: common warts and verrucae. Common warts appear on any part of the body, but they may be removed by applying the latex, or milky sap, of a dandelion root or stem. This treatment should be continued until the warts disappear. Verrucae, or plantar warts, occur on the soles of the feet, and they are often acquired by athletes who walk barefooted in a dressing-room. They are more resistant than common warts and can be very painful, for they grow into the skin. They should be kept dry because they thrive on moisture. They may be removed surgically, but dandelion latex is effective here if one is patient. The milky juice from unripe figs is also an effective treatment if applied as a lotion. A wart should not be confused with a naevus, or mole. See **naevus**.

water There is a preponderance of water on the earth – in the oceans, lakes, rivers, clouds and the atmosphere – and all living tissue contains water. About 90 per cent of a cabbage and 70 per cent of a human being consists of water. Therefore, it is hardly surprising that the philosophers in the ancient world regarded water as an elemental substance that is contained in all matter. But, modern chemistry informs us that water is not an element, but a compound of hydrogen and oxygen; and, though it exists in great abundance, it does not exist in all matter. TCM physicians have always regarded water as a precious commodity, which indeed it is, for it is vital to our existence and that of all living organisms. Although it is not a food, for it contains no nutrients, a regular intake of water provides rigidity to the body and facilitates the digestion and assimilation of food and the transport of various substances – nutrients and waste – to and from the tissues. Therefore, it is important that it should be pure and sufficient in amount. Whatever its source, all water intended for drinking, even spa water, should be boiled. The water that is available to us on tap is not always as potable as the authorities would have us believe, and though the sparkling spring water coming to us in attractively labelled bottles may contain mineral salts that are beneficial to the health, it may also contain pathogenic micro-organisms. In fact, bottled water may be less safe to drink than tap water. It is a mistake to assume that bottled spring water is absolutely pure, though it will have passed a test that guarantees a standard of purity which the authorities deem to be acceptable. Boiled water is a good start to the day if it is drunk immediately before breakfast. It offsets the dehydration caused by perspiration during the night, it has a cleansing effect on the bowel, it provides a solvent for the food that is to follow and, being water in a fairly pure form, it is easily assimilated by the alimentary canal. Boiling will have killed the micro-organisms contained in the water, and so there will be no biological perils. However, boiling does not eradicate the chemicals contained in the water. The pollution of water by nitrates from fertilizers, together with industrial waste and sewage, is one of the several reasons why the more enlightened governmental bodies are striving to clean up the environment. Water can be used medicinally. A frequent intake of water promotes frequent urination, which helps to eliminate toxic waste products from the bloodstream, and so aids in relieving arthritis, gout, eczema and many other ailments. Drinking a large amount of water is probably the most effective treatment for a hangover. When we have influenza or a cold, we drink large quantities of fluids in order to eliminate waste products and prevent dehydration. But, since tea, coffee and beer, etc., contain impurities, boiled water is the best liquid for this purpose. Boiled water, and not tea, is the favourite drink of the Chinese, which is hardly surprising. But, to the TCM physician, water is something more than one of man's basic needs and the 'universal solvent'. It is one of the five symbolic elements of Chinese philosophy and medicine. It is yin and is associated with the kidneys and the emotion of fear. To some extent, health depends upon the correct balance of water within the body. Where there is an excess of water, as with oedema, the Chinese physicians will use diuretic herbal medicines, which induce urination. Where a water loss could have a cooling effect, as with a fever, he will use diaphoretic herbal medicines, which induce perspiration. There are also medicines which have a drying effect or a moistening effect. See **element** and **environment**.

water-buffalo *Bubalus bubalis* Medicine. Distribution: China, India, Middle East. Parts: gallstones. Character: cool, bitter-sweet. Affinity: heart, liver. Effects: diuretic, sedative, anti-spasmodic, antipyretic, cardiotonic. Symptoms: fever, spasms, sore and swollen throat, irritability, abscesses. Treatments: conditions due to an excess of internal heat, throat infections. Dosage: 0.15–0.2 g. This medicine is costly and hard to come by, but there are suitable alternatives, such as the gallstones of the domestic cow, *Bos taurus domesticus*, and an extract from the gall-bladder of a pig. See **pig's gall-bladder**.

watercress *Nasturtium officinale* With the Chinese, watercress is a favourite item of diet, and is usually consumed in a soup. It is rich in vitamins A, B_2, B_9 and C, and is also a good source of calcium and potassium. It is helpful in the treatment of iron-deficiency anaemia. Chewing fresh watercress is a treatment for bleeding gums.

water-melon See **pimples and spots**.

water pills These are the simplest form of pills used in TCM, for neither a binder nor a buffer is required, and the pills are held together by moisture and the natural adhesive substances in the herbal ingredients. A flat bamboo basket is soaked in water, powdered herbs are sprinkled on to the inside surface, and the basket is then rocked and rotated until small pills begin to form. More water and powdered herbs are added, and the process is repeated until pills of the desired size are formed.

water plantain *Alisma plantago-aquatica* Herbal medicine. Temperate regions of Asia, Europe and North America. Parts: tubers.

Character: cold, sweet. Affinity: kidneys, bladder, female genitalia. Effects: diuretic, refrigerant. Symptoms: difficult and painful urination, diarrhoea, dark and cloudy urine, excess mucus. Treatments: leucorrhoea, vaginitis, conditions of heat excess. Dosage: 4–14 g.

water pollution This form of pollution has a variety of causes, which include the run-off from the fertilizers, pesticides, silage and other substances used in agriculture, the toxic chemicals in industrial waste, and the phosphates in detergents. This pollution can lead to skin disorders, birth deformities, miscarriages, cancer and death. Some people are allergic to the chlorine which is added to water as a sterilizing agent. Another source of water pollution and a great health hazard is the large quantities of untreated sewage which are being discharged into the sea in the hope that it will be rendered harmless by infinite dilution. But, in fact, it contaminates the water and the shellfish which live near the shore. Swimming in polluted sea water or eating contaminated shellfish can result in stomach upsets, hepatitis, ear and eye infections or something worse. See **water**, **environment** and **chemicals**.

water retention See **oedema**.

water therapy See **hydrotherapy**.

wax pills In making these pills, beeswax is used as a binder. This ensures that the ingredients are absorbed very slowly, which is highly desirable when the ingredients are very toxic. Wax pills are sometimes coated with another ingredient to either provide protection or impart an agreeable flavour. See **'putting on the overcoat'**.

'way of long life' See **Yang Shen**.

'way of yin and yang' This is a Taoist concept of how longevity may be achieved sexually by using tonic medicines and exercises to nurture the semen-essence. See **jing** and **Yang Sen**.

weakness A TCM dietary treatment for a person with a weak constitution is a soup made by slowly simmering knotty yam, *Discorea opposita*, with pork for over two hours. Lotus seeds, fox nuts, dried longan fruits and bitter almonds could be added. However, bitter almonds should be added only in small quantities, for they contain traces of prussic acid, which is poisonous. A traditional remedy for weakness in the hips and thighs is a soup made by first boiling and then simmering 250 g mutton bones or a pork hock and 15 g vinegar in a litre of water for two hours. See **stamina**.

weak pulse In TCM, ginseng is sometimes recommended as a treatment for a weak pulse. But a weak pulse is not an illness but a symptom, and so it would surely be sensible to identify and then treat the underlying condition, which is likely to be one that is yin, internal, cold and empty. See **pulse diagnosis**.

wealth See **health**.

weaning In TCM, powdered Glauber's salt (sodium sulphate), which has a slightly bitter taste, is rubbed on the nipples to wean children off breast-feeding.

weather In TCM, it is perceived that there is some relationship between illness and general climatic conditions and changes in the weather. Persons of low bodily resistance are likely to be adversely affected by coldness, dampness and dryness. In Western medicine, it is also understood that weather conditions can have a considerable influence on health. People who live in tropical countries are susceptible to intestinal disorders, prickly heat, heat exhaustion, heat stroke and those diseases, such as malaria and sleeping sickness, which are transmitted by some of the insects that thrive in a hot climate. At the other extreme, there are those people who live in very cold countries, and who are susceptible to hypothermia, frostbite and chilblains. Where there is a combination of warmth and humidity, as in crowded public places without adequate ventilation, disease germs breed and spread very quickly. Colds are often caught where there is low humidity because the mucus membranes become dry, and so are more liable to infection. Sunshine provides a psychological boost, and also assists in making vitamin D. Arthritis and rheumatism often worsen when the weather is cold and windy, and bronchitis worsens in misty or foggy conditions, especially if there is heavy pollution. On the other hand, asthma may improve when it is misty, for the lungs need moisture. Headaches, tension and moodiness may occur where there is a high concentration of positive ions – positive electrical charges – in the air. See **climate**, **sunlight** and **six excesses**.

weeds Many of the Chinese herbal medicines are available in the West; but, unfortunately, some of them, which the Chinese use for culinary as well as medicinal purposes, such as the humble dandelion, *Taraxacum officinale*, are regarded by us as weeds, and so we ignore them or destroy them, thus wantonly wasting one of nature's bountiful gifts to mankind. The wolfberry, or boxthorn, *Lyceum chinese*, an ageing-inhibitor, and the burdock, *Arctium lappa*, an antipyretic and diuretic, are further examples of excellent medicines which, in the West, are commonly regarded as weeds.

weeping golden bell See **golden bell**.

weight gain A sudden gain in weight can be due to one of a variety of causes. Generally, it is a consequence of a change in life-style, particularly in regard to diet and exercise. People who transfer from an active occupation to one that is sedentary, athletes who give up their athletic pursuits and people who take less exercise because of an incapacitating illness will be inclined to put on weight. The hormonal changes associated with the menopause may cause a temporary weight gain, but this is not harmful provided it is not excessive. See **menopause** and **obesity**.

Weil's disease An infectious disease caused by the bacterium leptospira, which is carried by rats, and which is transmitted to humans by contact with water or other substances contaminated by rats. The disease in its mild form is characterized by fever, headaches, vomiting and weakness. In its severe form, it may cause jaundice, kidney problems and bleeding in various parts of the body. Rats which inhibit sewers are the most likely to carry Weil's disease. In China, as elsewhere in the world, it seems that the most effective way to deal with Weil's disease is to deal with its carrier. See **vector** and **rodents**.

wei qi 'Protective-*qi*'. See **qi**.

welfare Clearly, health and welfare go hand in hand, and where there is a decline in living standards and a lack of security, or what we, in the West, would describe as social services, there will inevitably be a decline in health. Since ancient times, the Chinese have recognized that a person's state of health is closely linked to his standard of living, and his position and responsibilities in the community, for a healthy and wealthy person is a product of a healthy and worthy community – and vice versa. It could be said that China has had a welfare state for nearly 3,000 years, but one provided more by its traditions and the philosophical influences of Taoism and Confucianism than by administrative procedures of the state, though Confucianism was the state religion at the time of the Han dynasty (206 BC–AD 220). Chinese society has been held together by the Confucian emphasis on care and respect for one's neighbours, the affection and security provided by the family unit, and the Taoist emphasis on health and harmony with nature. Another important feature of the Chinese way of life is respect for one's ancestors, which creates a sense of continuity within the family and the community, so that no one may feel that he is living in isolation or without purpose. It also ensures that the young and the old are not neglected. Additionally, there are the racial characteristics of the Chinese, who are patient, kindly and honest by temperament, which make for social harmony and peace of mind. See **ancestor worship**, **Taoism** and **Confucianism**.

Welsh onion See **cong bai**.

west See **direction**.

Western medicine Although TCM retains its essential character in its principles and philosophy, it does make use of the equipment which has been made available by Western medical technology. There are also benefits in speed and accuracy to be derived from Western-style standardization, as with the metric system of measurements and the binomial nomenclature used in the classification of plants and animals, and so now, by adoption, the metric system is as official in China as it is in the Western world, and Chinese herbal medicines have Linnaean-style names as well as their traditional Chinese names. What is more, the TCM physician practising in the West will use, as a matter of convenience, those abbreviations of Latinized instructions contained in Western-style prescriptions: a.c. – 'before food', o.d. – 'every day', etc. See **New Medicine**, **Linnaean** and **Latin**.

'wet dream' See **nocturnal emission**.

wheat *Triticum aestivum* Herbal medicine. Distribution: temperate regions. Parts: grains. Character: neutral, sweet. Affinity: heart. Effects: cardiotonic, sedative. Symptoms: sleeplessness. Treatments: hypertension. Dosage: 14–28 g. As an item of diet, the whole wheat grains are a good source of protein, starch and dietary fibre, and they contain iron, calcium, manganese, phosphorus, thiamin and niacin, but most of the micronutrients are lost when the grains are ground to make flour. The bran, or husks, of wheat grains, is very rich in dietary fibre, and is preventive of constipation if it is a regular item of diet. Nutritionally, the most valuable part of a wheat grain is the germ, or embryo. It is rich in protein, unsaturated fat, vitamin E, B-complex vitamins, iron and phosphorus. However, very little wheat is consumed in the south of China, where rice is the staple. See **bread** and **perspiration**.

wheat bran See **wheat**.

wheat germ See **wheat**.

whiplash injury Damage to the neck vertebrae or tissues which is due to the sudden jerking forwards or backwards of the head. It is commonly associated with car accidents and athletic activities. The treatment will be determined by the nature and extent of the damage, but TCM would recommend massage and acupuncture or moxibustion to be applied to the meridians of the gall-bladder, small intestine, lungs, bladder and large intestine. There are some suitable remedial exercises in the *Chinese Exercise Manual*.

white fish See **fish**.

white meat Pork, veal, poultry, hare, rabbit, etc. In the Chinese view, white meat is not damaging to the health, as is red meat. See **meat** and **red meat**.

white mulberry See **mulberry**.

white peony See **peony**.

white rice porridge This porridge is generally effective as a remedy for nausea, loss of appetite, flatulence, diarrhoea, constipation and other conditions which result from over-indulgence in food or drink. In the West, it is regarded as a Chinese-style cure for a British-style hangover. Smoothly protective, it does not irritate the bowel, and is a very nourishing dish for invalids and elderly people with an impaired digestion. The recipe is as follows. Ingredients: 8 tablespoons rice, 1 tablespoon chopped dried orange peel or longan fruits. Put the ingredients into a wok/pan, add a litre of water, and then boil vigorously until the porridge assumes a milky appearance. Serve boiling hot, and consume slowly in gentle sips. After two days of this diet, all the symptoms of sickness should disappear, and then the appetite will improve. White rice porridge is a *fan* dish. It absorbs any excess of acids and grease in the digestive tract, and speeds their evacuation from the body.

white sugar Refined sugar. See **sugar**.

White Tiger In Chinese mythology, the White Tiger, who is a female, and the Green Dragon, who is a male, are disruptive and malevolent influences. In the past, some Chinese attributed illnesses and other misfortunes to the activities of these two creatures.

white vinegar Vinegar made from white rice. In the West, this term is applied, somewhat inaccurately, to synthetic vinegar, which is colourless. See **vinegar**.

whole food This is a food which has not been refined or processed in some way, and which is consumed in its natural state. A good example is wholegrain, or wholemeal, flour. It is made from grain from which the husks have not been removed by attribution. Whole foods are often grown without fertilizers, pesticides or hormones. Chinese food tends to be of this kind, for the Chinese are averse to the use of additives, and have a preference for food that is natural and fresh. Rice is a notable exception, for most of the rice consumed in China is the white, or polished, type. A diet consisting essentially of whole foods is thought to assist in preventing cancer and many other conditions. See **rice, wheat** and **organic farming**.

wholegrain See **whole food**.

wholemeal See **whole food**.

whooping cough See **pertussis**.

wild lettuce *Lactuca virosa* Herbal medicine. Distribution: North China, Western Europe. Parts: leaves. Character: warm, bitter. Affinity: heart, liver, stomach, spleen. Symptoms: sleeplessness, irritability, indigestion, anxiety, muscular aches and pains. Treatments: insomnia, weak digestion, neuroses. Dosage: 1.5–8 g. Unlike its cultivated relatives, which are eaten in salads, wild lettuce is NOT suitable as an item of diet, and it must be used with care as a medicine. An overdose can result in stupor, coma or even death. See **lettuce**.

wild turmeric See **turmeric**.

willow A tree of the genus *Salix*. See **traditional medicine** and **aspirin**.

will-power An important factor in recovery from an illness is the effort of will which the patient makes himself. When a patient gives up the fight for life, perhaps because the pain or distress are unbearable, he will have a tendency to succumb. Will-power is an important component in such therapies as hypnosis, auto-suggestion and meditation. It is certainly the case that the main factor in the recovery of a person suffering from a nervous breakdown is the effort he makes himself. See **nervous disorders**.

wind This is one of the six excesses of TCM. See **climate** and **six excesses**. Wind should not be confused with inner-wind, which is not associated with the weather, and which is an energy imbalance arising in the liver, heart or kidneys. The word *wind* is used colloquially in the West to mean 'flatulence'. The Chinese word for flatulence literally means 'gas', which is apt. See **flatulence** and **pig's feet**.

wind-cold This is a combination of the excesses of wind and cold, and it will produce the symptoms associated with both excesses: headaches, coughing, sneezing, dizziness, aches in various parts of the body, cramps, etc. See **wind, cold** and **excess combinations**.

wind-damp This is a combination of the excesses of wind and dampness, and it will produce the symptoms associated with both excesses: headaches, coughing, sneezing, dizziness, aching limbs, languor, etc. See **antirheumatic, wind** and **damp**.

wind-drying This is a Chinese food-preservation technique whereby foods are dried by exposing them to the atmosphere, especially where there are currents of air. It has the merit that none of the constituents are destroyed, as some of them are by pickling. See **preserved food** and **dried herbs**.

wind-dryness This not a common excess combination. The two commonest forms of dryness are hot-dryness and cold-dryness. See **excess combinations**.

wind-heat This is a combination of the excesses of wind and heat, and it will produce the symptoms associated with both excesses: headaches, coughing, sneezing, dizziness, heavy perspiration, dry mouth and throat, palpitations, constipation, etc. An infusion, taken internally, of 4–9 g flowers of chrysanthemum, *Chrysanthemum morifolium*, is an effective treatment for wind-heat conditions. See **wind**, **heat** and **excess combinations**.

wind-injury Here, *wind* is used in the sense of 'harming', not 'wounding'. It refers to those conditions which are brought about by an excess of wind. Headaches, colds, fevers, sore throats and muscular aches and pains are usually wind-injury conditions.

wine *Jiu*, as the Chinese call wine, is drunk extensively throughout China, both as a source of pleasure and for its medicinal benefits. Chinese wines are characterized by great quality and much variety, but they rarely feature in family meals, and they are generally reserved for special occasions, such as weddings, banquets and the Chinese New Year and other feast days. The Chinese never drink on an empty stomach, and so food is always served with wine. Nor do they mix their drinks. Excessive drinking of wine is regarded with disfavour, and since a Chinese person's face becomes flushed after he has taken alcohol, he will not want to drink to excess, for his greed would be readily advertised. But wine is also regarded as a health remedy if it is drunk in moderation. Chinese wines are made from a wide variety of materials: rice, wheat, millet, sorghum, chrysanthemum flowers, ginger and pears, pomegranates and other fruits. Rice wine is also called *shaojiu*. *Baijiu*, or 'white wine', which is made from grain, is the most popular wine in China. *Kaoliangjiu*, or 'sorghum wine', is similar to gin or vodka in flavour and colour, and is used to flavour and preserve food. *Shaoxingjiu*, or 'Shaoxing wine', from Shaoxing, in the Zhejiang province, in the east of China, is made from glutinous rice. *Huangjiu*, or 'yellow wine', is made from glutinous millet. *Sanshao*, which is distilled from the wine made from glutinous millet, is the Chinese equivalent of brandy. A liquor fermented from the seeds of Job's tears, *Coix lacryma-jobi*, is used to treat rheumatic pains. It has been suggested that a regular intake of wine might prevent heart and circulatory disorders by lowering cholesterol levels, and now, in the West, some research is being carried out in this connection. See **alcohol**, **fermentation**, **medicinal wine**, **spring wine** and **hangover**.

wine vinegar See **vinegar**.

wing-chun See **martial arts**.

winter melon Called *donggua* by the Chinese, the winter melon is a gourd which attains the size of a pumpkin. The Chinese regard it as a valuable health food, for it is diuretic, antitussive, antipyretic, refrigerant and of benefit to the intestine. It is generally simmered with pork, chicken or pigeon and black mushrooms and shellfish, and then consumed as a soup.

winter mushrooms Called *dongku* by the Chinese, winter mushrooms are consumed in large quantities in China. They have a blackish-brown, leathery appearance, and are obtainable at Chinese grocery stores in the West. They are always purchased in the dried state, and need to be well soaked before use. When cooked with meat, they provide a highly nutritious and perfectly balanced meal. They are rich in vitamins, especially those in the B-complex of which cobalamin, niacin and riboflavin are predominant. They are a tonic for the nervous system and are preventive of anaemia and cancer. They also reduce hypertension and give some immunity against viruses and epidemic diseases generally. See **fungi**.

wisdom and age One of the several reasons why the Chinese respect, and even revere, elderly people is that they also value wisdom, which comes with age, for experience is a good teacher. According to legend, Lao Zi, the founder of Taoism, on which much of Chinese medicine is based, was born with the silver hair and all the wisdom of an elderly man. See **Lao Zi**.

wisdom tooth The third molar tooth, which erupts during youth. See **teeth**.

withdrawal *Coitus interruptus*. This is a method of contraception which requires that the penis be withdrawn before ejaculation. One would think that this procedure is both unreliable and unsatisfying to the two parties concerned. But a similar technique, which even precluded ejaculation, was practised in ancient China. See **Yellow Emperor** and **birth control**.

withdrawal symptoms The unpleasant physical reactions which generally accompany the process of ceasing to take addictive drugs and which are described colloquially as 'cold turkey'.

woad *Isatis tinctoria* Herbal medicine. Distribution: Europe,

China, Japan. Parts: leaves. Character: cold, bitter. Affinity: heart, stomach. Effects: antipyretic, antiphlogistic, antiseptic, antidote. Symptoms: fainting, heat rash, sore and dry throat, abscesses, delirium. Treatments: erysipelas, encephalitis, conditions due to internal heat excess. Dosage: 6–14 g. At one time, woad was a source of a blue dye, but it has been superseded by indigo.

wolfberry *Lycium chinense* Herbal medicine. Distribution: China, Japan. Parts: skin of roots. Character: cold, plain-sweet. Affinity: kidneys, lungs. Effects: antipyretic, refrigerant, antitussive. Symptoms: fever, coughs, blood in sputum or urine. Treatments: asthma, conditions due to heat excess in lungs, yin-deficiency conditions, hypertension. Dosage: 9–14 g. Parts: fruits. Character: neutral, sweet. Affinity: liver, kidneys. Effects: tonic to kidneys and liver, nurtures semen, improves eyesight. Symptoms: headaches, blurred vision, giddiness, back aches and pains. Treatments: conditions due to liver-yin and kidney-yin deficiency, lumbago, spermatorrhoea, mild conditions of diabetes. Dosage: 3–9 g. The wolfberry is one of those herbs which occupy a respected place in Chinese tradition as both medicines and culinary items. For thousands of years, its fruits, which are believed to be supportive of *qi*, or 'vital energy', have been used as a health food to inhibit the ageing process, lengthen the life-span, increase virility and calm the nerves. Although the wolfberry is indigenous to China and Japan, it has been cultivated in Europe, but it has escaped from gardens and become naturalized. In Britain, where it grows wild in the hedgerows and is regarded as a weed, and so is generally ignored, it is known as the Chinese wolfberry, boxthorn or Duke of Argyll's tea-tree. Its bright-red fruits are about the same size and shape as small peanuts. When the fruits are used as a remedy for the mild form of diabetes which occurs in elderly people, they may be combined with white rice porridge. Added to soups, they strengthen the bones, muscles, teeth and hair, and also relieve aching joints. Steamed or boiled with fruit or vegetables, they make a tonic food that is suitable for persons of all ages. The fresh roots, as well as the fruits, reduce blood sugar, and so they, also, may be used as a treatment for diabetes in elderly people. In the Chinese language, the fruits of the wolfberry are generally called *gouguzi*, but they are also called *chiehlautze*, which means 'repel-old-age berries', and is an indication of the esteem in which they are held as an inhibitor of ageing. See **white rice porridge**.

wolfberry wine The fruits of the wolfberry, *Lycium chinense*, are a remedy for many ailments. In fact, the Chinese regard them as an ageing-inhibitor and a panacea for many ills, and so it is hardly surprising that they use them as an ingredient in a medicinal wine, for which the recipe is as follows. Ingredients: 90 g dried wolfberries, 600 ml white wine or rice wine, 90 g honey. Put all the ingredients – do not wash the berries – into a large, clean jar, cover, seal and store in a place that is cool, dry, dark and undisturbed. After 12 months, strain the wine, keeping back the berries, and transfer it to a clean bottle. It is now ready for drinking. The berries may be used again, but no more than once, in the following year. The usual dosage is one small glass (30 g) per day. See **wolfberry**.

wolfsbane Monkshood. See **aconite**.

womb See **uterus**.

wood One of the five elements of Chinese philosophy and medicine. It is yin and is associated with the liver and the emotion of anger. See **element**.

woodbine See **Japanese honeysuckle**.

wood ears See **mukyi**.

wooden ladle See **eating utensils**.

wood garlic See **ramsons**.

wood liquorice See **liquorice**.

wood spirit See **alcohol**.

woolly grass *Imperata cylindrica* Herbal medicine. Distribution: South China, India, Africa. Parts: roots. Character: cold, sweet. Affinity: stomach, lungs. Effects: diuretic, antipyretic, haemostatic, demulcent. Symptoms: nausea, vomiting, cough, blood in urine or sputum. Treatments: all conditions of heat excess, internal haemorrhage, bruises. Dosage: 10–30 g.

World Health Organization An agency of the United Nations established in 1948 with the aim of promoting the highest levels of health in all communities. Its many activities include medical research and the training of medical workers. A valuable facet of its work is research in regard to the efficacy of traditional Chinese herbal medicines. One could hope that, eventually, this will make it possible for everyone to benefit from the oldest and safest system of preventive medicine in the world. See **birth control**.

worms See **anthelmintic and parasite**.

wormwood There are several species of wormwood in the *Artemisia* genus, or wormwood family. The ones commonly used in TCM are sweet wormwood, *Artemisia annua*, moxa weed, *Artemisia capillaris*, and mugwort, *Artemisia vulgaris*. Another member of this genus is absinth *Artemisia absinthium*, which was once commonly used for flavouring drinks, but its use for this purpose is now illegal in most countries. In Western herbal medicine, absinth is used medicinally as an antipyretic, anthelmintic and tonic, but it causes hallucinations and injury to the heart if it is taken in excess.

wound In TCM, powdered cuttlefish bone is used as a styptic in treating an external wound that is bleeding severely. The Chinese use the word *wound* in two senses – actual physical injury or damage to the emotions and well-being – as we do in the West. Ko Hung, a Taoist scholar, wrote in a work called the *Nei Pien* about those vices and bad habits which can wound, or damage, one's peace of mind, and which, in turn, can damage one's physical body. 'Sadness, disquiet, ambition without talent, greed, jealousy, excessive joy, idleness, drunkenness, decrepitude, oversleeping and over-strenuous activity are wounds; and when they have amassed to the highest level, exhaustion and death will soon follow. Therefore, to keep alive, one must not listen, look, sit, drink, eat, work, rest, sleep, walk, exercise, talk or dress too much.' Clearly, Ko Hung had perceived that there is a relationship between health and personal habits. But he goes on to say: 'Do not overdo the five tastes when eating, for too much saltiness injures the heart, too much bitterness injures the lungs, too much pungency injures the liver, too much acidity injures the spleen, and too much sweetness injures the kidneys.' Ko Hung had established an important principle, and one which had gone largely unobserved by the physicians of the West until recent times. See **moderation**, **morality** and **psychosomatic**.

woundwort Another common name for betony, *Stachys betonica*, and one which is misleading, for all the species in the genus *Stachys* are called woundworts: wood woundwort, marsh woundwort, alpine woundwort, field woundwort, etc. See **betony**.

wrinkles The connective tissue which forms the inner layers of the skin loses its elasticity and moisture-retaining capability with age, and so, to some extent, one must accept wrinkles just as one must accept age. However, with care, one can attain a vigorous and youthful old age, and so with care, one should also be able to attain an old age without too many wrinkles. In general, those Chinese-style foods, medicines and exercises which inhibit ageing will, as a by-product, also prevent wrinkles. It is important to keep out of the sun, for its radiation can damage the skin. Also, one should avoid continual frowning and puckering the lips and on-and-off dieting sessions, which result in the formation of loose folds of skin. One should not put too much faith in those advertisements for lotions which, so it is claimed, will do wonders for the skin. One treatment for wrinkles is to apply, as a lotion, an infusion of 10–12 g leaves and stems of bedstraw, *Galium verum*. According to Chinese tradition, the inclusion of soya-bean sprouts in the diet helps to prevent wrinkles. See **ageing** and **complexion**.

Wu The first Zhou king (*c.* 1100 BC). See **Pa Kua**.

wu chin hsi See **wu qin xi**.

wunyi See **silver wood ears**.

wu qin xi Also written as *wu chin hsi*. 'Five animal play'. A system of therapeutic exercises devised by the physician Hua Tuo, and which are based on the movements of five animals: the bear, deer, tiger, monkey and crane. These exercises tone up the circulation and respiration, relieve constipation, aid digestion, reduce fatigue and depression, loosen joints and invigorate the vital organs. They are fully explained in the *Chinese Exercise Manual* See **Hua Tuo**.

wushu See **martial arts**.

wu zang See **solid organs**.

X

Xia dynasty Also written as *Hsia dynasty*. By tradition, the Xia dynasty (*c.* 2100–1600 BC) is regarded as the first imperial system of China, but little is known about it, and its emperors and heroes are legendary figures. See **legendary emperors** and **past history**.

xian 'Immortals of the Mountains'. Hermits of the period of the Zhou dynasty (*c.* 1100–221 BC) who, in the seclusion and safety of the mountains, experimented with medicinal herbs and practised the 'way of long life', which included kungfu, meditation, breathing exercises and a diet of herbs. They believed that the mountain mists contained *qi*, the 'vital energy' of life. They also sought for an elixir which would confer immortality upon them. Their activities gave a considerable impetus to the development of Chinese medicine.

xiangqi Chess. See **games**.

Xien Qin Fang See **Tsien Chin Fang**.

Xi Ji See **Shi Ji**.

xing yi (*hsing-I*) 'Form of will'. One of the soft, or internal, styles of kungfu, whose forms of attack are characteristic of the five elements – metal, water, wood, fire and earth.

xi xin See **toothache**.

x-rays Electromagnetic radiation of short wavelength. They are used to make radiographs, which are photographs showing the denser structures of the body. X-ray equipment is used in Chinese hospitals and by Chinese doctors who practise Western medicine, but physicians in the rural areas still use the remarkably accurate traditional techniques, such as pulse-taking and listening by a stethoscope, in making diagnoses. See **meridian meditation**.

xue Blood, which is one of the four humours of both TCM and traditional Western medicine. See **blood**.

Y

yam There are several species, which belong to the genus *Dioscorea*. The tubers of the yam, together with those of the taro, which are very rich in starch, were the staple food of the Chinese before rice began to be cultivated. Yams are a valuable crop in time of food shortage. The yam has the appearance of a large and ugly potato, but it should not be confused with the sweet potato, which belongs to an entirely different family of plants. Some species of yam are used medicinally. See **knotty yam**.

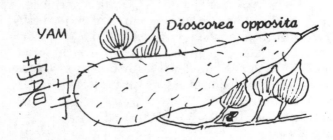

YAM — Dioscorea opposita

yang Symbolized by fire, yang is the positive, active and masculine principle, pole or force in nature, including the human body. It signifies such things as vitality, strength, day and birth. Yang medicines have a stimulating or warming effect. Equilibrium between yang and yin, the negative principle, maintains harmony within the human body and elsewhere. See **Tai Chi**. Although the various individual aspects of a person's temperament and physique may be yang or yin, overall he will be predominantly a yang-type or a yin-type. A yang-type will tend to be tall, well-built, strong, virile, active, sociable, impetuous and outgoing. He is what we, in the West, would describe as an extrovert.

yang-deficiency See **yang tonics**.

yang meridians *Qi*, or 'vital energy', flows down the yang meridians on the body from head to foot, and from fingers to shoulders when the arms are held above the head. The positions of the yang meridians and the organs which they complement, and to which they connect, are as follows: small intestine, outside arm; large intestine, outside arm; triple-heater, outside arm; bladder, back of body; gall-bladder, side of body; and stomach, front of body and side of leg. As an example, this diagram shows the positions of the yang meridians on a person's right arm (rear view). See **vital organs** and **meridian**.

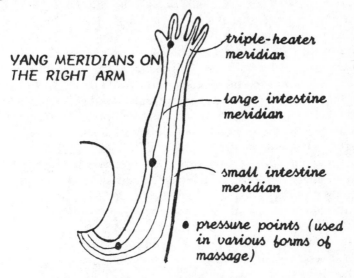

YANG MERIDIANS ON THE RIGHT ARM

triple-heater meridian

large intestine meridian

small intestine meridian

● *pressure points (used in various forms of massage)*

Yang Sen A Chinese general from the Sichuan province, who died only a few years ago, Yang Sen is a good example of how a long and healthy life of vigorous youthfulness can be achieved by following Taoist principles – the 'way to a long life' – in matters of health and medicine. He took regular exercise and was careful with his diet, supplementing it with tonic herbs and medicinal wines. He had numerous wives and mistresses and countless children. For the latter part of his life, he lived in Taiwan, where he engaged in many sporting activities. It is reported that he was physically, mentally and sexually active right up until the day of his death at the ripe old age of 98. See **spring wine**.

yang symptoms Those symptoms of illness which indicate stimulation of the vital organs, and are usually accompanied by warmth and fullness, are regarded as being yang, and suggest that yin remedies should be applied. Typical yang symptoms include excess bodily heat and feverishness, great thirst, constipation, hard stools, hot urine, a flushed face, a bright-red tongue, laboured breathing and a heavy pulse.

yang systems In TCM, the yang vital organs, or hollow organs, are the stomach, large intestine, small intestine, bladder, gall-bladder and triple-warmer. However, in the West, the triple-warmer, or triple-heater, which consists of the openings to the stomach, bladder and small intestine, would not be regarded as an independent organ, and so it is best to regard these organs as functional or energy systems dealing with the transfer of food and liquids. That, after all, is their essential function, which clearly indicates that the physicians and sages of ancient China were not lacking in perspicacity.

yang tonics Those ailments which are regarded as yin, and which are indicated by coldness, emptiness, urinary incontinence and sexual impotence, are what we, in the West, might describe as debility, and what Chinese physicians would describe as yang-deficiency, which requires yang tonics to replace the energy lost. These yang tonics could include horny goat weed, *Epimedium sagittatum*, longan fruit, *Euphoria longan*, angelica, *Angelica sinensis*, and Chinese wolfberry, *Lycium chinense*. It is important to know that yin tonics, which have the opposite effect, should not be used in these cases. It is reasonable for yang-deficiency to be equated, in part, with what the physicians of the West regard as a deficiency of vitamins or minerals. See **tonic**.

yang treatments Where the symptoms of illness are yin – weakness, coldness, fatigue, low breathing, paleness and loss of appetite – yang treatments are required. They include remedies which are stimulating, warming and toning. See **yang tonics**. Ginseng, *Panax ginseng*, and *tienchi*, *Radix pseudo-ginseng*, which are reputed to have healing and health-giving properties that border on the miraculous, would be helpful here. Ginseng also has aphrodisiac properties.

yao The Chinese word for 'medication'. It originated during the time of the Zhou dynasty (*c.* 1100–221 BC).

yarrow *Achillea millefolium* Also called milfoil, nosebleed or staunchgrass. For centuries, this herb has been used to treat nosebleeds and staunch wounds. Its leaves are sometimes used as a substitute for tobacco and snuff. An infusion taken internally of 3–12 g yarrow flowers is a treatment for cramp, poor digestion, fever, irritability and menstrual bleeding. A decoction rubbed on the scalp may delay balding.

ye See **jin ye**.

yeast Single-celled fungi of the genus *Saccharomyces* used in brewing and baking. See **bread**. Brewer's yeast is a rich source of protein, amino acids, B-complex vitamins, minerals and trace elements. As a food, it improves the complexion, increases stamina and inhibits the ageing process. It is thought to be preventive of cancer. The Chinese would regard it as a yang food or tonic. It is a natural inhabitant of the alimentary canal, but an excess of it, brought about by the ingestion of too much sugary food, on which it feeds, may cause digestive or vaginal infection. See **Candida albicans** and **fermentation**.

yee chin ching Popular in ancient China, and still popular today, *yee chin ching* is one of the many systems of massage-cum-exercise therapy that are available to the Chinese. It develops muscular strength and helps in the recovery of people with bone-related ailments. See **healing exercises**.

Yellow Emperor Huang Di. One of the legendary emperors who lived during or prior to the time of the Xia dynasty (*c.* 2100–1600 BC). His exploits prompted the preparation of sexual manuals which perpetuated the belief that, for men, sexual intercourse without ejaculation and the discharge of semen – something difficult to achieve one would think – is good for the health and leads to longevity. Women were not restricted, for it was held that they have unlimited supplies of what was quaintly described as 'yin essence'. The Yellow Emperor is regarded as the father of Taoism, which is the philosophy and science of life and longevity, and the *tao of revitalization*, which is a system of movements to improve mental and physical health and retard the ageing process. See **legendary emperors**.

yi The Chinese word for 'medicine', which originated during the time of the Zhou dynasty (*c.* 1100–221 BC). In the written language, the character for *yi* was derived from the character for 'wine'. The connection is obvious, for rice wine was commonly used as a base for herbal medicines.

Yijing See **I Ching**.

yin Symbolized by water, yin is the negative, passive and feminine principle, pole or force in nature, including the human body. It signifies such things as inertia, delicacy, night and death. Yin medicines have a suppressive or cooling effect. Equilibrium between yin and yang, the positive principle, maintains harmony within the human body and throughout the universe. See **Tai Chi**. Although the various individual aspects of a person's temperament and physique may be yin or yang, overall he will be predominantly a yin-type or a yang-type. A yin-type will tend to be short, small, frail, inactive, unsociable, timid and restrained. He is what we, in the West, would describe as an introvert.

ying qi 'Nourishing-*qi*'. One of the many forms of *qi*, or 'vital energy'. See **qi**.

yin meridians *Qi* energy flows up the yin meridians on the body from feet to head, and from shoulders to fingers when the arms are held above the head. The positions of the yin meridians which they complement, and to which they connect, are as follows: heart, inside arm; heart-constrictor (pericardium), inside arm; lung, inside arm; liver, front of body; spleen, front of body; kidney, front of body. The diagram below shows the positions of the yin meridians on the front of a person's body. See **vital organs**.

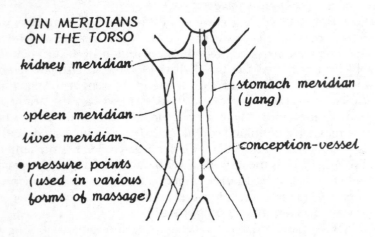

YIN MERIDIANS ON THE TORSO

kidney meridian

spleen meridian

liver meridian

• pressure points (used in various forms of massage)

stomach meridian (yang)

conception-vessel

yin symptoms Those symptoms of illness which indicate suppression of the vital organs, and are usually accompanied by coldness and emptiness, are regarded as being yin, and suggest that yang remedies should be applied. Typical yin symptoms include cold sensations, a desire for hot drinks, loose stools, clear urine, a pale face, a swollen and white and furry tongue, shallow breathing and a weak pulse.

yin systems In TCM, the yin vital organs, or solid organs, are the heart, liver, kidneys, spleen, lungs and heart-constrictor (pericardium). However, in the West, the heart-constrictor, or pericardium, which is a membraneous sac enclosing the heart, would not be regarded as an independent organ, and so it is best to regard these organs as being functional or energy systems.

yin tonics Those ailments which are regarded as yang, and which are indicated by warmth, fullness, thirst and headaches, are what Chinese physicians would describe as 'yin-empty ailments', which require yin tonics to cool and soothe. These yin tonics could include Chinese wolfberry, *Lycium chinense*, lower shell of turtle, *Chinemys reevesii*, and carapace of tortoise, *Trionyx sinensis*. It is important to know that yang tonics, which have the opposite effect, should not be used in these cases. But there are a few exceptions. The Chinese wolfberry, for example, which is neutral in its effects, may be used as either a yang tonic or a yin tonic. See **tonic**.

yin-yang diagnosis The symptoms of illness, as determined by the four methods of diagnosis – consultation, observation, hearing and feeling (see **diagnosis**) – are classified as yin or yang. Some typical yin symptoms are as follows: coldness, desire for warmth and hot drinks, poor appetite, loose stools, clear and profuse urine, pale face and lips, tiredness, swollen and white furry tongue, shallow breathing, weak pulse, cold hands and feet, cramps, abdominal aches. Typical yang symptoms include: warmth, excessive thirst, hard stools, constipation, hot and scanty urine, flushed face, nervousness, irritability, bright-red tongue with yellow fur, talkativeness, laboured breathing, heavy pulse, abdominal pain. Yang symptoms indicate stimulation of the vital organs, and yin symptoms indicate their suppression. But this is an over-simplification, for an ailment may be characterized by a mixture of yin and yang symptoms, and it sometimes happens that a yin symptom will mask a yang symptom. and vice versa. In these cases, the Chinese physician will draw on his long experience.

yin yang huo See **goats**.

yin-yang illnesses Ailments are classified as yin or yang, the former being empty and internal, and the latter being full and external. They will need to be treated with a medication of an opposite character in order to produce the desired effect, as this table shows:

SYMPTOMS	AILMENT	MEDICINE	EFFECT
hot	yang	yin	cooling
cold	yin	yang	warming
full	yang	yin	sedative
external	yang	yin	suppressive
empty	yin	yang	toning
internal	yin	yang	elevating

yin-yang principle This principle of complementary opposites (see **Tai Chi**), which indicates how harmony is produced by maintaining a balance between yin and yang forces, applies as much to Chinese medicine as it does to all else. Thus, symptoms, ailments, medications, the effects of treatments, energies, elements, flavours and directions are all classified as yin or yang, as the table shows. Yin is considered to be superior to yang, though one may wonder why this should be, for fire, which is symbolic of yang, is suggestive of brightness and energy, whereas water, which is symbolic of yin, is suggestive of dullness, coldness and inertia. But water extinguishes fire and is certainly more enduring than fire. See **element**.

YANG
Symptoms: hot, full, external
Ailments: warm, stimulating
Medications: ginger, liquorice
Effects: warming, toning yang
Energies: hot, warm
Elements: metal, earth, fire
Flavours: hot, sweet, plain
Directions: ascending, elevating

YIN
Symptoms: cold, empty, internal
Ailments: cool, suppressive
Medications: boxthorn, sour plums
Effects: cooling, sedative
Energies: cold, cool
Elements: wood, water
Flavours: sour, bitter, salty
Directions: descending, suppressing

yisheng The Chinese word for 'physician'.

yoghurt This sourish and curd-like food is prepared from milk fermented by the addition of bacteria. It is a rich source of protein, calcium and a few of the B-complex vitamins, and the bacteria it contains assist in the proper functioning of the digestive tract. It has acquired some considerable importance as a health food among the people of the Western world. However, their enthusiasm for this milk product is not shared by the Chinese, who, for various sound reasons, contend that milk and its products are not quite as healthy as they might appear to be. See **milk and milk products**.

youth Like health, youth is a precious commodity, and the

Chinese have discovered from long experience that a full and healthy life of vigorous youthfulness can be attained by a sound diet, an adequate amount of exercise, moderate habits, preventive medicine, including herbs which inhibit the ageing process, and a wise philosophy of living, as is contained in the teachings of Taoism and Confucianism. They would contend that it is a big step in the right direction if one thinks youthfully and does not miss out on laughter and sleep, and avoids the vices of old age, which include irascibility and sedentary habits. We, in the West, could quote the proverb 'All work and no play makes Jack a dull boy'. But the Chinese could counter this by saying 'All play and no work makes Chang an unhealthy boy.' Few Chinese have sedentary habits. Even when very old, they still occupy themselves in arduous physical labour. See **ageing**.

yuan qi 'Primordial vital energy'. This is the original and perfect state of a person's total vital energy, which slowly deteriorates until the last day of his life. The rate of deterioration determines his life-span. To the Western mind, this concept may seem to be somewhat far-fetched, but one should not allow oneself to be confused by language barriers and the symbolism employed in Chinese philosophy. Is it not the case that the human body, like a machine, wears out quickly if it is ill used? And does not this constant ill use produce a deterioration in functions?

Yu Fu Over 2000 years ago, the physician Yu Fu used stone needles in his acupuncture treatments. See **acupuncture needles**.

Yunnan bai yao A white herbal powder which is powerfully haemostatic, both externally and internally. It is also called *shan qi*, which means 'mountain varnish'. Its main ingredient is *san qi*, *Panax notoginseng*, which grows mainly in Yunnan Province, though some is grown in Sichuan and Japan. See **jin bu huan**.

Yu the Great See **legendary emperors**.

Z

za fu pei See **tsa fu pei**.

za-zen The daily meditation practised by the Zen Buddhists, and in which the meditators sit uncomfortably erect and cross-legged, counting from one to ten over and over again, and disciplining their thoughts. See **zen meditation**.

Zen Buddhism The Japanese form of Buddhism, which has been developed from the Buddhism introduced into Japan from China during the twelfth century. One of its aims is to achieve *satori*, or 'deep insight', by meditation. See **Buddhism**.

Zen garden A garden devised by Zen Buddhists to provide an ideal setting for meditation. It can be simple or elaborate, its essential characteristics being a rock or a small number of rocks to serve as a focal point which, when viewed, transports the mind into a state where thought may proceed without hindrance, and a setting which separates the focal point from the wider surroundings. See **Zen meditation**.

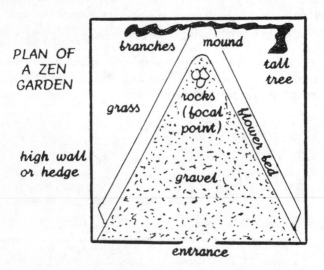

PLAN OF A ZEN GARDEN

branches · mound · tall tree · grass · rocks (focal point) · flower bed · high wall or hedge · gravel · entrance

Zen meditation Zen Buddhists maintain that moral attitudes and intellectual activities are of no value without *satori*, or 'deep insight'. They seek this through meditation, in which they consider the meaning and purpose of life and those paradoxical issues which seem to give the lie to conventional logic and scientific thought. They would contend that there are gaps in our knowledge because our systems of reasoning are inadequate. We have limited knowledge because we have limited minds. Zen meditation could be helpful to those who have become the victims of the problems of materialism and egocentricity, which are often manifested as stress, anxiety and depression. See **za-zen** and **Zen Buddhism**.

Zhang Zhongjing One of the most renowned physicians of ancient China. About 200 BC, during the time of the Han dynasty (206 BC–AD 220), he wrote *Shang Han Lun*, or 'Discussions on Febrile Conditions'. This work contains 113 prescriptions based upon 100 medicines, most of which are herbal. He studied many ailments, but devoted much of his attention to typhoid and other fever-related diseases. He put ailments into six classes, three yin and three yang, and endeavoured to correct the imbalances between yin and yang by inducing or reducing vomiting, elimination or diaphoresis. He also devised a 'map' to show the positions of the meridians as used in acupuncture. See **meridian**.

Zheng He See **Ming dynasty**.

zhi mu *Anemarrhena asphodeloides*. Herbal medicine. Distribution: North China. Parts: stems, rhizomes. Character: cold, bitter. Affinity: lungs, kidneys, stomach. Effects: antipyretic, demulcent, tonic to kidneys. Symptoms: heat, thirst, irritability, sleeplessness. Treatments: bronchitis, pneumonia, yin-empty ailments. Dosage: 3–6 g. Incompatible with preparations containing iron.

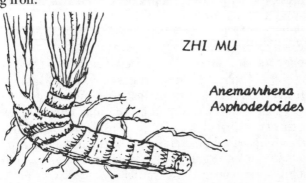

ZHI MU

Anemarrhena
Asphodeloides

Zhou classics A number of great literary works, more generally described as Confucian classics, came into being during the period of the Zhou (Chou) dynasty (*c.* 1100–221 BC). One of these, the *Shijing*, or 'Book of Odes', makes frequent reference to medicinal herbs, which is an indication that, during this period, the Chinese were becoming more health conscious and a study of medicine was developing.

Zhou dynasty Also written as *Chou dynasty*. This period (*c.* 1100–221 BC) was one of political and social turmoil and internecine warfare, but it was also one of intellectual development. It was the Golden Age of Chinese philosophy, when Taoism began to emerge, herbal medicine became more sophisticated, and herbalists and alchemists strove to find an elixir which would confer immortality.

zhunzi 'Superior man'. This is the Confucian concept of a true gentleman, who behaves correctly in all situations. For the Chinese, a superior man – or woman – is a person of high morality and insight who is striving to attain the Confucian virtues of wisdom, justice, sincerity, benevolence and propriety. Confucius realized that social friction and instability are productive of stress, anxiety and other forms of mental ill health.

zinc A trace element that is a vital constituent of many enzymes and necessary for growth and sexual maturation. Its deficiency causes loss of appetite, poor circulation, increased susceptibility to infection, pains in the joints, degeneration of the skin and general fatigue. Zinc occurs in large amounts in eggs, liver, fish, shellfish, vegetables, wholegrains, pulses and nuts, which items constitute a major part of the Chinese diet. Oysters are a particularly rich source of zinc, which probably accounts for their reputation as an aphrodisiac. Centuries ago, Chinese physicians knew nothing of trace elements as chemical substances; but, from experience, they would have been aware of those foods containing health-giving and health-protective components, which they would probably have categorized as *ying qi*, or 'nourishing-*qi*', and *wei qi*, or 'protective-*qi*'. See **mineral**.

zodiac exercises A set of 12 exercises, devised by the Taoists, by which each of the 12 vital organs can be treated with the appropriate exercise during the astrological two-hour period of the day when its activation will be at a maximum intensity. The Taoist theory is that there can be no function without an organ and *qi*, or 'energy'. Thus, an organ without energy is dead, and energy without an organ is of a spectral character, and has no meaningful existence. This rather contradicts the long-held

Christian belief that the soul, or personality, can exist separately from the body. The regulation of the energy balance within the organs of the body itself and external influences is of a fluctuating nature, and so the sum total of the activities of the organs creates the impression that there is a 'body clock', or 'biological clock'. Modern research in the West has shown that these biological fluctuations, more properly called biorhythms, do exist, and are related to solar and lunar influences and time measurements. Old age has been likened to the running down of the 'body clock', and it could well be that biorhythms account for the dawn chorus of the birds. A zodiac exercise will benefit the organ for which it is designed if applied at any time of the day, but the maximum benefit will be derived only if it is applied during the designated two-hour period. See **circadian rhythm**, **insomnia** and **jet lag**.

ZODIAC EXERCISES

1– 3 a.m. liver	1– 3 p.m. small intestine
3– 5 a.m. lungs	3– 5 p.m. bladder
5– 7 a.m. large intestine	5– 7 p.m. kidneys
7– 9 a.m. stomach	7– 9 p.m. heart-constrictor
9–11 a.m. spleen	9–11 p.m. triple-warmer
11– 1 p.m. heart	11– 1 a.m. gall-bladder

zone therapy Reflexology, a form of massage which originated in China over 5000 years ago, was introduced into the West in 1913 by Dr William H. Fitzgerald, an American consultant. Originally, he called it zone therapy, for he had divided the body into ten zones, or energy channels. He applied healing pressures to points on these channels. See **reflexology**.

zoology Scientific study of animals. The Chinese have always had great respect for both animal and human life, and so they have always been averse to dissection, vivisection and the wanton destruction of animals. And the Buddhists, who believe in reincarnation, would certainly not countenance these practices. Therefore, until recent times, the zoological knowledge of the Chinese would have tended to be more physiological than anatomical, and limited to that derived from observations of habits and external features. See **anatomy**.

zoonoses Diseases of animals which may be transmitted to humans. See **vector**.

zymase Enzyme in yeast which converts sugar into alcohol and carbon dioxide. Until recent times, the Chinese would not have isolated zymase as a chemical substance, and would probably have concluded that yeast contains *jing*, or 'vital essence', and *qi*, or 'vital energy', which is transferred from yeast into sugar and water to produce wine. It is likely that they regarded yeast, which occurs naturally as the bloom on grapes, as merely a plant product, and not as a plant. In modern chemistry, the production of alcohol may be briefly described by equations.

glucose (simple sugar) → alcohol + carbon dioxide
$$C_6H_{12}O_6 \rightarrow 2C_2H_5OH + 2CO_2$$
sucrose (cane sugar) + water → alcohol + carbon dioxide
$$C_{12}H_{22}O_{11} + H_2O \rightarrow 4C_2H_5OH + 4CO_2$$
See **fermentation** and **yeast**.